Diagnosis and Evaluation in Speech Pathology

Ninth Edition

Rebekah H. Pindzola
Auburn University

Laura W. Plexico
Auburn University

William O. Haynes
Auburn University

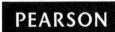

Boston   Columbus   Indianapolis   New York   San Francisco   Upper Saddle River
Amsterdam   Cape Town   Dubai   London   Madrid   Milan   Munich   Paris   Montréal   Toronto
Delhi   Mexico City   São Paulo   Sydney   Hong Kong   Seoul   Singapore   Taipei   Tokyo

Vice President and Editorial Director:
  Jeffery W. Johnston
Executive Editor: Ann Castel Davis
Editorial Assistant: Janelle Criner
Executive Field Marketing Manager: Krista Clark
Senior Product Marketing Manager: Christopher Barry
Project Manager: Kerry Rubadue
Program Program Manager: Joe Sweeney
Operations Specialist: Deidra Skahill
Text Designer: S4Carlisle Publishing Services

Cover Design Director: Diane Ernsberger
Cover Image: Shutterstock
Media Producer: Autumn Benson
Media Project Manager: Tammy Walters
Full-Service Project Management: S4Carlisle
  Publishing Services
Composition: S4Carlisle Publishing Services
Printer/Binder: : LSC Communications
Cover Printer: LSC Communications
Text Font: Palatino LT Std

Library of Congress Cataloging-in-Publication Data

Pindzola, Rebekah H. (Rebekah Hand), author.
  Diagnosis and evaluation in speech pathology/Rebekah H. Pindzola, Laura W. Plexico, William O. Haynes.—Ninth edition.
    p. cm.
  Preceded by: Diagnosis and evaluation in speech pathology/William O. Haynes, Rebekah H. Pindzola.—8th ed. c2012.
  Includes bibliographical references and index.
  ISBN 978-0-13-382390-5
  ISBN 0-13-382390-3
  I. Plexico, Laura W., author. II. Haynes, William O., author. III. Haynes, William O. Diagnosis and evaluation in speech pathology. Preceded by (work): IV. Title.
  [DNLM: 1. Speech Disorders—diagnosis. WL 340.2]
  RC423
  616.85′5—dc23

                                                          2014048546

2   18

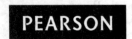

Traditional Book ISBN 13: 9780-13-382390-5
                  ISBN 10:   0-13-382390-3
E-text ISBN 10:   0-13-408664-3
           ISBN 13: 978-0-13-408664-4

Preface

With this ninth edition of *Diagnosis and Evaluation in Speech Pathology*, we welcome a new coauthor and invite a new group of students and practitioners to consider the complex and fascinating arena of assessment in communication disorders. For over 40 years, this text has introduced diagnosis and evaluation as a *process* conducted in the context of an *interpersonal relationship* between clinicians and clients. This interesting and challenging process is a curious blend of science and art. On the science side, each case requires the clinician to think, solve problems, form hypotheses, gather data, and arrive at conclusions. Assessment, however, is much more than the simple administration of a few psychometrically adequate tests or scales, which takes us into the more artistic side of the process.

The diagnostician is much more than a neutral conduit through which test scores pass, and he or she must interact with clients to determine the real effects of communication impairment on their lives. The clinician must be able to interpret scores and measurements in the context of an individual client's circumstances. Thus, in this edition, we again remind readers that most communication disorders have functional consequences for a person's life. The World Health Organization continues to emphasize the role of functional effects of disorders in its International Classification of Functioning, Disability and Health (ICF). Third-party coverage in the United States, be it through Medicare or other insurers, also emphasizes functional outcomes, and so our assessment baselines are of critical importance. Another emphasis of the current edition is the ongoing nature of assessment. We must move beyond the notion of a single diagnostic session and think of assessment as gathering baseline data, monitoring treatment progress, determining if generalization has occurred from training, and documenting functional gains in communication in a client's life.

Many readers of the prior editions have commented that they found the book to be both readable and clinically relevant. They have also made insightful suggestions, which we have endeavored to address in the present edition. Since the first edition appeared in 1973, the field of communication disorders has gone through many changes. With each successive revision of the text, we have attempted to reflect theoretical, clinical, and technological advances that have taken place in the field. The ninth edition is no different. The reader will notice that we have attempted to maintain the strong points of the former edition while including new research and clinical tools in this new edition.

NEW TO THIS EDITION

We have made every effort to modernize assessment practice patterns in this book and have done so for a more expansive array of speech, language, and swallowing disorders. Here is a summary of these changes and additions:

- Expansion of assessment tools available for each disorder, many with insightful critiques and procedural guidelines

- Additional chapter (Chapter 10) dedicated to assessing adult dysphagia and pediatric feeding and swallowing disorders
- Expansion of clinical interviewing to include ethnographic and motivational interviewing
- Expansion of child speech-language assessment issues, including phoneme awareness and literacy
- Additional chapter (Chapter 13) dedicated to head and neck cancer and the ongoing assessment of alaryngeal speakers
- Addition of sample sections of diagnostic reports showing writing attributes covering a wide array of communication disorders
- Expansion of billing and coding issues inherent in diagnostic evaluations, including coverage of the new ICD-10 system
- Addition of an appendix (Appendix A) dedicated to the oral peripheral examination
- Addition of an appendix (Appendix B) offering various assessment resources, such as information on developmental milestones, transcription symbols, hearing screening guidelines, hearing-related case history questions, and a selection of reading passages for clinical use
- Inclusion of learning tools for the reader in each chapter, such as learning outcomes and end-of-chapter self-assessment questions

ACKNOWLEDGMENTS

We would like to express appreciation to our students, clients, colleagues, and past teachers who helped to mold our thinking about the assessment process. We would also like to acknowledge Dr. Lon Emerick, who provided the initial impetus for this work. His basic philosophy, sensitivity, and enthusiasm still echo through the text. We also thank the reviewers of this book: Beverly Henke-Lofquist, SUNY Geneseo; Karen Harris Brown, University of West Georgia; Rosemary Lubinski, University of Buffalo.

Many of their helpful suggestions have been incorporated into the ninth edition of *Diagnosis and Evaluation in Speech Pathology*.

Finally, we should remember that the diagnostic session is our initial contact with clients; we never get a second chance to make a first impression. Every evaluation is unique, and each client deserves the best we can offer in terms of our ability, knowledge, judgment, and interpersonal sensitivity. We hope that this text can communicate to our readers both the method and the magic of this challenging task.

Contents

CHAPTER**10** *Adult Dysphagia and Pediatric Feeding and Swallowing Disorders*   298

CHAPTER**11** *Laryngeal Voice Disorders*   318

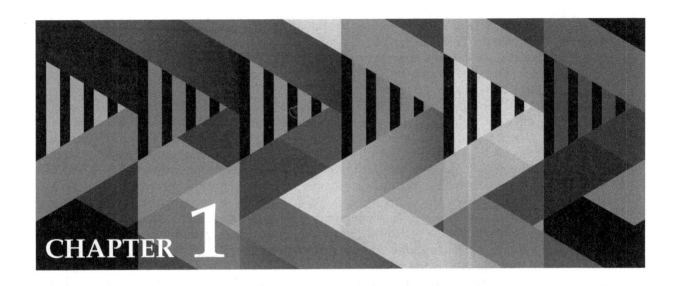

CHAPTER 1

Introduction to Diagnosis and Evaluation

Philosophical Issues and General Guidelines

LEARNING OUTCOMES

After reading this chapter you will be able to:

1. Define and describe the difference between the terms *evaluation* and *diagnosis*.
2. Describe the two major reasons evaluations are performed.
3. Define the three levels of diagnosis and evaluation.
4. Describe the three parts of evidence-based practice.
5. Describe response to intervention and how it is used for evaluation.
6. Compare and contrast the differences between dynamic and static assessment.
7. Describe the guidelines described by the World Health Organization that drive the American-Speech-Language-Hearing Association's preferred practice patterns.
8. Describe the three components in determining a communication disorder.
9. Distinguish among predisposing, precipitating, and perpetuating factors.
10. Describe how the diagnostician is a factor in the evaluation process.
11. Describe factors that require consideration when making prognoses.

Speech-language pathology is a wonderfully diverse profession that requires a practitioner to possess a wide range of skills, knowledge, and personal characteristics. A speech-language pathologist (SLP) works as a case selector, case evaluator, diagnostician, interviewer, parent counselor, teacher, coordinator, record keeper, consultant, researcher, and student. Because the boundaries for these various duties are not clearly defined and because the clinician must move continuously from one area to another, no one person can expect to be equally competent in all areas. The ultimate goal is to maximize one's strengths in all aspects to provide the best possible service to individuals with communicative disorders.

Diagnosis is one of the most comprehensive and difficult tasks of the speech-language pathologist. The diagnosis of a client requires a synthesis of the entire field: knowledge of norms and testing techniques, skills in observation, an ability to relate effectively and empathetically, and a great deal of creative intuition. Because communication is a function of the entire person, the diagnostician must try to scrutinize all aspects of behavior. We must remember that we are not simply working with speech sounds, fluency, vocal quality, or linguistic rules but rather with changing people in a dynamic environment. The ambiguous findings that sometimes culminate in a diagnostic evaluation must be dealt with in a fashion that perpetuates the evaluative undertaking rather than closes the door on further probing and a greater understanding of the presenting problem(s). Diagnosis is a continuous and open-ended venture that results in answers or partial answers that themselves are open to revision with added information. The experienced diagnostician does not look at objective scores of articulatory skill, point scales of vocal quality, or standard scores as ends in themselves but rather as aspects of an individual's communication ability—we diagnose communicators, not just communication. That revelation is a major factor in the transition from a technician to a professional clinician.

DIAGNOSIS AND EVALUATION DEFINED

Some clinicians, at first glance, may consider the words *diagnosis* and *evaluation* to be synonymous. It is our intent in this text that the term *diagnosis* refer to the classical Greek definition of distinguishing a person's problem from the large field of potential disabilities. The term *diagnosis* in Greek means "to distinguish." The prefix *dia-* means "apart," and *-gnosis* translates as "to know." To distinguish a person's particular problem from the many possibilities available, we must know the client thoroughly: how he or she responds in many conditions and how he or she performs a variety of tasks. *Evaluation* refers to *the process* of arriving at a diagnosis. Thus, informal probes, trial therapy tasks, and gathering generalization data are part of evaluation. In standard dictionary definitions, the term *diagnosis* is generally described as "the use of methods or processes to identify or determine the nature and cause of a disease or problem. This process is accomplished through an analysis of patient history, examination of signs and symptoms, administration of special tests, and a review of data." Our conception of diagnosis, then, includes a thorough understanding of the client's problem and not merely the application of a label. It is relatively simple to call a child "language impaired," but it is a more difficult matter really to understand how this child deals with linguistic symbols in a variety of tasks and situations. *The latter* is diagnosis in our view. We would also like to expand the notion of diagnosis to include distinguishing the nature and evolution of a person's problem at different points in time. Thus, diagnosis and evaluation are ongoing processes. We perform evaluation activities to arrive at an initial diagnosis, and we also examine the client repeatedly during the course of treatment. A client's diagnosis and the nature of the client's difficulties often changes over time. For example, a child may initially present with language delay and, after a period of language treatment, be characterized as primarily demonstrating a phonological disorder. A neurogenic patient may initially be diagnosed with aphasia but may experience further neurological damage and be re-diagnosed with aphasia and dysarthria. Another major thrust of this text is that the diagnostic process need not be confined to a 2-hour block of time in a university setting or a 30-minute period in a medical facility. The competent clinician will continue evaluation activities until the client's performance is understood to the extent necessary to determine an effective treatment approach.

We perform evaluation tasks with two major goals in mind. First, we evaluate to arrive at a good understanding or diagnosis of a client's problem. Arriving at a diagnosis is a complex task. It requires problem solving, reasoning, and the ability to recognize patterns (Richardson, Wilson, & Guyatt, 2002). Sometimes these evaluation activities will be confined to an assessment period, and at other times they will be performed well into the beginning of treatment. Often we must begin therapy with a client before arriving at a firm diagnosis. This approach is not optimal, but it is justified as long as we realize that (1) *any* treatment approach is experimental to a certain degree in the beginning, (2) most initial treatment goals will generally be "in the ballpark" in terms of appropriateness (e.g., we probably would not engage in voice therapy for a stuttering client), and (3) beginning treatment does not mean that we have abandoned our efforts to define the parameters of the client's problem and arrive at a diagnosis. We can always fine-tune a treatment program based on an increased understanding of a client's problem and capabilities.

A second major reason to perform evaluation activities is to monitor the client's progress in treatment and describe changes in the communication disturbance. In this use of evaluation activities, we are not necessarily trying to diagnose the problem but to document treatment progress and determine possible changes in the course of treatment. In the chapters of this text that deal with disorders, we will suggest evaluation tasks often used for these purposes that are not in the formal test category. Formal tests are designed more for categorizing clients as exhibiting certain disorders, whereas nonstandardized evaluation tasks are used to gain insight into specific client abilities and to gauge treatment progress. We will now discuss some of the purposes of diagnosis and evaluation in more detail.

BROADENING THE NOTION OF ASSESSMENT

Most people tend to think of diagnosis and treatment as two separate parts of the clinical process. We schedule clients for an "assessment" and then, if they evidence a problem, we arrange for them to receive "treatment." This distinction between assessment and treatment is somewhat arbitrary and nothing more than an administrative dichotomy made by school systems, medical settings, and insurance companies. In reality, we perform evaluations at the beginning of a clinical relationship with a client in order to determine the existence of and nature of a communication disorder, but the assessment does not stop there. Figure 1–1 shows a process in which diagnosis, to determine the existence of a problem, is only the first step in assessment. We diagnose the problem typically by using a combination of norm-referenced standardized tests coupled with nonstandardized communication tasks. Once the problem is confirmed, many additional evaluation tasks are performed to determine a client's baseline performance on very specific aspects of communication. These tasks are often performed after the initial diagnostic session and become part of measurements taken during the treatment phase of clinical work. We continue to evaluate in order to understand the client's baseline performance levels for specific treatment goals, functional communication, and communicative effectiveness in the natural environment. We must also continue to evaluate in order to monitor treatment progress. Thus, even though treatment may have been going

FIGURE 1–1
Diagnosis and Evaluation Involve Determining the Existence of a Problem, Taking Baseline Performance Data, and Monitoring Treatment Progress

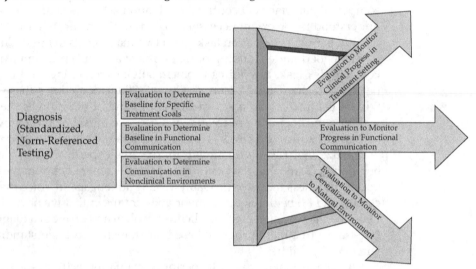

on for months, we continue to gather assessment data on the client's performance in the clinic, his or her changes in functional communication abilities, and the generalization of these abilities to other environments. These three levels of diagnosis and evaluation form a continuum ranging from diagnosis on one end, moving through establishing baseline performance data, and finally ending at measurement of treatment progress.

ILLUSTRATING THE IMPORTANCE OF MEASUREMENT IN CURRENT TRENDS

The assessment activities that take place after the initial diagnostic session have taken on increased importance in recent years with the emergence of three important influences in the field of communication disorders. These three influences have had and should continue to have far-reaching effects on our field in terms of research, theory, and clinical practice. The areas of which we speak are evidence-based practice (EBP), the response to intervention (RTI) initiative in public education, and research in dynamic assessment. You will soon see that the three areas overlap and in many ways deal with the same underlying construct of ongoing assessment or measurement of treatment progress. The three areas are illustrated in Figure 1–2. We will briefly discuss each of these important influences in the following sections.

Evidence-Based Practice in Speech-Language Pathology

The Joint Coordinating Committee on Evidence-Based Practice of the American Speech-Language-Hearing Association (ASHA) produced a position statement (American Speech-Language-Hearing Association, 2005). Among the recommended skills for speech-language pathologists, we emphasize following:

- Ability to perform screening and diagnostic procedures to gather information in a cost-effective manner; the SLP, then, must be aware of assessments as well as their efficacy.
- Ability to evaluate the efficacy, effectiveness, and efficiency of assessments as well as ongoing treatment.

FIGURE 1–2
Three Overlapping Areas in Current Literature Where Measurement Techniques Are Critical

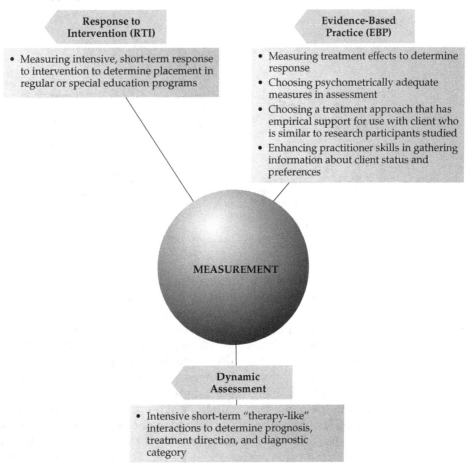

Response to Intervention (RTI)

- Measuring intensive, short-term response to intervention to determine placement in regular or special education programs

Evidence-Based Practice (EBP)

- Measuring treatment effects to determine response
- Choosing psychometrically adequate measures in assessment
- Choosing a treatment approach that has empirical support for use with client who is similar to research participants studied
- Enhancing practitioner skills in gathering information about client status and preferences

MEASUREMENT

Dynamic Assessment

- Intensive short-term "therapy-like" interactions to determine prognosis, treatment direction, and diagnostic category

These skills suggest two major implications of evidence-based practice. First, in selecting diagnostic measurements, it is our responsibility to choose those that have the most scientific support and psychometric adequacy. The second implication involves the notion that assessment is ongoing, and it is only through such continued evaluation that we can monitor treatment progress on the goals we have selected as targets. In short, what is the "evidence" in evidence-based practice? In many ways it all boils down to measurement of one type or another.

Evidence-based practice was initially developed in the medical profession as a means of promoting ". . . the integration of best research evidence with clinical expertise and patient values" (Sackett, Straus, Richardson, Rosenberg, & Haynes, 2000, p. 1). Obviously, this implies a three-part model with research evidence, clinical expertise, and patient values at each point, presumably each contributing significant importance to making clinical decisions. Figure 1–3 depicts the relationships in this model to the assessment process. This model has been recently applied to many other professions, including education, social work, psychology, and communication disorders.

It is important to discuss how the three parts of the model in Figure 1–3 apply to assessment in communication disorders. The part of the model that deals with research evidence is critical in selecting both norm-referenced assessment instruments and

FIGURE 1–3
Three Classical Components of Evidence-Based Practice

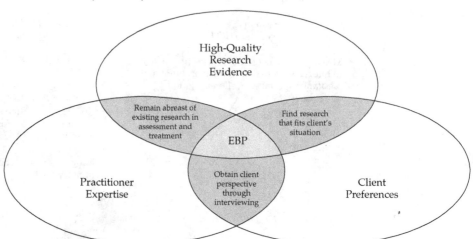

nonstandardized measurements of client behaviors. As we will discuss in Chapter 3, all standardized tests should have been carefully developed so that they have psychometric qualities that make them both valid and reliable. These tests should have been normed on populations that make them applicable to clients from a variety of social and cultural groups. A clinician must be very careful to use standardized tests that meet exacting psychometric criteria and have been scientifically shown to identify clients with communication disorders adequately. When a clinician chooses a nonstandardized method of examining client communicative behavior, research evidence is even more critical. We should not simply design our own methods of gathering data on clients, but we should use nonstandardized methods that research has shown to be reliable and valid. For example, measurements such as mean length of utterance, type–token ratio, maximum phonation time, and percentage of disfluency are nonstandardized procedures that have well-documented definitions, procedures for sampling/calculation, and data on reliability/validity from many scientific investigations. It is almost always preferable to use a technique that has been implemented in research rather than develop an idiosyncratic approach with no empirical support.

Another way that knowledge of research evidence comes into play is in selecting a treatment procedure. There is no shortage of manuals and programs that tell the clinician how to do therapy. However, not many scientific studies actually document treatment effects on clients who underwent specific therapy procedures. The implication here is that clinicians should choose treatment methods that have scientific support in research literature and not use untested techniques when others are available with evidence that shows effectiveness. Thus, research evidence is an extremely important component of the EBP model and applies to both assessment and treatment enterprises in communication disorders.

The second part of the EBP model includes the clinical expertise of the practitioner. Clinical expertise is important for several reasons. First of all, one cannot be clinically competent unless he or she keeps up with the current research literature in the field. This is where the second part of the EBP model intersects with the first, research evidence. We assume that a competent clinician is familiar with the latest developments in assessment and treatment. We also assume that if a practitioner uses new clinical methods, then he or she will study and practice them so that they are used appropriately with the client. The practitioner is responsible for choosing appropriate assessment and treatment methods and knowing how to use them.

The third part of the EBP model involves the values and perspective of the patient with whom we are working. It is the responsibility of the practitioner to evaluate the client as a person rather than merely a communication disorder. Every person has perceptions, values, and preferences that should be taken into account in a clinical relationship. For example, in the field of medicine, a person who has been diagnosed with cancer has many treatment options, ranging from surgery to chemotherapy and radiation. Each treatment has research data associated with it; these results can be communicated so that the patient and physician can make the decision that is best for the patient and family. Note that patients are not simply told which option to take; they have a choice. Sometimes they may choose to have a shorter survival chance but a better quality of life. The decision is up to the patient. Although this choice is not as dramatic in communication disorders, there are many possible ways of dealing with most speech and language disorders. For example, it may be preferable for a family to receive an intense parent training program instead of having to make frequent visits to a clinical setting, which may be more of a strain on finances and scheduling. Again, the patient's view should always be taken into account and his or her preferences should be included in the clinical decision-making process. This part of the EBP model interacts with practitioner expertise because a good clinician will be able to assess the values and preferences of the family and take them into account when arriving at a clinical decision. In Chapter 2 we discuss interviewing, which is the mechanism by which we get to learn about patient concerns, preferences, and goals. There is also an interaction between the patient perspective and research evidence. As a clinician chooses assessment and treatment techniques, he or she must determine if the technique has been used effectively on patients who fit the profile of the current client. That is, we should select treatment and assessment options that have been successful with clients similar to our patient.

It is easy to see from Figure 1–3 how research evidence, practitioner expertise, and patient preferences are not only important as individual entities but also in how they interact in carrying out the clinical transaction, both in assessment and in treatment. ASHA recently developed practice portals to help speech-language pathologists identify the best existing evidence and resources with credibility that are available. The content contained within the practice portals includes information on a variety of professional issues and clinical topics. To date, professional issues included are bilingual service delivery, caseload/workload, classroom acoustics, cultural competence, speech-language pathology assistants, and telepractice; clinical topics include aphasia, autism spectrum disorder, dementia, pediatric dysphagia, social communication disorders, and speech sound disorders. Evidence maps are provided within the practice portals to guide clinicians through an evidence-based clinical decision-making process and highlight the three components of EBP within each professional issue or clinical topic. You can search for the practice portals and the information contained within each portal at www.asha.org.

The Response to Intervention (RTI) Model

Authorities in the field of education and learning disabilities have recently postulated a procedure for identifying and treating students with disorders using a model called *response to intervention (RTI)*. The National Association of State Directors of Special Education (2005) defines RTI as "the practice of (1) providing high-quality instruction/intervention matched to student needs and (2) using learning rate over time and level of performance to (3) make important educational decisions." The legal groundwork for RTI was laid by PL 108-447: IDEA 2004, which states: "In determining whether a child has a specific learning disability, a local educational agency may use a process that determines if the child responds to scientific, research-based intervention." No Child Left Behind (NCLB) advocates the use of scientifically based research, which is described as "research that involves the application of rigorous, systematic, and objective procedures to obtain reliable and valid knowledge relevant to education activities and programs." These two legal perspectives seem to be quite compatible. Justice (2006) and Ukrainetz (2006) detailed how the SLP would fit into this type of approach to assessment and intervention for language, reading, and literacy disorders. We discuss RTI here only as an example of the important role that ongoing assessment plays in any program that involves continuous monitoring of client progress.

It is important to provide some perspective on why RTI is a novel approach to evaluating students. Historically, students with learning disabilities, the majority of which are language/literacy based, were given special education services after being diagnosed with a particular learning problem. In most cases this was done by using outdated discrepancy formulas, which showed a disconnect between a student's potential as measured through intelligence and aptitude testing and the student's performance on tests of specific abilities such as reading, writing, or oral language. Often, such evaluations were not completed until the end of second grade and, at this point, remediation is difficult and the social/psychological effects of failure may have already begun. The historical scenario described above has been called the wait-to-fail model. Currently, most authorities do not support the sole use of discrepancy models in diagnosis.

In an effort to be more proactive, educators have posited that variables other than just test scores could be used to determine the existence of a learning or language disorder. One such variable involves placing the student in a limited, intense period of treatment to determine if he or she can benefit from additional assistance. Proponents of RTI characterize the approach as having a number of tiers that provide progressively more specialized and intensive treatment. The number of tiers varies depending on the specific RTI model considered. Figure 1–4 illustrates a general four-tier model of RTI. Movement through the tiers depends on monitoring student response to treatment as revealed by continuous assessment. Those students who benefit from the assistance could continue to be served in the general education classroom on a consultative basis by the SLP. The students who do not benefit from the intense treatment regimen could then be declared eligible for special education services by the speech-language pathologist. In this way, a student's actual learning response can be a significant consideration in the decision to enroll him or her for specialized services instead of just using arbitrary cutoffs and test scores. Enrollment in specialized special education services often involves pulling the student out of the classroom, which could contribute to further academic problems caused by missing critical material. If a student can be served adequately in the general education setting in Tiers 1 to 3 without having to be admitted to a special education program, such additional academic problems might be avoided.

RTI involves prevention and intervention goals in an outcomes-driven system. For RTI to be successful, it must include a team approach involving parents, educators, special educators, administrators, and related service providers (e.g., SLPs). The American Speech-Language-Hearing Association has developed guidelines regarding the role of the SLP in RTI (Ehren, Montgomery, Rudebusch, & Whitmire, 2007). Most of the early work with RTI concerned children who have learning disabilities, but currently it has been applied to all children receiving services in early childhood. According to Jackson, Pretti-Frontczak, Harjusola-Webb, Grisham-Brown, and Romani (2009, p. 425), "Common principles of RTI include (a) many tiers to insure maximum support for each child, (b) instruction implemented with high quality, (c) a core curriculum that encompasses a research base, (d) a data collection system consisting of both formative

FIGURE 1–4
The Importance of Monitoring in RTI: Ongoing Assessment Determines Whether More Intensive Intervention Is Needed

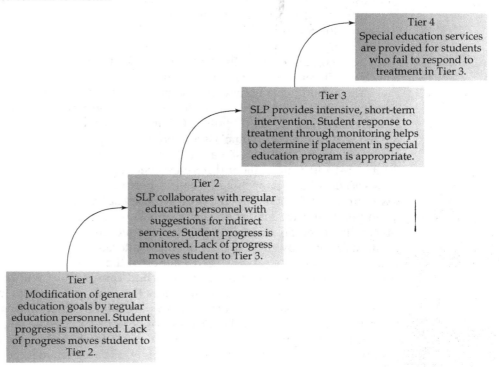

Tier 4
Special education services are provided for students who fail to respond to treatment in Tier 3.

Tier 3
SLP provides intensive, short-term intervention. Student response to treatment through monitoring helps to determine if placement in special education program is appropriate.

Tier 2
SLP collaborates with regular education personnel with suggestions for indirect services. Student progress is monitored. Lack of progress moves student to Tier 3.

Tier 1
Modification of general education goals by regular education personnel. Student progress is monitored. Lack of progress moves student to Tier 2.

and summative sources of information, (e) interventions that have an evidence base, (f) procedures for identifying the selection and revision of instructional practices, and (g) measures to monitor the fidelity of implementation." It is clear from this statement that assessment and evaluation procedures are intimately related to almost every principle. Jackson et al. (2009) go on to point out that preferred methods of assessment should include naturalistic observation, family preferences, and functional outcomes. When monitoring treatment progress, some allowance should be made not only for pre- and postintervention measures but also on more frequent assessments on a daily or weekly basis to determine if the program needs modification. For some SLPs this may require an adjustment. For example, Jackson et al. (2009, p. 429) indicate: "Although SLPs have specific knowledge in the area of communication and language, the challenge is to shift their focus from the discipline's traditionally 'clinical,' norm-referenced assessment approaches to engagement in collaborative assessment practices that are authentic and focus on all areas of child development."

So what does this have to do with assessment? It should be abundantly clear that evaluating a student's baseline abilities and then continuing to monitor his or her performance during an intensive, short-term treatment regimen involves copious measurements. In the RTI model, such assessment is very important because it can be used in the decision-making process to determine eligibility for special education services.

Dynamic Assessment

If diagnosis is to be of utmost benefit, it must be goal-oriented. Diagnosis is an empty exercise in test administration, data collection, and client evaluation if it fails to provide logical suggestions for treatment. Most clinicians would like to believe that there is a magic or set procedure that will work for each client to improve communication. In almost every disorder area (fluency, voice, language, articulation), however, there is a multitude of procedures from which to select. Not only are there different types of treatment in terms of philosophy, entry level, and targets trained but there are also differences in the nature of the delivery system (e.g., highly structured, behavioral, client directed, cognitive, etc.). Thus, the SLP is faced with a number of avenues from which to choose in terms of making treatment recommendations.

The notion of using time in a diagnostic session to gain insight into performance on treatment tasks is known as *dynamic assessment* (Gutierrez-Clellen & Pena, 2001; Johns & Haynes, 2002; Lidz, 1991; Miller, Gillam, & Pena, 2001; Pena, 1996; Wade & Haynes 1989). We feel that dynamic assessment is an important part of any diagnostic venture because, from these tasks, learning processes and a direction for treatment emerges. Table 1–1 illustrates salient differences between dynamic and static assessment. *Static assessment* is like a snapshot of a child's performance at a given moment in time. When we administer a standardized test, we are capturing a child's performance at a certain point, and we may characterize this behavior as a number or score. Static assessment, however, does not address how the child may be able to perform more effectively with assistance by the clinician or under altered circumstances. Dynamic assessment relies heavily on Vygotsky's (1978) notion of the zone of proximal development, which defines a range of performance that a child can produce with assistance from adults or peers. Standardized tests do not allow the clinician to assist a child or ask the client why he or she answered a question in a particular manner. In dynamic assessment, the clinician can determine a client's range of performance, given help by the clinician, and can find what types of circumstances result in improved performance. Almost every communication disorder area has a variety of variables to experiment with during a diagnostic session. We are of the opinion that treatment should be viewed rather like a single-subject experimental design. No one really knows which type of treatment will be effective for a given client or which variables will have the most impact on performance. This is typically learned during the first stage of treatment as the clinician begins to fine-tune the management program. However, the diagnostic session can easily be used to gain some insight into client tendencies and preferences. Clients with aphasia may respond more favorably to certain combinations of cues in word retrieval. Clients

TABLE 1–1
Comparison of Static and Dynamic Assessment

Static Assessment	Dynamic Assessment
Passive Participants Child does task without help	**Active Participants** Child participates with adult help; can ask questions and get feedback
Examiner Observes Scores test; typically right/wrong responses	**Examiner Participates** Gives feedback; helps child develop strategies
Results Identify Deficits Test results profile deficits, what child can and cannot do	**Results Describe Modifiability** Results profile how responsive the child is, given help; describe strategies
Standardized Administration Given in standardized manner; no deviation from standard format	**Administration Fluid, Responsive** Nonstandardized administration; examiner responses contingent on child's behavior

Source: Adapted from Pena, Quinn, and Iglesias (1992).

with fluency disorders may become more fluent with one particular technique than with a second method. A child with a language impairment may respond better to a structured task as opposed to a child-directed one, or vice versa. A nonverbal child may show a marked tendency to learn a few gestures during a diagnostic session rather than to master vocal productions or words.

We could continue with examples of ways in which the clinician can use a portion of the diagnostic session to learn about the client's response to certain treatment variables. Although the diagnostician should never make treatment recommendations based only on hunches, the judicious use of evaluation tasks in the assessment can suggest a reasonable starting point for treatment in many cases. Of course, these recommendations should be treated as working hypotheses and should be stated as such in the diagnostic report. The initial selection of a treatment option is in most cases only an educated guess and is always subject to change based on client performance, which is why we view evaluation as an ongoing process throughout the treatment experience.

THE IMPORTANCE OF FUNCTIONAL MEASUREMENTS: THE WORLD HEALTH ORGANIZATION, U.S. DEPARTMENT OF EDUCATION, AND AMERICAN SPEECH-LANGUAGE-HEARING ASSOCIATION

Over the years, the World Health Organization (WHO) has developed various conceptual frameworks to draw attention to the functional sequelae of an illness or disorder. WHO's International Classification of Functioning, Disability and Health, better known simply as ICF, provides a standard way of describing a person's health and health-related states (World Health Organization, 2002). The ICF is a multipurpose classification system that helps healthcare professionals describe a person's changes in two ways. The first concerns body function and structure: what the person can do in a standard environment. Such levels of capacity are often assessed through standardized testing. The second addresses what the person can actually do in his or her usual environment. These levels of performance are often assessed via nonstandardized probes and indexes of daily activity and participation. This ICF classification system is a radical change in healthcare diagnosis and evaluation—rather than emphasizing a person's disability, the focus is shifted to the level of health. Said another way, the focus is shifted from cause to impact. We see this change echoed in recent clinical research literature. The speech-language pathologist also no longer diagnoses and evaluates only a client's communication deficit. Rather, attention is also directed toward assessing a client's communicative functioning in his or her environment. What can the client do? What impact do the client's communication abilities have on her or his socialization? Psychological state? Education? Vocation and avocations? Clearly, the modern SLP is concerned with the concepts of functioning and social disability as espoused in the ICF (World Health Organization, 2002). In each chapter of this text, we will present this ICF model as a reminder of our professional concerns with both functioning and disability in our realm of diagnosis and evaluation.

Beginning in 2008, the U.S. Department of Education required all states to submit accountability data regarding programs that serve young children with disabilities. Hebbeler and Rooney (2009, p. 451) state, "Across professional organizations, the recommendations related to assessment contain similar themes, emphasizing the use of multiple sources of information, focusing on the child and family, and highlighting the use of assessment data for program planning and monitoring . . . . A balanced assessment, according to ASHA, includes gathering child-centered, contextualized, performance-based, descriptive and functional information from families, teachers and other service providers." The specific areas of interest involve social-emotional skills, acquiring and using knowledge/skills, and abilities of clients to make their needs known to others. Functional outcome assessments, as mandated by the U.S. Department of Education, typically take the form of a 7-point rating scale—7 being age-appropriate skills and 1 being lack of foundational skills to accomplish the task. All of the seven levels carry operational definitions, and the scale values can be used to determine functional response to treatment. Such rating systems are prevalent in healthcare settings (e.g., Functional Independence Measures; FIM) and in the ASHA National Outcomes Measurement System (NOMS). Thus, there seems to be a convergence of the various professional organizations and governmental agencies on the value of initial and ongoing assessment, no matter what the age group or disability.

Diagnosis and evaluation of communication disorders require significant input from speech-language pathologists, so it is important to review briefly the guidelines put forth by ASHA regarding assessment. First of all, ASHA develops what are called preferred practice patterns (PPPs) that generally define acceptable clinical approaches to assessment and treatment of communication disorders. Specifically, the PPPs "represent the consensus of the members of the professions after they considered available scientific evidence, existing ASHA and related policies, current practice patterns, expert opinions, and the collective judgment and experience of practitioners in the field. Requirements of federal and state governments and accrediting and regulatory agencies also have been considered" (American Speech-Language-Hearing Association, 2004, p. 3). It is easy to see that such guidelines can have a far-reaching effect on the knowledge and skills required in speech-language pathology training programs and also on clinical practice in the field. The ASHA document on PPPs is driven in large part by "fundamental components and guiding principles," which are based on guidelines from WHO mentioned earlier. According to these fundamental guidelines, the evaluation must first of all be comprehensive, which means that several important areas must be addressed:

1. *Body structures and functions.* Clearly, medically based problems are implicated in body structures (e.g., neurogenic disorders, cleft palate). Functions include "mental functions such as attention as well as components of communication such as articulatory proficiency, fluency and syntax" (p. 4). Thus, this first component would involve making a thorough diagnosis and defining the nature of a client's communication problem, similar to what professionals do in the assessment of any health-related condition. Obviously, we can accomplish the goal of a thorough diagnosis by administration of standardized and nonstandardized tests.

2. *Activities and participation.* This component deals with the client's ability to participate in daily social, communicative, and self-help activities and perform tasks that may be relevant to educational and/or vocational enterprises. Essentially this means that part of an effective assessment must involve looking at how a communication disorder may affect a client's daily activities and ability to perform in the real-life environments of society, work, or education. Clearly, the use of tests is likely not the most efficient way to gain this information because there is no substitute for case history information, clinical interviewing, observing the client in the natural environment, and rating his or her functional abilities in communication and related activities.

3. *Contextual factors.* These factors can include personal attributes of culture, education, social status, and environmental variables that may present obstacles or facilitate communication. Again, standardized testing may not be the most efficient vehicle for gaining this information. Rather, nonstandardized approaches such as interviewing, patient rating scales, and observation in natural settings may provide the most relevant clinical data.

The ASHA PPP document also provides other diagnostic and evaluation guidelines of a more general nature. Following are some selected principles that are especially pertinent to the present text:

1. *Measuring outcomes.* According to the guidelines, "Outcomes of services are monitored and measured in order to ensure the quality of services provided and to improve quality of those services" (p. 5). As we have stated previously, assessment is not confined to a diagnostic session but rather continues throughout treatment as well.

2. *Going beyond static assessment.* An emphasis of the present text is that diagnosis and evaluation are far more than simply administering a battery of standardized tests. While standardized tests can tell us if a problem exists, they rarely describe the nature or complexities of the problem. The ASHA PPP document states: "Assessment may be static (i.e., using procedures designed to describe structures, functions, and environmental demands and supports in relevant domains at a given point in time) or dynamic (i.e., using hypothesis testing procedures to identify potential for change and elements of successful interventions and supports)" (p. 5). We will be covering both static and dynamic assessment in this text.

3. *Approaching assessment scientifically.* The ASHA PPP recommends that "services are consistent with the best available scientific and clinical evidence in conjunction with individual considerations" (p. 5). This notion is essentially what has become known as EBP. ASHA and other disciplines are emphasizing EBP and following the lead of the medical profession in applying research to clinical practice. We will discuss selected aspects of EBP that apply to assessment later in this text.

The American Speech-Language-Hearing Association has also been involved in examining functional outcomes of treatment for communication disorders. Since 1994, a variety of ASHA task force groups have been active in developing NOMS, which includes functional communication measures (FCMs) for most speech, language, and swallowing disorders for children to adults. The FCMs are composed of 7-point rating scales that rate the patient from the least functional (level 1) to the most functional (level 7). The ratings are based on clinical observations by the SLP and do not necessarily rely on any formal assessment procedures. To date, FCMs have been developed for adults and prekindergarten children in the following areas: articulation/intelligibility, alaryngeal communication, attention, augmentative-alternative communication, cognitive orientation, fluency, memory, motor speech, pragmatics, reading, problem solving, spoken language comprehension, spoken language expression, swallowing, voice, voice following tracheostomy, and writing. Currently, ASHA releases the FCMs only in the context of NOMS, and the scales are used mainly in this ongoing research. Eventually, the FCMs will be useful for widespread clinical use. It is important to note, however, that in most healthcare settings worldwide, professionals in speech-language pathology, physical therapy, occupational therapy, and other disciplines have routinely used functional independence measurements (FIMs) to gauge client progress in the rehabilitation process. Such scores are typically on a 7-point scale, just like the FCMs described above; the scale runs from total assistance (level 1) to total independence (level 7). The scales are used for abilities such as ambulation, communication, grooming, bathing, dressing, memory, and social interaction. These FIM scores are used for many purposes, ranging from discharge decisions to reimbursement guidelines. Anyone working in a medical setting will tell you that FIM scores are one of the most important determiners of the effectiveness and efficiency of rehabilitation programs and a favorite tool of healthcare administrators.

It can be seen from this discussion that functional outcome measurements are important components in initially assessing clients and in monitoring progress through treatment. We want clients not only to improve their abilities on chosen methods of assessment but also to be able to master functional abilities that will affect their lives. The term *activities of daily living(ADLs)* refers to practical behaviors related to common activities such as eating, communicating, and ambulation. These ADLs are often selected as targets for treatment and measured in terms of functional gains. Thus, assessment is not only about testing; it also includes educated clinical observations and functional estimates of a client's performance.

DIAGNOSIS TO DETERMINE THE REALITY OF THE PROBLEM

One function of diagnosis is to determine whether the presenting communication pattern does indeed constitute a handicap. Before this determination is possible, however, it is necessary to have a clear idea of what constitutes a communication disorder. Van Riper's classical definition of a speech disorder is widely quoted: "Speech is abnormal when it deviates so far from the speech of other people that it calls attention to itself, interferes with communication, or causes the speaker or his listeners to be distressed" (Van Riper & Emerick, 1984, p. 34). Figure 1–5 depicts three components that must be considered in determining a communication disorder.

1. *Speech difference.* Speech difference refers to whether the speech signal calls attention to itself and when this might occur. We can quantify the physical characteristics of the speech signal through recording, measurement, and observation. In other words, we must scrutinize the physical characteristics of the speech signal and judge its quality. But these data are of limited value unless it can be determined what *difference* a particular speech parameter makes.

In most areas of communication disorders, the state of the art has not progressed to where we can simply take the quantified data, compare them with established numerical norms, and determine the correctness of the speech sample. Rather, each diagnostician must use professional judgment and develop a personal frame of reference. Vocal qualities are subject to individual impressions; although a clinician may *know* that the voice is awry, evidence of the difference may often elude the algorithms of our high-tech instrumentation. The question of whether the presenting speech difference is different enough to be of concern thus becomes a matter of human judgment. This judgment involves filtering incoming data through the clinician's many synaptic junctions, whose thresholds may have been worn thin by bias and experience. An inordinately critical or uncritical ear is a hazard with far-reaching implications.

FIGURE 1–5
Three Components of a Definition of a Speech Disorder

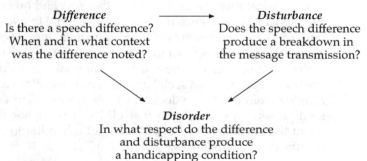

What constitutes normal behavior? Several definitions are available, but we will discuss only two, representing the diverging philosophies with which each clinician must contend in establishing his or her own concept. The first theory we shall call the concept of *cultural norms*. The assumption is that society considers some behaviors aberrant in terms of group characteristics. According to this model, each bit of behavior can be judged against a real or theoretical standard, the nature of which is independent of the individual's personal idiosyncrasies. The second theory we shall call the concept of *individual norms*. Advocates of this model assume that each individual has made a unique adjustment to life based on previous experiences, physical limitations, and the environment's reactions. Any judgment about the normalcy of a bit of behavior must be contingent on individual characteristics such as age, intelligence, and experience. Taken to the extreme, the latter model would assert that each person is normal no matter what he or she does because the behavior is the end product of all that plays upon the person. Within this theory the concept of individual norms loses meaning. But some case examples may help to clarify and give perspective.

The audiologist who examines the hearing of the 70-year-old individual and who obtains the typical presbycusic audiometric curve could make a case for the judgment that this person has "normal" hearing. According to individual norms, this is average or normal behavior for a person at age 70; according to cultural norms, however, the individual's hearing level is below the average for the total population. Follow-up procedures would thus be based on the practical matter of getting a more efficient communication system for the individual and also on providing counseling so that the person will understand the nature of his or her hearing. Therefore, both cultural and personal norms play a part in diagnostic judgments and rehabilitative programs. A 10-year-old child with severe cognitive delays and an unstimulable distortion of the /r/ phoneme may not be judged to have seriously defective speech, whereas an 8-year-old presenting a similar speech pattern but a different intellectual potential may be recommended for treatment. Such judgments have implications for case selection, and the clinician must reconcile the variances between the physical differences in the sounds involved and the individual variables in conjunction with what is normal for the population as a whole. Each clinician must continually use both concepts of normalcy in diagnostic work.

A speech signal can call attention to itself in all sorts of ways and yet be perfectly appropriate. For example, an African American English (AAE) speaker may alter aspects of speech and language when style-shifting between members of one culture and another. Although Standard American English (SAE) speakers may notice the differences in AAE, these variations certainly would not be viewed as evidence of a communication disorder. Another example might be when speakers alter their rate, loudness, and vocal quality in order to tell a funny story or relate a particular experience in a dramatic way. Age is another variable. If the speaker is a child of 2 who exhibits many articulatory substitutions and omissions, does this difference constitute a problem? The answer can only lie in an examination of these errors against the context of normal 2-year-old communication. Thus, a difference is not enough to constitute a communication disorder if the context suggests normality. This underscores the importance of the SLP knowing the contextual effects on communication and the contributions of age and the wide variety of cultural, ethnic, and geographical dialects on the speech signal.

2. *The intelligibility of the message.* The second component of determining a communication disorder involves the perception of disturbance in the signal that is transmitted. Is the signal distorted, or is its intelligibility affected? If the message transmission is adversely affected, there is a high probability of the existence of a problem. Many factors play a part in both the encoding and decoding processes, and the diagnostician must be capable of representing the standard for society when listening and making judgments.

We have mainly been content with clinical insight and intuitive estimates when we have judged the impact of speech differences on intelligibility. The clinician is able to count the phoneme errors, quantify the number of disfluencies per sentence, and establish various quotients of language ability, but it is still a challenge to assess the intelligibility of the message with any degree of reliability. In most cases the clinician resorts to scaling techniques to mark the impact of the disorder on intelligibility, and we do not really know what specific speech or language components contributed to the overall signal distortion. Clearly, severe disfluency can interrupt a message, intermittent cessations of phonation and poor vocal qualities can distort transmission, inappropriate phoneme selection or production can lead to unintelligibility, and ambiguous vocabulary or sentence structure can lead to misinterpretations. Whatever the cause of the communication failure, we must document that it occurs. At present, however, we have no widely accepted system to use in this documentation for most areas of communication disorders.

3. *Handicapping condition.* The final component in defining a disorder involves the determination of handicap in the life of the client. Emerick (1984) suggests:

> In the final analysis this third aspect justifies the existence of our profession. If the speech difference has no discernible impact on the child's behavior, and ultimately on his adjusting abilities and learning potential, there is little justification for concern on the part of the speech clinician. Although it is not feasible to compile a listing of all of the possible conditions under which a communication difference would become handicapping, it is generally agreed that communicative differences are considered handicapping when: (1) the transmission and/or perception of messages is faulty; (2) the person is placed at an economic disadvantage; (3) the person is placed at a learning disadvantage; (4) the person is placed at a social disadvantage; (5) there is a negative impact upon the emotional growth of the person; or (6) the problem causes physical damage or endangers the health of the person.

There are numerous examples of famous people who are highly successful and seemingly content with their lives despite manifesting a communication disorder. Some famous personalities have happy, fulfilling lives even though an SLP would have classified them as having a handicap. On the other hand, a minor deviation in a teacher or business executive may mean a significant handicap in terms of credibility and evaluation of job performance. Two people with hearing impairment can have identical audiograms and yet report significantly different effects that hearing loss has on their lives. If a person does not view his or her communication disorder as a handicap, it is difficult to justify clinical work or to motivate the client to improve communication skills.

DIAGNOSIS TO DETERMINE THE ETIOLOGY OF THE PROBLEM

Far too many clinicians view diagnosis simply as a labeling process; however, the actual labeling, or categorizing, is only a small part of the total assessment. Classification systems within our profession are poor at best, and high-level abstractions (e.g., stuttering) tend to emphasize the similarities within populations rather than the individual differences. The keen diagnostician regards classifications as communication conveniences to be viewed with suspicion. Of course, the convenience factor is important, and each clinician who makes a determination of the reality of the problem must be willing to label it. This necessity must, however, follow an orderly description of the characteristics of the disorder so that it can be clear what route the diagnostician took in arriving at the final classification. A diagnosis that only describes the characteristics of the problem, without judging its type or class, is a dead end. Nelson (2010, p. 102) points to three major difficulties with categorization: "(1) lack of recognition of complexity of human differences, (2) unnecessary stigmatization, and (3) not enough benefits to overshadow the limitations." She goes on to say that categorization will not be abandoned in the real world because it is helpful in qualifying children for special services, funding, and admission to special programs run by state and federal governments.

The opposite path is also dangerous; the diagnostician who is willing to begin an evaluation by labeling the problem has reversed the orderly sequence of acquiring knowledge and often effectively closes his or her mind to factors that may later point away from the premature diagnosis. Nelson (2010) applies an old metaphor to the diagnostic process. If a clinician focuses only on the macrolevels of diagnosis such as applying a label to a client, he or she is likely to miss the trees for the forest. On the other hand, if the focus is only on microlevels, such as memory or auditory processing, the forest is missed for the trees. This is a wise notion to remember as we engage in diagnosis and evaluation. If we concentrate on macrolevels, we do not become familiar with the individual needs of the client; if we focus on microlevels, we may not see how the client's abilities or impairments represent a broader syndrome.

The notion of "cause" has different meanings depending on its distance from the problem. As you look at a client in a diagnostic session, you search for reasons for the presenting behaviors. In fact, many of these reasons may be buried in the past and can be revealed only by painstaking effort. In many cases, cause and effect may be layered in complex patterns. Not only must we search through the client's past experience in order to uncover events that may help us alter current behaviors but we must also guard against looking for causes in only one dimension of behavior. A child's brain damage, once identified, is probably not the only etiological factor because communication is a complicated human function. Social, learning, motivation, and many other factors enter into the total process. Paul (2001) illustrates the complexity of determining causation in an example of babies who were exposed to cocaine because their mothers used the drug during pregnancy:

> Cocaine was usually not the only risk to which they were exposed. Mothers who abused cocaine during pregnancy also tended to abuse other street drugs, as well as alcohol. Alcohol itself is known to be a serious teratogen and could cause many of the problems thought to be present in these babies, even without any other substance abuse. Further, mothers who abused cocaine and other drugs during pregnancy frequently continued to do so after the child was born. These mothers would not be very available to their infants for either basic care or for social interaction . . . . Finally, mothers who abuse cocaine and other drugs tend to live in poverty. Poverty itself affects both general and communicative development through the tendency for poor children to have been born small and prematurely and to have poor nutrition, inadequate medical care and incomplete or absent inoculation against disease. (p. 99)

Thus, determining the etiology of a problem is not always straightforward, and we must be cautious about attributing the cause of a disorder to a particular event or factor. Classically, etiology has been defined in terms of predisposing, precipitating, and perpetuating factors. Predisposing factors are generally thought to be important because of their potential link with a third agent. A classic example of predisposing factors is the apparent genetic predisposition to stutter. We know that stuttering tends to run in families; however, it could be that environmental factors cause it to surface. The wary diagnostician must watch for factors that occur with high regularity in association with certain communication disorders. Such data could ultimately be instrumental in uncovering some basic information regarding the nature of the disorder.

Precipitating factors are generally no longer operating and, as such, may or may not be identifiable. For example, a child with a language disorder may have begun to lag behind in linguistic development during a period of recurrent ear infections that occurred when language was being learned. If the otitis has long since disappeared and the language disorder remains, it is difficult for the diagnostician to observe or even pinpoint the true cause of the disability. Even if the child did have recurrent bouts with ear infections, it can never be truly substantiated that these infections actually precipitated or played a role in language delay, especially because many children experience frequent ear infections and manage to develop language normally. In many cases the precipitating factors are clear, as in instances of stroke, vocal abuse, structural abnormalities, and certain congenital conditions.

The perpetuating factors are those variables currently at work on the individual. Almost without exception, habit strength is a prime perpetuating factor in many disorders because the client has made various compensations for the problem in terms of cognitive/linguistic strategies and motor adjustments. Other factors are also crucial, however, and it is the diagnostician's task to uncover the environmental and physical factors that are reinforcing and thus perpetuating the disorder. A hearing loss may be a precipitating and a perpetuating factor in a child's language delay. This child needs a thorough audiological evaluation and possibly amplification, if indicated, or else the problem will perpetuate. We must always work to identify and, if possible, remove or reduce any factors that maintain a communication disorder.

DIAGNOSIS TO PROVIDE CLINICAL FOCUS

Although it is important to know the causes of the disorder, it is substantially more important to gain some insight into the possible ways to improve the client's communication. At this point, diagnosis and clinical management overlap. This is also where the importance of knowing a host of evaluation techniques becomes significant in the diagnostic enterprise. The diagnostician must ask a series of questions, such as the following:

1. What do I know about this condition?

   What are the usual etiologies?

   What are the usual effective treatment procedures?

   What is the typical prognosis?

2. What do I know about this person?

   What is the impact of the condition on the person?

   What are the person's strengths and needs?

   How is this person like others I have worked with?

   How is this person different from others I have worked with?

3. What do I know about my own skills in the treatment of this disorder and this type of person?

   How have I approached similar problems effectively?

   How have I worked effectively with similar people?

4. What do I know about the services of other professionals available for this person?

   What referrals need to be made?

   What consultations do I need to make?

5. What factors need to be removed, altered, or added to improve the prognosis?

    What inhibiting environmental factors exist?

    What organic factors need alteration?

    What can enhance the person's motivation?

    How can the family be involved in treatment?

Note how many of these questions address components of evidence-based practice discussed earlier.

DIAGNOSIS: SCIENCE AND ART

Diagnosis demands a unique blend of science and art (Silverman, 1984). The scientific method is applicable to our work as diagnosticians, both in guiding our procedures and in focusing our attitude of operation. The scientific method directs the diagnostician to observe all of the available factors, to formulate testable hypotheses by using clearly stated and answerable questions, to test those hypotheses to determine their validity, and to reach conclusions based on the tested hypotheses. The method demands rigorous adherence to standardized procedures and has as its favorable characteristics objectivity, quantifiability, and structure. The scientific diagnostician tends to rely on tests, test data, and other procedures that lend themselves to quantification. As an attitude of operation, the scientific method implies that the diagnostician has not predetermined the test findings and that there is no bias in seeking the proof or disproof of hypotheses. The diagnostician sees hypotheses as something to be tested rather than something to be defended.

The self-fulfilling prophecy is a lethal but almost universal human characteristic; it must be counterbalanced by a scientific approach to testing. We are familiar with parents of children with language impairment who have traveled all over the country in search of a diagnostic explanation for the linguistic delay. Often these children are victims of the "fat folder syndrome," in which a case file has accrued over the years with reports from various authorities and clinics. Each report often reveals more about the examiner than the child because it cites facts in support of a theory of etiology congruent with the diagnostician's particular specialty. For example, in the same client, the audiologist finds auditory processing disorder, the autism specialist diagnoses an autism spectrum disorder, the psychologist discovers attention-deficit disorder, and the speech-language pathologist finds language impairment. Finding what you want to find is not always in the realm of the scientific method. Diagnosticians often use their pet test instruments, to use a famous saying, as the drunk uses the street lamp—more for support than illumination!

The strict adherence to fact that is demanded by the pure scientific method is often a bit confining. That may explain in part why we all practice the art of diagnosis at times. The artistic approach has several specific characteristics. The artist is less dependent on specific observations than on casual and nonstructured scrutiny for the formation of hypotheses. This type of clinician is perfectly willing to disregard formal test results or standard testing procedures in favor of what appears obvious on the basis of clinical experience and expertise. The hunch, or clinical intuition, plays a significant part in such evaluations. This diagnostician will contend that facts can be approached from several directions and that we are capable of assessing the same kinds of behaviors that are measured on formal tests by using nonstandardized evaluation tasks. Such contentions are disconcerting to the test-bound person who has come to expect that the only valid way to gain information is through standardized procedures. One of the emphases in this text is that these informal, nonstandardized evaluation procedures are valuable indeed in defining a client's problem and the potential response to treatment. In many ways these procedures may be more valid than standardized tests, as we will discuss in Chapter 3.

It is obvious that, in the extreme, there are weaknesses in both approaches. The scientist may tend to become so dependent on objective methods of measurement that he or she fails to see the client through the maze of percentiles and standard scores. The whole is greater than the sum of its parts, and every diagnostician must guard against simply measuring the isolated characteristics without getting a full picture of the individual. The possibility of a diagnostician projecting more than a modest amount of personal bias into the evaluation is greater when a less scientific approach is used. Clinical intuitions are often simply clinical biases, and it is very easy to make new evidence fit old categories. The diagnostician must find the proper mix of each philosophy in establishing assessment procedures.

DIAGNOSIS VERSUS ELIGIBILITY

As our legal system, medical settings, and public school systems have become more complicated, clinicians are faced with increasing pressure to conduct their clinical work within parameters that are set by administrators. The resulting procedures for case selection, testing, and determining eligibility for services many times fall short of the ideal professional criteria used to make these decisions.

The influence of administrative decision making on our profession has blurred the distinction between diagnosis, on the one hand, and determining eligibility, on the other. While we cannot always do everything optimally for a client in certain work settings, we need to be very careful in our decisions to streamline services and not make arbitrary decisions for administrative purposes that undermine our profession. For example, it is not unusual for private practitioners and community clinics to provide services to children who have clear language/phonological disorders but who are ineligible for such services in the local school system. Similarly, it is not unusual for private practitioners and university clinics to provide services to medically involved patients whose insurance carriers will no longer pay for treatment. Ehren (1993) nicely describes how caseloads are often influenced by eligibility. And the art of diagnosis has, in essence, been traded for the process of determining eligibility. The process of evaluating and describing what a child's communication needs are has been lost. She urges the community to return to its diagnostic clinical roots and the traditional process of first making a diagnosis, followed by treatment or service recommendations. Only after the diagnosis and service recommendations are made should eligibility be determined.

THE DIAGNOSTICIAN AS A FACTOR

What skills are necessary to develop in order to become an effective diagnostician? How do you develop them? What makes one diagnostician better than another? There are no easy answers to these questions. Experience in the diagnostic process is an absolute necessity, but experience in number of clients seen is not enough. A pompous clinician once bragged, "I've had over 20 years of experience." The unfortunate thing, however, is that this person had the first year of experience repeated 19 times, which is altogether a different matter. The diagnostician must be able to gain from new experiences, and this demands *flexibility*. The stereotyped, dogmatic, and stagnant diagnostician learns little from increased exposure to people and new situations. Diagnosticians who use their experience as a pattern to be compared against, rather than as a mold into which all new experiences must fit, will continue to grow and learn. The diagnostician must be flexible enough within the testing situation to shift from predetermined plans to new modes of evaluation as the client presents unpredicted behaviors. The examiner who fails to recognize that a client presents some interesting new behavior or exhibits valid instances of communication ability in nontest contexts will miss an important opportunity to gain insight into the problem. It is not atypical for beginning clinicians to panic in the face of unanticipated performance or behaviors. There is the tendency to become uncompromising in the application of a series of formal tests because there is a certain degree of comfort in known processes and sticking with the initial plan. Continued experience in diagnosis may provide the flexibility needed to move freely to other avenues of information.

Another characteristic of a good diagnostician is a *healthy skepticism* and ability to *evaluate critically* new clinical techniques. Practicing clinicians often eagerly accept new and novel techniques as they become available. New techniques must not be accepted or rejected carte blanche but rather must be scrutinized for their merit. We must learn to keep up with new developments by participating in an active continuing education program, both personal and professional. On the other hand, the beginning student must guard against the "recent article" or "new test" syndrome to which we all fall prey on occasion. Typically, the behavioral pattern goes something like this: You read an article that depicts a particular syndrome and explains the distinctive characteristics of a disorder; for a few weeks thereafter every child you see appears to fall into the pattern described in the publication. The way to overcome the "recent article" syndrome, of course, is to be aware that it exists and to have a thorough understanding of the nature of human perception. With regard to new tests, some clinicians get into the "new test" syndrome and use the most popular test of the day simply because it is new. Many forms of assessment have stood the test of time and should not be discounted for their age or dated packaging.

A clinician must possess many important *interpersonal relationship attributes.* Empathy, congruency, and unconditional positive regard are necessary characteristics of the clinician, and they most certainly apply to the diagnostic process as well. In many studies of clinical competence and outcome, the interpersonal or therapeutic relationship is a major factor contributing to successful treatment (Norcross & Wampold, 2011). Generally these qualities must be nurtured by consistent effort and proper guidance in training programs through analysis by clinical supervisors and review of session video recordings by clinicians in training.

The development of an *evaluative attitude* and *sensitivity* is often a rather difficult task for the beginning clinician. We are, to a large extent, slaves to our experience; each clinician tends to bring a social attitude into the test setting. Rather than look on the client's performance as having meaning for the evaluative process, we consult our own responses and formulate our own points of view in the give and take of the conversation. The critical, questioning attitude must be developed so that the clinician looks on the behaviors in terms of their meaning rather than in terms of the response expected. Social interaction lends itself to superficiality, whereas the flow of the diagnostic interaction must, by design, lend itself to uncovering the meaning of the incorporated behavior. Effective diagnosticians tend to question the surface validity of behaviors and search for motivations, explanations, and interpretations that are not readily apparent. Sensitivity may be defined as a keenness of sense or a heightened awareness of incoming sensory data. When viewed in this manner this term then has meaning for the diagnostician. The clinician must be able to detect subtle physical, psychological, or interactional changes in a client's behavior because these small changes may have significant meaning in the diagnostic process.

Closely allied with the concept of the evaluative attitude and sensitivity is the idea of *persistent curiosity*. The diagnostician must develop an inquisitiveness that will make him or her persistent in searching for explanations. Answers are seldom apparent at first, and continuous effort is imperative. The curious and persistent clinician continues to place the client in situations that will permit additional scrutiny. In an attempt to give each student a variety of clinical experiences, training institutions often tend to sever clinical undertakings with a client at each semester's end. It would be ideal, albeit probably unworkable in training programs, for students to follow their clients over longer periods of time so that the students could see how diagnosis is an ongoing process and an integral part of treatment as the client changes.

Objectivity comes from practicing the art of controlled involvement. The diagnostician must cultivate objectivity because everyone is subject to human errors. We must be warm, understanding, and accepting, on the one hand, and objective, evaluative, and detached, on the other. Without some degree of balance between the two extremes, the diagnostician may distort the interaction with the client so severely that little information of value is obtained. Objectivity demands more than simply guarding against undue emotional involvement. To grow as a diagnostician, the examiner must be objective about his or her skills, knowledge, and personal characteristics and must take an objective attitude toward the client.

Rapport may be defined as the establishment of a working relationship, based on mutual respect, trust, and confidence, that encourages optimum performance on the part of both client and clinician. Rapport is developed over a period of time and is not easily established in a single session or during a few minutes at the initiation of one diagnostic encounter. Rapport must not only be developed, it must also be maintained, and this calls for continued effort. We have known for decades that, especially with children, performance on formal tests varies with clinician familiarity (Fuchs, Fuchs, Dailey, & Power, 1985). Children tend to perform better if they have had an opportunity to become familiar with an examiner. While the reasons for this phenomenon are not totally clear, the concept of rapport is obviously involved.

It is important that our *focus* be on the client as much as possible instead of on our own performance and internal states. Diagnosticians are people too, and we often forget that they occasionally have a bad day. They too can experience the influence of pervasive personal problems and physical frailties that sometimes make them feel as though they should have stayed at home in bed. The most knowledgeable and skillful diagnostician, however, may fail to achieve adequate results if he or she lacks the inquisitiveness necessary to encourage continuous effort and if there is no professional drive to serve each individual to the maximum potential. Each of us is subject to individual variations in daily behavior (physical problems, depression, stress, etc.) that can have a direct effect on performance; however, it is incumbent upon every professional to control those variations to provide each individual with the best service available.

THE CLIENT–CLINICIAN RELATIONSHIP

Although much standardization is possible through strict adherence to test routines, the lowest common denominator in diagnostic evaluations is the examiner. Test results are the product of the subject, examiner, test, and test circumstances, and each has a certain influence. Examinations are clearly selected as a result of the experiences and biases of the examiner. Just as the answers we receive to questions are in part a function of the questions we ask and how we ask them, the diagnostic findings we obtain are in part a function of the tests we administer and the way they are administered. An impaired communication pattern may be partially due to a defective testing pattern or an incompetent tester.

The most crucial factor in conducting a successful diagnostic session is the client–clinician relationship and the establishment of a working alliance. When one person works with another, there is always human impact. No matter how well prepared and rehearsed an examiner may be, if his or her approach to people is poor or if his or her approach is incongruent with that of the clients, failure will result. All tests, all examinations, all so-called objective diagnostic procedures are mediated by person-to-person contact.

Impersonal, test-oriented clinical examination sessions can make assessment more difficult because there is no absolute division between diagnosis and therapy. The first contact with a client initiates treatment. During a diagnostic session, the client is forming opinions and conceptions about the clinician and the total clinical situation. Not all clients will require the full impact of this interpersonal dimension. Indeed, some individuals simply want to find out what is wrong and then rectify the situation. The point is, however, that the clinician should be able to discern what the client needs and then adjust his or her style appropriately.

THE CLIENT AS A FACTOR: CHILDREN, ADOLESCENTS, AND OLDER ADULTS

Although all age levels present unique diagnostic problems, three groups in particular—young children; adolescents; and, to a lesser extent, older or elderly clients—require special effort and expertise. The present chapter is generic in nature, so we will talk mainly about the general business of relating to the different age groups seen in diagnostic evaluations. Subsequent chapters will provide additional and more specific suggestions for dealing with the different age groups in the context of evaluating particular disorders. A major reason for including this generic section is that many readers of the present text are students in training to become speech-language pathologists. It is often difficult for a young person to capture the ephemeral guidelines for relating to people of different ages. It is not as simple as just "being yourself" or talking one way to a child and another way to an adult. Students have made certain common errors over the years that we can at least alert you to so that you may avoid them. These precepts, of course, are drawn from the experiences of the authors, and obviously many more guidelines could be added.

Young Children

Preschool and kindergarten children are often difficult to test and examine. Unlike most older children and adults, they just do not see the payoff for all the questioning and prodding. Often a major problem is dealing with the child's fear of the clinical situation. This apprehension may stem from one or more of the following related factors: (1) inadequate preparation for the examination by parents, (2) uncertainty about what will be done to or with the child by the clinician, (3) vivid memories of trauma during visits to dentists and physicians, (4) the contagious anxieties and uncertainties experienced by the parents, and (5) stress and conflicts engendered by past listener reactions to the communication impairment. Children confront the clinical examination in a variety of ways, but the two most trying responses are shyness and withdrawal and, at the other extreme, aggressiveness and hyperactivity.

In many cases with very young children, it is possible to have the parent participate in the interaction, and this avoids any separation anxiety on the part of the child. The parents are typically willing to cooperate, the child is happy, and the parents can often get the child to participate in many ways that the clinician would take several sessions of rapport building to accomplish. Parents can even be used to administer some formal tests that just involve turning picture plates and reading the cues on the backs of the pictures, while the clinician scores the child's responses. We have to choose our battles very carefully, and fighting an obstreperous child in a diagnostic session mainly leads to unsatisfying results for all concerned. In dealing with the children in the birth-to-age-2 age range, *most* of the pertinent information will be gleaned from parents, both from interview data and by observation of parent–child interactions. Not many 1-year-olds do well with an unfamiliar clinician, and we need to focus on the parent–child dyad anyway because treatment will doubtless involve the entire family.

Obviously many other considerations could be discussed; additional suggestions will be offered in the chapters concerning various disorders. For the present, here are several basic precepts on the management of preschool children in a clinical examination:

- Help the parents prepare the child for the diagnostic session. The parents can tell their child what will transpire and maybe even bring along some stimulus items favored by the child (toys, picture albums, books, etc.).

- Play, rather than small talk, is the natural medium of expression for children. This is especially important when dealing with youngsters who may have a communication impairment. While we have all known children in the 3-year-to-5-year age range who are impressive conversationalists, most children referred for communication disorders are not on this end of the conversational continuum. Try to arrange the diagnostic tasks with this in mind.

- As a general rule, ask less and observe more. Children usually lack the insight and cooperation necessary to analyze their problem rationally and objectively. Naturalistic observations—assessing a child's behavior in natural environments—yield more useful information.

- Learn everything possible about typical children in order to provide a baseline for observations of youngsters presenting problems. This can be done by taking courses, studying relevant norms, and most of all by extensive scrutiny and interaction with children in daycare and preschool facilities. You should have a good idea of the typical or modal behavior for children at various age levels.

- Limit the choices you offer a child. Don't ask if he or she would like to go with you, or do this or that, unless the alternatives do not conflict with the examiner's goals. The child will invariably say "No!" Also, refrain from saying "Okay?" after your utterances ("I want you to name these pictures, okay?"). This question suggests that there is an option available to the child.

- Be flexible in your use of tests and examinations. If you cannot employ the rigid standardized format for administration, use the test to obtain all the data you can. If the child refuses to name the test pictures or objects, you may be able to get a language sample from other items. Also, if there is no standard order for administration of tests and tasks, use items the child appears to be interested in at a particular time. For example, if a test has some objects associated with it and the child is attending to these items, start this examination even if you had initially planned it for later in the session.

- Absolute honesty and candor is important in working with children. Do not make promises unless you can keep them.

- The whole assessment does not have to be done in one session; marathon diagnostics tend to be counterproductive. Remember that all we can hope to obtain in one time frame is a sample of a child's behaviors. It is better to terminate (preferably on a pleasant, successful note) than to continue an unproductive session until the child is fatigued or upset.

- Watch your language complexity when talking to children. For obvious reasons, the examiner should avoid sarcasm, idiomatic expressions, ambiguous statements, and indirect requests.

Adolescents

Experienced clinicians frequently report that adolescents, especially those in grades 7 through 11, are often difficult to examine and resistant to treatment. The main problem seems to be getting through to the adolescent. There is no magic formula, but we would like to offer the following suggestions that we have found helpful in guiding our work with adolescent clients:

- Acquire an understanding of the myriad pressures and changes the teenager is experiencing: rapid physical growth, sexual maturity, conflicts between dependence and independence, the development of self-confidence and interpersonal skills necessary to make decisions, a search for identity and life work, intense group loyalty and identification, and many more. It is a turbulent, trying period of behavioral extravagance and excess. It is little wonder that teenagers are often overloaded with personal concerns and do not always welcome an overture of clinical assistance. Empathy that flows from understanding is a powerful force in establishing a working relationship.

- There is an intense desire to be like others, not to stand out from the group in any way that would suggest frailty. Hence, the adolescent may find it extremely difficult to reveal a communication impairment, even if help is desired. Often teenagers are simply sent for evaluation or treatment by parents. In some instances, the teenager with a chronic problem may have been in treatment for a long time and is weary of the idea of more therapy. Many tend to cover up true feelings with a sullen bravado or a dense "it-doesn't-bother-me" shell. Denial is a particular forte. "Coolness" and image are very important. You can neither beat this down nor simply dismiss it with a shrug, nor is silence a particularly effective tool in dealing with adolescent resistance. We advocate a straightforward approach: Acknowledge the forces that are bearing on the individual, point up objectively the paths that others have taken, and provide information about the economic and social penalties that accrue to the person with a communication disorder. Basically, try to demonstrate by your demeanor and what you say that you care about the client; a growing person needs lots of nourishment, and personal involvement and commitment are key factors.

- Do not abandon your professional role for that of a teenager. Be yourself. As Will Rogers pointed out, if they don't like you the way you are, they are sure not going to like you the way you are trying to be.

- Approach adolescents with tolerance and good humor. Do not be shocked or annoyed by their overstatements and superlatives; do not overreact to expressions of hostility or tempests of other emotions. Sometimes adolescents, in order to uphold their protective armor, resort to all sorts of strategies to confuse, defeat, or anger the clinician. The ability to laugh at yourself and to use humor in a gentle manner is an asset. Remember, though, to always treat the adolescent with honesty and dignity—don't make fun of intense or idealistic views.

- Explain the diagnostic process as much as possible by explaining what we are about, the reasons for the various tests and examinations, and how we will use the information. We encourage the adolescent to challenge and question what we are doing. Finally, we usually give the client an idea of the route we would follow when therapy commences, or we even do some trial treatment activities.

- If the client is highly critical of parents or school officials, we must keep the person's confidences and not act in a judgmental manner. We do not enter into the criticism or side with the client against others, nor do we try to defend the institution or retreat to moralisms.

- Discuss the results of the evaluation with the client before talking with the parents or school personnel. Be sure to let the client know exactly what you intend to tell parents and teachers and determine any feelings the client has about these suggestions.

These recommendations have been distilled from our clinical experience and are not presented as magical touchstones for all diagnosticians or all clients, nor do these recommendations represent the full range of possibilities for successful interaction with teenage clients. We present them here to encourage other workers to develop clinical generalizations on the basis of their experience.

Older Adults

Older clients may present some rather special problems for the diagnostician, or they may need no particular special handling. Although the concept of "older" is relative, we refer here to persons in their 60s or older. A word of caution: Although certain generalizations are useful for planning and conducting evaluations, older people are not any more "all alike" than are children or adolescents.

The clinician should be alert to fatigue, disorientation, failing eyesight, and hearing loss. With advanced age, the person may find it more difficult to focus attention on a task and generally may have trouble remembering directions because of possible short-term memory decline. Many of these potential problems are exacerbated when the person has experienced a neurological insult, as can happen in a good number of elderly clients. Therefore, we need to explain each step of our clinical procedures at greater length and repeat instructions when necessary to ensure understanding. Our pace should be geared to the client's abilities—if necessary, to a slower pace. Organize the testing sequence carefully to reduce distractions, noise, or interference. Older people are often more cautious and have a greater need to be certain before they respond, so adapt the tasks with this in mind; following standard procedure may not be as important as providing an environment in which the person is able to perform at an optimal level.

Because many older clients tend to feel useless and discarded in our youth-oriented culture and resentful that their bodies are betraying them, we may find it important to spend some time listening to their memories of past achievements. Older clients should always be treated with respect and not referred to by their first names unless they request that you do so. The clinician should also guard against using a louder vocal intensity and increased pitch range, as if talking to a child. It is grossly offensive to infantilize an adult client. Many of our older clients come to us with neurologically based disorders, serious vocal pathologies, and other medically related problems. There is a tendency among many to talk about medical issues because older clients' problems have originated from this area. It is important for the diagnostician to be patient with these clients and listen to their concerns while not allowing conversation about medical issues to interfere with the testing.

In most cases, clinicians will find older clients to be interesting, socially adept individuals to be treated with courtesy and respect. The number of people over age 60 composes a significant proportion of the population, and we cannot afford to perpetuate the stereotype that old people are expendable or that they should be relegated to demeaning idleness. As with children and adolescents, the diagnostician should know as much as possible about aging. Many references pertinent to communication disorders are readily available (Kirkwood, 2000; Morrison, 1998; Shadden & Toner, 2011; Sheehy, 1996).

PUTTING THE DIAGNOSIS TO WORK

Perhaps the most demanding of all diagnostic ventures is the ultimate synthesis of findings into a coherent statement of the nature of the problem. The skilled clinician draws the findings together by using the data available, past experience, knowledge, and intuition to formulate a total picture of the condition. At this point, textbooks, research findings, and academic lectures fail to provide all of what is needed to succeed. Maturation of skills develops only in an extensive practicum under the close supervision of a knowledgeable diagnostician. The essence of the synthesis process is a comparison of what is observed with what we expect to observe from our knowledge of the normal process. The incongruities between the observed and the normal provide the building blocks for completion of the picture. Figure 1–6 identifies a model of diagnosis as a synthesis of findings and shows a number of outcomes to which the synthesis might lead.

Figure 1–6 points out several important concepts. First, the bedrock of the entire model is the clinician's knowledge and skill base. Without adequate training and experience, the administration of tests and tasks becomes meaningless.

A second important point in the model is the series of six boxes immediately above the clinician's knowledge and skill base. These boxes highlight the diversity of information that the diagnostician should ideally obtain in order to make a principled judgment about a client's disorder (case history, prior reports, observation, interview, informal

FIGURE 1–6

Components of an Effective Diagnosis/Evaluation

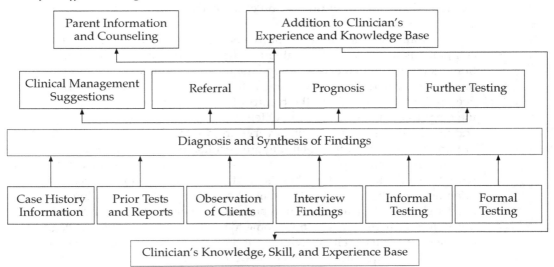

testing, and formal testing). It is not unusual for prior reports and tests to be missing, case history information to be returned by the client at the time of evaluation instead of prior to it, the case history forms to be incomplete or lost, and the interview cut to a 10-minute conversation because of time pressure. It is also not unusual for the clinician to spend the entire assessment time giving tests, with little opportunity left for informal testing or observation of clients in relevant situations. While it is difficult to obtain information from all six boxes in the model, we must try to get as close to the ideal as possible. In many settings, the evaluation does not take place unless the client has submitted all pertinent information and unless reports from other agencies have been received. This practice is certainly the case in many other professions (medicine, psychology, etc.). We must ask ourselves about the quality of the diagnostic evaluation that is done with incomplete information. What is the efficacy of performing an evaluation if we do not have access to critical information and are not willing to spend the time to carry on a decent interview and do informal testing and client observation? Remember that a crucial part of evidence-based practice is to understand the client's disorder and perspectives as fully as possible.

A third area, in the center of the model, is the synthesis of findings. This is where we begin to see overlaps in the data from case history, interview, reports, observations, and testing results. We should look for common threads among all these information sources and tie them together in the synthesis and diagnosis. Often, this is where certain informational components begin to disagree with one another, which is also informative. For example, the parents indicate intense concern over their child's articulation in the case history and the interview. They also bring a host of prior reports that indicate the child has no clinically significant problem, and they look to you for guidance. If your own test results, informal task performance, and observations indicate that the child is performing within normal limits, the discrepancy between these components and the parents' perceptions is obvious. The prior reports also now gain significant importance in terms of counseling the parents and pointing out the disparity between their views and the perceptions of many professionals. Another example may point out the foibles associated with one or more of the sources of information. For instance, a child may not perform within normal limits on formal tests of language ability, yet that same child communicates well in informal tasks and observations of play interactions with caretakers and peers. The clinician must question the formal test results if the child's communication exceeds that which these measures suggest he or she is capable of.

The fourth box in the series of five boxes in the model points out some important components of a diagnostic evaluation that are present after the synthesis of information. As we mentioned earlier, a good diagnostician will make suggestions for treatment in terms of which goals may be logically selected for initial intervention. The parents need to be counseled about the results of the evaluation, and any problems or feelings they express must be dealt with. Often we are so zealous in performing the evaluation and in scheduling time for doing everything we feel is necessary that we give the client or parents short shrift in explaining our results. In many cases, the results we report to parents and clients represent a significant affective burden. For example, even though parents usually know in their hearts that their child has a communication disorder, they often hold out the hope that their child really is typically developing and will grow out of a language or articulation difference. Telling parents that their child is indeed showing an impairment forces them to come to terms with this problem. Diagnosticians may experience parents or clients who cry at the culmination of the evaluation session when they are told something that confirms the idea of a disorder or commits them to an undetermined length of time spent in rehabilitation. Other emotions also emerge, such as anger and denial, which must sometimes be dealt with at the end of the diagnostic session. Emotions aside, it is enough of a challenge simply to communicate the complex evaluation results to parents of different educational levels and abilities. A skilled diagnostician has the ability to summarize assessment results and recommendations on the correct level of abstraction for different parents and clients. Another aspect to deal with after synthesis is the possibility of referral. Many cases require a consultation by other professionals, such as audiologists, laryngologists, neurologists, special educators, psychologists, and others. Often the assessment raises more questions than it answers, and this is perfectly acceptable. We need to know the parameters of the patient's problem, and many times this insight can be gained only from professionals who have expertise in areas with which we are not totally familiar.

Prognosis is another variable depicted in Figure 1–6. *Prognosis* may be defined as a prediction of the outcome of a proposed course of treatment for a given client: how effective treatment will be, how far we can expect the client to progress, and perhaps how long it will take. Inasmuch as diagnosis is a continuing process, prognosis should, like treatment planning, have both long-range and immediate facets. Immediate prognosis covers what the person can do now, what steps in therapy are possible, and what is the best route to take. Prognosis for specific communication disorders will be discussed in subsequent chapters; in this section we present some generic purposes and a possible danger involved in predicting a client's response to treatment.

Patients and families want to know what they may expect in terms of progress. Some general factors that the clinician must consider when making predictions are as follows:

1. *Age*—The chronological age of the client is a gross predictor of treatment success. In general, the younger the client, the better the treatment outcome. For example, the earlier the intervention is begun in childhood disorders, the more progress can be made prior to the start of school. The earlier we involve children in treatment, the more likely we are to prevent the formation of secondary problems (Shine, 1980; Starkweather, Gottwald, & Halfond, 1990), such as social, psychological, and educational penalties. In adult cases, it is well known that patients who develop neurogenic disorders at younger ages (40–60) are generally given better prognoses than patients who develop these problems at later ages (70–90) (Rosenbek, LaPointe, & Wertz, 1989). This, of course, is due to a variety of factors, including psychological, motivational, and physical. Thus, age is a macrovariable that, in and of itself, is not a potent variable, but it subsumes many factors that do have an influence on prognosis.

2. *Length of time the impairment has existed*—The length of time a client has had a communication impairment may relate to prognosis. Obviously, if the impairment has a component of habitual activities (motor patterns, processing strategies, etc.), these are more difficult to alter in clients who have performed them for a lengthy period. In addition to the habit patterns developed over time, the client has also learned complex ancillary adjustment patterns to compensate for the communication impairment that may involve social, psychological, and motoric activities. These compensatory patterns eventually become part of the problem and often must be eliminated, as in the case of operant behaviors learned by people who stutter (head jerks, timing devices, etc.).

3. *Existence of other problems*—It is axiomatic that the more problems a client has, the more difficult it will be to deal with the disorder. A client with aphasia who is also hearing impaired will be more difficult to treat than one with the language disorder alone. A child with a cleft palate and articulation problems will be more difficult than one with the articulation problem alone. A child who is language delayed and cognitively impaired is different from one who presents only a language disorder.

4. *Reactions of significant others*—A child with a communication disorder will make better progress in treatment if the parent takes an active role in the intervention. Many parents are interested in participating in treatment and will carry on home programs. On the other hand, if a child is brought to the clinic by a social worker and the parents do not appear interested in treatment, this child will probably take longer to succeed in remediation. If the spouse of a patient with aphasia is disinterested in facilitating communication, the client may make slower progress. The same can be said about the cooperation of teachers, aides, daycare providers, siblings, peers, and anyone else who comes in significant contact with the client and is in a position to help with treatment. Generally, the more assistance available from significant others, the better is the prognosis.

5. *Client motivation*—While we have no reliable way to measure motivation in a client, most diagnosticians can recognize it when they see it. If the client appears enthusiastic, interested, and anxious to begin treatment, it is clearly a plus. If the client is an adult, was he or she self-referred? Self-referral may be a positive indication compared to referral by an employer or teacher or being dragged to the evaluation by a domineering spouse. There may also be some positive prognostic value in cases where the client has something to gain from successful treatment (better social life, higher-paying job, etc.). Motivation is always difficult to quantify, but few would totally disregard the importance of this admittedly hard-to-define construct.

Accurate prognoses can help establish our credibility with other professions. The ability to predict with reasonable precision is perhaps the highest form of scientific achievement. Needless to say, however, these predictions should be based on something more than clinical intuition. Impressionistic conclusions, especially when made by experienced workers, can often be startlingly accurate, but they should always be labeled as impressionistic: A prognosis should be supported by a substantial amount of information. We never say that "the prognosis is favorable" without some documentation, both impressionistic and scientifically based. It is much better to say the following: "The prognosis is good because the child is stimulable for all error sounds, trial therapy has indicated good attention and a cooperative attitude, parents have committed to a home program, the client has stated he wants to change his speech, the client has normal hearing, and language problems are not evident."

In what sense might a prognosis be dangerous? First, no one really knows the future. A client's prognostic variables might soon change with unforeseen circumstances (e.g., the uninterested parents become involved, the client develops motivation, the client makes a breakthrough in the ability to perform certain functions). Prognosis as a construct is thus dynamic, not static. A second danger is that the prognosis may well influence a client's performance and perceptions. If a clinician has certain expectations regarding the case's potential performance, this could be inadvertently communicated to the client or the family and could negatively affect the course of therapy. It could also influence the level of effort exhibited by the clinician. The old notion of a self-fulfilling prophecy is still alive and well. We must always be willing to alter prognostic judgments in light of new data and, perhaps more important, we must be willing to refrain from making prognostic statements in the first place if we do not know what we are talking about. It is better to say, "I don't know how he will do in treatment; let's see what happens" than to jaundice the whole enterprise with a negative prognosis that has no real basis, or to disappoint all concerned with a positive prognosis that is never realized. This is *not* an exact science!

CONCLUSION AND SELF-ASSESSMENT

In this chapter we have presented some suggestions for general conduct of the diagnostic session. We dislike diagnostic formulas, and our purpose has not been to give out recipes but rather to describe some way of approaching various problems without going too far astray. By way of summary, we now present a list of interrelated and overlapping precepts regarding the clinical examination:

- We examine persons, not communication problems. Our primary concern is with communicators, not just communication.

- The clinical examination is conducted interpersonally; the catalyst of a diagnostic session is the person-to-person relationship between clinician and client.

- There is an element of magic in every transaction between people. A diagnostic session can, in some instances, ameliorate a problem situation by engendering hope, or it can be deeply disappointing to a client who hopes that a test or examination will resolve a difficulty.

- A most important requisite for conducting a clinical examination is a thorough understanding of normalcy.

- Diagnosis is the initial phase of treatment. The very first contact with a client—the manner in which he or she is treated during a clinical examination—is a crucial determining factor in response to therapy.

- Diagnosis is not necessarily confined to a single session.

- Treatment is often diagnostic; we often discover the nature of a client's problem in the initial stages of therapy.

- The clinical examination is performed to provide a working image of the individual; it is accomplished by interviewing, examining, evaluating, and testing.

- An important aspect in acquiring a working image of an individual is determining the person's self-perception and situation.

- An individual makes certain adjustments to a problem (attempts to solve the difficulty), which may include a protective cover of defenses. These defenses may be part of the problem, but they must not be confused with the problem.

- Behavior is a function of the individual and the situation. We should be aware that our test results reflect not just the client's abilities but also performance in the diagnostic setting rather than the natural environment.

- Our diagnostic activities should include an assessment of a client's larger social context (home, family, peers, job, school, etc.).

- Tests are only tools to provide a systematic guide for our observations. They enable the clinician to scrutinize a client in a structured manner.

- Although, for the examiner, the testing situation may be very familiar and routine, it is a novel experience for the client.

- Examination and testing can be iatrogenic: They can suggest problems to the client that he or she had not previously considered.

- Simply because a testing device is made up of a series of precisely defined tasks, administered and scored in a rigidly structured manner, does not mean that a client's responses are similarly precise.

- It is as important to observe *how* the client responds during a testing procedure as it is to obtain a score. Informal evaluation tasks are as important or more important than formal, standardized procedures.

- The needs of the client, not the work setting in which the clinician labors, should determine the scope of diagnostic activities. A good diagnostic is over when sufficient information about a client is gathered and should not be short-circuited because of administrative red tape, arbitrary guidelines of a facility, or government regulations. A good clinician will find ways to obtain critical information even if the evaluation extends into the realm of treatment.

This chapter has served as a general introduction to diagnosis and evaluation. The following chapters will focus more closely on important parameters of this interesting process with specific areas of communication disorders. We hope that students can see that this is an exciting enterprise that combines instruments with interpersonal relationships, testing with talking, and measurement with personal magnetism. The assessment process is the portal through which real people with real problems come to us for help. We must offer them the best of scientific as well as human resources.

After reading this chapter you should be able to answer the following questions:

1. How do the terms *evaluation* and *diagnosis* differ from one another?
2. What are the two major reasons that evaluations are performed?
3. What are the three levels of diagnosis and evaluation?
4. What are the three parts of evidence-based practice and how do they contribute to the clinical decision-making process?
5. What is RTI and how is it incorporated into the evaluation process?
6. How do dynamic and static forms of assessment differ from one another?
7. How did the WHO contribute to the development of ASHA's preferred practice patterns?
8. What three components require consideration when determining whether a communication disorder is present?
9. What is the difference among predisposing, precipitating, and perpetuating factors when considering etiology?
10. How does the diagnostician contribute to the evaluation process?
11. What factors must the clinician consider when making prognoses?

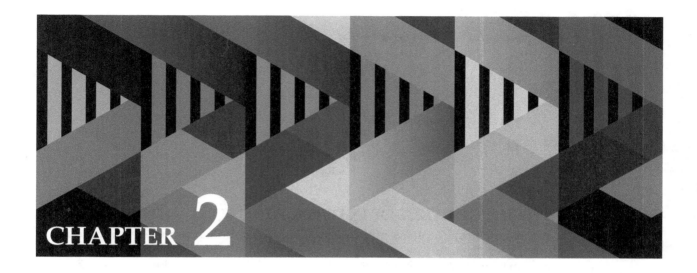

CHAPTER 2

Interviewing

LEARNING OUTCOMES

After reading this chapter you will be able to:

1. Describe the potential disadvantages of relying solely on paper-and-pencil techniques for collecting client information.
2. Describe three common barriers to interviewing.
3. Describe the seven general topics or areas of inquiry that are useful in any diagnostic session.
4. Provide the three basic goals in diagnostic interviews.
5. Describe the types of behaviors and questions to avoid during an interview.
6. Describe the types of questions that are commonly asked during an interview.
7. Distinguish among different types of listening.
8. Describe three popular techniques used in clinical interviewing.

The clinician sets in motion the process of recovery at the very first contact with a client. This is accomplished through the vehicle of the spoken word—in short, by means of the initial, or intake, interview. Because the intake interview ushers the client into treatment, it is the key link in the evaluation process. To assess and treat persons with communication disorders, it is essential that we know how to talk with them in a manner that reflects our expertise, inspires confidence, fosters trust, and sets the stage for a fruitful working alliance.

FIGURE 2–1
Interviewing Is Central in Speech Pathology

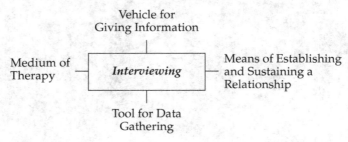

THE IMPORTANCE OF INTERVIEWING

Although clinical evaluation obviously involves more than proficiency at conducting interviews, the interview is central to the role of the diagnostician. By means of verbal exchange, we gather data about the individual, deliver information, and establish and sustain a working alliance. The interview is also the means by which treatment is carried out and, as such, serves both as a therapeutic tool and as a relationship (see Figure 2–1). For the clinical speech-language pathologist, interviewing and professional communication in general are extremely important activities (Burrus & Willis, 2013).

Although widely used, interviewing is often one of the least understood aspects of the clinician's role. Prospective clinicians are expected to acquire an impressive array of knowledge, but it is often presumed that they know how to communicate effectively with clients. The mastery of interviewing is either taken for granted or expected to accrue somehow as an artifact of required coursework and practicum experiences.

Some clinicians consider interviewing to be secondary; they use paper to replace personal interaction. An elaborate case history form containing a plethora of questions is mailed to the clients, and they are asked to fill it out and return it before the diagnostic appointment. The rationale for this procedure is that it saves the clinician time and reveals problem areas that can then be explored in the personal interview. Although the clinician certainly should get some idea of the problem before the diagnostic examination, there is no substitute for an in-depth interview. An approach that uses only paper-and-pencil techniques has several disadvantages:

1. The questions on forms are often generic—they cover all possible respondents—and thus are ambiguous or not applicable to any particular type of client. Therefore, a client or caregiver may not understand the relationship between the questions posed and the communication problem. Face-to-face interviews permit greater flexibility in formulating precise and germane inquiries.

2. Clients may ignore certain questions, forget to address important information, or omit important information. Clients or caregivers may not be able to remember the specific information requested or understand the relevance of the questions asked.

3. The queries may be misinterpreted, may be perceived as threatening, or may engender guilt, and the clinician is not present to observe the respondent's reactions or to explain, support, and assist the respondent as he or she searches for an answer. A large percentage of our communication is visual, and a face-to-face interview provides gestural and other visual cues that are not available in written format.

4. It is difficult to determine cause-and-effect relationships from questionnaire data because it is impossible to account for all influential variables in a single questionnaire.

5. Does the mailed questionnaire allow time for the respondent to plan a defense? Is it more likely that we end up with a view of what the respondent wants us to see, a view that he or she perceives as being more socially acceptable? More often than not we are able to obtain more complete information through an interview, where primary questions may be followed up with pertinent secondary inquiries.

Do not imply from this list of disadvantages that the present authors are opposed to obtaining information by having clients complete *well-designed* case history forms. Such data are critical for understanding the client's perspective. Our emphasis is that one should not rely *exclusively* on paperwork in assessment. In fact, see the section in Chapter 4 on preassessment as a valuable part of planning an evaluation.

THE NATURE OF INTERVIEWING

An interview is essentially a process, not an entity—a process of verbal and nonverbal communication between a trained professional and a client or parent who is seeking services. More specifically, an *interview*, in a clinical and diagnostic sense, is a *purposeful* exchange of meanings between two persons, a directed conversation that proceeds in an orderly fashion to obtain data, to convey certain information, and to provide counseling. The professional, by reason of his or her position and clinical expertise, is expected to (and usually does) lead and direct the verbal exchange. Thus, an interview is not just an ordinary conversation in terms of a desultory exchange of opinions and ideas but rather a specialized pattern of verbal interaction directed toward a specific purpose and focused on specific content. The roles of interviewer and respondent are more highly specified in a professional interview than in a conversation. The *clinician* knows that an interview is a unique and distinct mode of verbal exchange. But does the *client* need to know? Probably not. Indeed, we typically advise students to refer to an interview as a "talk" or "a chance to share information" when they contact clients or parents to request an appointment time. An "interview" can sound rather ominous and frightening.

An interview differs from a social conversation in that the time and location of an interview is specified formally and the inquiries are generally unilateral. That is, the clinician may ask about the parents' relationship with their child, but it is not expected that the client will reciprocate with questions about the clinician's children. The clinician also does not necessarily avoid unpleasant topics in the interest of social propriety. Perhaps for the first time, the respondent can talk freely, without fear of criticism or admonishment.

In a good diagnostic interview, the clinician and client must develop a working alliance, multiplying their efforts by creating a mutual feeling of cooperation. The term "alliance refers to the quality and strength of the collaborative relationship between client and therapist" (Norcross, 2011, p. 120). It is futile to expect straightforward answers to simple questions. A good diagnostic interview and the establishment of a good working alliance always involve more than making queries and recording answers. It also involves skillfully navigating the human elements of personality and the personal culture that *both* you the clinician and the client bring to the interaction. Egan (2014) suggests that demonstrating behaviors that show empathy and respect for clients is foundational to the ability to develop and maintain a working alliance. Empathy is "the ability to understand the client from his or her own point of view and, when appropriate, to communicate this understanding to the client" (p. 48), whereas respect refers more to the regard, esteem, or way in which we view another.

In summary, a *diagnostic interview* is a directed conversation, carried out for specific purposes such as fact finding, informing, or altering attitudes and opinions. The clinician's efforts are directed toward the creation of mutual respect and team effort in the understanding and solution of the communication problem.

COMMON INTERVIEWING CONSIDERATIONS

Several factors can prevent the establishment of effective communication and a working alliance between a speech clinician and those whom the clinician interviews. Although the list could obviously be expanded, we have picked three aspects that, in our experience, are the most common interviewing barriers: the clinician's fears, lack of specific purpose, and failure to consider the client's cultural background. We will discuss each of these factors next.

The Clinician's Fears

At two points in a student clinician's career, anxiety can rise to very high levels: the confrontation with his or her first therapy case and the first diagnostic interview. It is—and should be—an awesome responsibility to undertake the professional treatment of another human being. There is always an element of risk in offering help.

Perhaps the most common fear expressed by the beginning clinician is that clients will not accept the clinician in a professional role because of the clinician's youth. The clinician doubts that he or she can bridge the age gap, especially when the clinician deals with parents: "Who am I to be asking questions and giving suggestions to them when they are older and more experienced? Won't they look down on me if I don't have children?" Most of this is pure projection on the clinician's part (Haynes & Oratio, 1978). If the clinician indicates deep concern for the welfare of the client, then nearly every parent and client will respond in a positive manner, without scrutinizing the clinician for wrinkles, or gray hairs, or looking for photographs of children on the clinician's desk. The clinician, of course, should not communicate any uncertainty during the interview; otherwise, he or she will never establish competence or inspire confidence.

Another common fear among beginning clinicians—and one that is also largely projected—is that the client will become defensive or resentful during questioning. We have seen students omit a whole series of important questions when a client, especially a parent, responded curtly or showed mild annoyance. While it is not uncommon for parents to think of their child's communication disorder as an outward and visible sign of their own failure, in our experience few parents are resentful or defensive about the clinician's sincere efforts to determine the nature of the child's problem. Again, the important point is to make the clients and their families feel that they have done the best they could do, and now, with some assistance from the clinician, they can do better. The clinician should *always maintain a nonthreatening posture in the clinical transaction.*

Many beginning clinicians are leery of questions directed at them. "What do you do when the client starts asking *you* questions?" the beginning clinician frequently despairs. "Will I be able to explain to the client adequately what he or she needs to know? How will I know if I have communicated properly if the client just sits there and nods?" We shall return to this important topic of client questions in a later section of this chapter.

Lack of Specific Purpose

Many beginning clinicians either have purposes that are too broad and general or interviewing goals that are too nebulous. It is important to write out carefully and rather explicitly the purposes for an interview before meeting with the client. We must know *why* we want the answers to the questions we ask. Specifying the purposes of an interview is also an effective way to reduce the interviewer's uncertainty and anxiety. Kadushin (1972) summarizes the importance of planning in this way: "To know is to be prepared; to be prepared is to experience reduced anxiety; to reduce anxiety is to increase the interviewer's freedom to be fully responsive to the interviewee" (p. 2). The clinician should keep in mind, however, that thorough planning does not mean the application of an inflexible routine.

Failure to Consider the Client's Clutural Background

When the client and clinician represent differing cultural or racial backgrounds, there is an additional potential obstacle to overcome. Some clients may not feel as comfortable when they must reveal certain information to a stranger, and this discomfort may be intensified when the clinician represents a different race or culture. The solution is clearly not to make certain that clients and clinicians are culturally homogeneous. Given the diverse nature of our society, this would be impossible from a scheduling standpoint and unwise from a philosophical one. The best way to approach cultural diversity in clinical situations is to make certain that, as clinicians, we have consideration and sensitivity for cultural differences, and knowledge of multicultural issues in assessment and treatment. The American Speech-Language-Hearing Association (ASHA) has mandated that every accredited training program in communication disorders infuse multicultural information into each area of academic preparation and clinical practicum. A major implication of multicultural issues on assessment concerns the diverse belief systems of the various cultural groups regarding disabilities and communication. Some cultures believe that a handicapping condition is a situation that nothing can or should be done about, or that the help for this condition is spiritual rather than clinical (Cheng, 1989). If the clinician charges into the initial interview with a client and makes a host of recommendations without addressing cultural attitudes toward remediation, the suggestions may fall on unsympathetic ears. The clients may also be offended and not return for treatment.

AN APPROACH TO INTERVIEWING

We now present an interviewing approach, an eclectic product of our clinical experience together with an intensive study of relevant bibliographic materials. No doubt the reader will want to modify our approach in order to suit individual settings. It is desirable for you to do so: Only through critical self-evaluation and modification can any clinician acquire an interviewing procedure that is uniquely personal.

Diagnostic interviews have three basic goals: to obtain information, to give information, and to provide counseling. For the purpose of discussion, each goal will be considered separately in the next sections.

Goal One: Obtain Information

Although it may seem obvious, it is worth restating that, as clinicians, we must actively listen before we speak. There are essentially three reasons for this: (1) It gives clients an opportunity to talk about problems, to express fears and feelings, thus enabling them to benefit more from the guidance that the speech clinician offers; (2) it gives the clinician an idea of the nature and scope of the information the client will need; and (3) it allows the clinician to formulate hypotheses concerning the individual's communication disorder.

Setting the Tone

The first important task of the clinician is to set the right tone for the interview, to get a structured conversation initiated and channeled in the proper direction. How does one go about setting the right tone? We find that defining the roles is an effective procedure:

> Ms. Taylor, I want to talk with you before we start our evaluation with Larry. I know you filled out the case history form we sent you, and that provided a lot of important information. I did have a few questions about some of the things you said about Larry's early development and I also wanted to ask you about some of the speech and language he uses at home. It's hard for us to get an accurate picture of a person just by reading paperwork, so if we can talk a bit about Larry and get some examples of his communication from you, it will help us to do a more effective evaluation.

It is helpful to think of the interview as a kind of role-playing situation. As the clinician, you define the roles for the client and indicate the rules and responsibilities for these roles. You tell who you are, what you intend to do, and what you expect of the client. In other words, you structure the situation by explaining the purposes of the interview—why the information is needed and what will be done with it. Initially, of course, the client accepts the respondent role because of the nature of the situation and the official sanction of the interviewer's position. Then it is up to you to demonstrate your empathy and clinical expertise in order to engender further cooperation.

Two problems sometimes arise here. First, some clients may be inhibited by such explicit role definitions; respondents from lower-middle or lower social classes may have had little experience in holding directed conversations. In this case, a clinician can prolong the small-talk phase, emphasize the nature of the interview as chatting, and gently ease into the more structured situation as the relationship develops. When two or more people get together, even for serious purposes, a certain amount of social and small talk seems to foster positive attitudes toward continued interaction.

Second, many cultural and socioeconomic variables, as they relate to clinical interactions, deserve consideration. We have indicated that much of the information exchanged in a clinical interview is of a highly personal nature and possibly charged with considerable affect. Many cultures (e.g., Native Americans and certain Asian groups) find it difficult to share personal information with unfamiliar people. Thus, in the interview it may be extremely uncomfortable for them to reveal some types of data. The clinician must be sensitive to such cultural beliefs and not press the client to provide information too soon. In some cases it will be necessary to conduct multiple interviews and establish a strong relationship with the clients before they will give information or take advantage of clinician suggestions for treatment. This issue alone is a strong indictment of some rigid policies in which an evaluation is expected to be completed in an hour or two or in which Individualized Education Plan (IEP) goals must be written in limited time frames. We must learn that different cultures may require alterations in our methods if we are to serve them optimally.

Another multicultural influence is the possibility of working with children and adults from bilingual backgrounds. In some cases, the clinician must be bilingual, and in others the interviewer must provide interpreters. The use of an interpreter, however, is a very specialized operation, and the clinician must be certain that the person has adequate knowledge and experience to perform this specialized task. In some areas of the country, there is an increased likelihood that the speech-language pathologist (SLP) will encounter a bilingual population, and he or she should reflect on how these clients will be served appropriately in assessment and treatment. It is not possible to provide adequate services to these populations without a knowledge of and sensitivity to multicultural issues. Lynch (1998) describes the ideal interpreter as someone who (1) is proficient in the language (including specific dialect) of the family as well as that of the interventionist, (2) is trained and experienced in cross-cultural communication and the principles (and dynamics) of serving as an interpreter, (3) is trained in the appropriate professional field relevant to the specific family–interventionist interaction, and (4) can understand and appreciate the respective cultures of both parties and convey the more subtle nuances of each with tact and sensitivity. Lynch (1998) cautions against the use of family members as interpreters because they rarely meet these criteria and could inject significant bias and family difficulties into the clinical situation. Most authorities on the use of interpreters emphasize the importance of thorough preparation of the interpreter prior to the clinical encounter in terms of the goals and purposes of the evaluation, potentially sensitive clinical and family issues, the format of the interview, and any technical terms and paperwork to be used in the conference. It is helpful to introduce all people present and clarify the goals and purposes of the interview so family members will know what to expect. Diligent clinicians may take the time to learn several social phrases in the language of the family so that greetings, saying thank you, and leave-taking can be done in a manner comfortable to the clients. This demonstrates respect for the family and shows that the clinician is making an attempt to understand and appreciate cultural differences. During the interview it is customary for the clinician to address remarks and questions to the family, not the interpreter. Also, while listening to the family, it is appropriate to look at the person who is speaking, not just at the interpreter. In this situation it is clearly beneficial to avoid technical jargon and figurative language that not only is difficult to translate but may also be confusing to the clients. As the interview progresses, especially in the portion where information is provided to the clients, it is wise periodically to check the families' understanding of facts presented and any recommendations given by the clinician. Finally, most experts on the use of interpreters recommend a debriefing session in which the clinician and interpreter can discuss the information collected, any difficulties encountered in the conference, any problems with the interpreting process, and any subtle impressions gleaned by the interpreter that go beyond the literal translation of the client's utterances (e.g., anger, hostility, fear, etc.). Although such impressions are subjective on the part of the interpreter, they may represent important information about the family's acceptance of the problem, perceptions of the clinical situation, and possible compliance with a treatment program. It is vital that you convey sincere interest in the situation as the client sees it. Demonstrate to the client that you are genuinely trying to comprehend what the problem is and what it means to the client personally.

Part of setting the tone is the establishment of rapport and hopefully a working alliance. Rapport, of course, is not a separate substance you can pour into a session; it is mutual respect and trust, a feeling of confidence on your part, and a large measure of understanding. Empathy, warmth, and acceptance are also crucial aspects; strive for the ability to understand sensitively and accurately the interviewee's situation. Also try to be genuine, not contrived, with a professional demeanor. In addition to the words spoken, a number of forces shape the interview. For example, the setting and the clinician's dress, manners, and nonverbal expressions all influence the tone or nature of the interview. In professional interviewing, the goal is to provide an atmosphere that fosters communication between client and clinician.

Asking the Questions

You should use an interview guide or outline rather than read prepared questions. The questions should be worded in a manner that is in keeping with your understanding of the individual's situation. This will result in an interview that is much more spontaneous and meaningful. In most cases, formal preestablished questionnaires operate as another type of barrier or crutch for the insecure interviewer.

The specific content of the queries addressed to a respondent depend on the age of the client, the nature of the problem, and the purposes of the interview, among other factors. Most clinicians find that the younger the client being evaluated, the more important the parent interview. Because we intend to focus on style of interviewing in this chapter, we will not include lists of questions that pertain to particular disorders of communication. Many examples from specific areas are provided in later chapters. Seven general topics or areas of inquiry are useful, however, in any diagnostic session:

1. *What is the respondent's perception of the problem?* Here, the clinician seeks a global description of the communication disorder. In a parent interview, for example, we frequently open the session with an open-ended question: "Tell me why you brought Jamie to the clinic" or "What concerns do you have about Jamie?"

2. *When and under what conditions did the communication disorder arise?* The purpose of this question is to determine the onset and developmental history of the problem. An example of when the etiology of the problem would be especially important is in the development of a voice disorder. (e.g., rapid versus gradual onset, occurrence of vocally abusive behaviors, changes in medication).

3. *In what ways has the communication disorder changed since its onset?* The goal of this question is to determine whether the problem has lessened, worsened, or changed in form since its onset. When interviewing the parents of a child who is exhibiting early signs of stuttering, for example, we are interested in how the speech disfluency has changed since it was first noticed.

4. *What are the consequences (handicapping conditions) of the problem?* In what manner—socially, educationally, occupationally—does the communication disorder affect the person's life? In what ways has he or she adapted to the disorder?

5. *How have the client and family attempted to cope with the problem?* What lay remedies have been tried by the client and family to resolve the problem? How has the client responded to the families' efforts to resolve the problem?

6. *What impact has the client's communication disorder had on the rest of the family?* When a family member has a disability, it creates fertile ground for familial conflict (see Featherstone, 1980). To obtain a description of a child's ongoing behavior and how he or she fits into the family regimen, ask the parents to describe a "typical" day, from the time the youngster gets up until he or she goes to bed.

7. *What are the client's (or parents') expectations regarding the diagnostic session?* The client or caregivers often come to a helping professional with an agenda (hidden or otherwise) and set expectations. The client may want the problem finally diagnosed after months of wondering about it. The parents may want a recommendation for treatment because they already know that their child has a communication problem. Sometimes parents have been agonizing over some hypothesis that has been advanced by a relative ("He's tongue-tied" or "We're afraid he is behind in his development") and their biggest concern is that the clinician address this issue. Whatever the expectations, do your best to determine what those expectations are and to manage those expectations in a way that is solution-oriented and continues to foster a positive working alliance. Although it may sound counterintuitive, managing expectations does not always mean having all the answers or providing the resolution to the client's communication problem. You need to be honest with your clients from the start. Some problems can't be fixed, some don't have easy solutions, and generally too many factors are at play to make grandiose promises.

A good diagnostic interview is characterized by a shifting of styles: objective questions that ask for specifics, subjective queries that deal with feelings and attitudes, and finally the indeterminate questions, like "Tell me more," to keep the respondent going. The interviewer should start with the least anxiety-provoking queries, mostly objective questions that have high specificity, and then proceed to more subjective questions as the relationship develops. Quite often, however, we find it useful to employ a "funnel" sequence of inquiry during the course of a diagnostic interview—starting with broad, open-ended questions and then progressing to more specific or closed questions. An "inverted funnel," used less often, would be just the opposite: starting with the tougher, more specific questions first, followed by the broader, more open-ended questions. The approach used depends on the amount of time you, as the interviewer, have. If you have ample time, use the funnel approach. If time is limited and you need to get to the meat of the interview quickly, however, use the inverted funnel. Here is an example of a funnel sequence for questions from a parent interview:

- How does Jimmy function in the family setting?
- How does he get along with his brothers and sisters?
- How does his older sister "help" him communicate?
- Can you describe an instance in which she talked for him?

It is best to avoid the checklist or long series of "tunnel" questions that call for information on one level of specificity, all of which are asked in a similar style (e.g., "Did your child have earaches, fevers, head injury?").

The Presenting Story

Most persons who anticipate visiting a helping professional will mentally rehearse what they intend to say. Often you will have to contend with events that occurred prior to the session—the family car's failing to start, a burned breakfast, absence of a convenient parking place. A few words to reveal your understanding of the distracting antecedents will generally assist the respondent in shifting to the topic of the interview. In some cases, the client may even have a pseudoconversation with you while he or she is driving to the appointment: A person often rehearses, en route, how to describe his or her symptoms. We must allow this story to be unraveled, or the respondent will be left with a sense of frustration. A question such as "What seems to be the problem?" or "What brings you here today?" will permit the flow of conversation to begin. Remember that the client's description is how the *client* perceives the problem—it is the client's unique way of looking at the situation. The client's description may be grossly inaccurate, but you should hear it out; nothing turns a respondent off more quickly than for the interviewer to suggest by word or action that the respondent's views are silly or misguided. Sometimes the presenting story will become a motif that occurs again and again during the course of the interview.

This is generally a crucial point in an interview. The interviewee may cautiously extend a portion of him- or herself verbally, carefully scan the interviewer's response, and then decide whether to reveal more or tell the whole story. Sometimes a respondent may even set up a straw man to see how the interviewer deals with it.

This is not the proper time to debate an issue with the client. The story can be accepted initially on the level of feeling, and later in the interview—when rapport is stronger—an issue can be discussed more fully. We feel very strongly that these initial stories, these primitive theories, should be respected as the best possible answer that clients have been able to think of. It does not mean that you agree with a client's conclusions; it just means that you accept a client's perceptions and judgments with understanding so that you can form a basis for further communication.

Actually, the presenting information can be a very rich source of clinical hypotheses to be explored during the course of the interview. How do the client and parent present themselves—as long-suffering, anxious, diffident? How do they associate ideas or items of information sequentially? What priorities do they assign to issues they raise? Do they seem to be realistic in their expectations regarding the diagnostic session and treatment? Do they express likes or dislikes that can be capitalized on or that should be avoided during the diagnostic session or treatment?

Nonverbal Messages

The clinician and respondents do not communicate by words alone, and the discerning clinician attends to the client's as well as his or her own bodily behavior and oral language during an interview. The nonverbal messages we convey with our posture, degree of eye contact, facial expression, and physical appearance can carry significant weight during silence or when combined with a verbal message. As a matter of fact, some observers suggest that a large portion of the total message—particularly messages involving strong feelings—is carried by nonverbal cues. They are considered harder to disguise because they are often less likely to be under conscious control. However, resist the urge to interpret a client's every twitch; each instance of nonverbal behavior should be related to the *content* of the oral message and to the *context* in which it occurs. For example:

> If a parent leaves her coat on during an interview, it may mean she feels vulnerable and the garment provides a bit of protective armor. It may also mean that she has a spot on her dress, or that all the hangers in the waiting room were taken again by forgetful students, or that the room is chilly. However, if she shifts her chair away from the clinician, sits with her arms and legs tightly crossed, avoids eye contact, and responds to questions with one-word answers, then it may be possible that she is defensive and guarded in the clinical setting.

The issue here is to avoid making one item of nonverbal behavior the sole basis for interpretation; be on the lookout for patterns. The most important thing to look for may be lack of congruence between the respondent's verbal and nonverbal messages; in cases where the two conflict, body language is generally a more accurate indicator of how a person feels about an issue. Nonverbal behaviors often give insight into what a client may be thinking or feeling but not saying.

During the interview process, nonverbal behaviors require close consideration when interviewing an individual from another culture. Nonverbal behaviors vary considerably across cultures, and what is considered or perceived as appropriate and desirable for one culture could be perceived as disrespectful and inappropriate for another. Here are a few examples:

- *Touch* In the United States patting a child's head is considered an affectionate or friendly gesture. However, the Asian culture considers it inappropriate because it is believed to be a sacred part of the body. And in Muslim cultures, touch between individuals of opposite genders is generally inappropriate.

- *Eye contact* In mainstream U.S. culture, eye contact is desirable and interpreted as an act of attentiveness. In many other cultures like Hispanic, Asian, Middle Eastern, and Native American, it is perceived as rude or disrespectful.

- *Physical space* The acceptable physical distance between one person and another can vary significantly across cultures. The acceptable distance for Latin American and Middle Eastern cultures is generally shorter than that of European and American cultures.

Things to Avoid in the Interview

Beginning interviewers commit several common errors. The following list is not meant to be exhaustive, but it does cover the most glaring mistakes:

1. *Avoid questions that may be answered by a simple yes or no.* Open-ended questions produce longer responses, encourage clients to start talking and include more detailed information. Such questions often start with the words *what, why,* or *how.* When an interview is loaded with closed-ended questions, the number and type of answers are limited. While they should be used sparingly, closed-ended questions are useful for fact checking.

2. *Avoid asking questions that are "double barreled."* This mistake occurs when a question is asked in a manner that addresses two or more questions at one time before giving the client a chance to respond. Generally, if a client is required to answer more than one question, he or she will often answer only one of the questions: the easiest or the one he or she was asked last.

3. *Avoid phrasing questions so that they inhibit freedom of response.* Leading questions lead another to a predetermined conclusion or insight. Do not say, "You don't have any difficulty with ringing in your ears, do you?" or "You don't tell Billy to stop and start over again, do you?" Such leading questions are not effective interviewing and can be perceived as manipulative, judgmental, and/or dishonest. The beginning interviewer tends to be anxious about asking open-ended questions, fearing that silence will result and that this will damage his or her relationship with the client. So the interviewer will ask an open-ended question and then close it with a closed-ended leading question: for example, "How do you feel about David's stuttering? Does it bother you?" Leave questions open! Although open-ended questions consume more time and may produce some rambling and irrelevant responses, they have many advantages.

4. *Avoid abrupt transitions or topic shifts.* Try to avoid abrupt shifts in your line of questioning. For example, if you are exploring the client's feelings or attitudes on a particular issue (subjective questions), don't suddenly ask a question on a different topic. Inexperienced interviewers tend to jump around. If you are interested in learning about a child's play, ask all your questions pertaining to the child's play together. Do not skip around from play to language, to book reading, to medical history, and so on. The interview should flow so that one question logically links or flows into the next. When the client causes the interview to wander, avoid abrupt transitions to bring it back to the point. Most of the clients you will interview have had little experience in directed, orderly conversation. They tend to follow chance associations and wander far afield. The experienced interviewer has the ability to make smooth transitions. The best way to get the interview back on track is by building a bridge to the respondent's previous statements: for example, "That's interesting, Ms. Davis. Maybe we can come back to that in a little while. Now earlier you were mentioning that your child's loss of hearing occurred suddenly. . . ." The goal here is to use respondent antecedents—what the client has said earlier in the interview.

5. *Avoid talking too much.* This is perhaps the most common mistake of the beginning interviewer, who feels that every pause must be filled with verbiage. It is much better to rephrase what the respondent has said or make some comment like "I see," "Tell me more," or "Anything else?" Sometimes a smile and an understanding nod are effective when it seems that the client has more to say but needs some silent time to collect his or her thoughts. If there is a positive attitude—a good rapport—and if the client feels comfortable in the situation, then these encouragements increase the length of the response. If the topic or situation is neutral, these comments tend to expand the message. As a general metric, about 80% of the talking should originate with the client.

6. *Avoid concentrating on physical symptoms and etiological factors to the exclusion of the client's feelings and attitudes.* There is a little bit of physician in all of us; we yearn to play the role of omniscient healer. The interviewer should remember to distinguish between items of information that are simply interesting and background information that is really important.

7. *Avoid providing information too soon.* There will be plenty of time to clear up misconceptions later in the interview. The surest way to cut off the flow of information is to stop a parent, for instance, after he says, "I just tell Michael to stop, take a deep breath, and start all over again," and counsel him on the proper responses to nonfluency. It is best to take note of areas that need clarity and address those areas when you are providing information rather than gathering information.

8. *Avoid qualifying and hemming and hawing when asking questions.* Ask questions in a straightforward fashion and maintain eye contact. Rather than asking, "Did you find that, well, you know, when you were, uh, shall we say . . . with child, did you experience any untoward conditions?" say, "Did anything unusual happen during your pregnancy?" Instead of inquiring, "Did you discover, hmm, I mean, well, after your father, uh, passed away, did your stuttering problem increase?" say, "What impact did your father's death have on your speech?" Beating around the bush and qualifying questions can result in the perception of discomfort or a lack of confidence.

9. *Avoid negative, judgmental, or moralistic responses, verbal or nonverbal, to the client's statements.* The flow of information will stop abruptly and the relationship will be impaired severely if the client senses that a clinician finds him and/or his behavior distasteful. Avoid even the response "Good" because it implies a value judgment. We do not have to subscribe to a person's values or code of behavior for us to show compassion for and understanding of his or her situation. Use inquiries that begin with "Why . . .?" very sparingly because beginning a question with the word *why* is often perceived as a challenge or threat; this line of questioning is too reminiscent of disciplinary sessions ("Why were you late for class?" "Why can't you behave properly?"). In a clinical setting, we must not let our values obscure our perception of the client's frame of reference. An interview is not the place to push the clinician's personal points of view. This can immediately alienate or offend clients if they do not share the clinician's point of view.

10. *Avoid allowing the interview to produce only superficial answers.* We need to get deeper, more significant responses from our clients. Several interviewing devices, termed *probes,* can be helpful to the clinician. Clinicians who are skillful at probing can stimulate the client to provide more information without leading the client or injecting themselves into the process. Several different types of probes can be used.

Crosshatch, or *interlocking,* questions are useful when we need to elicit more detail about a topic that has been glossed over. Often discrepancies must be resolved. To elicit more detail, ask the same question in different ways and at different points during the interview. For instance, the father of a young child who stuttered responded in a superficial manner to our query about his relationship with the child. He assured us that he had a "loving relationship" with his son and then complained at length about his working conditions. Later in the interview, when we asked him to describe the sorts of activities he did with the child, he was unable to mention a single one. We don't mean to imply that the clinician should attempt to catch the client lying and then demand an explanation. The clinician must examine discrepancies, however, in order to enhance understanding of the problem because such discrepancies could have a significant effect on the mode of treatment.

Pauses, or silent probes, can be very helpful. When there is a lull in the interview, it may mean simply that the client has exhausted his or her store of information, that a memory barrier has prevented further recall, or that he or she senses lack of understanding by the clinician. It can also mean, however, that a sensitive area has been touched on. Do not feel that pauses harm the interview. Much significant information can be forthcoming if we keep quiet and indicate with a smile or a nod that we expect more.

The *summary probe* is one of the best ways to keep the interview moving smoothly. The clinician summarizes periodically what the client has said, ending perhaps with a request for clarification or further information. Incidentally, this procedure also demonstrates to the interviewee that the interviewer is listening and is indeed trying to understand the problem. We generally use "minisummary probes"—echo questions—all the way through an interview, for example:

Respondent:	After my husband's stroke, my whole world collapsed.
Interviewer:	You were overwhelmed by the sudden change in your life.
Respondent:	Yes, one day he was happily planning our trip to Sanibel Island . . . and then, in just a moment, he was paralyzed and couldn't talk. Now all our plans are up in the air . . . the new car, the checking account, he took care of all that.

The *stumbling probe* is a variation of the summary probe; we have found it helpful, especially with the reticent respondent. The interviewer rephrases a portion of the respondent's communication and then, attempting to interpret or comment upon it, the interviewer pretends to halt or stumble. For example, when interviewing the mother of a child allegedly beginning to stutter, the clinician might say: "Now, you were saying that Bruce first started to repeat and hesitate after he caught his finger in the car door. Under these conditions, it would be natural for you to . . . uh . . ." The respondent's need for closure may elicit additional significant information and, perhaps more important, significant insights.

Finally, an interviewer can use the *assuming probe*. If the client has avoided an important area, leaving much unsaid regarding the speech or hearing problem and what it means to him or her, then it is up to the interviewer to bring this out. One adolescent boy, who had been vehemently denying that his stuttering bothered him, unburdened himself when we said, "It bothers you so much that you don't want anybody to know, do you?" While the assuming probe can be very powerful; it should be used sparingly and with care because the client could become put off or offended.

11. *Avoid letting the client reveal too much in one interview.* Sometimes a beginning interviewer makes the mistake of trying to get everything in one sitting. The client, sensing perhaps that this is the first person who really understands him or her, may want to provide more personal details than are necessary. Later, however, the individual will feel embarrassed and foolish, perhaps even exposed and guilty, at revealing so much to a comparative stranger.

12. *Avoid trusting to memory.* Record the information as the interview progresses. Tell the client that you will take some notes during the interview so that you can plan the treatment program more effectively and make recommendations for other services. Such note taking, or even recording devices, is rarely questioned. Indeed, we have found that clients expect you to write down some of the information they are giving you; they doubt that you would be able to remember all of their answers. You obviously would damage or lose the client relationship, however, if you scribbled furiously while the client was revealing some sensitive information. It is also self-evident that the client's confidence will be respected, but this is often not explicitly stated to the client. The clinician's manner should suggest that all information received is to be held strictly confidential.

Prepare a report of the interview as soon as possible. Commit your observations to paper while the encounter with the respondent is still fresh in your mind (see Chapter 14 for information on writing reports).

Goal Two: Give Information

No one likes uncertainty. All too frequently any information that is not supplied by the professional will become distorted by input from other sources. We can do an admirable job on our evaluation, but if we drop the ball on communicating the results to our client, we have not been successful. When not correctly informed, clients and parents can become misinformed, and this misinformation leads to confusion and misunderstanding, and further compounds the problem. It is our responsibility, therefore, to provide accurate, unemotional, objective information of the status of the individual's problem. This forwarding of information is generally accomplished during the postdiagnostic conference.

Summarize the findings of the clinical examination in simple, nontechnical language, and use common terms compatible with the client's background. We prefer to commence, if possible, with results that show a client's area of normal functioning and thus review findings that indicate what is good before describing deficiencies. Relate comments to normative values whenever possible. Clarify and help the respondent ask questions by using examples and simple analogies. If you are in doubt concerning the client's understanding of the diagnostic material (clients will rarely ask if they don't understand), talk more slowly, employ longer descriptions, and use many examples and more redundant language.

The Questions Clients Ask

An interview is much more than a clinician posing questions and recording the client's answers. It is an important forum for *exchange*—a reflexive, dynamic experience of sharing between the diagnostician and the informant. Indeed, we find that a client—especially a parent of a young child being evaluated—frequently is eager to probe the clinician's expertise. The clinician must evaluate the client's or parent's inquiries and determine, What is the person *really* asking? Is there an unstated concern behind the questions? Luterman (1979) divides the questions that clients ask into three categories: *content, opinion,* and *affect.* We will describe and illustrate these three types of inquiries with excerpts from an initial interview with the mother of a 3-year-old child brought to the clinic because she was concerned that her child was beginning to stutter.

1. *Questions dealing with information or content.* In this instance, the client seeks an informative or factual response from the clinician. The inquiry usually takes the form, "I want to know about something, and I hope you have the right information."

Ms. Bell: The type of choppy speech [disfluency] Jesse has—is it common among children his age?

Clinician: It sure is. Most children between the ages of 2 ½ and 5 do a lot of repeating and hesitating.

2. *Questions with predetermined opinions.* Here the client has an opinion regarding a particular subject and wants to determine if the clinician agrees with it. The clinician must be careful not to dismiss the client's opinion until the clinician understands *why* and *how strongly* the client holds it.

Ms. Bell: Um, on TV a couple of times, I've seen a demonstration of the airflow technique for stuttering. What do you think of it?

| **Clinician:** | Those demonstrations are very dramatic, aren't they? What's your impression of the technique as it applies to Jesse? |

3. *Questions that are a "faint knocking on the door."* In this case, the client is not asking for information or to determine the clinician's opinion but rather for emotional support and reassurance. The question conceals a feeling that the client either is unaware of or is reluctant to reveal.

| **Ms. Bell:** | Do you think my divorce and remarriage had anything to do with Jesse's speech problem? |
| **Clinician:** | It's pretty common for parents to feel guilty about something they might have done to cause their child to begin stuttering. |

You may have already detected a flaw in the triad: On the surface, each question posed by Ms. Bell could be classified in any of the three categories. How does a clinician know *what* the client means? The clinician doesn't know in every case, but he or she tries to determine the purpose of a question by scrutinizing *how* a client asks it—by vocal inflection and body language—and by examining the context in which the inquiry appears. As long as the clinician is *trying to understand,* a client will not be alienated by an inaccurate interpretation.

In our experience, beginning clinicians, probably because the bulk of their training focuses on information, do a good job of responding to content questions. However, many clinicians in training find it difficult to respond appropriately to a client's expression of emotion. Avoid superficial statements of reassurance. The client's anxiety and uncertainty will be better relieved once he or she begins to understand his or her particular speech problem; the best antidote to fear and uncertainty is knowledge. Do not use terms or suggest consequences that will precipitate more stress for the client. Do not communicate any negative expectations regarding the outcome of therapy to the client. It is possible that such statements could influence the client's performance in treatment.

The following six basic principles are addressed to the beginning clinician. We have found them useful for imparting information to clients.

1. Emotional confusion may, and often does, inhibit the client's ability to understand cognitively what you are trying to say. Just because you have once reviewed the steps of therapy is no reason to expect that their importance will be grasped.

2. Refrain from being didactic; do not lecture your clients. Focus on sharing options rather than giving advice.

3. Use simple language with many examples and illustrations. Err on the side of being too simple rather than too complex. And repeat, repeat, repeat the important points—rephrasing each time.

4. Try to provide something that the client—especially a parent—can do. Action reduces the feelings of futility and anxiety. The activity should be direct and simple and should require some kind of reporting to the clinician.

5. Say what needs to be said pleasantly—but frankly. Do not avoid saying something that must be said on the assumption that the client cannot take it or that you will be rejected. People often display an amazing reserve of courage in difficult situations.

6. Remember, however, that the one who finally communicates what the client may have been dreading to hear is often hated and maligned. If you are the first to say the feared words, you may become the focus for all the hostile, negative feelings thus aroused. As a professional, you will have to be strong enough to be the lightning rod for these emotions.

Clients and parents expect to receive help from the clinician but often will resist change. No matter how maladaptive a client's behavior may seem from an objective point of view, it represents the client's best solution. In fact, the client will often resist attempts to alter his or her equilibrium, precarious as it may appear to others. Change is stressful. Diagnosis and treatment imply change; therefore, assessment and therapy are stressful.

We must listen for two aspects of our clients' utterances: a *cognitive* aspect (the content) and an *affective* aspect (the feelings). For genuine understanding to take place, both aspects must be included in the interviewer's response to the client's statement. If you are successful in crystallizing both aspects of your response, you provide an *interchangeable base* that allows the interview to move forward to levels of helping that involve direct action. Here are some examples taken from diagnostic interviews:

Client:	(In response to a query regarding his marital status) No, I'm single. . . . Who would want to marry someone who stutters like me?
Clinician:	You feel rejected because of your speech problem, is that right?
Parent:	We tried to be good parents, we really did . . . but somehow we messed up in helping Peter learn to talk.
Clinician:	You feel a sense of failure, perhaps even guilt, that your child has a speech problem.
Client:	I stutter so badly that life is worthless. . . . I can't get a job. . . . The business of living just doesn't seem to meet expenses.
Clinician:	You feel thwarted and frustrated by your speech problem. Sometimes you wonder if you can go on.

Note the clinician's responses carefully. The clinician does not simply repeat the client's comment but attempts to restate it in clarified form. Observe that the interviewer used the second-person singular "you" in referring to the client's affect. Feelings are commonly stated first because they are more important than content. We sometimes add a tag question ("Is that right?") to check on the client's intake of our responses.

Goal Three: Provide Counseling

The clinician does not, of course, wait until the end of the interview to provide release for the frustrations and fears of the client. Most parts of the interview already discussed will serve this purpose. By helping the client talk about his or her problems, the clinician is providing an excellent escape for pent-up feelings. We maintain that our purpose is not just to remove discomfort but also to promote a state of comfort and well-being.

More than advice is needed during interviews for the purpose of helping a client take some specific action or move in a particular direction. The client needs help in sorting out confusing choices and recognizing opportunities that they may not be able to see at the moment. To support a respondent's real strengths, we need to make it clear that we understand what the situation means to him or her and that we uncritically sympathize with his or her feelings and attitudes. We can restore the client's self-esteem and ability to function more appropriately if we convey our interest in him or her as a person and our solid acceptance of the client's importance.

Client counseling has an unfortunate tradition of "sweetness and light." A person has a problem. The person is sad and depressed, and we try to cheer that person up. Sometimes this degenerates into a debate, with the interviewer attempting to persuade the person not to feel miserable. A person who feels depressed, anxious, and fearful does not want to count his or her blessings. That person wants you to feel miserable, too, and to share and identify with him or her on the same level. Thus, you are given a basis for communication with the person. Start where he or she is, accept it as the proper place to start, and agree that it is a sad state of affairs that would make anyone sad and depressed. This bond of identification becomes a basis for communication, and you can use this bond to assist in solving the problem. The main ingredient is *empathy*, the capacity to identify with another's feelings and actions. The best way to demonstrate an attempt to understand a client's point of view is by listening creatively. In our judgment, of all the skills inherent in effective interviewing, the most important is the ability to listen carefully and empathically. This skill can be learned, although beginning clinicians find it difficult to listen and respond in ways that facilitate a client's expression of feelings. One of the best ways to increase your active listening skills is to recognize when you are engaging in a poor form of listening. Egan (2014) describes four forms of poor listening:

Nonlistening occurs when your mind wanders. While it may appear that you are listening, you are truly not engaged. You also would not be able to restate the provided information reliably.

Partial listening occurs if you are able to pick up part of the message but the depth of the message is being lost. Egan describes this as "phony" listening.

Tape-recorder listening may appear like listening on the surface because you are able to repeat the words of the client, but in reality there is a lack of psychological and emotional presence. In this scenario the clinician can relay the content of the message but fails to identify or realize the corresponding meaning and relevance.

Rehearsing occurs when the clinician prepares his or her response to the client rather than remaining in the state of active listening.

How does one handle emotional scenes? They are bound to arise at some point in your interviewing experience. Some clinicians excuse themselves from the room and allow the respondent to recover his or her dignity alone. Others try to change the subject to something less emotional. Both of these approaches may, with certain clients, give the impression that you are rejecting their feelings. It is more effective to indicate understanding of the feelings that are being expressed and accept them as natural human reactions: for example, "That's okay to let it come out, Ms. Cobb. You have been holding it back too long. Sometimes it helps to get it out in the open."

Not all clients seen by the speech clinician will need or even want extensive supportive interviewing. In some cases, the procedures discussed here would be grossly inappropriate. Visualize an interview as ranging along a continuum from affective concern, such as feelings and attitudes, to objective matters, such as goals and advice. Some respondents simply need objective information so that they can take over and modify their behavior. The clinician's role in some interviews may consist of simply listening to and supporting a client. A good relationship is a *necessary* but not a *sufficient* condition for good interviewing. Although it may sound trite, it is true that the secret of care *of* a client is caring *for* the client. The sense of being understood by a helping professional is a powerful stimulant to the client's growth.

USING INTERVIEWING SKILLS BEYOND THE DIAGNOSTIC EVALUATION

As we mentioned in Chapter 1, evaluation is not confined to a 2-hour block of time in a university or a 1-hour session in a school district. The speech-language pathologist constantly gathers data on clients as treatment progresses in order to determine if the remediation is successful or if goals should be adjusted. In many types of cases seen by the SLP, the treatment plan is formulated jointly by the clinician, parents or family members, and other professionals. In such instances, the amount of information gathered in the diagnostic evaluation is not sufficient to generate a meaningful treatment plan that takes into account both the clinician's and the family's perspectives. Thus, more extensive interviewing is necessary to discover information on family strengths, concerns, and needs. More interviewing of related professionals is needed to determine how the client is performing in a variety of contexts. We will briefly illustrate this notion with the following three popular clinical techniques:

1. *Ethnographic interviewing.* As clinicians, we often need to attend to potential sources of cultural bias during the interview process because the families we treat often come from backgrounds and/or lead lives that are very different from our own. That is, we need not only to understand the presenting problem but also to understand the problem through the same lens of our clients. Ethnographic interviewing provides the structure for accomplishing this task. This kind of interviewing requires that a clinician have the ability to develop relationships with others and the ability to embrace the unfamiliar. This is accomplished through an empathic understanding and having a genuine curiosity and interest in the differences we encounter in the way people and families go about their daily lives (Schensul, S. L., Schensul, J. J. & LeCompte, M. D. (2013).

   An ethnographic interview has three phases (Spradley, 1979). The first phase entails defining or explaining the *specific purpose* of the interview to the client. During the second phase, you as the interviewer explain, through *ethnographic explanations,* how the purpose of the interview will be achieved. That is, during this process you describe to the client what topics or areas will be covered during the interview, the methods you will use to record responses, and how you would like the participant to respond to the questions that are raised during the interview process. Finally, after the stage for the interview is set, the interviewer will ask a variety of *ethnographic questions* to guide the client through the interview process. Ethnographic questions include grand-tour, mini-tour, structural, and contrast questions. *Grand-tour questions* are used to get a verbal description that captures the essential features associated with the goal of the interview. More specifically, these questions are designed to capture the client's experience with the problem, the daily routine, and who the client interacts with in his or her daily life. For example, a typical grand-tour question could be "Walk me through the routine of a typical day." *Mini-tour questions* are used to get more details about information that comes about from the grand-tour question. For example, "Tell me more about the structure of a typical school day." *Structural questions* are asked when you need to understand the organization of the information provided. *Contrast questions*, on the other hand, are asked when events or descriptions need to be set apart or further differentiated.

   Especially in cases where the SLP is working with infants, toddlers, and preschool children, the law requires that families be an integral part of treatment planning and monitoring. In fact, the clinician, along with other professionals and the family, must generate an individualized family service plan (IFSP) that states specific information related to the treatment program (see Chapter 4 for more details) (Nelson, 2010). If you were to use ethnographic interviewing, the focus would be on the parent and the goal would be to obtain the parent's perspective of the problems, goals, and approaches used in treatment. The clinician asks both broad-based grand-tour questions and more specific mini-tour questions that are not meant necessarily to lead the parent but just to guide the conversation and explore the problem. The goal is to let the parent set the direction of the interview toward what is important to him or her; ideally, the parent will do most of the talking, with encouragement and structure from the clinician. This type of in-depth interview is used to understand the family situation and its goals and aspirations for the child with a communication disorder. Parents are encouraged to tell the clinician what goals are most important to them and which ones they would like to see incorporated first into the remediation plan. If you consider the wealth and depth of possible information to gather in such a case, it should be no surprise that ethnographic interviews take hours of conversation to complete effectively.

2. *Motivational interviewing.* For cases where intrinsic motivation for change needs to be explored or developed and ambivalence needs to be overcome, the method of motivational interviewing might be ideal (Miller & Rollnick, 1991). *Motivational interviewing* is client-centered. Through expressed empathy, the clinician is able to help clients recognize and take some sort of action to resolve a problem. The goal is to foster change from within by developing the client's intrinsic motivation rather than suggesting changes that can come across as imposed. Motivational interviewing is not advice giving. Clients are encouraged to think about their current situation or problem and how life would be if they did or did not incorporate changes. Through weighing the pros and cons, the client is able to explore and resolve any ambivalence. Miller and Rollnick (1991, 2002) provide five clinical principles on which motivational interviewing is based:

    • *Expressed empathy* through reflective listening is viewed as an essential component of motivational interviewing. This process requires an attitude of acceptance and a belief that ambivalence is normal. That is, you must understand and have tolerance for the concept that people resist change even when change is desired.

    • *Identification of discrepancy* requires that the clinician amplify and create opportunity for the client to self-identify discrepancy between behavior and stated goals. You want the client to develop the argument for change through the use of reflective listening and objective feedback.

    • *Avoid persuasive arguments* and develop a facilitative, mutual working relationship. Direct persuasion is viewed as counterproductive to the motivational interviewing process because an argumentative or persuasive demeanor can lead to increased resistance and defensiveness. The more a client verbally defends or argues her or his position, the more likely it is that the client will talk her- or himself out of changing a behavior. It is ultimately the client's responsibility and decision to change.

    • *Accept and roll with resistance* rather than confront it or oppose. Resistance should be acknowledged and explored.

    • *Support self-efficacy* because the client is viewed as an instrumental resource and partner in the process of finding a solution. The goal is to enhance the client's degree of optimism and confidence so he or she can adequately cope with and succeed during the change process.

    The emphasis in motivational interviewing is that it is often best for the client, rather than the clinician, to develop an argument for change. It has been found to be more efficacious than traditional advice giving with regard to the treatment of a variety of health-related problems (Burke, Arkowitz, & Menchola, 2003; Rubak, Sandbaek, Lauritzen, & Christensen, 2005). It is often perceived as effective when used by itself or when combined with other forms of intervention.

3. *Curriculum-based assessment*. In cases where a school-age student is being treated for a language disorder, many considerations in planning therapy go beyond the diagnostic evaluation. Curriculum-based assessment is concerned with finding out the demands placed on a child by the educational environment in which he or she must use language and literacy skills (Nelson, 2010; Paul, 2007), and developing a plan where the child can experience success within her or his educational environment. For this to happen, the child is evaluated to determine the functioning level of instruction where the child can succeed within the general education curriculum. Teachers are given instructional placment information, which is valuable for planning and advancing the child's skills in a manner that can reduce feelings of failure and frustration. To determine the types of communication, language, and literacy skills necessary to compete in the classroom environment, the SLP must interview teachers and examine curricular materials. This, again, requires conversation with other professionals to design treatment programs and monitor progress and generalization of the skills focused on in therapy.

Telepractice

In many geographical areas, access to an SLP is limited. Barriers to service access can include distance, impaired mobility, and the lack of an available SLP or specialist. To overcome the barriers of access to service, *telepractice* (as ASHA prefers to call it) is now accepted as an appropriate service delivery model for the evaluation, diagnosis, and delivery of treatment (American Speech-Language-Hearing Association, 2005a, 2005b). Telepractice involves the use of telecommunication to establish a real-time audio and video connection with a client to create an experience that will simulate and be equivalent to a traditional in-person encounter. Technology requirements include a secure videoconferencing platform, Internet access, headphones, scanners, and printers.

IMPROVING YOUR INTERVIEW SKILLS

You can see that interviewing never stops, from the beginning to the end of our clinical relationships. The same types of skills that we use in our initial intake interview are used again or are modified as we gather and disseminate information through therapy and dismissal. The more practice and experience in talking with families and clients you can obtain, the better your clinical skills will become. We have included a series of activities and projects for your own practice. Let them serve as the beginning steps in a continual learning effort toward improved interviewing. You will find that the time devoted to such training exercises is well spent. Now, consider these steps for improving your interviewing skills:

1. *Read widely from a variety of sources.* Find out what people are like by reading in sociology, psychology, anthropology, and philosophy. This is, of course, a lifetime project, which we feel is delightful because there is always a new frontier, an open horizon toward which we can set our sails.

2. *Listen to all sorts of people.* Listen to their dreams, their rationalizations, their insights—or lack of them—and their gripes. Get acquainted with the way people think and talk by following the example of others (Least Heat-Moon, 1982; Terkel, 1980, 1993, 2001).

3. *Form small heterogeneous groups of students majoring in speech pathology and audiology.* Conduct some sensitivity and values clarification training, particularly as it relates to your self-concept, assets and liabilities, responses to people, and your relationship with your own parents and other older adults (Kaplan & Dreyer, 1974). To provide assistance

to others, we must know our own foibles and potential blind spots and have them under reasonable control.

4. *Evaluate your degree of self-awareness.* To understand the way our actions will affect those we are trying to help, we have to acquire the skill of self-awareness. Self-awareness is an attitude toward interaction that helps you understand the impact that your personal thoughts, behaviors, and actions will have on others. Through self-awareness, you can build rather than burn bridges and develop better relationships with your clients. Self-awareness can be developed (because it is a skill) through being open-minded and engaging in self-introspection. It will take a conscious effort. The power and courage behind knowing yourself and how you affect others, and then letting that understanding guide your interactions with others should not be underestimated.

5. *Role-play to prepare for interviewing.* Set up several typical interview situations in front of a class and play, for example, the roles of the reluctant parent, the spouse of a patient with aphasia, or a hostile father. Discuss the interaction and replay the situations with others, assuming different roles. Write interview purposes prior to the role-playing and determine, or have the class determine, how effectively the interviewer accomplished the stated purposes. Whenever the viewers feel that the interview went wrong or the responses were ineffective, see how many different ways the interview could have been handled. This builds up the beginning interviewer's repertoire of adaptive responses. You can do a surprising amount of intrapersonal role-playing in your spare time. While we are waiting for a class to begin or for a light to change, we frequently imagine ourselves in various interviewing situations and then explore alternate statements, probes, and so forth.

6. *Record your first few interviews, then analyze them carefully with your clinical supervisor or a colleague.* Evaluate your diagnostic interviews by using the checklist of interviewing competencies (see Figure 2–2). Obviously, no beginning clinician will remember, let alone exhibit, all the skills in the checklist; practice only a few at a time, and provide constructive feedback for each other.

We would like to end this chapter with a challenge: Utilize the interviewing approach delineated in the chapter, find the errors, the things that just don't work for you, and then develop your own methods. We have given you the foundation blocks. Can you use them to make stepping-stones?

FIGURE 2–2
Checklist of Interviewing Competencies

Interviewer: _____ Date: _____

Client/Respondent: _____

I. *Orienting the Respondent*
   A. Attends to comfort (coats, seating, and so on)
   B. Engages in appropriate "flow" talk
   C. Explains purposes, procedures
   D. Structures roles
II. *Engendering Communication*
   A. Attending behaviors (demonstration receptiveness)
      1. Relaxed, natural posture
      2. Appropriate eye contact
      3. Responses that follow the client's comments (restating, overlapping the client's message)
   B. Open invitation to share (open-ended questions)

(continued)

FIGURE 2–2   (*continued*)

C. Nondistracting encouragement to continue talking
   1. Verbal ("Yes," "I see," and the like)
   2. Nonverbal (nodding, shifting posture toward client)
D. Obtains an overview of the presenting problem
III. *Use of Questions and Recording*
  A. Orderly, sequential questions
  B. Nondistracting note taking
IV. *Active Listening*
  A. Reflects feelings (empathic statements)
   1. Matches affect
   2. Matches content
  B. Periodic summarizing of affect and content message
V. *Monitoring Nonverbal Clues*
  A. The diagnostician's
  B. The respondent's
VI. *Skills in Presenting Information*
  A. Transmission of information
   1. Content
   2. Style and language
  B. Responds to questions appropriately
  C. Appropriate use of humor, "flow" talk
VII. *Closing the Interview*
  A. Summary, review of findings
  B. Recommendations
  C. Supportive comments
VIII. *Analysis of Information*
  A. Major themes in the client's presentation, association of ideas, inconsistencies and omissions
  B. Descriptive report

Note: This checklist is designed to help monitor the performance of beginning interviewers. It can be used as a self-rating device or as a format for supervisory feedback.

CONCLUSION AND SELF-ASSESSMENT

We hope the material in this chapter will be useful to students majoring in clinical speech pathology and to our colleagues working in various settings. However, no one ever became proficient in interviewing solely by reading about it. Nor, it seems, are interviewing skills enhanced by increasing knowledge about communication disorders. It took us many years of constant searching and experimenting to evolve the interviewing approach presented here. And with the indulgence of our clients and parents, we continue to explore for better ways.

After reading this chapter you should be able to answer the following questions:

1. What are some potential disadvantages to using only paper-and-pencil techniques for collecting client information?
2. What is a diagnostic interview?
3. List and describe three common barriers to conducting an effective diagnostic interview?
4. What are the three basic goals in conducting diagnostic interviews?
5. List and describe the different types of questions that are commonly asked during an interview.
6. What types of things should be avoided while conducting a diagnostic interview?
7. What are three popular techniques used in clinical interviewing? Describe how they are distinct from one another.

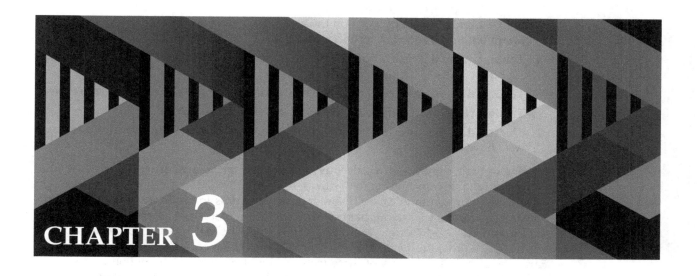

CHAPTER 3

Psychometric Considerations in Diagnosis and Evaluation

LEARNING OUTCOMES

After reading this chapter you will be able to:

1. Identify the differences between norm-referenced and criterion-referenced assessments.
2. Define validity and distinguish among the different types of validity.
3. Define reliability and distinguish among the different types of reliability.
4. Describe measures of central tendency.
5. Distinguish among the different types of scores found on formal tests.
6. Describe the relevance of evaluating the sensitivity and specificity of a standardized assessment.
7. Identify four common mistakes made in the use of standardized assessments.
8. Describe factors that require consideration when evaluating a client from another culture.

Consider the following sales pitch.

Let us interest you in purchasing a standardized test to use in assessing communication disorders. It has the following characteristics:

1. Test administrators have trouble agreeing on whether or not a response on the test is correct.
2. Clients seem to perform differently on the test each time they take it.

3. The test really does not focus on the aspects of communication that are relevant to treatment or diagnostic decision making.

4. The test manual is vague about how to administer the instrument and how to interpret the results.

5. The test does not really examine the true process that you are attempting to assess.

6. The test was normed on 200 typical white children from Idaho.

7. The test does not discriminate adequately between clients with disorders and those who have none.

No one in their right mind would buy this instrument because it would provide little valid and reliable information to use in assessment.

Do tests for communication disorders ever have this many shortcomings? Unfortunately, *many* formal tests in our field suffer from the problems just listed (Huang, Hopkins, & Nippold, 1997; McCauley & Swisher, 1984a, 1984b; McFadden, 1996; Muma, 1983, 1984, 2002; Muma, Lubinski, & Pierce, 1982; Plante & Vance, 1994; Spaulding, Plante, & Farinella, 2006)! The authors of these tests no doubt begin with the notion of designing a useful instrument; however, when conceptual and psychometric limitations manifest themselves, the test designer is typically reluctant to scrap the whole enterprise. Usually, the test is submitted, warts and all, to a publisher because, even though it suffers from inadequacies, it represents a significant amount of work in its development. It is therefore up to the consumer to evaluate carefully any instrument in terms of its psychometric adequacy before purchasing it. We must become educated in evaluating instruments because purchasing an inadequate test is a waste of money and, more important, a waste of time. It also affects our clients because they must spend money paying for the administration of these tests and also must invest their time to take the tests. Clients can also be misdiagnosed, mislabeled, and mistreated on the basis of testing with psychometrically poor instruments. One can readily see that psychometric adequacy of standardized tests is a significant issue, one that we must deal with in a text on diagnosis and evaluation.

When a client comes for a speech and language evaluation, we must remember that the primary goal of the evaluation is to diagnose whether the client has a problem that would lessen or be alleviated with intervention. Therefore, we need to know whether the tests we select, formal or informal, will evaluate what the client states to be the presenting problem and identify the strengths and weaknesses in the area of the presenting problem. It is also important to remember that, during the evaluation process, we are only testing or sampling our client's behaviors. Testing is the process of using a set of systematic procedures to sample or observe behaviors of interest (Anastasi, 1997). It would be nearly impossible to test behavior in its entirety and in all given contexts. That is why our evaluations would be considered more of a sampling or observation of specific behaviors, skills, or abilities. And it is our job, as the speech-language pathologist, to make sure that the observations and samples we get during the testing process are representative. For example, it would be inappropriate for me to assume that one 300-word conversation sample obtained from a fluency client in the diagnostic room would be representative of that client's fluency with all people and across all situations. In reality, we have only obtained a small glimpse of what that client's fluency behavior could include because it could vary dramatically across different communicative contexts.

COMMON TYPES OF TESTS

One way we often try to capture or sample behavior is through the use of standardized and nonstandardized tests. A test is considered a *standardized test* if it is administered and scored in the same manner across all individuals tested. A test would be considered *nonstandardized* when the manner in which the test is given and the scoring differs across individuals tested. The benefit of standardization is that the consistency in the administration and scoring procedures allows for a more reliable comparison across clients because each client's performance would be more likely to reflect differences in the behavior being evaluated versus differences resulting from variable scoring and testing procedures.

There are two types of standardized tests: norm-referenced and criterion-referenced. Most textbooks on psychometric issues focus on norm-referenced tests. Often norm-referenced tests are called standardized tests or formal tests, depending on the designer's preference. Just because a test is standardized, however, does not mean that it is norm referenced. Standardization implies only that the *procedures* for test administration are standard, not that norms are provided with the instrument. In developing norm-referenced tests, the designers have created some tasks they feel are relevant (valid) and have administered the instrument to large groups of subjects who, one hopes, represent the population on whom the test is to be used. From these large-scale administrations, the designers are able to calculate normative data that reflect the performance of the large sample. When an individual is given the test, his or her score is compared to the performance of the normative sample, and it is determined how this person performed relative to the large group. The purpose of *norm-referenced tests* is to determine if an individual obtains a score similar to the group average or, if not, how far away from average the individual's score is. Generally, if the individual scored within 1.5 to 2 standard deviations above or below the mean, he or she is said to reflect performance within "normal limits." If the score was more than 2 standard deviations above or below the mean, the performance is said to be exceptional because only about 5% of the normative population scored in a similar manner. Thus, norm-referenced tests have the major purpose of determining if there is a problem, or a significant enough difference from standard performance, to warrant concern with regard to normalcy. Examples of commonly used norm-referenced tests in speech-language pathology include the Goldman-Fristoe Test of Articulation, Second Edition (Goldman & Fristoe, 2000); Clinical Evaluation of Language Fundamentals, Fifth Edition (Semel, Wiig, & Secord, 2013); and the Western Aphasia Battery–Revised (Kertesz, 2006). We will have more to say in a later section of this chapter regarding some qualifications that must be taken into account when considering this purpose of standardized tests.

The other type of test typically mentioned in psychometric texts is the criterion-referenced instrument. *Criterion-referenced instruments* also appear under other terminologies such as mastery testing, domain-referenced testing, objectives-referenced testing, and competency-based testing. These measurements are designed to distinguish specific levels of client performance in a clearly specified domain. The client's performance can be interpreted using raw scores because the goal is to determine performance in relation to a particular performance standard instead of determining how an individual scores in relation to a normative group. Functional outcomes are often criterion-referenced behaviors that describe what a person can do after treatment that he or she could not do prior to treatment. We mentioned functional outcomes in Chapter 1 when we discussed the initiatives of American Speech-Language-Hearing Association (ASHA) and the World Health Organization (WHO) in developing measures that reflect patient progress in real-world activities.

The criterion-referenced test serves a different purpose compared to a norm-referenced instrument. It is clearly more related to defining specific skills in assessment and treatment and emphasizes individual performance, while the norm-referenced test focuses on group similarity. McCauley (1996) provides guidelines for the evaluation, selection, and development of informal criterion-referenced measures in communication disorders. Unfortunately, there are precious few formal criterion-referenced measures in our field. Some examples include the Rossetti Infant–Toddler Language Scale (Rossetti, 2006); the Hodson Assessment of Phonological Patterns, Third Edition (Hodson, 2004); and the Functional Communication Profile–Revised (Kleiman, 2003). Current emphases on evidence-based practice and functional outcome measures promote the development of more criterion-referenced tests in the near future. Most of our formal instruments are norm-referenced, so the focus of the rest of the chapter will be on these types of tests.

THE FOUNDATION OF THE TEST OR MEASURE

It is important for us to know that a test described as adequately normed and standardized does not mean it has adequate or desirable psychometric properties. That is, it is possible to have a test with very sound administration procedures and norms and it is of poor quality. So how do we determine whether the test is a quality test, or is a "sound measure" of the behavior we are trying to sample? We need to consider the test's validity and reliability. We would also like to point out that it is not only standardized instruments that require some measure of psychometric adequacy. Although many clinicians associate psychometric principles only with standardized, norm-referenced tests, it is the feeling of the present authors that most of the informal or descriptive measures that we use in communication disorders are also susceptible to considerable error. Just because we are not using a standardized test does not relieve us of the responsibility of checking our validity and reliability. The same psychometric rigor applied to standardized examinations could easily be applied to our informal evaluation procedures. Informal measures can also vary in the degree to which they are valid and reliable.

VALIDITY

Validity basically refers to the degree to which a procedure actually measures what it purports to measure. Validity is highly related to the purpose for which the test is used, and a particular test can be valid for one purpose and invalid for another. If we say we are going to measure a child's language comprehension, we should select a test that can accomplish this goal. If the test is measuring something other than the child's language comprehension, then the test is invalid. So many of the behaviors we assess in communication disorders are extremely complex and involve multiple systems. Language, for example, has many areas (semantics, syntax, morphology, phonology, pragmatics), and it is influenced by other systems (cognitive, social, psychological, neurolinguistic, etc.). If we develop a test of "language ability" that can be administered and scored in 20 minutes, and this test has the child imitate, name pictures, and point to photographs, we have not really looked at language ability in its entirety. We have taken a few tasks and we are willing to make judgments about a very complex linguistic system based on the child's ability to perform these operations, which are totally unnatural and unrelated to normal language use. This is tantamount to a cardiologist's making a clinical judgment about a significant heart condition only by feeling the patient's pulse; such a judgment is just not valid, especially when we have the technology available to do a thorough evaluation of heart function. The major point here is that without validity for a test, we are fooling ourselves if we use the test to look at complex behaviors. Even if we can demonstrate that the items on the test are reliable, it does not matter because we have only developed a reliable way of looking at irrelevant facts. This point is made painfully clear by several authors who raise ethical concerns about the administration of tests that lack validity (Messick, 1980; Muma, 1984). If we use such tests, we not only waste time and money, but we can arrive at erroneous judgments about our clients, which results in incorrect goal selection or, worse, placement in inappropriate programs.

Discussions of validity focus on three types: construct, content, and criterion-related validity. *Construct validity* is "the extent to which the test may be said to measure a theoretical construct or trait" (Anastasi, 1997, p. 126). To obtain this type of validity "the test author must rely on indirect evidence and inference" (Salvia, Ysseldyke, & Bolt, 2010, p. 68). Thus, a test in any area of communication disorders must ideally reflect the underlying construct it is attempting to assess.

A second type of validity is content validity. Typically, *content validity* is derived by "a careful examination of the content of a test. Such an examination is judgmental in nature and requires a clear definition of what the content should be. Content validity is established by examining three factors: the appropriateness of the types of items included, the completeness of the item sample, and the way in which the items assess the content" (Salvia & Ysseldyke, 1981, p. 102). Typically, expert judges are included to examine the content of the test in order to make the determination of content validity.

A final type of validity is *criterion-related*, which takes into account the degree to which a test associates with a similar measure (i.e., criterion) of the same behavior. There are two types of criterion-related validity: concurrent validity and predictive validity. *Concurrent validity* is a measure of how an individual's current score on one instrument can be used to make an estimate of his or her current score on some other criterion measure, typically another test in a related area. *Predictive validity* is a measure of how an individual's current score on one instrument can estimate scoring on a criterion measure taken at a later time. A critical variable, however, is the validity and reliability of the criterion measure selected for use in criterion-related validity. The instrument you design must be valid, and so must the criterion measure.

The three types of validity mentioned above would ideally be used in concert to determine the overall validity of a test instrument. There is, however, a tendency among some test designers to believe that only one or two types of validity are required to validate an instrument and that perhaps the three types of validity are equally powerful and thus interchangeable. This is *not* the case. The most potent type of validity is construct validity. Construct validity is viewed by most authorities as the *keystone* of test development (Messick, 1975, 1980; Muma, 1985). Muma (2002) provides an excellent summary of construct validity and reviews many contemporary language tests to show that most of these instruments are found lacking in construct validity. We agree that this is a serious problem with the standardized tests (especially in language and phonology) in our field. This once again shows that there is no substitute for a thorough analysis of real communication in assessment. We have separated this section on validity from the rest of the psychometric background in this chapter and discuss it first because it is probably the most important issue in psychometric adequacy. It does not matter how popular a test is, how easy it is to administer, or how much statistical hocus-pocus is found in the examiner's manual. If the test lacks validity, it is nothing more than a wasteful, empty exercise.

Validity also requires consideration in informal procedures. For instance, we can ask a person with velopharyngeal incompetency to blow a pinwheel, and we can time how long it spins to get an indication of velopharyngeal closure. This measure may have good reliability in that two clinicians could time the pinwheel with a stopwatch and agree on how long the wheel spins. Perhaps the client could even be reliable in terms of blowing the wheel in a similar fashion over several trials and making the wheel spin for a fairly consistent length of time each trial. The problem, however, is validity. We know that blowing a pinwheel may not relate at all to the ability to maintain velopharyngeal closure during speech production. Reliability is useless if the measure being taken is not valid.

RELIABILITY

The notion of reliability is critical to formal as well as informal measures. If one were to develop a valid norm-referenced test, it would be useless if the test developer could not demonstrate that different examiners could use it with similar facility and that clients performed consistently from one occasion to another. Many of the behaviors that we informally observe, count, or time are often not clearly defined, and this imprecision contributes to a lack of reliability. For good agreement, two examiners would have to be looking for the same behavior and coding it in a similar manner. The difficult aspect of informal assessment is that many behaviors that we examine are transient (phonemes, disfluencies, facial grimaces, laryngeal tension, slight head jerks, etc.), while others may be ill defined and subjective (pitch changes, topic changes, cohesive adequacy, voice quality changes, stress alterations, intelligibility, severity, etc.). Clinicians must devote the same attention to these issues if they use informal measures so that these measures can be replicated over time as indications of treatment progress. Without validity and reliability, informal measures are nothing more than the subjective judgments of one person that may tell us little about client performance. Several types of reliability are discussed in the following sections.

Interjudge Reliability

Interjudge reliability refers to the agreement of two independent judges on the occurrence and type of responses performed by a client. Almost every clinician has had the experience of asking another speech-language pathologist (SLP) to look at a difficult case. We often question our abilities to judge aberrant qualities. We want another opinion about factors like vocal quality, intelligibility, or pragmatic abilities. Clients who stutter often present with many complex avoidances and timing devices that we ask our peers to scrutinize, just to make sure we are on the right track. Sometimes, even in standardized tests, we ask the opinions of others to check some arbitrary scoring convention that we have used because the manual did not tell us what to do in enough detail. All of these factors have to do with interjudge reliability.

The types of responses that we ask children and adults to make in diagnosis and evaluation tasks are many and varied. Some responses are relatively straightforward and easily agreed upon by two independent judges. For example, if we ask a client to point to one of four pictures in response to an auditory model (e.g., "Point to 'running'"), most judges would agree on the correctness of the client's response. Other types of responding may not be quite as clear. For instance, judges may not be able to agree on the occurrence of a distorted /s/ or /r/ phoneme.

Judges may have difficulty determining whether a response was correct if the client initially makes the wrong response and then self-corrects it. Does the test provide guidelines for examiners in terms of accepting a self-corrected response as correct? In informal tasks, it is often difficult for judges to agree on certain behaviors, such as the amount of time spent in symbolic play. An adequate operational definition of symbolic play would be necessary, and criteria for when such play begins and ends would be required if two judges are to agree on time sampling of behavior. Thus, we can see that the behaviors that judges must agree on vary in terms of their observability, definition, and subjectivity. If judges cannot agree on what they are observing, then the test or procedure is unreliable. Here are some obvious contributing factors that decrease interjudge reliability:

- *Incomplete or ambiguous definitions.* If a behavior is to be counted, timed, observed, or interpreted, there must be an adequate definition of the behavior so that independent judges can agree on behavioral occurrences. For example, if one goal of treatment is to reduce behavior problems in a client with language impairment, the measurement of this construct (behavior problem) must be guided by a specific definition. Do behavior problems include only tantrums, or do actions such as pushing the materials away, whining, repetitive vocalizations, and refusal to participate in tasks also constitute behavior problems? One can readily see that two examiners could experience major disagreement on this measure unless the definition was quite precise. The two judges need to know what to count or time and what behaviors to exclude from the concept of behavior problems. Sometimes the operational definition selected by an examiner may not be universally agreed on, and this may affect the *validity* of the measure. Even if the definition is somewhat incomplete, however, reliability can be increased by limiting the behaviors under scrutiny so that everyone can agree when they occur. Regardless of whether the measure is a formal standardized test or an informal evaluation measure, interjudge reliability is critical to the psychometric adequacy of the test. Formal tests should include data on interjudge reliability. Test manuals should include detailed definitions of the behaviors to be scored and as many guidelines as possible about potential response modes that may be difficult for the examiner to interpret as a correct or incorrect response. Some tests (Porch, 1981) have multidimensional scoring systems in which the client's response is not merely judged for correctness but also for the way the response occurred and for levels of acceptability. If the scoring system is complex enough, the test developer may even recommend taking a training course in test administration. This training is routinely done for tests of intelligence that require many judgment calls about client responses and some consistency in these decisions.

- *Training.* For any procedure to be reliable, the judges need to receive similar training in the observation, coding, and interpretation of the data. Most researchers put reliability judges through training periods, sometimes lasting several hours, prior to actual computation of the reliability scores. It makes good sense that, prior to using any procedure, a clinician will have adequate exposure to the methods and some practice using them.

- *Practice.* Reliability is a function of practice. Both formal tests and informal evaluation measures require practice to administer and score efficiently. If one judge has much experience with a particular test or measurement and another judge has had none, lack of reliability can be expected. The more we perform procedures, the more systematic and consistent our decision making becomes.

- *Response complexity.* Generally, the more complex the response, the greater the lack of reliability. If the system you are using to examine teacher–child interactions has a host of teacher and child variables, it will be more difficult to use than one with fewer variables to examine. Another common example is the poor reliability associated with narrow phonetic transcription. The more narrow we become in what we test, the more difficult it is to obtain adequate reliability. In this age of writing generative phonologies from children's spontaneous samples, you can imagine how many specific disagreements could occur between two clinicians. First, error occurs in just transcribing the sample, and there is the opportunity for many disagreements. Second, error occurs in detecting the specific errors within the transcript. Third, error occurs in trying to arrive at a list of phonological processes or idiosyncratic rules that account for the child's sample. Finally, error occurs in determining the frequency or percentage of occurrence of each rule derived from the sample. The result could be a catalog of chaos. The more guidelines that clinicians have in making decisions, the better the reliability; in addition, the less complex the decisions, the better the reliability. This is why some authors have developed specific guidelines and definitions to use in phonological analyses (Ingram, 1981; Shriberg & Kwiatkowski, 1980).

- *Live scoring versus recording analysis.* Scoring behaviors during test administration is always more difficult than being able to replay video or audio recordings for second and third opportunities to examine a behavior. Video scoring probably tends to be more reliable simply because it is difficult to observe behaviors in rapid sequence accurately and to take the time to note their occurrence on an observation form (which also takes away from one's ability to observe).

Reliability can be computed in several ways. One method involves statistical procedures known as reliability coefficients or correlation coefficients (Hegde, 1987; Salvia, Ysseldyke, & Bolt, 2010). Typically, for formal tests, such correlations are judges to determine if the scores they derive are in general agreement, compared to moving up and down together. It is preferable for standardized tests to have inter-judge reliability coefficients of .90 or above to show good agreement among examiners. For example, if Judge A scored a series of tests as 89, 62, 53, and 36 and Judge B scored the same tests as 90, 60, 50, and 35, there would be general agreement and a possible correlation of .99. The closer a coefficient of reliability is to 1.0, the more reliable the scoring. Some reliability coefficients take into account variance in the examiner's judgments (e.g., intraclass correlation, Winer's coefficient of reliability). Other test developers have used a simple correlation coefficient (e.g., Pearson product moment), which is far less effective in evaluating reliability (Bartko, 1976). In the example above, Judge A and Judge B did not agree exactly on any of the test scores, but there was a general trend for the two judges' scores to go up and down together. There was also a tendency for the scores to be rather close (within 3 points of each other). This type of reliability may be acceptable for general responses, but if we want to gain insight into more specific behaviors, the correlation coefficient is too general a measure.

Let's say that we want to count specific articulatory errors; it would be important to agree on the type of error produced. It would also be important for the judges to be counting the *same* errors. The following scenario is possible. A child is asked to produce 10 words for two judges who are going to count misarticulations. Both judges come up with five misarticulations. If the two judges made these kinds of responses over many subjects, they would appear to represent perfect agreement (1.0 in a correlation). Further analysis reveals, however, that Judge A found errors in the first five words and Judge B found errors in the last five words. In essence, they did not agree on *any* of the misarticulations but came up with the same total number.

This example underscores the importance of a different type of reliability measure called *point by point* or *percent exact agreement.* In this type of reliability, a formula such as the following is used:

$$x = \frac{\text{Agreements}}{\text{Agreements} + \text{Disagreements}} \times 100$$

Thus, one takes the total number of specific agreements and divides this number by the total number of agreements plus the disagreements, multiplies the result by 100, and arrives at a percentage of exact agreement. In this way, we get a good idea of the behaviors that judges rate in exactly the same way. Any clinician can compute such a simple formula and determine interjudge reliability for almost any clinically relevant behavior in a diagnostic or treatment context. Often it is a good idea to check our perceptions occasionally to see if we are fooling ourselves with regard to the occurrence of client behaviors. This type of reliability is especially important in behaviors that lend themselves to error because of subjectivity. Unfortunately, this includes many of the relevant measures in communication disorders.

Test-Retest Reliability

Some behaviors are highly stable over time. We would hope that most of the responses we assess to gain insight into various processes underlying communication are of this variety. If we are attempting to examine language comprehension, we assume that client performance on one day will be similar to client performance on another day. Vocal differences found one week would hopefully be observed the next week. If it were not for these behavioral consistencies, we really would have difficulty justifying treatment. A person's voice is either disordered or it is not. Clearly, behavioral fluctuations exist in some disorders (e.g., stuttering, voice problems that vary with fatigue, etc.), but in others one can expect a fairly consistent occurrence (e.g., articulation errors, language errors). Tests are supposed to be designed to probe a particular error so that they show consistent problems with a client's communication. If a patient with aphasia showed drastically different performances from week to week, it would be impossible to formulate a treatment program because the targets would always be changing. If a laboratory test for cancer varied from day to day in its diagnosis of tissue samples, it would be unusable. It is easy to see that test-retest reliability has much to do with the behavior being evaluated and also with the test items chosen to reveal the skill you are testing. Test-retest reliability is a measure of consistency that requires administration of a test at two different points in time. Through this process, the stability of scores between *test* and *retest* conditions can be evaluated. The closer the scores are to each other, the more reliable the test. Reliability coefficients, as described, are used to examine test-retest reliability, and those coefficients close to 1.0 indicate stability or repeatability in performance on a particular task. A shortcoming of test-retest reliability is the *practice effect,* where individuals become familiar with the test and answer based on their memory of the answers to the last test. The practice effect can inflate reliability estimates. One can also use the point-by-point procedure to determine if the errors made on one day are similar to those made at a later time. It depends on how detailed the clinician wants to be in examining client performance.

Split-Half Reliability

Many formal test developers want to evaluate the internal consistency of the items on their instrument. This is achieved by splitting in half all the items on the test. In essence, they want to determine if both halves of the test tend to be reliable, or agree, in terms of scores obtained.

SOME QUANTITATIVE BACKGROUND FOR TEST INTERPRETATION

Some basic concepts in measurement are necessary in order to appreciate most standardized tests. Many traditional quantitative aspects will not be covered because they are rarely found on tests we use (e.g., mode, median, semiquartile range, types of curves, kurtosis, and skewedness). Although we are omitting these topics, we are certainly not suggesting they are of diminished value. We simply want to discuss aspects that are useful for interpreting most tests in communication disorders. For more detailed accounts of these concepts, consult other sources that provide more in-depth coverage (Anastasi, 1997; Salvia, Ysseldyke, & Bolt 2010).

CENTRAL TENDENCY, VARIATION, AND THE NORMAL CURVE

Whenever someone takes a test, he or she earns one or more scores. Part of test interpretation involves placing the score(s) of an individual in the context of others who have also been administered the instrument. The most frequently encountered measure of central tendency in formal tests is the *mean* or arithmetic average of the normative sample. This is computed simply by adding all the scores of the standardization sample and dividing by the total number of scores. As a clinician, you will probably not have to compute many mean scores on clients you test. You will see means in formal tests that have been used to examine differing age groups on a particular skill, and you will use this information as a reference point to compare the score of a specific child or adult you have tested. For example, if you have tested a 4-year-old on a vocabulary test, you are interested in how his or her score compares to the normative sample of 4-year-olds who took the same test as part of the standardization procedure. While some tests report data on other measures of central tendency (e.g., mode, median), the most frequently reported scores are means, and they are perhaps the most meaningful to a clinician.

The other important score we must deal with in order to make sense of normative data is some measure of variability (variance) in the standardization sample. The *variance* is "a numerical index describing the dispersion of a set of scores around the mean of the distribution" (Salvia, Ysseldyke, & Bolt, 2010, p. 35). In computing the variance, the statistician first derives the amount by which each person's score deviates from the sample mean (e.g., if the score is 70 and the test mean is 60, the deviation is 10). After this is done for each subject in the sample, the deviation scores are all squared. These squared scores are added and then divided by the total number of subjects minus one. This results in the variance. One can easily see that we are essentially obtaining a very gross measure of the average amount of variation from the mean (squared) by computing the variance. The variance is not particularly meaningful in test interpretation so its square root, the *standard deviation,* is used because it is a more interpretable measure of variation. Thus, if the variance is 25, we take its square root, or 5, which is the standard deviation. This measurement is more interpretable because it is in the same units as the mean instead of in squared values, as in the variance. If the mean on a test is 50 points and the standard deviation is 5 points, one can actually use these numbers together to gain a picture of variability. If we used a mean of 50 points and the variance of 25, we are no longer talking about the same types of numbers (points) because the variance is the average number of points of deviation squared.

In most cases, whenever researchers gather data on a particular skill from a large sample of people, the scores tend to form what statisticians call a *normal curve.* This means that there will be a tendency for most of the scores to fall around an average value, and some scores will be scattered toward very high and very low values. If researchers weighed a random sample of 2,000 adults between the ages of 20 and 40, they would probably find an average weight, with most people clustered around this value, and a much smaller number of people who were overly obese and very thin and thus deviated markedly from this value. In this situation, means and standard deviations are helpful in describing the performance of a given population of subjects.

Figure 3–1 shows a normal bell-shaped curve that could theoretically depict the performance of a sample of people on any variable. For our purposes, let's say that the curve represents scores on a vocabulary test. Several details are important to note. First, the line in the center of the normal curve at the score of 45 represents the mean performance or the average score in the distribution. Notice that it is the tallest line in the curve because height represents the largest number of people (9) who earned this score. The lines on either side of the mean are shorter and represent smaller numbers

FIGURE 3–1
Example of Normally Distributed Data

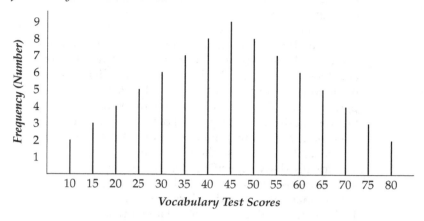

of subjects (8) who earned the respective scores (e.g., 40 and 50). The lines becoming shorter indicates that fewer subjects earned the scores as they moved progressively higher and lower than the mean of 45. The two subjects scoring 10 and the two subjects scoring 80 are in the tails of the normal curve and are called outliers.

Look again at Figure 3–1, which depicts vocabulary scores. Previously, we said that the mean was 45. If we said that the standard deviation was 10, this would mean that +1 standard deviation would be located at 55 and −1 standard deviation would be located at 35. Taking the example further, +2 standard deviations would be at the score of 65, and −2 standard deviations would be at 25. Now look at Figure 3–2, which depicts the percentage of cases under portions of the normal curve and the standard deviations at the bottom. We can see that about 68% of cases in the sample would probably score within −1 and +1 standard deviations from the mean. This means that, on the vocabulary test, about 68% of the subjects would earn scores somewhere between 35 and 55. If we considered the cases scoring between −2 and +2 standard deviations, about 96% of the subjects would earn scores in this range, somewhere between 25 and 65. Finally, if we looked at cases scoring between −3 and +3 standard deviations, around 99% of the cases would earn scores between 15 and 75.

Thus, the use of means and standard deviations helps researchers and test developers to determine scoring patterns that are characteristic of the majority of a particular

FIGURE 3–2
Percentile Ranks and Standard Scores under the Normal Curve

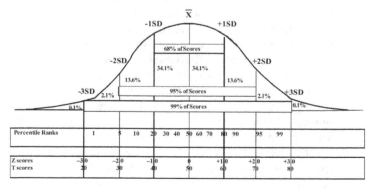

population. It has often been stated in the assessment literature that scores falling at or below −1.5 to −2.0 standard deviations from the mean are thought to be abnormal enough to be clinically significant (Ludlow, 1983; McCauley & Swisher, 1984b). This, of course, indicates that the score in question was lower than some 95% of the population included in the standardization sample. Thus, it should be clear that we use the means and standard deviations of the normative sample as a context for comparing an individual client's score on a standardized test. If the client's score falls below a particular standard deviation level (e.g., −2.0), we may decide to make a judgment about lack of normality in performance. This example demonstrates why it is important to understand some basic facts about means and standard deviations. Although many authorities advocate the use of cutoff scores, as mentioned earlier, others (Plante & Vance, 1995; Spaulding, Plante, & Farinella, 2006) dispute the use of such arbitrary guidelines and suggest that clinicians empirically derive specific cutoff scores for each test they use on local populations. This suggestion is based on research that shows variability in the ability of specific tests to discriminate normally developing children from those with disorders (Plante & Vance, 1995). If tests will be used to establish whether a child has a problem, the tests should have demonstrated discriminant validity. All distributions, however, are not normal. Some are skewed positively (many low scores) or negatively (many high scores); others have much variation (*platykurtic*) or very little variation (*leptokurtic*). It is significant that most standardization samples tend to be normally distributed, which is important for the statistical analyses that are applied to them. Abnormally distributed data present many problems that are beyond the scope of the present text. It is enough if we are clear about normally distributed data and about the ways of describing these distributions.

Types of Scores Found on Formal Tests

The diagnostician will encounter several kinds of scores when dealing with standardized, norm-referenced tests. The first type of score we will mention is the *raw score*. The raw score is the actual number you arrive at when grading the client's test. Many times the raw score amounts to the number of correct responses that the client gave to the test items. If the test has 75 items on it and the client got 50 of them correct, the raw score might be 50. On some tests, the raw score is not simply the number correct but is some other number (e.g., maybe each test item is worth 2 points). To achieve the raw score, the basal and ceiling rules for the given assessment must be taken into account. The *basal* is the starting point for a test and represents the point at which it is assumed a client would answer all previous items correctly. For this reason, the items prior to the basal are not administered and are assumed to be correct. Once the basal is determined, a test is administered until the client reaches a ceiling. The *ceiling* is the end point where the client has made a predetermined number of errors and serves as the stopping point of assessment. It is assumed that the client would incorrectly answer the remaining items on the test once the ceiling has been reached. For example, when starting at the established starting point for a test, the client might have to answer two consecutive items correctly to establish the basal. If a basal is not established at the starting point, the clinician will need to administer items prior to the starting point to establish the basal. To achieve the ceiling, the same client may need to miss three consecutive items to stop testing. The basal and ceiling rules vary from test to test and can be found in the test's manual. Once the basal and ceiling have been established, score the test and arrive at some number that the test manual typically refers to as the raw score.

Most standardized, norm-referenced examinations include a manual to be used by the diagnostician in scoring and interpreting the test results. These test manuals typically contain a series of tables that are designed to convert raw scores into more interpretable numbers. Raw scores by themselves are not readily meaningful. For instance, the raw score of 50 out of 75 does not tell us anything about how our client's score compares to the performance of the normative sample. Perhaps this is normal performance for the client's age group and perhaps it is not. Thus, we must convert the client's raw score into a more meaningful type of number to allow comparison with the normative sample. Another reason to convert the raw scores to some other type of derived score is that one cannot compare the results of two different tests by using raw scores. For instance, if a child obtains a raw score of 50 out of 75 on a vocabulary test and then earns a raw score of 125 out of 200 on a metalinguistics test, it would be difficult to compare these two results. If the raw scores were converted to some derived score, however, we could generally compare the performances on the two measures.

One type of converted score is called the *percentile rank*. Percentile ranks reflect the percentage of subjects or scores that fall at or below a particular raw score. For example, if a child scored in the 20th percentile, this means he or she scored as well as or better than 20% of the children of the same age in the normative sample. Likewise, if a child scored in the 90th percentile, the score was as good as or better than 90% of the children taking the test. Another way to look at it is that only 10% of the normative population scored higher than a child who performed in the 90th percentile. If you look again at Figure 3–2, you will see that percentile ranks are arranged under the normal curve. The 50th percentile rank basically represents the middle or median performance of the normative sample. A percentile rank of 10 is slightly more than −1 standard deviation below the mean. Remember from the prior discussion that some authorities view performance below −1.5 or −2.0 standard deviations to constitute clinical significance or abnormality. Some authorities (e.g., Lee, 1974) suggest that consistent performance below the 10th percentile is cause for clinical concern because this is between −1 and −2 standard deviations. One can see that conversion of the raw score into a percentile rank allows the clinician to put an individual client's performance into the context of the normative sample. It is meaningless to say that the client got a raw score of 90, but it is much more valuable to be able to say that a client scored in the 90th percentile.

Another way to derive more interpretable data from a client's raw score is to convert it into a *standard score*. The diagnostician will encounter a number of different standard scores on formal tests; however, we will discuss only the two most common types: *z-scores* and T-scores. Standard scores transform the raw scores into sets of scores that have the same mean and standard deviation. A z-score has a mean of 0 and a standard deviation of 1. One can see from Figure 3–2 that the z-scores are exactly equivalent to the standard deviations in the normal curve. Thus, a z-score of −1.0 is in the same place on the curve as a standard deviation of −1.0. A raw score can be converted to a z-score by subtracting the raw score from the mean of the normative sample and dividing the resulting number by the standard deviation of the normative sample. Test manuals typically include tables for the conversion of raw scores into z-scores so that the clinician will not have to perform the mathematical operation just described. It is easy to see that when a client's raw score is converted to a z-score, it is much more interpretable. For instance, it is meaningless to that say a client had a raw score of 59 on a test because it does not relate to the normative sample. If the client has a z-score of −2.0, however, we can look at Figure 3–2 and see that this is equivalent to performing at −2.0 standard deviations, which is a clinically significant abnormality according to the criteria mentioned earlier. The T-score operates basically the same way as the z-score except that the mean is 50 and the standard deviation is 10. Thus, the performance of a client with a T-score of 30 would be equivalent to −2.0 standard deviations.

A final type of standard score is the *stanine.* Tables for converting raw scores to stanines are not found as often in standardized tests. Stanine scores range from 1 to 9, have a mean score of 5, and have a standard deviation (SD) of 2. For stanine scores, the normal distribution is divided into nine parts. The lowest 4% of scores that are greater than or equal to −1.75 standard deviations below the mean are given a stanine of 1, whereas the highest 4% of scores that are greater than or equal to +1.75 standard deviations from the mean are given a stanine of 9. Stanines 2 through 9 are each .5 standard deviations in width. As a result, for the mean stanine of 5, the standard deviation ranges from −.25 below the mean to +.25 above the mean.

It can be seen from this discussion that standardized, norm-referenced tests provide the diagnostician with a variety of possible scores to use when interpreting a particular client's performance. Remember that although standard scores are useful to the diagnostician, they are valid only if the score distribution in the normative sample is normal. Percentiles do not require a distribution to be normal and can be computed on any distribution shape; thus, they have fewer requirements than standard scores for accurate use and interpretation.

The Age and Grade Score Trap

Many formal tests include tables for converting raw scores into age-equivalent or grade-equivalent scores. Thus, a 9-year-old child who earns a raw score of 50 might be said to have an age-equivalent score of 7.5 (7 years, 5 months). A fourth-grader might earn a grade-equivalent score of 2.2 (second grade, second month). It is easy to be seduced into using these types of scores because they appear to relate to development. On the surface, these age and grade equivalents seem to place the child in a developmental context with peers who took the test. It is tempting to say that the 9-year-old mentioned above is really at the 7½-year-old level, or the fourth-grader is performing at the second-grade level. All of these assumptions could be wrong. Most authorities who focus on psychometric interpretation indicate that age-equivalent and grade-equivalent scores are the *least* useful and *most dangerous* scores to be obtained from standardized tests because they lead to gross misinterpretations of a client's performance (Lawrence, 1992; McCauley & Swisher, 1984b; Salvia, Ysseldyke, & Bolt, 2010). Basically, age-equivalent scores indicate that the client's raw score approximated the average performance for a particular age group. In the example above, the 9-year-old earned a raw score that was the average of the children in the 7½-year-old group of the normative sample. A similar relationship holds for grade-equivalent scores.

McCauley and Swisher (1984b) discuss two common difficulties with age- and grade-equivalent scores. First, differences observed in age-equivalent scores result from progressively smaller raw score differences as a child increases in age, thus causing the reliability of the age-equivalent scores to be more questionable with increased age. For example, you have a younger and an older child who are both 1 year behind their chronological age. While they are both delayed by 1 year, this outcome may have resulted from 10 missed items for the younger child and only 3 missed items for the older child. Second, age-equivalent scores are often determined indirectly rather than directly from evidence generated by children of a given chronological age. The scores are sometimes indirectly determined through interpolation or extrapolation between age groups for which data are available in the normative sample. Therefore, it is possible for a child to receive an age-equivalent score that reflects an age that does not match that of any child contained within the normative sample. The psychometric problems above lead to a number of misinterpretations of age-equivalent scores. First, as Salvia, Ysseldyke, and Bolt (2010) indicate, it leads to "typological thinking." As they say, "The average 12-0 child does not exist. Average 12-0 children represent a range of performances, typically the middle 50 percent" (p. 41).

A second misinterpretation is that laypeople and some professionals may believe that a 9-year-old child who earns an age-equivalent score of 7-0 is *performing like* a 7-year-old. This is probably not true. While the 9-year-old may have earned the score obtained by the average 7-year-old, the test items that were correct and those that were missed may be totally different in the client and the normative sample of 7-year-olds. As McCauley and Swisher (1984b) state: "Similarly, a 60-year-old suffering from aphasia might receive an age-equivalent score of 10 years on the vocabulary test. It is unlikely, however, that such a client would make the same kind of errors as the 10-year-old or that he would exhibit similar communication skills" (p. 341).

A final danger in using age-equivalent scores is their use in attempting to define impairment in a client. The assumption is often made that a child exhibits a disorder if his or her age-equivalent score is lower than his or her chronological age (e.g., a 4-year-old earning an age-equivalent score of 3.0). It is important to understand that these age-equivalent scores do not take into account the variation in performance expected in a particular age group. If a child performs below the average score for his or her age group, it may be within the range of normal variation for that group and not an indicator of impairment at all (McCauley & Swisher, 1984b).

It is almost universally agreed that the least useful and most perilous types of scores are the age-equivalent and grade-equivalent scores just discussed. They tend to distort a client's performance and lead to misinterpretations by laypeople and professionals alike. Yet many state departments of education mandate use of age-equivalent scores for purposes of determining eligibility for services (Lawrence, 1992). Most authorities advocate the use of percentile ranks and standard scores for test interpretation because these do not suffer from the problems mentioned in relation to developmental scores. Perhaps the percentile rank is the easier of the scores to use in communicating with parents and spouses because most people can understand this concept readily. Clinicians who are consumers of formal, standardized norm-referenced tests would be wise to refuse to purchase examinations that offer only age-equivalent scores and that omit standard scores and percentile ranks.

Standard Error of Measurement and Confidence Intervals

Two final concepts that we will deal with regarding standardized tests are the notions of *standard error of measurement (SEM)* and *confidence intervals*. When used with the concepts previously discussed (mean, standard deviation, standard scores), these measurements give the diagnostician some very powerful quantitative tools to use in evaluating test performance.

Even though a standardized test may be developed very carefully, a client's responses to test items may not really reflect the underlying ability that the examination is attempting to measure. Statisticians realize that *any* measure is susceptible to error. Error is ubiquitous—it is in everything we measure, especially in measuring human performance. Thus, we know that no test is perfectly reliable (1.0) and that some distortion is present in any measurement device. Some statisticians use the terms *observed score* and *true score* to refer to the actual raw score that the test taker earns and to the "ideal" score that the person would have earned if there were no error in the measuring instrument. The true score, then, does not really exist; it is only hypothesized. We would like the observed score to be highly similar to the true score, and this is the case in using tests that have high reliability. As the reliability of a test decreases, the disparity between true and observed scores increases.

A statistic called the *standard error of measurement (SEM)* is an index of expected variation in the observed score that has been developed to increase our precision in determining whether the observed score of a client is reasonably close to his or her possible true score. SEM is expressed in standard deviation units. Although one could calculate SEM and associated confidence intervals from one of several statistical formulas, most tests provide tables from which to arrive at this information. We should be able to look up SEM in a test manual and find a table that indicates the confidence intervals around the client's true score. The *confidence interval* is an estimation of the likelihood that a score would fall within a range of scores centered around the true score. The level of confidence chosen and expressed as a percentage (e.g., 68%, 90%, 95%) indicates how confident we can be that the true score will fall in the given range. Thus, if a subject had an observed score of 50 on a test, and we calculated the true score as 53, there would be a pretty good correspondence between the observed and true scores. If we look up the 95% confidence interval in a table included in the test manual, we might find that the confidence interval is 5. Next, we subtract 5 from the subject's true score, arrive at 48, add 5 to the true score, and get 58. Thus, we have a range from 48 to 58, with the subject's true score in the middle. We can have confidence that the subject's true score would fall in this range 95 times out of 100 test administrations.

McCauley and Swisher (1984b) point out the importance of using confidence intervals, especially when attempting to determine cutoffs for abnormality. This problem becomes especially important in cases where psychometrists are attempting to determine if a child is cognitively impaired. If an IQ below 70 is indicative of significant impairment, it would be important for the client's true score *and* confidence interval to be well below 70 to make a judgment. If the confidence interval overlaps the cutoff, it is possible that the true score could lie in the area above the cutoff, even though the observed score is below it. Important decisions about whether an impairment exists should not be dealt with lightly, and clients should be given the benefit of the doubt, especially where program placements are concerned.

SENSITIVITY AND SPECIFICITY: KEY CONCEPTS IN EVIDENCE-BASED PRACTICE

When a diagnostic test is developed, it is critical that the instrument be able to distinguish people who have the disorder from those who do not. In the process of test development, researchers have used the concepts of *sensitivity* and *specificity* to characterize the ability of an instrument to "fail" the people with disorders and to "pass" the people who do not have the disorder. In Chapter 1, we mentioned evidence-based practice (EBP) and the importance of using scientifically sound assessment instruments. Specificity and sensitivity are critical concepts in evidence-based practice. Imagine that you have a group of 83 people. Of the 83 people, 21 have a particular communication disorder and 62 have normal communication. Ideally, a standardized test would fail all 21 of the people with disorders and pass all of the normal communicators. Most tests, however, are not ideal. Figure 3–3 illustrates four possible scenarios, depicted in the figure's four boxes, for administering this examination.

One outcome of testing (box a: *true positive*) is that the instrument would accurately identify people who have the disorder. That is, the people with the disorder would fail the test, that is, test positive for the impairment. Another outcome could be that people who are normal fail the test (box b: *false positive*). In this case, you have identified people who have no problem and you now must spend time doing further evaluation to determine whether or not they should be added to your caseload. A third scenario could be that some people who have the disorder actually pass the test, that is, test negative for the impairment (box c: *false negative*). In this case, you would be missing people with the disorder, and they might not be eligible for services. A fourth outcome might be that

FIGURE 3–3

Sensitivity and Specificity Values for Standardized Tests: The Concept and an Example

Target Disorder

	Present	Absent	
Positive (failed the test)	True Positive (People with disorder failed the test) a Ex: 19	False Positive (People who were normal failed the test) b Ex: 12	a + b
Negative (passed the test)	False Negative (People with disorder passed the test) c Ex: 2	True Negative (People who were normal passed the test) d Ex: 50	c + d
	a + c	b + d	

Test Result

Sensitivity = a/(a + c), or the percentage of people with the disorder who failed the test

Specificity = d/(b + d), or the percentage of people who were normal who passed the test

Example Sensitivity: 19/(19 + 2) = 90%

Example Specificity: 50/(50 + 12) = 80%

people who do not have the disorder pass the test (box d: *true negative*). This, of course, is exactly what one would want to happen; normal speakers are actually identified as such. Because no diagnostic test is without error, it is most often the case that all four scenarios occur simultaneously with test administration. Test developers and clinicians should be interested in the rates of true positives, false positives, false negatives, and true negatives associated with any particular instrument. Thus, the terms *sensitivity* and *specificity* are used to characterize two of the most important scenarios: the percentage of true positive scores and the percentage of true negative scores.

The notions of sensitivity and specificity would be simple indeed if people with disorders and those with normal communication performed so that there was a clear demarcation between their performances on a test instrument. The top half of Figure 3–4 illustrates the "ideal" situation in which people with disorders have a distribution of scores on a test that does not overlap at all with the normal speakers. Deriving a cutoff score to use in identifying people with a disorder from those who are normal would be quite easy. In the real world, however, the distributions tend to overlap to a considerable degree, and choosing a cutoff results in the errors (false positives, false negatives) just discussed. The sensitivity and specificity depend on where the test developer sets the cutoff score. In the bottom half of Figure 3–4, we illustrate the consequences of choosing a cutoff in terms of committing false positive and false negative errors.

Figure 3–3 illustrates an example in which the sensitivity was 90% and the specificity was 80%. This example test is not as good at identifying normal speakers (80%), and one would expect that more people without disorders than acceptable would tend to "fail" the test. However, the test can identify people with disorders fairly well, at 90%.

FIGURE 3–4
Illustration of Idealized Nonoverlapping Distributions of Normal and Abnormal Populations (Top) and the Typical Overlapping Distributions (Bottom)

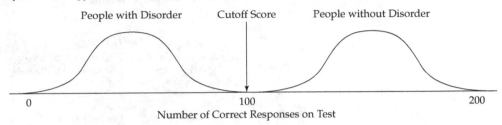

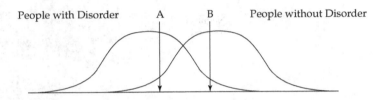

Cutoff "A" misses many people with disorders and passes most people without the disorder (poor sensitivity)

Cutoff "B" identifies most people with disorders, but fails many people with normal communication (poor specificity)

When test developers design diagnostic instruments, they should use a reference standard to identify initially people who have disorders. This reference standard should be independent of the test being developed, and the assumption is that it is a gold standard for identifying the particular disorder. Thus, sensitivity and specificity are always viewed in juxtaposition to the reference standard. Most authorities would expect sensitivity and specificity measures to be over 85% for a test to be of clinical use, and most test developers strive for figures in both sensitivity and specificity to be over 90%. When you are planning to purchase a test, it is important to examine the test manual for data showing the sensitivity and specificity of the instrument.

CRITERIA FOR EVALUATING STANDARDIZED TESTS

This section is intended for consumers of standardized tests. Every year clinicians in most work settings may be lucky enough to be given a budget for purchasing new materials. Among these new acquisitions are standardized tests. If you have had the occasion recently to peruse publishers' catalogs containing new tests, you have doubtless found that these instruments are quite expensive. It is rare to find a test for less than $100, and many examinations may sell for between $200 and $500. Even new packets of test response forms are expensive to replace each year for the examinations already owned by a facility. Thus, if your budget is $500, you can easily spend all of it on a single test. For economic reasons alone, clinicians need to evaluate seriously any test they consider for purchase and not make the decision lightly.

The expense, however, is just one consideration in deciding whether to purchase a particular test. Another major issue is whether the test was developed using rigorous scientific standards. Does the test have good reliability and validity? Can it adequately discriminate clients with disorders from those who have normal communication? If you purchase a test that does not have good psychometric qualities, you have wasted your money. Administering a test that lacks good psychometric qualities is, at best, a waste of your client's time and money; at worst, it is an ethical problem. We wish that we could tell you that all tests advertised by publishing companies are of high quality. Unfortunately, there is wide variety in the psychometric adequacy of tests available on the market. While some companies pay careful attention to the science of test development, many instruments advertised in catalogs are not psychometrically adequate. Therefore, it is up to the consumers of test instruments to examine carefully the process by which a test was developed prior to purchasing it. In Chapter 1 we talked about the importance of evidence-based practice (EBP). A major tenet of evidence-based practice is that we should use measurements that have been developed using correct scientific methods. We need to be assured that a test instrument can, in fact, do what the publisher indicates it can do in the test manual.

What are the most important psychometric considerations in evaluating standardized tests? The criteria have been reported by many authors (Andersson, 2005; Hutchinson, 1996; McCauley & Swisher, 1984a; Salvia, Ysseldyke, & Bolt, 2010), but the criteria are basically presented in the *Standards for Educational and Psychological Tests* compiled by the American Psychological Association (APA). Figure 3–5 shows selected psychometric qualities usually associated with standardized tests. We will discuss those considerations here briefly, but the reader should know that the actual APA standards go into much more detail.

FIGURE 3–5
Selected Critical Psychometric Qualities Associated with Standardized Tests

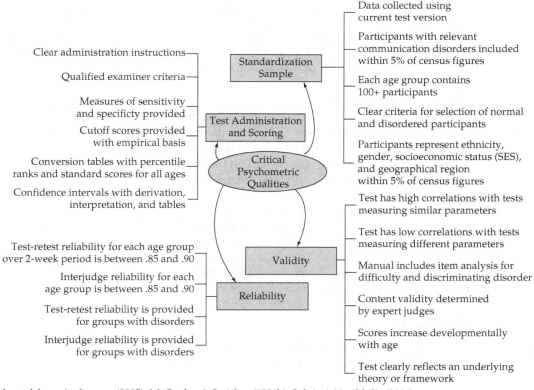

Source: Adapted from Andersson (2005); McCauley & Swisher (1984b); Salvia & Ysseldyke (2004).

Test Administration and Scoring

Some clinicians wonder why every test comes with a fairly extensive manual that goes into painful detail about (a) the rationale behind the test; (b) the psychometric development of the instrument; (c) the specific purposes for which the test is to be used and not used; (d) qualifications of the test administrator; and (e) detailed instructions for administering, scoring, and interpreting the test. It is the tendency of most students and beginning clinicians to skip the part of the test having to do with the development of the instrument. Some students read just enough of the manual to be able to administer the test, and then revisit it when it is time to score it.

Manuals are detailed for several reasons. First, the portion dealing with psychometric qualities of the test should be read in detail prior to purchasing the test. This is where you see the information on reliability, validity, sensitivity, specificity, the normative sample, and all sorts of other important information. There is no point in purchasing a test that is psychometrically inadequate. The part of the manual that talks about its rationale and purposes lets the consumer know if the instrument is well grounded in current theory about the disorder. In some cases, examiners may require training or specific educational background in order to administer and interpret a test. In the field of psychology, for instance, one has to have highly specific training in order to administer and interpret tests of intelligence. Because the test has been standardized, it is important that it be administered to an individual client in exactly the same manner as it was given to the normative sample. If you administer the test to a client without regard to the instructions, then you cannot compare his or her score to the norms for the instrument. The larger the number of questions about administration that cannot be answered by the test manual, the more idiosyncratic decisions must be made by the clinician. For example, if you ask a client to point to a particular picture and he says "Huh?" are you allowed to tell him the name a second time? The manual should address concerns such as this, or else the test will have a large amount of error associated with its administration.

Similarly, the manual should include detailed scoring instructions because we do not want clinicians making individual judgments about what is or is not correct. It should all be spelled out as clearly as possible. One way that test manuals assist clinicians is that they provide detailed tables to be used in converting raw scores to percentile ranks and standard scores. Tables should also be provided for confidence intervals. You can easily see how much error would be injected into the testing process if each clinician had to put raw scores into a formula of some type and crunch numbers to arrive at standard scores. Even with tables, there is error in clinicians running their fingers down the wrong row or looking up conversion factors in tables for the wrong age group. The tables help to reduce error to an acceptable level, however, and are indispensable to a good test instrument.

A good test manual should provide information to aid clinicians with interpreting the scores. If there is a cutoff score that defines the existence of a problem, it should be explained in the test manual. Measures of sensitivity and specificity should be provided to show that the test can discriminate adequately between people with disorders and those who exhibit normal communication. Earlier in this chapter, we indicated that it is ideal for these two measures to be above 90%.

Reliability

We have already discussed the importance of reliability in developing a standardized test. It is important that the test manual reports both test-retest and interjudge reliability scores for the normative sample. The test-retest reliability for each age group over a 2-week period should be between .85 and .90. The desired coefficients for interjudge reliability should also be near .90. Some test developers report reliability across an entire age span of the normative population; that is, if the normative sample is for children between the ages of 5 and 10 years, they report a single reliability coefficient. Ideally, reliability coefficients should be reported for each age group and separately for groups with communication disorders. It is quite possible for reliability to change with age and with the presence and absence of disorder.

The Standardization Sample

If a client is to be compared to norms on a standardized test, it is important to know about the makeup of the normative sample. It was not that many years ago that test developers normed standardized tests on groups of white, middle-class, Standard English speakers. The result, of course, was that people from different ethnic and cultural backgrounds who were dialect speakers "failed" the test, and our caseloads contained a disproportionate number of clients who did not exhibit real communication disorders. More recently, test developers have tried to take into account socioeconomic and ethnic considerations in selecting participants for the normative sample to which people will be compared. Generally, participants should represent ethnicity, gender, socioeconomic status (SES), and geographical region within 5% of national census figures. Thus, if African Americans represent 15% of the population, the normative sample should also have 15% from this cultural group. Another consideration in addition to culture is the size of the age groups represented in the normative sample. Historically, it was not unusual for individual age groups to be represented by fewer than 50 participants in the normative sample. We now know that the number of participants is an important factor in adding stability and strength to the normative data. A contemporary instrument should have age groups that contain a minimum of 100 participants. If the test focuses on communication disorders, participants with relevant communication disorders should be included in the normative sample within 5% of the current census figures. Also, there should be clear criteria for selecting the participants who represent normal and disordered groups. This is the reference standard referred to earlier in the chapter.

Validity

We have already discussed the importance of validity and some common measures test developers use to confirm whether an instrument measures the parameters it is designed to assess. First, the examination manual should detail the underlying theory or framework upon which the test is based. Second, there should be some measure of content validity as determined by expert judges. Thus, if a test is purported to measure cognitive development in Piaget's sensorimotor period, judges should be able to examine the test items and link those to the pertinent theory of cognitive development. A third type of validity reports how well the instrument correlates with other known tests of the same construct. Therefore, a new instrument should have high correlations with tests measuring similar parameters, and low correlations with tests measuring different parameters. So a test of receptive vocabulary should correlate highly with other receptive vocabulary tests, and less of a relationship might be found with tests of syntax or phonology. Test developers should also include an item analysis by which test items are evaluated statistically for difficulty level, changes in scores with age, and the ability of particular test items to discriminate between people with and without disorders.

It should be clear that selection of a standardized norm-referenced test should not be just an arbitrary decision on the part of a diagnostician. Purchasing one of these instruments is significant in terms of cost and, more important, in terms of serving our clients well. Try to examine these tests at conferences and conventions, read reviews in professional journals, and examine the *Buros Mental Measurements Yearbook* for critical reviews (Spies, 2010). Many libraries have online access to the *Buros Mental Measurements Yearbook*. Although it is published only every few years, an online database includes reviews for upcoming issues, and the Internet resources may be more timely than bound volumes.

Test brochures and catalogs may not tell you enough to make an accurate judgment. If possible, order a test "on approval," and pay for it only if you are satisfied with its psychometric adequacy and what it will actually tell you about a client. Most reputable publishers allow a customer to return an instrument that he or she is not satisfied with.

COMMON ERRORS IN THE USE OF NORM-REFERENCED TESTS

With very few exceptions, norm-referenced tests are designed to help the clinician determine if a client is performing within normal limits on a particular behavior. We compare an individual's score to the normative data and decide if our client is impaired or not. Muma (1973b) has said that the purpose of formal tests is to solve the "problem/ no problem" issue. Often, the clinician could do this just by observation alone, but many institutions (e.g., school systems) may require some formal test score to include in a client's record instead of relying solely on clinical judgment. The Individuals with Disabilities Education Act (IDEA) requires that a standardized test be used in assessment. At any rate, solving the problem/no problem issue is a rather narrow payoff for taking the time to administer and score a standardized test. As a result, some clinicians try to make more of the test results than they should. Formal tests are designed to go only so far; if we make other judgments about our clients based on these data, we are violating the assumptions of the tests. The following are some of the common ways in which clinicians misuse standardized tests:

1. *Measuring treatment progress with norm-referenced tests.* We mentioned earlier that the purpose of norm-referenced tests is to determine if a client is performing in a way that is similar to a large standardization sample. The tests were not designed to measure progress in treatment. If the clinician administers a formal test at the beginning of treatment and re-administers the test (or even an alternate form of the test) after a period of treatment, the resulting scores can lead to gross misinterpretations. First of all, the formal test samples a broad range of behaviors and may sample the behavior trained in therapy only in a few trials. Thus, much of the time spent in test administration would be devoted to assessing behavior that is unrelated to therapy. It would be much more logical to examine the trained behavior in detail by using an informal format that focused more fully on the particular behavior of interest. Second, a child who scores abnormally low on an initial administration of an instrument will tend to score higher on a subsequent administration of the same test. This well-known phenomenon is called *statistical regression*, which states that subjects earning extreme scores (either high or low) tend to regress toward the mean of the sample population on subsequent administrations. Thus, a client may receive a higher score not because of treatment effects but because of statistical regression. Third, clinicians may unconsciously "teach to the test" and prepare the client to do well on a second administration by practicing items in a format similar to the formal test. Fourth, all tests include elements of unreliability. It is quite possible that an increase in an overall score on a formal test is simply the result of chance. We urge clinicians never to use standardized, norm-referenced tests as measures of progress. Criterion-referenced tests and informal probe tasks are the best way to gauge treatment progress.

2. *Analyzing individual test items for treatment target selection.* After administering a norm-referenced test, it is always tempting to examine the client's responses to particular test items and to try to determine some pattern of impairment. For example, on a receptive vocabulary test, one might find that particular prepositions are in error. A natural tendency would be to include the understanding of prepositions in a treatment program based on the analysis of the formal test performance. This approach presents several problems. Clients cannot be expected to take tests that are of an inordinate length. As a result, a formal test must be relatively brief in order to be practical. On the other hand, most formal tests are fairly broad-based in that they cover a number of areas (e.g., syntax, morphology, vocabulary) or one area that has several facets to it (e.g., assessment of all relevant, bound morphemes). This characteristic creates a dilemma for the person who is developing a test instrument. To cover all the areas of interest, or even all aspects of one area, the test developer must be very selective in deciding how many items to include and how many times a particular behavior will be sampled. In assessing bound morphemes, for instance, the test developer must determine how many times each morpheme of interest will be sampled and in what contexts. Often, a particular form will be sampled only two or three times in order to make the length of the test manageable. Herein lies the trade-off: Making a test of reasonable length necessitates the use of small samples of each behavior of interest. Thus, it would be difficult to make a judgment about a particular grammatical morpheme (e.g., plurals) based on only two or three occurrences. This observation is especially true when client responses on formal tests can be due to a variety of reasons. As much as test developers would like to believe that an incorrect response indicates lack of ability on a particular item or that a correct response suggests mastery of an item, it is well known that test takers are human. Clients make lucky guesses, are distracted during test administration, do not fully understand instructions, and experience a variety of internal states (fatigue, boredom, pain, need to use the bathroom, etc.), all of which can affect test performance. Research has clearly indicated that use of individual standardized test items targeting specific structures for treatment planning is not advisable (McCauley & Swisher, 1984b; Merrell & Plante, 1997; Plante & Vance, 1994). Be wary of selecting treatment objectives from any norm-referenced test.

3. *Forgetting that formal tests almost always distort what they are designed to examine.* Almost every construct one might desire to measure in communication disorders is highly complex. Whenever we deal with human behavior and try to translate a complex activity into a single score, there is a considerable amount of information lost in the process. Is it valid to say the child's vocabulary is a 74 because he or she earned this score on a test? Does this tell us how many words are in the child's lexicon or are understood by the child? Does it tell us how words are retrieved? Does it tell us if the child's internal definition of the word is equivalent to an adult's? Do we know how the word is used for communication? Do we know how the word will be used in sentences or written language? We could continue to ask questions about how deeply we have examined the child's vocabulary by obtaining a formal test score, but you probably have the idea by now that such a score is quite superficial. In designing a test, developers have competing goals that make it almost impossible to create the perfect instrument. Figure 3–6 illustrates this dilemma. As the test becomes more specific and controlled, it becomes more unnatural. As we move toward a naturalistic task, we lose control over stimuli, tasks, and responses. Standardized tests tend to distort the constructs that we wish to examine in a number of ways.

First, almost all tests that are standardized imply a circumscribed method of administration. The testing must be done in a particular setting, specific instructions must

FIGURE 3–6
Competing Goals of Measurement: The Test Developer's Dilemma

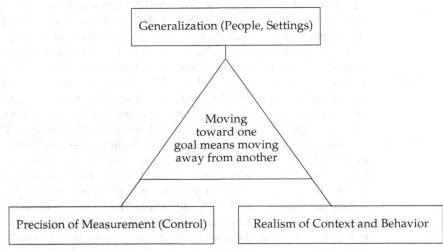

Source: Adapted from Sabers (1996).

be given, and items must be administered in a particular order. In addition, the client's responses must be graded as pass or fail, based on the criteria set forth by the test developer (some tests do not classify client responses as pass or fail, but these are few in number). The vast majority of formal test scenarios involve a highly artificial, regimented way of assessing performance.

A second reason for distortion is that most of these tests designed to assess communication rarely examine *real* communicative efforts. The interactions are typically artificial. The client has no real communicative intent, communications are often about trivial topics (e.g., telling the examiner what is going on in a picture while both client and clinician look at it), and the topic of each task is constantly changing as the clinician flips the test plates. Thus, we must *always* remember that we have not examined real communication until we have analyzed the client's communication in a natural situation.

A third source of distortion is the fragmentation of integrated systems often seen in formal testing. As Muma (1973b) points out, many systems interact with one another in communication, and to single out a particular area to analyze is in many cases ludicrous. For instance, how can one separate semantics from cognition, syntax from semantics, syntax from morphology, phonology from syntax, motor speech skills from language, intonation from meaning, or structural language from pragmatics? Although this can be done on the formal test level, it certainly cannot be done on a construct validity level. We cannot evaluate a system or subsystem independently of the context in which it typically operates. If we do, we have not really evaluated the system of interest. Always be aware that when we use an artificial task as found on most formal tests, we are always a dimension or more away from looking at the reality of communication.

MULTICULTURAL CONSIDERATIONS

If birthrates and immigration trends continue as predicted, the population of the United States will become increasingly diverse by the middle of the 21st century. Specifically, there will be significant increases in African American, Hispanic, and Asian groups, and the population of citizens with white, European backgrounds will remain relatively

FIGURE 3–7
Population of the United States by Race

	Total Population	Percentage of Population
White	223,553,265	72.4
African American	38,929,319	12.6
American Indian/Alaska Native	2,932,248	0.9
Asian	14,674,252	4.8
Native Hawaiian/Pacific Islander	540,013	0.2
Other	19,107,368	6.2
Two or more races	9,009,073	2.9
Hispanic or Latino	50,477,594	16.3
Total population	308,745,538	100.0

Source: 2010 Census.

stable or even decrease. By 2050, it is predicted that white Americans with European ancestry will no longer be the predominant segment of the population. In some states (e.g., Texas, California) where there are large groups of Hispanic and Asian citizens, this is already the case. This trend is not just a wild prediction or theory but is based on data from the Bureau of Labor Statistics. Figure 3–7 shows the United States population by different cultural groups using the 2010 U.S. census figures.

It has been well known for some time that standardized testing presents a serious threat to fair assessment of children from diverse language groups (Kamhi, Pollock, & Harris, 1996; Taylor & Payne, 1983; Vaughn-Cooke, 1986). As a result, children from diverse linguistic and cultural backgrounds tend to score lower on these measures, and these lower scores could result in a disproportionate number of minority children being placed in special education programs. A number of factors or types of bias require consideration because they can have a negative impact on the collection and interpretation of data on standardized tests (Fagundes, Haynes, Haak, & Moran, 1998; Wyatt, 1998). The commonly observed types of bias include situational bias, directions bias, value bias, linguistic bias, format bias, stimulus bias, and cultural misinterpretation. *Situational bias* occurs when the communication styles or pragmatic expectations between the client and clinician are not congruent with one another. This mismatch can be observed in relation to the "rules of who may speak to whom, appropriate elicitation procedures, appropriate language behaviors, what behaviors serve as communication, and rules of production and interpretations" (Taylor & Payne, 1994, p. 97). *Value bias* results when the client is asked to respond to test items that require moral/ethical judgments that differ from their own. For example, problem-solving questions such as those that begin with "What should you . . . " or "Why should you . . . " are more susceptible to value bias. Both value bias and situational bias can result in *cultural misinterpretation,* which occurs when a clinician negatively interprets a client's behavior as inappropriate when it is culturally appropriate.

Directions bias occurs when the directions given by the clinician can be misinterpreted by the child. *Linguistic bias* results when the client is being tested with a test that was derived from a language system that differs from the client. Currently, the majority of standardized assessments used within our field are based on the Standard American English (SAE) dialect. As a result, linguistic bias can and often does result when we administer these tests to clients who speak another dialect (e.g., African American English) or language (e.g., Spanish). *Format* and/or *stimulus bias* can occur when clinicians use

FIGURE 3–8
Selected States and Their Cultural Makeup (as a Percentage)

State	African American	Other Nonwhite	Hispanic
Alabama	26.2	3.8	3.9
Arizona	4.1	19.5	29.6
Arkansas	15.4	5.6	6.4
California	6.2	31.4	37.6
Colorado	4.0	14.6	20.7
Florida	16.0	7.4	22.5
Georgia	30.5	7.6	8.8
Hawaii	1.6	50.1	8.9
Illinois	14.5	11.6	15.8
Louisiana	32.0	3.7	4.2
Maryland	29.4	9.6	8.2
Michigan	14.2	4.5	4.4
Mississippi	37.0	2.7	2.7
Montana	0.4	7.6	2.9
New York	15.9	15.3	17.6
North Carolina	21.5	7.9	8.4
South Carolina	27.9	4.3	5.1
Texas	11.8	15.1	37.6
Wyoming	0.8	6.3	8.9

Source: 2010 U.S. Census.

procedures, stimuli, vocabulary, or topics that are unfamiliar to or inconsistent with the client's cognitive style.

In the area of standardized language testing, the importance of the population tested in the development of the instrument cannot be overemphasized. It is not only important to see how children from different cultures respond to the test stimuli but also how the scores they make on the test contribute to the standardization sample or "norms" of the test. It is axiomatic in the psychometric literature that norms are not valid if the standardization sample differs significantly from the local population tested. Although many test instruments that are currently used have included children of different cultural groups in their norming samples, the percentage of these children may not be reflective of the proportion of such children in many local areas. For example, the general population of the United States is composed of approximately 13% African Americans; however, the concentration of this cultural group in many cities and states may be several times this proportion. Figure 3–8 shows selected U.S. states and their percentage of cultural makeup mainly for African American and Hispanic residents (the "other" category includes American Indian, Pacific Islander, and Asian individuals). It is clear from this table that many states have significantly more than the national average of African Americans (e.g., Georgia and Maryland). If we turn to a more powerful lens and focus on cities in the United States (see Figure 3–9), you can see that the percentages of the various cultures change drastically. The 2010 census shows that more than half of the U.S. population lives in the 39 largest metropolitan areas. It is questionable, at best, to use a test that included only 9% African American children in its standardization sample if one is working in a community where over 60% of the children represent this cultural group. A second problem with the standardization samples in their reflection of cultural differences may surface in a lack of specific description of the

FIGURE 3–9
Selected Cities and Their Cultural Makeup (as a Percentage)

City	African American	Other Nonwhite	Hispanic
Albuquerque	3.3	22.3	46.7
Atlanta	54.0	5.5	5.2
Baltimore	63.7	4.5	4.2
Boston	24.4	17.7	17.5
Charlotte	35.0	12.3	13.1
Chicago	32.9	19.4	28.9
Cleveland	53.3	6.5	10.0
Dallas	25.0	21.7	42.4
Denver	10.2	16.8	31.8
Detroit	82.7	4.5	6.8
El Paso	3.4	13.0	80.7
Fresno	8.3	37.1	46.9
Houston	23.7	22.5	43.8
Los Angeles	9.6	35.9	48.5
Memphis	63.3	5.8	6.5
Miami	19.2	5.5	70.0
New Orleans	60.2	5.1	5.2
New York	25.5	26.5	28.6
Philadelphia	43.4	12.7	12.3
San Francisco	6.1	40.8	15.1
Tucson	5.0	21.0	41.6
Washington, DC	50.7	8.0	9.1

Source: 2010 U.S. Census.

groups in the norming sample. For instance, saying that 120 African American children were included in the norming sample does not provide any information on their socio-economic level or whether they spoke African American English (AAE). If the children were not dialectal speakers, then their scores may have no relevance for evaluators who want to compensate for language bias on the test or to compare these scores to a population in an inner city where dialectal usage is a prominent feature. If a clinician uses a standardized test on dialect speakers and scores it differently from the procedure used with the normative sample, the norms should not be used because the test was not scored the same way as it was during test development.

There is some question, however, that scoring a test differently would even make a difference in some cases. For instance, Rhyner, Kelly, Brantley, and Krueger (1999) used the Bankson Language Screening Test 2 and the Structured Photographic Expressive Language Test-Preschool on 99 preschoolers who represented low-income SES. They state: "Presently, there are no standardized language screening tests that include normative data on African American children or children of any social class who do not speak the SAE [Standard American English] dialect" (p. 50). In this study the children had very high failure rates, even with scoring modifications that took into account AAE dialect. Evidently, administration of standardized tests, even with alternative scoring, is not the ultimate solution to cultural bias in assessment. Recently, however, a new standardized testing procedure has been developed (Seymour, Roeper, DeVilliers, & DeVilliers, 2005). Preliminary studies have shown it to be valid and nonbiased for African American and Standard English children and that it can distinguish African American dialect speakers from African American children with language impairments. The test is called the *Diagnostic Evaluation of Language Variation* (DELV) and it has a screening test, a criterion-referenced edition, and a norm-referenced edition available. The norms are based on U.S. census figures and are demographically adjusted for children ages 4 through 9. The test examines syntax, phonology, semantics, and pragmatics. Because phonological development in African American English and mainstream American English have been shown to have different developmental trajectories, it is recommended that only features that share similar developmental patterns between the two language groups be used in diagnosis of language impairment.

The concept of *local norms* has been discussed for years in the psychometric literature (Adler, 1990; Evard & Sabers, 1979; Omark, 1981; Popham, 1981; Seymour, 1992). Owens (2004) states:

> Often the norming sample does not represent the population with which the speech-language pathologist is using the assessment procedure. In this situation, the norms are inappropriate and should not be used. This situation occurs most frequently with minority or rural children or with children from lower socioeconomic groups. In these cases, local norms should be prepared by following the norming procedure described in the test manual. Some tests, such as the Test of Language Development–Intermediate (TOLD-I) and the CELF, explain this process in detail. (p. 65)

Generating and using local norms does not mean clinicians can ignore national norms in evaluating a client. It is useful to obtain both national and local perspectives, however, in order to discover test biases and the most discriminating types of norms for identifying disorder versus cultural difference in performance. Recently, clinical research has suggested that a variety of tools and standard score cutoff levels may be useful in differentiating language difference from disorder. For example, Oetting, Cleveland, and Cope (2008) found that use of a standardized subtest of language comprehension could identify only 56% of school-age children with language impairment using a cutoff of -1 standard deviation (SD), but when a cutoff of -0.5 SD was used, the percentage of those correctly classified rose to 81%. When a nonword repetition task was added to the classification scheme, the correct identification increased to 90%. This suggests that when judicious use of locally determined cutoffs instead of arbitrary global cutoffs such as 1.5 SD are coupled with other nonbiased measurements such as nonword repetition tasks, our ability to diagnose effectively is increased. Stockman's (2010) recent review of assessment in African American populations also suggests use of multiple tools and procedures for unbiased evaluation.

CONCLUSION AND SELF-ASSESSMENT

Some students and clinicians feel frustrated when confronted with the type of information presented in this chapter. This frustration can be felt more keenly if the clinician has emphasized formal tests in his or her approach to diagnosis and evaluation. Others also may feel a bit guilty if they have misused norm-referenced tests or have used instruments and techniques uncritically without ensuring the validity and reliability of those instruments or techniques. These practices, however, are probably the rule rather than the exception. Others might feel lost if all of their traditional tools are suddenly taken away from them, and they may ask, "What are we supposed to do without our tests?" There is no simple answer. One obvious response would be that we can still use tests for the purposes they are intended to serve, but we need to tighten our criteria for test selection, use, and interpretation. Another response is that we need to develop and use more informal methods for diagnosis and evaluation that will give us insight into the nature of a client's problem and the means for treating it. In many areas of communication disorders, we are beyond the basic question of the problem/no problem issue. We need ways to describe client performance and gain insight into individual differences, dynamism, ecological relevance, processes, and patterns of behavior (Bates, Bretherton, & Snyder, 1988; Bronfenbrenner, 1979; Chafe, 1970; Donaldson, 1978; Muma, 1978, 1981, 1983, 1984, 2002). The field of communication disorders is moving more toward descriptive and criterion-referenced measures rather than toward norm-referenced tests. This trend does not absolve each of us, however, from the ultimate responsibility of incorporating sound scientific principles into our measurements. An informal probe or task used to describe client behavior is just as susceptible as a norm-referenced test to psychometric and examiner error. Students, professors, and working clinicians should adhere to high standards of measurement and should refuse to use inadequate test instruments or descriptive procedures that cannot be effectively replicated.

After reading this chapter you should be able to answer the following questions:

1. How do norm-referenced and criterion-referenced assessments differ?
2. What makes a test valid, and what are the different types of validity?
3. What makes a test reliable, and what are the different types of reliability?
4. What are measures of central tendency?
5. What types of scores are found on formal tests, and how do we use them to interpret performance?
6. Why would it be important to consider the sensitivity and specificity of a standardized assessment?
7. What are four common mistakes made when using standardized assessment?
8. What factors require consideration when evaluating a client from another culture?

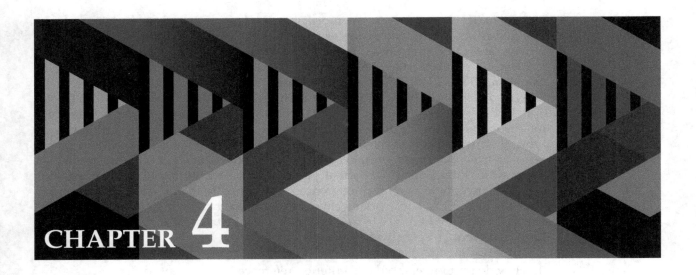

CHAPTER 4

Assessment of Children with Limited Language

LEARNING OUTCOMES

After reading this chapter you will be able to:

1. Describe the developmental progression children follow to become effective communicators.

2. Describe the three general categories of children with limited language and corresponding assessment parameters.

3. Identify the challenges and difficulties encountered in language assessment.

4. Describe six diagnostic precepts that can inform one's approach to language assessment.

5. Describe preassessment and the process of obtaining pertinent case history information for a child with limited language.

6. Describe the relevance of obtaining a caretaker–child interaction and parameters to be assessed during this interaction.

7. Identify parameters to consider when evaluating a child's adaptive behavior.

8. Describe the relevance of assessing play and the factors to consider in play assessment.

9. Describe how to evaluate communicative intent and function.

10. Describe methods used in the assessment of single-word utterances.

11. Describe methods and forms of assessment used to evaluate multiword utterances.

12. Identify confounding factors in the assessment of language comprehension.

13. Identify how to use and when to incorporate measures of utterance length.

14. Describe the factors to consider when assessing the language of children from culturally and/or linguistically different backgrounds.

Our discussion of evaluation of child language disorders will be divided into two chapters. This chapter considers clients whose language does not exceed simple multiword combinations. Because most clients with limited language are children, we will refer to them as such in this chapter. Chapter 5 focuses on children who are using longer sentences and are typically school age or older.

THE PROCESS OF BECOMING A COMMUNICATOR: GETTING THE BIG PICTURE

MacDonald and Carroll (1992) have presented a useful conception of the developmental progression children must follow on their way to becoming effective communicators. The steps are deceptively simple yet elegant. The following steps should be easy to remember, and they are important to consider in development, assessment, and treatment:

- *Play partners (Implication: cognitive assessment).* Does the child play with objects appropriately? A child's play tells us about his or her conceptions of objects, events, and relationships in the world. A child who exhibits primitive play strategies with objects (e.g., mouthing, banging, sensorimotor exploration) is likely to have quite different cognitive abilities than a child who engages in functional object use and symbolic play. A child who does not know how to play with objects in productive ways is unlikely to learn to communicate about objects and events appropriately.

- *Turntaking partners (Implication: social assessment).* After children learn some appropriate play strategies with objects, they begin to involve adults in their play interactions. This social development is a critical prerequisite for communication. The development of reciprocity is important because communication involves social turntaking between partners.

- *Communication partners (Implication: assessment of communicative intent and gesture system).* The initial communications of children are gestural in nature. They point, pull, push, give, take, and reach while looking at adults and objects. These initial nonverbal communications precede the use of words to regulate adult action and attention. Nonverbal communicative intents or functions such as declaratives and imperatives are included here. These communicative acts may or may not be accompanied by vocalizations.

- *Language partners (Implication: language model analysis and language structure analysis).* After the flow of communication is established through the use of gestures, children begin to approximate word productions that are modeled by their caregivers.

- *Conversational partners (Implication: pragmatic analysis).* When the use of language is firmly established, the child gradually learns the pragmatic rules for taking into account listener perspective, topic manipulation, and appreciation of social context in participating in dialogue.

One can easily see that the five areas mentioned above build on one another, and in assessment we can locate a child on this continuum. Each step implies a different evaluation focus and different treatment implications.

FOCUSING ON THE CHILD'S LANGUAGE LEVEL: NONVERBAL, SINGLE-WORD, AND EARLY MULTIWORD COMMUNICATORS

In talking about children with language disorders, it is not uncommon for authorities to refer to children's presenting linguistic-development level (Carrow-Woolfolk &

Lynch, 1982; Paul, 2007). Often, training programs in speech-language pathology offer one course that deals with language disorders in infants/toddlers and another course that focuses on language disorders of school-age children and adolescents. It is not the chronological age per se that is important here because a client with limited language can be from any age group (e.g., there are nonverbal teenagers and adults with cognitive impairments). Thus, it is unlikely that a single assessment procedure would be appropriate for *every* 4-year-old because some of these children could be using advanced syntax while others could be using nonverbal communication. It is much more meaningful to discuss techniques that would be useful for a client who is communicating at the single-word or early multiword level regardless of his or her chronological age. For example, Tager-Flusberg et al. (2009) propose recommendations for defining spoken language benchmarks for children with autism.

> They recommend ". . . moving away from using the term functional speech, replacing it with a developmental framework . . . [T]hey recommend multiple sources of information to define language phases, including natural language samples, parent report and standardized measures. They also provide guidelines and objective criteria for defining children's spoken language expression in three major phases that correspond to developmental levels between 12 and 48 months of age" (p. 643).

These recommendations are similar to the developmental phases recommended for assessment in this text, which rely on developmental language levels (nonverbal, single word, early multiword, syntax). Assigning such developmental benchmarks can be used to track clinical progress in treatment and can also be used by researchers to equate groups for empirical study rather than exclusively using standardized tests.

For purposes of assessment, it is useful to consider children with limited language in three general categories. First, there are children who are largely nonverbal. They use vocalizations and perhaps gestures, but their caretakers report no real use of language to control the child's environment. Obviously, in dealing with a nonverbal child, a "test of language ability" would be too advanced. Therefore, the clinician must often focus on more informal assessment procedures. McCathren Warren and Yoder (1996) identify four proven predictors of later language development in prelinguistic children: (1) use of babbling, (2) development of pragmatic functions, (3) vocabulary comprehension, and (4) the development of combinatorial/symbolic play skills. Unfortunately, most available formal assessment instruments do not measure these variables adequately. Notable exceptions are the *Communication and Symbolic Behavior Scales* (CSBS) (Wetherby & Prizant, 2002a) and *Assessing Prelinguistic and Early Linguistic Behaviors in Developmentally Young Children* (ALB) (Olswang et al., 1987).

A second group of children consists of those who speak largely at the single-word level (Nelson, 1973). According to some authorities, the child may accrue a lexicon of about 50 words before starting the use of word combinations for generative language. A third type of child is one who is using early multiword combinations. For this type of child, it is clear that some basic cognitive capacity for using a symbol system exists because the child is, in fact, using one. In studying an early multiword child, it is more important to focus on the types of word combinations used and the functions for which the child uses the utterances. The phonetic inventory and phonological-process analysis also become important for this type of case because a child's oral language can be functional only if it is intelligible to listeners. Thus, for the child who uses early multiword utterances, we must examine the language but not necessarily in the same way as we would a language sample of a child who has a longer length of utterance.

The clinician's first step is to determine in which category the client is placed based on preponderant communication behaviors. The next step involves considering the high-probability diagnostic areas associated with the category. Table 4–1 provides a

TABLE 4–1

Assessment Areas to Consider at the Nonverbal, Single-Word, and Multiword Levels

Assessment of Nonverbal Children
General developmental level
Adaptive behavior
Biological prerequisites
Case history
Caretaker–child analysis
Communicative intent inventory
Vocalization analysis
Gestural analysis
Cognitive analysis
Lexical comprehension

Additional Assessments for Single-Word Child
Length measures from spontaneous sample
Form/function analysis of productions
Analysis of presyntactic devices
Analysis of lexical production
Phonological analysis

Additional Assessments for Multiword Child
Analysis of semantic relations
Specific language development test
Comprehension of simple commands
Assessment of emerging literacy skills

list of assessment areas that are especially important to consider in the evaluation of nonverbal, single-word, and multiword communicators. Clearly, the assessment of a single-word or multiword child is both similar to and different from that of a child who is nonverbal. In terms of similarities, we are still interested in general developmental levels, biological prerequisites, case history, caretaker–child interaction, communicative intent, the phonetic inventory, cognitive development, and understanding of semantic elements. At the single-word and multiword level, however, additional areas of assessment require consideration. Finally, the clinician can use some of the specific procedures referred to later in this chapter, which will allow evaluation of the pertinent areas.

Most of the assessment targets cannot be evaluated by using formal test instruments (Wetherby & Prizant, 1992). Crais and Roberts (1991) provide a useful conceptual framework for the clinician in the form of decision trees to help generate assessment questions, select procedures, and link these procedures to intervention recommendations. Nelson (2010) provides a useful flowchart of clinical questions the diagnostician must ask while moving from initial evaluation to setting goals and finally to monitoring progress.

CONSIDERING ETIOLOGY

Although we have characterized children with language disorders by their general linguistic development level, some readers may be tempted to describe those disorders by using etiology (e.g., autism spectrum disorder, cognitive impairment, or hearing impairment). We agree with those who suggest that classification of language disorder by etiology does not relate productively to assessment (Lahey, 1988; Nelson, 2010; Newhoff & Leonard, 1983; Paul, 2007). The various etiological groups themselves are highly heterogeneous; thus, to refer to a child as "intellectually disabled" really means little in terms of predicting what he or she might be like. In addition, the language disorders manifested by these various groups may not be significantly different. Therefore, the language samples gathered from children who are hearing impaired, cognitively impaired, learning disabled, autistic, and language delayed but with normal intelligence may be highly similar. Diagnostic grouping, then, does not necessarily provide the clinician with valid guidelines for assessing language skills. On the other hand, a focus on the language abilities of a child helps clinicians to understand the strengths and limitations of communication and to assist in the development of treatment objectives.

WHY IS EARLY LANGUAGE ASSESSMENT SO DIFFICULT?

Language assessment in children is one of the most difficult and challenging tasks faced by the speech-language pathologist (SLP), and many clinicians are insecure about their diagnostic ability in this area.

1. *Heterogeneity of the population.* One complicating factor for the diagnostician is that the population that exhibits a language disorder is extremely heterogeneous (Wolfus, Moscovitch, & Kinsbourne, 1980). In addition, children from a wide spectrum of etiological groups manifest language impairment, and the practitioner is faced with youngsters who are cognitively impaired, autistic, hearing impaired, or learning disabled, or who exhibit a variety of other organically based conditions. This heterogeneity appears to make diagnosis quite difficult, especially for the clinician who knows only one approach to language assessment.

2. *Highly varied severity levels.* A second variable that makes language diagnosis difficult is the difference in the degree of severity found in the language-impaired population. The children range from those who are nonverbal with a lack of social and cognitive bases for language, on the one hand, to youngsters who inconsistently misuse grammatical morphemes or exhibit subtle pragmatic problems on the other. Thus, for each evaluation, the clinician must be prepared to assess the broad representation of linguistic and prelinguistic behaviors.

3. *Language is a complex phenomenon.* A third variable that makes language assessment confusing is the complex nature of language itself. Most introductory courses discuss language as an area that is comprised of various domains. In fact, many textbooks are organized with reference to language areas such as semantics, syntax, morphology, phonology, and pragmatics. Any or all of these areas can be affected in a language disorder. Most theorists agree that these domains are not isolated from one another but have complex interactions. Complicating the problem further is the fact that authorities in the area of psycholinguistics are not in total agreement regarding exactly how these domains of language interact with each other in spontaneous communication.

4. *A multitude of assessment instruments and procedures.* Another variable that makes it difficult to know what to do in language evaluation is the proliferation of assessment devices and procedures available on the market. We are inundated with flyers and catalogs, many reputed to offer "the best language assessment device." How does one select a test? Is one test really enough? The fact that people have designed tests of language for children, often with very inclusive titles, suggests that it is possible to find out all one needs to know from a single test. Unfortunately, the disclaimers that some authors place in their test manuals regarding the shortcomings of the instruments are forgotten, and the perhaps overambitious title remains in the mind of clinicians and parents. Also, tests are based on different theoretical points of view or models. The differing theoretical

underpinnings result in dramatically different types of tasks and areas of emphasis on tests. The plethora of tests, then, is a source of confusion to many clinicians.

5. *Language is profoundly affected by multiple processes and domains.* It is also difficult to know what to do in language assessment because language development and disorders encompass so much more than just linguistic ability. In the literature on language acquisition, for instance, one routinely reads about cognitive development, neurolinguistics, linguistic theory, adaptive behavior, play development, social development, self-help skills, phonology, motor ability, emergent literacy, caretaker–child interaction, and other areas that may not appear to be directly related to linguistic symbols but are critical to language development. Because language itself has many domains (semantics, syntax, phonology, morphology, pragmatics, etc.) and the related areas mentioned above are numerous, language assessment may take on quite different guises, depending on the focus of the evaluation. This complexity is clearly a source of confusion for clinicians and requires a very broad base of skill and knowledge.

The difficulties just mentioned probably contribute to many clinicians' uncertainties in the area of language assessment. Models, as we indicate in the following section, are sometimes helpful in reducing the difficulties in understanding an area and in assisting diagnosticians to develop workable clinical procedures.

MODELS TO CONSIDER IN LANGUAGE ASSESSMENT

If we were to travel around the country and eavesdrop as SLPs evaluate children, we would find a confusing conglomeration of activities performed under the shield of linguistic assessment. Here are some examples:

A clinician has a child repeat sentences.

A child plays silently while the clinician takes notes.

A child is trying to obtain a toy, and the clinician resists.

A clinician is asking a child to point to one of three pictures.

A clinician is instructing a child to act out a scene with dolls.

A clinician is watching a child and her or his parents play.

A child is trying to complete open-ended sentences presented by the clinician.

What does it all mean? Are all these clinicians really performing language assessments? How does a clinician know which assessment to do with a particular child? One thing is clear: Language assessment requires the clinician to possess more varied skills and a more comprehensive educational background than ever before.

The clinician in a language evaluation must have some framework on which to gather and organize data. When a clinician has some sort of guiding principle to use in assessment and treatment, the model appears as a relevant clinical concept. You cannot operate effectively unless you have some organizational framework. Models, then, are organizing principles that help to make the clinician more operational. The way in which the clinician conceptualizes language and communication will largely dictate how language disorders are assessed and treated. For instance, a strict behavioral model of language and communication would not necessarily consider cognitive or social prerequisites. It may not deal with intent or other unobservable phenomena. If a clinician subscribes exclusively to this model, there may be no evaluation of the areas mentioned earlier. Models that emphasize modalities of input and output, such as Kirk and Kirk's (1971), do not particularly focus on linguistic aspects such as syntax, morphology, and pragmatics. Prerequisite areas (cognitive, social, biological) are ignored. These are just two examples of how the model of language that is adopted by a clinician can constrain thinking and clinical behavior. Thus, all models are not equally useful to a clinician, and certain important aspects of the language process can be missed.

There are some cautions. First, general semanticists have said for decades that the "map is not the territory." So it is with models. They are not the knowledge or behavior they represent. Clinicians should never forget that it is what they know, far beyond any model, that is important. Models are perspectives and guides for organizing clinical information, nothing more. If the clinician is confronted with a real child who is performing at odds with a model's prediction, the validity of the child's behavior is not questionable, but the applicability of the model in this case is certainly a bit dubious. A second caution is that, at the present time, no one knows for certain all the details of exactly how language is developed or processed, or how it is assessed most efficiently. Thus, any model is likely to be inaccurate or, at least, incomplete. Clinicians, like theorists, must be open to change their conceptualizations of language and its evaluation.

THEORETICAL CONSIDERATIONS IN LANGUAGE ASSESSMENT

Following the lead of Muma (1973b, 1978, 1983), we would like to echo some basic diagnostic precepts that we feel should underpin language assessment. First, the best language assessment device, as Siegel (1975) stated, is a well-trained clinician who keeps up with current developments. There is no "best" language test, just as there is no ideal language treatment program.

Second, language is a multidimensional process that has many facets of structure and use. The prerequisite areas (e.g., cognitive, social) discussed earlier must also be considered in evaluation. The existence of the multidimensional process makes it unrealistic to separate structure and function or syntax from semantics or pragmatics. The most ecologically valid methods of analyzing the process are preferable. Whenever we fractionalize the communicative process, we are no longer really looking at it. If we are interested in a child's communication abilities, we should look at real communication, not some artificial task from which we have to infer communication abilities.

Third, Muma (1978) has reminded us that whatever we do in assessment must apply to treatment of the language disorder. If we administer tests and then do not consider these results in planning our treatment, the time spent in assessment is wasted. Our assessment and treatment procedures should also be based on similar assumptions about the communication process.

A fourth important concept, also articulated by Muma, is that the diagnostic paradigm seems to have two levels or issues associated with it. The most basic issue is the problem/no problem issue. Standardized tests help to solve the problem/no problem issue by comparing a child's test performance to that of other children. This type of testing emphasizes group similarity and minimizes individual variability. The nature of the problem issue, however, must be addressed through description of the individual child's communicative performance. This assessment is best accomplished through nonstandardized, descriptive techniques that are more ecologically valid. Fortunately, the problem/no problem issue is solved by many parents when they have referred their children for evaluation. These parents typically know that something is wrong when they compare the communication of their child with that of his or her peers. A standardized test can confirm this, but it rarely can be prescriptive in terms of specifying treatment targets (Millen & Prutting, 1979).

A fifth important notion has to do with sampling. All we ever do in a diagnostic evaluation is obtain a sample of communicative behavior. Several important implications stem from the sampling idea. First, the samples we obtain should be representative of the child's communicative performance. The notion of representativeness has been with us for a long while, and we must not forget that a sample we obtain may or may not represent a child's typical or best performance. Second, speech pathologists have subscribed for years to the idea that an evaluation can and must take place within a 1- or 2-hour block of time. This kind of thinking can result in frustration when clinicians do not obtain the data they need in the allotted time, or if the child is uncooperative. Evaluation is ongoing, and there should be no pressure to find out all there is to know in a limited time frame. The medical profession does not feel compelled to diagnose in a limited time, with short, abbreviated procedures. Physicians order examinations that they feel are appropriate, and the diagnostic process takes place over as much time as is necessary. This is not to say that we should emulate the lengthy testing procedures of the medical profession; on the other hand, we should not become like purveyors of fast food. Third, whenever possible, the clinician should attempt to obtain multiple samples. Many children behave differently in the clinical setting than they do at home or in preschool.

A sixth basic premise of language assessment is that for every technique or test that the clinician uses, he or she must realize that certain assumptions are implied about child language. To use an instrument, you should accept the assumptions that underlie it. Whenever we receive the myriad flyers and announcements of new language assessment instruments, we should remember that each is based on assumptions. We should ask ourselves, "What do I have to believe about language to use this instrument?"

These suggestions should not be taken to mean that we are opposed to the use of standardized tests. We do, in fact, recommend the use of such instruments for the purpose they are most able to accomplish, namely, to determine if a child is performing similarly to other children of his or her age group. Standardized tests cannot make a principled clinical judgment, however; clinicians make decisions. Assessment has aspects of both art and science (Allen, Bliss, & Timmons, 1981). We advocate the use of a combination of standard measures coupled with nonstandardized tasks and more naturalistic sampling of communicative behavior (Lund & Duchan, 1988; Nelson, 2010; Paul, 2007). We believe that exclusive reliance on either type of procedure will not provide as complete a picture of a child's performance as the use of both types. School systems and other work settings typically require some form of standardized testing. Figure 4–1 illustrates the components, goals, and example procedures we recommend for the assessment of children with limited language. The areas of nonstandardized testing and evaluation of the relevant environment address pertinent aspects of the World Health Organization International Classification of Functioning, Disability and Health (ICF) model presented in Chapter 1.

Language Screening

Often speech-language pathologists will also be asked to conduct language screenings as a method for determining two details: whether or not a child could have a problem (answering the broad problem/no problem question) and whether the child would benefit from a comprehensive or more in-depth language evaluation. The formality associated with a screening varies; however, in our experience, screening is usually more of an informal approach to assessment. The decision of how and what to screen and what methods or tests to use for a screening are often influenced by the purpose of the screening and how efficiently and quickly a given screening protocol can be completed.

FIGURE 4–1
Critical Assessment Process in Limited Language

Examples of Assessment Procedures	Assessment Process in Limited Language	General Goals of Assessment Process
Audiometric evaluation, neurological evaluation, medical evaluation	Evaluate Biological Foundations for Communication	Determine if sensory, motor, and structural mechanisms will support verbal language
Interview, preassessment questionnaire, case history information, reports from other professionals	Obtain Background Information	Determine family perceptions of problem and family's strengths and needs; obtain relevant information from parents and other professionals
Administration of standardized tests	Perform Standardized Testing	Determine if a problem exists by comparing child's performance to normative data
Analysis of gestural communication and communicative intent, play analysis, language sampling, caretaker–child interaction analysis, analysis of infant cues, criterion-referenced testing, dynamic assessment	Perform Nonstandardized Testing	Determine child's modifiability and ability to respond with assistance from clinician; determine specific treatment goals by examining real communication
Curriculum-based assessment, examination of hospital environment, home environment analysis, assessment of preschool or school setting	Evaluate Relevant Environments	Determine environmental requirements for communication and language; resources for treatment; obstacles to success in communication, social, or academic areas

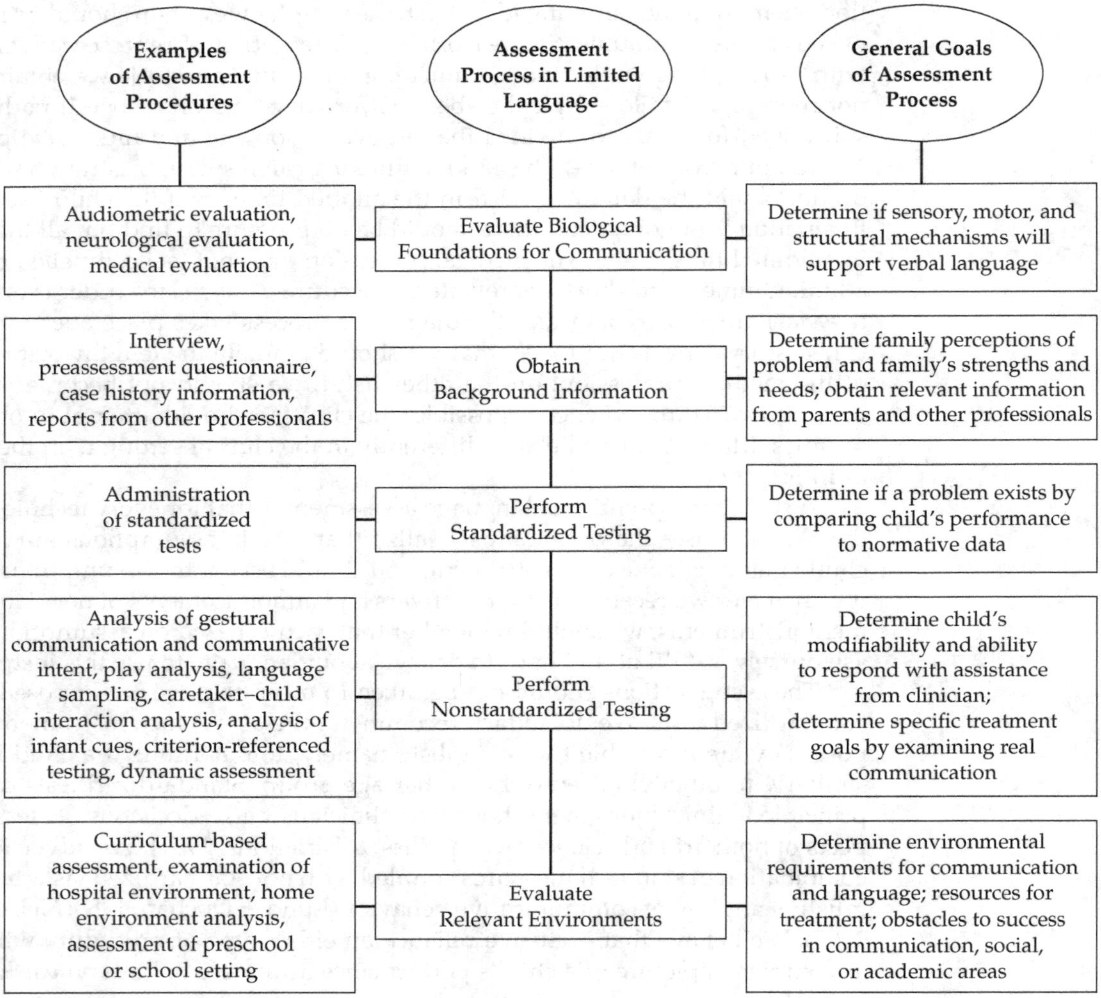

Typically, a screening will take less than 30 minutes to complete. A general screening needs to sample a range of language abilities and should not be too narrow in its focus. For example, we don't want to screen only a child's receptive language and miss a potential deficit in expressive language. Often screeners will also probe for whether broad criterion-based developmental milestones have been attained across several domains of development (see Appendix B for developmental milestones). This form of screening often entails using a checklist of skills and abilities that pertains to the age of the child being screened to document whether a particular skill or ability is present or absent at the time of screening. The following list is by no means exhaustive, but it does include some commercially available screeners that are used to screen developmental milestones and/or language:

Clinical Evaluation of Language Fundamentals Screening Test, Fifth Edition (Wiig, Semel, & Secord, 2013)

Preschool Language Scale–5 Screening Test (Zimmerman, Steiner, & Pond, 2011)

Fluharty Preschool Speech and Language Screening Test, Second Edition (Fluharty, 2000)

Early Language Milestone Scale, Second Edition (Coplan, 1993)

Ward Infant Language Screening Test, Assessment, Acceleration and Remediation (Ward & Birkett, 1994)

McArthur Communicative Developmental Inventory (Fenson, Marchman, Thal, Dale, Reznick, & Bates, 2007)

Ages and Stages Questionnaire, Third Edition (Squires & Bricker, 2009)

Language Development Survey (Rescorla, 1989)

Clinical Linguistic and Auditory Milestone Scale (Accardo et al., 2005)

As a word of caution, clinical judgment comes significantly into play during the screening process. The sensitivity and specificity of screeners, generally speaking, is often questionable. Following are some general recommendations for conducting and interpreting a language screening:

1. When conducting a mass screening that includes a large number of children, choose a screener that is cost-effective and efficient yet samples several domains of language. If conducting a screening on a select child, choose a screener that includes the domain of concern raised by the caregiver. For example, if the caregiver's concern is related to his or her child's pragmatic language abilities, choose a screener that includes the domain of pragmatics because not all screeners assess pragmatics.

2. If a possible language disorder is suggested, additional assessment is needed to determine whether a language disorder exists and to establish a diagnosis. The results from a screener should not be overinterpreted. It is strongly ill-advised to diagnose or put a child in therapy based on the results of a screener.

3. If a language disorder is not suggested and there is caregiver concern, it is still important to assess the child for other developmental problems that may be contributing to the initial concern. Screeners generally do not sample all domains of language and development and could therefore not include the area of weakness.

4. All children with language disorders will *not* be identified early by screeners. Given that the time at which a child experiences difficulty and symptom severity can vary, a full evaluation may be warranted if caregiver concerns persist or become apparent.

5. Parents should be counseled on the limitations of a screening. Some children who have a language disorder will pass a screening, whereas some children who fail the screening will not necessarily have a language disorder.

ASSESSMENT THAT FOCUSES ON EARLY COMMUNICATION AND VARIABLES THAT PREDICT LANGUAGE GROWTH

Wetherby and Prizant (1992) called for a new approach in evaluating early communicative competence. They were in the process of developing the *Communication and Symbolic Behavior Scales* (CSBS) and wanted to capture relevant features of early communication use. Wetherby and Prizant listed several features that they viewed as critical to such early assessment: (1) assessing communicative functions; (2) analyzing preverbal communication; (3) evaluating social-affective signaling; (4) profiling social, communicative, and symbolic abilities; (5) using caregivers as informants and as active participants in the evaluation; and (6) assessing a child's communication directly in spontaneous child-initiated interactions. When these authors examined the 10 most frequently used standardized test instruments for the limited-language population, it was clear that most of these examinations did not address relevant features or only addressed them in a limited manner. In most cases, there are no standardized tests that focus on the most relevant variables, and we must rely on nonstandardized approaches to evaluate domains such as communicative intent, play, social behavior, affective states, gestural communication, and caregiver–child interaction.

In the time since Wetherby and Prizant suggested this new approach to assessment of limited language, several studies have shown that many of the variables listed above have predictive value in terms of communication development. For example, McCathren, Warren, and Yoder (1996) reviewed literature to determine which variables in prelinguistic children were effective predictors of language development. They found four major areas that were important. First, the amount of babbling vocalizations and use of consonants in those vocal productions was an important predictor (the more the better). Second, the use of pragmatic functions in behavioral regulation (protoimperative), joint attention (protodeclarative), and social interaction (e.g., showing off, taking turns, social reciprocity) was another good predictor of language development. A third area that was predictive of language development was vocabulary comprehension as measured on the *MacArthur-Bates Communicative Development Inventories* (CDI) (Fenson et al., 2006). Finally, the combinatorial and symbolic play skills of children were predictive of later language development. Yoder, Warren, and McCathren (1998) studied 58 children with developmental delay and gathered a baseline sample of their communication. One year later, they divided the children into two groups based on their expressive language. Prefunctional speakers were those children with fewer than five different nonimitative spoken words in a language sample. Functional speakers were those children with more than five different nonimitative words in a sample. Three variables predicted 83% of the children in terms of group membership (functional or prefunctional): (1) number of canonical vocal communication acts (CVCV combinations), (2) CDI discrepancy score (number of words said divided by number of words understood and said), and (3) rate of protodeclarative production. Similarly, Calandrella and Wilcox (2000) examined relations between children's prelinguistic communication and language ability 1 year later. They found that nonverbal communication acts involving intentional gestural communication and social interaction signals predicted receptive and expressive language outcomes 1 year later. Brady, Marquis, Fleming, and McLean (2004) conducted a longitudinal study of 18 children with developmental disabilities who were between 3 and 6 years old and followed them for 2 years. The three most potent predictors of language outcome as revealed on the SICD-R were the initial level of gestural attainment, rate of communication, and parental response contingency. Many other studies of language prognosis in children described as late talkers have also found the variables mentioned earlier to be valuable in predicting language development. The CDI has recently been used to attempt predictions of language development for populations such as children with developmental delay and autism spectrum disorders (Luyster, Qiu, Lopez, & Lord, 2007). *Prelinguistic skills* are critical predictors of language development in many groups of children. For example, specific skills such as vocabulary size, verbal imitation ability, pretend play with objects, and use of gestures to initiate joint attention have been shown to be important predictors of vocabulary development in children with autism (Smith, Mirenda, & Zaidman-Zait, 2007).

The predictive variables for children with limited language have two important assessment implications. First, as indicated by Wetherby and Prizant (1992), the exclusive use of standardized tests with this population will miss most of the critical behaviors that are relevant to assessment and prognosis. McCathren, Warren, and Yoder (1996) examined the most popular prelinguistic assessment instruments and, similar to Wetherby and Prizant, found that those instruments ignored relevant areas or only examined them in a limited fashion. McCathren, Warren, and Yoder suggested that only two assessment procedures at that point in time addressed the four critical predictive areas of babbling, pragmatic functions, vocabulary comprehension, and combinatorial/symbolic play. One of the measures was the CSBS (Wetherby & Prizant, 1998) and the other measure was the ALB (Olswang, Stoel-Gammon, Coggins, & Carpenter, 1987).

A second implication of the research on predictive variables is that there is no substitute for communication sampling, play evaluation, caretaker involvement, gestural communication, and evaluation of communicative intent in limited-language cases. This sampling and evaluation can be done using a published procedure such as the CSBS, the ALB, or any number of nonstandardized procedures that focus on specific areas of interest. We will mention some of these nonstandardized approaches in the following sections.

SPECIFIC ASSESSMENT AREAS: PROCEDURES, CONSIDERATIONS, AND DIRECTIONS FOR FURTHER STUDY

In the sections that follow, we discuss specific techniques for assessing important areas related to the communication of a child with limited language. We try to provide guidelines and references for the clinician to use in learning about these various aspects of language assessment. In cases where we cannot adequately summarize a procedure (which is most of the time), we refer you to a primary source with the hope that you will critically evaluate and perhaps learn techniques that will be clinically useful.

At the beginning of most sections, we provide a brief sketch of some important developmental trends reported in the existing research. It is imperative to appreciate that each assessment technique mentioned is basically grounded in the research on communication development. While it is beyond the scope of this chapter to present an adequate view of any aspect of language acquisition, we would be remiss if we did not touch on some highlights of the process that are related to language assessment. Many fine textbooks are available that summarize research in language acquisition, and you should become familiar with this information before engaging in any language assessment.

Preassessment and Pertinent Historical Information

Preassessment

In most clinical settings, prospective clients are required to complete a case history before being seen by the speech-language pathologist or other professionals. It is especially unnerving to meet a client for the first time without first receiving the completed case history information because it is impossible to prepare for the evaluation otherwise. Especially in the area of language disorders, the client could be at levels ranging from totally nonverbal to a syntax level with only subtle language problems. Thus, it is crucial for SLPs in any work setting to avoid performing an evaluation without access to important historical information. Prior knowledge of historical information can allow the clinician to plan the evaluation to maximize the use of time and resources during the initial contact with the child and parents.

Gallagher (1983) suggested a preassessment procedure for use with language cases and outlined the advantages of such a process for the clinician in planning and conducting evaluations. *Preassessment* is more than the typical process of having the parents fill out a case history form. The notion of preassessment includes finding out some clinically useful data that could affect the way in which the initial evaluation is conducted. In our university setting, clients are sent and asked to complete and return a preassessment form before the day of the evaluation appointment. In cases where the parents cannot read or have difficulty completing the form, an interview session is scheduled before we see the child. The important point is that the clinician has a fairly good picture of the child's cognitive, social, play, and communicative behavior before the evaluation session. Typically, to provide additional information on noncommunicative behaviors that relate to cognitive, social, and language development, we also include a short adaptive-behavior scale that focuses on motor skills, self-help skills, and personal/social abilities.

The child's preferences and language-facilitating situations need to be explored prior to the day of the evaluation. The clinician can plan ahead and ask family members to bring specific stimulus items, toys, or interactants that would provide the best sample of a client's communication abilities.

The Parent Interview

Many questions will be raised by parent responses on the preassessment packet. The interview is a good place to clarify any missing information or inconsistencies in a parent's responses. The information obtained from caretakers of limited-language children is highly important. First of all, many of these children may not have the linguistic means or cognitive development to express themselves well, and the parent or guardian must be relied upon to provide pertinent background details and estimations of present skill levels. Second, recent research has suggested that expressive language disorders tend to run in families (Lahey & Edwards, 1995), and information regarding symptoms, treatments, and outcomes related to disorders in other family members is most easily obtained in the interview format, which allows for examples and follow-up questions. Third, the Individuals with Disabilities Education Act (IDEA) of 2004 mandates that families are critical team members and requires professionals to work closely with them when assessing and treating children with communication disorders. We will discuss this more specifically later in this chapter. The parent interview is an important information-gathering mechanism in this regard.

As mentioned in Chapter 2, we do not recommend that the diagnostician write specific questions prior to the evaluation. Appendix C contains an interview protocol for assessing the limited-language child. The interview protocol is divided into broad areas covering the prerequisites to language as well as the beginnings of linguistic development. Much of the specific information can be filled in from responses to the preassessment packet, and the interview can simply follow up on areas of interest to the clinician. The interviewer should ask questions in the broad areas, obtaining information in each subarea. The exact wording of questions is not provided because of the pragmatics of the interview situation. Parents represent differing levels of education, intelligence, socioeconomic status, and experience, and we have found it more feasible to tailor interview questions for each individual case. The interview protocol was designed only to jog the mind of the clinician, who, it is hoped, will ask questions in specific topic areas. When remarkable information is reported in any area, the interviewer should formulate appropriate follow-up questions to illuminate the area of interest. The major interview areas represent biological, social, and cognitive prerequisites to language as well as linguistic level, and were gleaned from a variety of child-language-acquisition and language-impairment sources. The interviewer should especially focus the interview on the most applicable portions of the protocol and not ask unnecessary questions. For instance, if a child is using a wide variety of multiword utterances and is communicating effectively in the environment, it would not be productive for the interviewer to spend a lot of time on cognitive and social attainments.

One of the most revealing questions about the child's home environment is the item in the interview protocol that asks a parent to describe a typical day in the life of his or her child. It is often surprising how much important information can be uncovered in the answer to this question. For instance, a parent may report that the child spends many hours watching television, or playing alone outside, or engaging in self-stimulatory activities—activities that have been allowed to continue despite their lack of productivity. Often, a pattern emerges that shows that the child spends little time in meaningful social interactions. Another pattern that reveals much about a child's problem is lack of a schedule or rules in the household. One mother reported that her nonverbal 3-year-old child typically went to bed at 11:30 P.M. after a late-night talk show and liked to sleep until 9:30 A.M. The child also ate all his meals while walking around inside the house, refused to wear pajamas, threw frequent tantrums, and was prone to writing on the walls. This scenario suggests that the parents and child may be in some need of counseling regarding behavior management. Much of this information would not have been gleaned from the preassessment packet or a formal test, but the information would be quite important when it comes to making recommendations for treatment. If, for example, we wanted these parents to begin to withhold desired items from this child in order to create communicative opportunity, they would have extreme difficulty with this procedure because there appear to be few existing rules in the home. Tantrums would inevitably increase, and the treatment plan would have a high probability of being aborted by the family.

Assessment of Social Prerequisites and Caretaker–Child Interaction

Language development takes place in a social context. From the moment of birth, a child interacts with his or her caretakers and is bombarded with visual, auditory, and tactile stimuli that occur in this relationship. As indicated previously, IDEA mandates the involvement of the family in both assessment and treatment, and it is especially important, for two reasons, in cases of nonverbal, single-word, and early-multiword-level children to observe them as they interact with their caretakers.

First, we want to observe the child with someone with whom he or she is familiar and feels comfortable. The best sample of the child's communication is often obtained in this portion of the evaluation. When unfamiliar clinicians attempt to establish rapport with a child in strange surroundings, it may be quite difficult to observe natural communication, especially in a limited time period. Occasionally, we have seen children who refused to interact with us in an evaluation. In these cases, the caretaker–child interaction is the only source of information available. When we started in this field, we were frequently told that the initial step in an evaluation was to separate the child from the mother. Often, this resulted in a catastrophic reaction on the part of the child, and little information was gained from the evaluation (other than the fact that the child did not separate well from the mother). We must not lose sight of our goal, namely, to observe the child's communicative and prelinguistic skills through talking and play. If the caretaker can provide a more effective demonstration of certain skills than the clinician can, then we must take advantage of this opportunity and not feel that we have failed as clinicians. Rather, we have succeeded in getting the data we were after as the result of making a sound clinical judgment. Establishing a relationship with a child can always be accomplished in the initial treatment sessions, where we are not under severe time constraints. In communication samples gathered by either the clinician or the caretaker, the caretaker should always be asked whether the child's communicative behavior is representative of his or her typical interaction.

A second goal of the caretaker–child interaction is to observe the quality of the language model provided by the parent. Research has shown that caretakers alter many aspects of their communicative behavior: They raise their vocal fundamental frequency, increase their pitch range, speak more slowly, and use double primary-stress patterns.

The caretaker is less disfluent when talking to an infant and pauses at major linguistic constituent boundaries. Linguistically, the mean length of utterance is reduced, and the vocabulary and syntactic complexity are simplified. Developing children, in addition to being exposed to a simpler language model, are given an introduction to the reciprocity of communicative interchange. Snow (1977) has shown that, with neonates as young as 3 months of age, mothers engage in turntaking, reciprocal behavior. Early on, the child's "turn" is a biologically programmed nonverbal action, such as smiling, sneezing, or burping. The mother simply responds to this with some sort of language response and often takes the child's turn for him or her linguistically. As the child develops, the caretaker demands that the youngster's turn more closely resemble the adult correct model.

As important as the model itself are the circumstances under which it is delivered. The youngster benefits cognitively from interacting with the caretaker. Mothers and fathers typically show the child "how the world works" by demonstrating the functional use of objects and body parts, the attributes of objects, and many other conceptual aspects of the environment. Children have been observed to follow a caretaker's line of vision (to look at an object a parent is focused on) very early in development (McLean & Snyder-McLean, 1978). Adults also show the child how to play with a variety of objects and even stimulate symbolic play. We see, then, that caretakers demonstrate language structure, language use, concepts, and the reciprocity of communication. Children are highly sensitive to their social environment, and they learn that language is a tool to be used for a variety of social and nonsocial purposes (Dore, 1975; Halliday, 1975). With young children, it is clear that their early exposure to language and their early use of it is highly social.

One important aspect of caretaker–child interaction involves book sharing. Parents share books with their children from infancy onward. This activity carries with it reciprocal roles and redundancy in language stimulation. The roles taken by parent and child change over time as the child develops language and cognitive abilities. Initially, the child just looks at the book with the caretaker and visually follows the caretaker's pointing behavior. Later, the child takes on the role of "pointer" as language comprehension develops, and the caretaker asks questions about pictures in the book (e.g., "Where's the kitty?"). During this time, the child is also becoming oriented to the nature of literacy activities such as page turning, book positioning, and the differences between text and pictures. When the child reaches the single-word period, the caretaker asks questions and the child names pictures in the book. Ultimately, when the child has connected speech, the caretaker asks more difficult questions about what events will happen next and how characters feel. Many authorities suggest sampling joint book reading as part of an evaluation to determine caretaker–child interaction strategies and get a sense of how both participate in literacy activities. Kaderavek and Sulzby (1998) developed a protocol for evaluating parent–child joint book reading behaviors and strategies, which would be a useful adjunct to assessment. Similarly, Rabidoux and Macdonald (2000) described caretaker–child interactive parameters during joint book sharing, including communicative styles, child roles/styles, and strategies for maintaining interactions. This taxonomy may be useful in assessing the climate of children's emergent literacy. One might assume that the nature of a child's language impairment itself would be the best predictor of emergent literacy. McGinty and Justice (2009), however, found that differences in language ability were not particularly good at explaining variability in print knowledge in children with language impairment. Instead, they found that the quality of home literacy experience was the best predictor of print knowledge, especially in language-impaired children with attentional difficulties. Factors such as degree of emotional support, sensitivity, responsivity, and the manner in which mothers engage their children in a book-reading task have been found to be predictive of degree of participation (Kaderavek & Sulzby, 1998; Skibbe, Moody, Justice, & McGinty, 2010). This again underscores the importance of examining the literacy experiences and opportunities available in the family for children when we are examining emergent literacy. Research has shown that teachers can also provide important information on preschoolers' emergent literacy skills, and it is wise to enlist their input to determine in which skills a child has strengths. Teachers have not necessarily been effective, however, in identifying or diagnosing children who are at risk for literacy difficulties (Cabell, Justice, Zucker, & Kilday, 2009).

The clinician needs to answer many questions about the caretaker–child interaction. Does the caretaker talk about the "here and now" (Holland, 1975) or about objects and events removed in time and space? What kind of joint referencing takes place in the interaction? Does the caretaker talk about and participate in things that the child appears to be interested in? Does the caretaker direct the child's play to things that the former feels are significant and disregard the child's preferences? Is there a balance between when the parent joint-references with the child and when the child joint-references with the parent? Regarding the uses of language, does the parent force the child into limited or respondent modes of communicative function? It is not unusual to observe parents of early language-disordered children who ask incessant questions (e.g., "What's this?" "What color is this?") or who ask the child to imitate constantly (e.g., "Say 'ball'"). We are not intimating that the parent's interactive style is in any way causally related to the child's language disorder. In fact, a parent's way of talking to a child could be a result of the disorder rather than a cause. Whatever the relationship, the caretaker's model as it presently exists may not be conducive to language development and should be changed. The only way to determine the quality of this relationship is through the observation of caretaker–child interaction. Evaluating and working with caretaker–child interaction is especially important when dealing with infants and toddlers who are at "high risk" for language disorder. Providing the best-quality stimulation for these children will go a long way toward preventing, or at least reducing, the severity of potential language disorders. Table 4–2 provides an example of a checklist that the clinician can use in examining caretaker behaviors during interaction in the evaluation session. The clinician's impressions of the caretaker modifications could lead to treatment recommendations involving work with interaction patterns.

It is also important to examine specific aspects of the child's social behavior in the caretaker–child interaction. Socially, the child's eye contact and willingness to participate in reciprocal nonverbal activities should be observed. A child who does not tolerate or seek out the participation of another person may not have any need for a communication system. Perhaps this child might need to work on some prelinguistic social skills along with the development of language. Recall that MacDonald and Carroll (1992) said that a child must first become a play partner and a turntaking partner before a communication partnership develops. Language is, after all, a social tool, and a child who is not "social" has little need of a code to use around people with whom he or she does not even communicate nonverbally. Children with autism spectrum disorders require close examination of social skills because these may play a major role in determining diagnosis and monitoring treatment. Parents are a rich source of information on social behavior and so are teachers because they spend many hours observing and interacting with the child. The input from these two groups, however, may not provide equivalent information. For instance, Murray, Ruble, Willis, and Molloy (2009) found that while there was general agreement between parents and teachers on overall social skills ratings, there was poor agreement on individual social behaviors. The implication is not that one group is more correct than another but that there can be contextual differences in a child's behavior, and multiple informants provide a more complete picture of social skill than relying on a single source. Bopp, Mirenda, and Zumbo (2009) followed children with autism over a 2-year period and tried to predict vocabulary production

TABLE 4–2
Caretaker–Child Interaction Attributes

Child: _____ Date: _____ Age: _____

Nature of interaction in terms of toys, room, and interactants:

General Parameters	**No**	**Yes**
1. Encourages communication by looking expectantly		
2. Responds to communication by reinforcing it with action or utterance		
3. Joint-references with child		
4. Alternates adult/child direction in joint referencing		
5. Talks about present context (here and now)		
6. Model is timed to coincide with joint referencing		
7. Talks at child's eye level		
8. Successful attempts at interpretation of child's utterances and communicative intents		
9. Creates communicative opportunities by using sabotage or pause time		
10. Does not anticipate child's needs ahead of time, thus reducing communicative attempts		

Language Model Parameters
1. Reduces sentence length
2. Reduces sentence complexity
3. Repeats utterances frequently (redundancy)
4. Paraphrases utterances ("throw the ball; throw it")
5. Uses exaggerated intonation patterns
6. Places stress on important words
7. Uses concrete, high-frequency vocabulary
8. Does not talk too much and dominate conversation
9. Does not use excessive questions and commands
10. Uses slower speech rate

Use of Teaching Techniques
1. Self-talk
2. Parallel talk
3. Expansion
4. Expatiation (enlargement)
5. Buildup/breakdown sequences
6. Recast sentences

and comprehension from an initial sample of behavior. Specifically, they found that high rates of inattentive behaviors such as not paying attention to the environment, distractiveness, failure to listen to instruction, and looking away from a joint task tended to predict less progress in vocabulary production and comprehension. The more socially unresponsive the child, such as not making eye contact, failing to respond to his or her name, and rarely smiling, the greater was the association with less language progress. Again, this suggests that the SLP should examine not only linguistic skills but also ancillary behaviors that are associated with social abilities. Some past investigations have suggested that about 50% of the population of children with language impairment has been reported to manifest behavior problems.

In some of the early research, however, the diagnosis of children with language disorders may not have been confined to those with specific language impairment. For example, children with developmental delay or pervasive developmental disorder might have been included. Rescorla, Ross, and McClure (2007) found that children with language delay did, in fact, show more total behavior problems, and language scores were significantly correlated. However, when the researchers eliminated children with neurodevelopmental delay and pervasive developmental disorder, total behavior problems and language scores were no longer significantly related. With this exclusion, only the variable of social withdrawal remained correlated with language ability. Harrison and McLeod (2010) gathered data on almost 5,000 Australian children to determine risk and protective factors related to language impairment. The variables considered spanned the child, family, parent, and community. They found that risk factors involved being male, having persistent hearing difficulties, and being more reactive in temperament. The major protective factors were having a sociable temperament and higher scores on maternal well-being. The implication of this study is that we must look beyond the child's test performance on language measures and into social/emotional and family contexts to understand prognostic factors.

Adaptive Behavior Scales

Adaptive behavior scales typically rate a child's development in motor skills, social behavior, self-help skills, and language ability. Children are given tasks to perform, or the parents are asked to respond to items on the interview protocol. The advantage of such scales is that they help to broaden the perspective of the SLP beyond exclusively examining language ability. Although we will assess social cognitive development as it relates to language, much of a child's adaptive behavior depends on cognitive and social attainments. We can obtain a better overall picture of the child's level of functioning, and this information, when coupled with our other assessment data, can be valuable. In addition, many conditions (e.g., cognitive impairment) may show that a child is generally low functioning in most areas and that language is only part of the problem. Knowledge of adaptive behavior will also be important to the clinician in making referrals. Language-treatment activities can also be designed to incorporate motor, social, and self-help areas so that the child is learning a variety of needed skills as well as the language associated with them. Several adaptive behavior scales are available: Adaptive Behavior Assessment System–2 (Harrison, & Oakland, 2003), Adaptive Behavior Scale–School, Second Edition (Lambert, Nihira, & Leland, 1993), and Vineland Adaptive Behavior Scales, Second Edition (Sparrow, Cicchetti, & Balla, 2005). In most work settings, including public schools and many medical settings, SLPs are part of a transdisciplinary or multidisciplinary team. Other professionals such as psychologists, psychometrists, occupational therapists, physical therapists, special education teachers, and medical personnel can provide valuable interpretations of the noncommunication domains included on such behavior scales, such as self-help, motor skills, and social adjustment (Haynes, Moran, & Pindzola, 2012). The advantage of such a team approach is not only in interpreting assessment findings but also in programming goals for multiple domains across the treatment regimen.

Assessment of Play to Gain Insight into Cognitive Attainments Associated with Communication

As mentioned by MacDonald and Carroll (1992) in the big picture of language acquisition provided at the beginning of this chapter, typically developing children first become play partners and turntaking partners. This involves learning how to joint-reference with the caregiver and manipulate objects together, both in exploration and in functional use of items. Play assessment helps us to determine if a child is capable of being a productive play partner and social participant with the adults in his or her environment. Evaluation of cognitive attainments is simultaneously simple and elusive. First, it appears that relationships between cognitive and linguistic skills change significantly with development. Although a particular cognitive attainment may relate strongly to a communication skill at one age, this relationship may disappear as the child continues to develop. If anything, there is a general as opposed to a specific relation between cognition and language. Yet when we see a prelinguistic child for an evaluation, we would like to get a sense of what he or she seems to understand about the objects, events, and actions in the world. Obviously, a nonverbal child cannot provide this information through language and speech. Many authorities have suggested that a child's play strategies reflect, to some degree, his or her concepts and understanding of the world. The main vocation of a child is play, and an examination of play routines can allow the clinician to make some general inferences about the child's worldview. It is unlikely that a child with primitive play routines that involve sensorimotor exploration, shaking, banging, and mouthing of objects has an understanding of objects and events that lends itself well to coding with a linguistic system. A child with no concept of functional object use (using an object appropriately, as in pushing a toy car) is unlikely to need language to code the name of this object (*car*) or the relationships this object enters into (e.g., *push, go, big*).

Conceptual holdings are thought to be important to linguistic acquisition for several reasons. First, language is a representational act. It represents reality or stands for objects and relationships in the world. Second, language is an abstract symbol system. To appreciate abstract symbols, we must be able to represent them mentally. Third, language is a tool that we use in social interactions. Tool use implies certain conceptual underpinnings, such as the apprehension of relationships like means–end. Fourth, language use involves talking about objects, events, and relationships in the world. It is necessary that one knows and can remember the properties of these objects and relationships before talking about them coherently. As Nelson (1974) said, we use words as *tags* for the concepts that we have.

Perhaps the best-known researcher in the area of children's cognitive development is Jean Piaget. A most significant period in language development occurs between birth and 2 years (Beard, 1969; Ginsburg & Opper, 1969; Morehead & Morehead, 1974). By the age of 2, a child is typically beginning to use multiword utterances and has clearly demonstrated the symbolic capacity for dealing with language. Piaget calls the period between birth and age 2 the *sensorimotor stage of cognitive development* because most learning takes place through active sensorimotor exploration of a child's environment. Piaget has divided his sensorimotor period of cognitive development into six substages (see Table 4–3). In typical development, a child attains at least stage 4 of the sensorimotor period to evidence gestural communication and stage 5 or 6 for expressive single- and early multiword constructions. In reviewing the cognitive development literature, however, there seem to be certain skills that are included on cognitive assessment scales and are often referred to by authorities as potentially being language-related.

Functional object use has been related to the development of communication (Steckol & Leonard, 1981). Using an object for its intended purpose (e.g., combing hair with a comb) requires the mental representation of both the object and its use. Also, when a child begins to talk about basic relations in the environment, utterances typically concern objects, their functions, and all the relationships an object enters into (Nelson, 1974).

Imitation and *deferred (delayed) imitation* also have been related to the development of language (Bates, 1979). Imitation requires mental representation of an act for a short time period, and deferred imitation requires holding onto an event for a longer duration. Both suggest at least an ability to represent reality for a length of time and not depending on immediate stimulus support.

TABLE 4–3
Piaget's Six Sensorimotor Substages of Development

Sensorimotor Substages	Age	Description	Example
1. Reflexes	Birth–1 month	Behaviors include innate reflexes, which are reflected as an automatic response to stimuli.	Sucking on a pacifier
2. Primary circular reactions	1–4 months	Focus on own body (i.e., primary) and repeat actions that occurred by chance (i.e., circular).	Repetitive open and closing of the hand; sucking on thumb
3. Secondary circular reactions	4–8 months	More responsive to outside world (i.e., secondary) and becoming object-oriented. Differentiation between means and ends.	Repetitive dropping of a toy after it is picked up and handed to the child
4. Coordination of secondary circular reactions	8–12 months	Establish goal-directed behavior, object permanence, and cause–effect relationships.	Hand–eye coordination; can retrieve hidden toys and combine behaviors to achieve a goal
5. Tertiary circular reactions	12–18 Months	New flexibility (i.e., tertiary) with acquired responses.	Finding a new possibility for an object
6. Mental representations	18–24 months	Development of symbolic thought and deferred imitation.	Mental prediction and planning, and the ability to recall and imitate another's past behavior

Source: Adapted from Piaget, J. (1952). *The origins of intelligence in children*. New York: International Universities press.

Symbolic play (pretend behavior) is frequently regarded as evidence of a child's general symbolic capacity. One can think of symbolic play on a continuum from playing with exemplars of an object that are physically similar to the real object (e.g., a box representing a car) to playing with exemplars that are dissimilar to the real object (e.g., a comb for a car), and finally to playing with no object at all (*pantomime*). The use of one object to stand for another is similar to the way that words represent objects in the real world. A basic symbolic capacity must be present in order to use a symbolic play routine, and these routines should be noted in a child's behavior as positive signs of increased symbolic capacity.

A primary reason to assess cognitive level is to determine a child's ability to represent reality and deal with symbols. An important notion to keep in mind when assessing cognitive attainments is that clinicians watch a child's behavior and *infer* his or her conceptual holdings. We should obtain as much information as possible about the child's typical play routines and object use. The preassessment questionnaire and parent interview are invaluable here. The child may exhibit evidence of more sophisticated play at home and not demonstrate it in the clinical setting. The failure of a child to perform a task that we set up to evaluate a particular cognitive attainment is not necessarily evidence of a lack of the concept. A child can fail a cognitive task due to inattention, disinterest, or some other reason that has nothing to do with his or her cognitive status.

With these admonitions in mind, how does one perform a play assessment, and what type of child undergoes the evaluation? We have found it productive to take note of cognitive attainments in children who are nonverbal and those who are at the single-word level. Children who currently use productive, early multiword utterances already demonstrate some representational ability and symbolic ability just by using language normally. It is not useful to administer a lengthy and complex cognitive test battery initially. We recommend that the diagnostician move from general analyses to more specific ones.

The first level of analysis can be a lengthy behavioral observation of the child engaged in play. In our experience, children whose cognitive levels are lower will exhibit primitive play routines and perseverative use of objects. Several scales are available for play assessment. Westby (1980) outlines some useful stages and a scale to use in assessing the developmental relationship among cognitive development, language, and play (see Table 4–4). The clinician can set up a play situation and watch the child interact

TABLE 4–4
Westby Play Scale

Stage	Age	Play	Language
1	9–12 months	Uses some toys appropriately and travels to get items. Can find hidden objects.	Appropriate toy use with performance sounds and words.
2	13–17 months	Explores toys and will seek adult help if unable to operate.	Use of single words and word production is context dependent.
3	17–19 months	Uses objects and toys appropriately and engages in autosymbolic play.	Words begin to have functional and sematic relations.
4	19–22 months	Symbolic play extends beyond self to include other people or items. Also combines items in play schemes using realistic items.	Beginning of word combinations; refers to people or items that are not present.
5	24 months	Play begins to represent daily experiences.	Phrases and short sentences. Plurals, present progressive, and possessive begin to appear.
6	30 months	Play extends to less frequently experienced schemes like going to doctor.	Responds to and asks who, what, and where questions. Why questions are still challenging.
7	3 years	Child begins to sequence play activities and engage in associative play.	Begins to use past and future tense.
8	3–3 1/2 years	Begins to engage in imaginative play and uses one object to represent another.	Descriptive vocabulary expands, engages in dialogue, and uses metalinguistic language.
9	3 1/2–4 years	Begins to plan ahead for events and can develop three-dimensional structures.	Communicates intentions and future events.
10	5 years	Fully cooperative play that can include a sequence of pretend events. Highly imaginative.	Relational terms are used.

Source: Adapted from Westby (1980).

TABLE 4–5
McCune Scale

Level	Age	Description	Example
1. Presymbolic play schemes	Less than 18 months	The relationship between the features/use of an object and associated actions are recognized.	Drinking from a cup or brushing hair.
2. Self-pretend	18–24 months	Child is playful and, with awareness, pretends to play. Can distinguish the real acts from play counterpart.	Pretending to eat from a spoon or drinking from a toy cup with exaggerated gestures and sound effects.
3. Other-pretend	2–3 years	Play that involves the activity of others agents or objects. Pretends behaviors observed in others.	Often includes maternal behaviors such as cleaning, pretending to read a book to others, or feeding a doll.
4. Combinatorial pretend	2–3 years	A scheme involves more than one actor and receiver of an action *or* several schemes are combined and related to each other within a sequence.	Child pretends to drink from a cup and then asks caregiver to drink from cup. Carries out a routine like dressing a doll, brushing the doll's hair, and then feeding the doll.
5. Hierarchical pretend	2–3 years	Internal representation for planning of pretend acts and multi-scheme acts.	Engages in preparatory acts before a routine by finding all necessary objects. Prepares to play out a home living routine by finding all the items needed to prepare a meal.

Source: Adapted from McCune (1995).

with objects and people. It is important to remember that the toys and objects provided give the child an opportunity to exhibit higher levels of play. Casby (2003) offers material suggestions for use in play assessment. For example, if only a car, ball, blocks, and a toy horse are provided, the child will be limited in his or her ability to demonstrate combinatorial symbolic play. On the other hand, if a doll, doll bed, spoon, bowl, baby bottle, comb, brush, and blanket are provided, the child will have the opportunity to show how he or she could pretend using these objects in combinations.

Carpenter's (1987) *Play Scale* was designed to evaluate symbolic behavior in nonverbal children but also has utility for children with emerging language. For this scale, the caretaker asks to play with the child and uses props to engage in four play scenarios: tea party, farm, transportation, and nurturing. The caretakers are to follow the child's lead and respond to the child in a natural manner. Behaviors broadly examined include toy use, nesting, and type of play episodes. McCune (1995) also offers a method for analyzing play behavior. Her system also requires an analysis of the caretaker engaging in play using a standard set of toys and items. She provides criteria for analyzing behaviors to determine the level of the child's play. The five levels of play and their descriptions are summarized in Table 4–5.

Regardless of the scale used, the most important point to determine is the child's *modal level of play*, which is the most frequently occurring type of interaction. The examiner should be looking for behavior that suggests functional use of objects, symbolic play, means–end, combinatorial play, sensorimotor exploration, imitation, and searching for hidden objects. It is optimal to video-record the play interaction for later specific analysis (Lund & Duchan, 1988). We recommend the following general steps as you analyze a video recording. First, divide the play session into play episodes that represent a particular theme. For instance, if the child is playing with a farm set, call the play episode "farm." Then look at each interaction the child has with the objects and people in each play episode. If a child picks up a cow and puts it in his mouth, this should be documented as mouthing or sensorimotor exploration. If the child makes the cow walk and jump into the back of a truck, take note of this behavior as possibly symbolic play because pretending is involved. If the child brushes a doll's hair, puts the doll to bed, and covers it with a blanket, this may be combinatorial symbolic play. A summary of behaviors in play episodes can easily result in a modal level of play in terms of sensorimotor exploration, functional object use, or symbolic play. In all cases, view the specific behaviors in terms of the context in which they occurred. For instance, pretending that a block is a car can qualify as symbolic play only if the clinician did not demonstrate this activity earlier in the session. At any rate, it is important to view children's nonverbal play behaviors contextually and, if possible, obtain some historical data on their play routines.

After observing play routines, consider whether a cognitive delay is suggested based on the quality of play exhibited. With the information collected, we should "triangulate" a child's chronological age, language stage, and play level to determine if there are discrepancies. For example, a 3-year-old child may exhibit a play level of 3 years of age but a language level of 1 year of age. This suggests that the child's language level is lagging behind his or her cognitive development, and this is likely to be more of a language problem than a cognitive one. If, on the other hand, a 3-year-old child is at the 1-year level for both language and cognition, it is possible that both cognitive and linguistic goals should be targeted in treatment. Sometimes there will clearly be no representational problem based on the sophisticated levels of observed play routines. Other times, behavior will occur that strongly suggests a rather primitive representational ability. Many cases fall between these two ends of the cognitive continuum, and these children may require further testing to determine which level of cognitive development they have attained.

A final level of analysis is to administer a more detailed scale such as the *Uzgiris-Hunt Ordinal Scales of Infant Development* (Uzigiris & Hunt, 1975). Dunst (1980) has developed some helpful procedures for use with the Uzgiris and Hunt scales that make the clinical administration of the tasks more streamlined. Such lengthy measures should be administered to a child who is strongly suspected of exhibiting cognitive deficits.

The speech-language pathologist should be careful when assessing cognitive attainments related to language and not allow other professionals or parents to perceive this evaluation procedure as the testing of a child's *intelligence*. We should make no judgments about how "smart" a child is or necessarily even his or her potential for cognitive growth. Children whose play behavior and performance on cognitive scales indicate that they lack some cognitive basis for language should be referred to other professionals (e.g., psychologist, special educator) for a program that includes many domains of child development, including cognitive, social, self-help, and motor abilities. SLPs examine cognitive attainments only because they appear to be related to the acquisition and use of abstract language systems. If we determine that a child does not possess the cognitive attainments for acquiring the abstract and arbitrary symbol system of language, we can then consider attempting to train cognitive goals (Kahn, 1984) or teaching a communication system that is less abstract, such as simple signs or augmentative communication devices that code concrete and frequently occurring activities. Cognitive assessment is not just smoke and mirrors; this information has practical clinical applications. Recall the earlier section in this chapter on prediction and prognosis in early language development. Among the strongest predictors of language development in children are the level of play, symbolic play, and use of combinatorial play. These are also potent predictors for discriminating whether a child is a late talker or is language impaired, as are other measures of language production, comprehension, communicative intent, phonology, and social behavior. Another practical aspect of looking at children's play is its relationship to social behavior. Some studies have shown that children with language impairment also exhibit social deficits. Children who play appropriately will be able to form social relationships with others, while those who are limited to sensorimotor exploration will have difficulty being accepted by their peers. Incorporating play/cognitive goals into language treatment is relatively easy and has a potentially large payoff for a child's social interactions.

The *Communication Symbolic Behavior Scales (CSBS)—Developmental Profile* of Wetherby and Prizant (2002a) is respected by many clinicians and researchers as a useful measure of early language development because it focuses on many aspects of communication, including cognitive, social, affective, phonetic, and linguistic domains. The CSBS uses a relatively natural sampling procedure for communication and play, and provides normative data on all areas examined. This is also a reasonable initial step in cognitive assessment. The CSBS has also been extended to include a shortened procedure that can be administered and scored in significantly less time than the entire CSBS battery (Wetherby & Prizant, 1998).

Assessment of Communicative Intent and Function

The third step toward becoming a communicator is to interact with caregivers as communication partners (McDonald & Carroll, 1992). It is important to realize that *communication* is not synonymous with speech and language. That is, children communicate gesturally long before they do so with words. A thorough analysis of a child's gestural communication is an important part of early language evaluation to determine if a child is, in fact, a communication partner. Gestures are actions that have communicative intent and are expressed with fingers, hands, arms, facial expressions, and bodily motions (Iverson & Thal, 1998). Gesture development can be divided into three primary categories: showing off, deictic, and representational (Iverson & Thal, 1998). Showing off is an early sign of communicative intent where the infant engages in repetitive behaviors to gain an adult's attention (Bates, Benigni, Bretherton, Camaioni, & Volterra, 1979). Deictic gestures are divided into contact and distal gestures, and typically emerge around 10 to 12 months (McLean, McLean, Brady, & Etter, 1991). Contact gestures require contact with an object or caregiver (e.g., pushing a hand away), whereas distal gestures do not (e.g., pointing). Representational gestures are symbolic gestures that are used to represent a social action (e.g., waving good-bye) or a feature of an item (e.g., hand to mouth to represent drinking) and emerge around 12 months. Bruner (1981) indicates that these early gestural acts have three communicative functions: behavior regulation, social interaction, and joint attention.

Crais, Douglas, and Campbell (2004) conducted a longitudinal study of 12 typically developing children between the ages of 6 and 24 months. They provide a detailed summary of gestural developments as they relate to Bruner's (1981) broad categories of regulating behavior, gaining joint attention, and social interaction. Within each category, means and variability data are provided for individual gestures, which would be valuable in assessment of gestural communication. The *Early Social Communication Scale* (ESCS; Mundy, Hogan, & Doehring, 1996) is also based on Bruner's theoretical framework and provides a structured method for evaluating early social communicative behaviors.

Preverbal communicative acts are fairly easy to see in children. They communicate profusely by pushing adults, pulling adults, pointing at objects or events, reaching for objects, giving objects to adults, and showing objects to adults. They also use gaze shifts as very important components of their preverbal communication. Children will point at an object and alternate their gaze between the caregiver and the object. They will also engage in visual checking to see if a caregiver is watching their gestural communication while they are pointing or reaching. We cannot emphasize enough that the analysis of communicative intent is critical to assessment of early language cases. There is a strong rationale for this notion. First, function/intent precedes form/structure in communicative development. Children exhibit intentional communication before they produce words. Second, training forms/structures in the absence of functions is not efficacious. That is, it is not particularly useful to train a child to say words when he or she has no reason to use them. This type of case probably needs a focus on training social reciprocity, communicative intent, and gestural communication in addition to learning words. In therapy we would much rather see a child who likes to pull, push, and point than one who has no intentional gestural communication with others in the environment. Standardized tests typically do not often examine communicative gestures, so the clinician must rely on nonstandardized communication sampling. Steigler (2007) showed that an in-depth analysis of interactions using conversation analysis and speech act analysis can provide important insight into variables such as conversational sequencing, diversity of speech acts, gazing, smiling, initiations, and communicative output of a child with autism. Such measurements are not often found on standardized tests and instead focus on actual social or clinical interactions.

Capone and McGregor (2004) outline the development of communicative gestures in early childhood in both typical children and those with language impairment. They discuss implications of examining gestural development for diagnosis, prognosis, and intervention. Determining a child's semantic representations is almost always a difficult task for the clinician. This is especially challenging when a child has a limited vocabulary. Some authorities have indicated that a frequent manifestation of early language disorder in children is their failure to use language (Fey, 1986; Lucas, 1980; Wetherby & Prutting, 1984). As mentioned previously, a prelinguistic or nonverbal child has no expressive language. This does not imply, however, that the child is not communicating. Any mother of a prelinguistic child will attest to the fact that her child communicates profusely about his or her desires, moods, and a variety of pleasing and noxious biological states. Bates (1976) studied the sensorimotor performances of young children and determined that those children have primitive forms of *imperatives* or commands by which they use adults to obtain access to objects in their environment. The goal is to gain access to the object. One can initially see the child physically manipulating the adult, as in putting the adult's hand on a jar to open it. Later, the child may use pointing coupled with vocalizations to indicate to the adult what he or she wants done. Bates also noted primitive forms of the *declarative* in which the child uses an object to gain adult attention as the goal. There appears to be a progression that begins with the child's showing and giving objects to adults. Ultimately, the child exhibits the declarative by pointing toward objects with an alternating gaze between the adult and object. Bates (1979) reported a gestural complex that may be related in part to language development. Thus, communication is taking place quite vividly in the preverbal child.

There is also preverbal evidence of the functions of language alluded to by Halliday (1975) and Dore (1975). That is, children use the greeting function nonverbally by waving, they question by exhibiting a quizzical look, and they regulate adults physically before they use language for these purposes. In preverbal children, the primary evidence for their communication ability is found in gestures, facial expressions, and/or vocalizations. These phenomena can be observed by a clinician in a diagnostic session, or caretakers can be asked in an assessment interview about how the child makes his or her needs known at home and at school.

Communicative intents can be realized on a gestural, vocal, or verbal level. Dore et al. (1976) noted that a prelinguistic child is not simply uttering "jargon" vocalizations. Dore et al. noted the presence of phonetically consistent forms, which Dore termed transitional phenomena, at a certain point in a child's development. *Phonetically consistent forms (PCFs)* are vocalizations that are stabilized around certain situations. They are not word approximations but are fairly stable phonetic productions typically consisting of vowel or consonant–vowel combinations. They are repeatedly associated with specific situations such as showing affect (emotion), indicating or pointing to aspects of the environment, or expressing a desire to obtain an object or event. Dore et al. observed that these PCFs seem to act as a transition to words wherein certain phonetic elements must be stabilized around a specific referent. Thus, it would be important in an evaluation of communicative function to determine not only which basic functions are present but also whether those functions manifest themselves on a gestural, vocal, or verbal level. Stark, Bernstein, and Demorest (1993) and Proctor (1989) report useful data on vocalizations produced for a variety of communicative functions and outline an orderly developmental sequence of vocal communication in the first 18 months of life.

According to Chapman (1981), the clinician may adopt an existing classification scheme or change these available systems so that functions that are of interest can be coded. Many systems might be useful clinically (Coggins & Carpenter, 1978; Dore, 1975; Folger & Chapman, 1978; Halliday, 1975; Tough, 1977). From examining the categories in these systems, it is clear that many of the terms overlap with respect to the functions they describe. McLean and Snyder-McLean (1978) have suggested that functions of language may be distilled into two basic uses. One use is to influence joint attention, and the other is to influence joint activity. These functions basically correspond to the imperative and the declarative, respectively, in English. The clinician should select a system that contains at least some basic declarative and imperative operations so that the child's initiation of a response to communications can be coded.

Some additional general guidelines should be discussed. The assessment of communicative function should, in part, be carried out in a naturalistic situation. It is sometimes difficult to contrive situations in which a child will express a genuine communicative intent. The clinician should have present in the room a wide variety of toys and stimuli that would elicit a number of different expressions of need or declarations. If there are other children or adults in the situation, the clinician must remember that the functions expressed by the child are inextricably related to the behavior and utterances of other conversational participants. In addition, functions are only interpretable in light of the nonverbal context of communication.

Some authors have suggested using standard elicitation tasks for basic communicative functions, which has been done for imperatives and declaratives (Dale, 1980; Snyder, 1978, 1981; Staab, 1983; Wetherby & Prizant, 1992; Wetherby & Rodriguez, 1992) but not as widely for more specific functions of communication. Generally, declaratives seem to be elicited most effectively by presenting novel or discrepant events and objects in the sampling situation. The child may then comment on the novel stimulus. For example, a clinician can allow a child to remove items from a bag. When an item is produced, the child will often comment or name the object. Imperatives are more reliably obtained than declaratives because the clinician can maintain control over the stimuli and activities in the sampling situation. The child will ask for access to toys or will ask the clinician to assist in certain operations (winding of toys, etc.). Ideally, communicative intent should be sampled using a combination of spontaneous play and use of elicitation tasks.

Wetherby et al. (1988) have contributed research that practicing clinicians will find most helpful. These researchers studied normally developing children at the preverbal, single-word, and early multiword stages of development to describe their intentional communication. Rate of communicative acts increased predictably as the children increased in mean length of utterance. The children tended to move from gestural modes in the prelinguistic stage to verbal modes in the early multiword stage. Wetherby, Yonclas, and Bryan (1989) used similar procedures on children with language impairment, Down syndrome, and autism, and indicate that some of these measures (e.g., rate of intentional communication) may have potentially useful clinical value in describing these populations. A rate of about one communicative act per minute seems to be related to the onset of single-word utterances (Wetherby et al., 1988).

Two standardized tools address gestural communication to some degree: the Communication and Symbolic Behavior Scales (CSBS) and the MacArthur-Bates Communicative Development Inventories, Words and Gestures (CDI). The Rossetti Infant-Toddler Language Scale (Rossetti, 1990) also has a large number of gesture items but lacks normative data, thereby requiring clinicians to make judgments about developmental appropriateness. Other tests, like the Preschool Language Scale, Fifth Edition (Zimmerman, Steiner, & Pond, 2011); Bayley Scales of Infant and Toddler Development, Third Edition (Bayley, 2006); and Receptive Expressive Emergent Language Test, Third Edition (Bzoch, League, & Brown, 2003), include a few gesture items.

These are good starting points in the evaluation of gestural communication; however, it is recommended that less formal measures also be considered in assessment. For example, Crais, Watson, and Baranek (2009) suggest that we obtain measurements on the frequency of gesture use. Data on frequency of communication for children at 12, 18, and 24 months suggest that they should be communicating at 1 time per minute, 2 times per minute, and 5 times per minute, respectively (Wetherby, Cain, Yonclas, & Walker, 1988). Other measures, such as the type of specific gesture used (e.g., distal point, reach, show, give), should also be inventoried, as should the communicative function of each gesture (e.g., imperative, declarative). Crais, Watson, and Baranek (2009) also recommend examining use of gestures in concert with eye gaze toward people and objects as well as the coordination of verbal productions with gestures.

More extensive normative data are available in the CSBS (Wetherby & Prizant, 1992). These scales examine the areas of communicative functions, gestural communicative means, vocal communicative means, verbal communicative means, reciprocity, social-affective signaling, and symbolic behavior. The data on this measure come from caregiver questionnaires, direct sampling, and some structured elicitation tasks. Standardization data on hundreds of children are available for use by the examiner. This test is a good example of how ecologically valid behaviors can be evaluated and put into a normative developmental framework. Standardized testing does not always have to be artificial. The *communicative temptations* used in the Communication and Symbolic Behavior Scales were piloted in the earlier work of Wetherby mentioned above. Videos are also available to demonstrate administration and scoring of the CSBS. This helps to increase reliability in the procedure. The *Autism Diagnostic Observation Schedule (ADOS)*, Second Edition (Lord, Rutter, DiLavore, Risi, Gotham, & Bishop, 2012) is another standardized instrument that uses communicative temptations for the evaluation of communication, social interaction skills, play, and behaviors that are necessary for a diagnosis of autism spectrum disorder.

In cases where the child is nonverbal or at the single-word level, it is feasible to analyze functions and target communicative functions in treatment (Wilcox, 1984). For example, the clinician may want to increase the number of regulatory attempts in a particular child or increase the verbal realizations of regulation in a client. Brunson and Haynes (1991) provide an example of an alternating-time sampling procedure that can be used in classroom contexts to monitor the use of communicative functions in naturalistic activities. This system can also track intentional communication of teachers for possible inclusion in the treatment program.

Use of Tests and Formal Procedures with Limited-Language Children

Only two decades ago, there were few assessment instruments available to the SLP for use on children with limited language. This is not necessarily because SLPs were uninterested in preschool-age children (SLPs have always dealt with youngsters of this age). Several influences on test development have increased the construction of instruments appropriate for the preschool, or limited-language, population. First of all, passage of IDEA mandates that preschool children between the ages of 3 and 5 years are dealt with by clinicians working in the public school setting. Many school systems are currently responsible for children between birth and age 3. With the enactment of federal legislation, test developers have increased their efforts in devising test instruments for preschoolers. The second influence on test development has been the significant strides that we have made in communication development research in the past 20 years.

We can divide the preschool tests that deal with communication into several categories. First, large test batteries include language or communication as one aspect of assessment. These standardized batteries include sections on motor skill, cognition, personal-social behavior, adaptive behavior, and communication. The portion dealing with communication is necessarily incomplete and superficial because the entire battery must examine so many different domains. This general battery, however, could suggest that a child's communication development may be delayed in comparison to the norming sample, and herein lies one value of the test (problem/no problem issue). Certainly, the test could never tell a clinician specific aspects of communication that are delayed or that suggest treatment objectives. There are many large batteries that include language as a subpart.

On another level are tests that focus more specifically on language and communication. These instruments may be helpful to the SLP in providing direction toward areas in need of probing through nonstandardized methods. Some of these instruments are standardized, norm-referenced tests; others may be criterion-referenced. These measures should satisfy any administrative requirements imposed by work settings on obtaining scores in assessment. The measures could also prove useful as a beginning point for naturalistic evaluation tasks. Crais (1995) reviews many of these instruments and discusses issues related to early assessment.

A list of some commonly used standardized tests available on the market for early child language disorders is provided in Table 4–6. There are literally hundreds of standardized tests in the area of child language; therefore this list is by no means exhaustive. Other useful references and descriptions of standardized assessments can be found in Paul (2012), Shipley and McAfee (2009), and Stein-Rubin and Fabus (2012). It is our view that such summaries should be used only as a starting place in locating particular tests that may be appropriate for child language assessment. It behooves you as a consumer to spend some time carefully examining these instruments at conventions or conferences before purchasing them. There is no substitute for reading a thoughtful and lengthy review of a test, scouring a test manual, and working the examination materials themselves to understand a test. The Buros Mental Measurements Yearbook Online (http://buros.unl.edu) provides in-depth reviews of most tests; however, there is a charge to access the information. Many libraries contain the *Buros Mental Measurements Yearbook,* which can be examined at no cost. Finally, much test information is readily available on publishers' websites and in those multiple brochures that arrive in your mailbox.

As stated earlier in this chapter, we urge you to remember that standardized tests represent only a very small part of understanding a child's language system; they confirm whether the child has a problem in comparison to his or her peers in a normative sample. This is the simplest level of diagnosis. Chapter 3, on psychometric issues,

TABLE 4–6
Assessments for the Evaluation of Young Children

Instrument Title	Author(s) and Year of Publication	Year	Age Range	Parent Report	Languages	Description
Ages and Stages Questionnaire, Third Edition	Squires and Bricker	2008	1–66 months	Yes	English, French Korean, Spanish	Parent-completed questionnaire that identifies children with developmental delays. Screens the following developmental areas: communication, gross motor, fine motor, problem solving, and personal-social.
Assessing Prelinguistic and Early Linguistic Behaviors in Developmentally Young Children	Olswang, Stoel-Gammon, Coggins, and Carpenter	1987	Birth–24 months	Yes	English	Family-based language diagnostic tool that assesses prelinguistic communication in children. This assessment includes both observational and structured scales. These scales are completed to describe a child's play, communicative intention, language production, and comprehension.
Assessment, Evaluation, and Programming System for Infants and Children (AEPS)	Bricker	2002	Birth–6 years	Yes	English	Curriculum-based, criterion-referenced assessment for children who have disabilities or are at risk for developmental delays. Assesses the following areas: fine motor, gross motor, cognitive, adaptive, social-communication, and social development.
Battelle Developmental Inventory, Second Edition *(BDI-2)*	Newborg	2004	Birth–7:11	No	English, Spanish	Developmental assessment that evaluates whether a child has reached early developmental milestones. Assesses the following areas: personal-social, adaptive, motor, communication, and cognitive ability.
Bayley Scales of Infant and Toddler Development, Third Edition *(Bayley-III)*	Bayley	2005	1–42 months	Yes	English	Norm-referenced scale used to assess a child's development. Comprised of five scales, three administered to the child (cognitive, motor, and language) and two conducted with a parent questionnaire (social-emotional, adaptive behavior).
Birth to Three Assessment and Intervention System, Second Edition *(BTAIS-2)*	Ammer and Bangs	2000	Birth–3 years	No	English	Criterion-referenced measure developed to assess children in the following areas: language comprehension, language expression, nonverbal thinking, social/ personal development, and motor development.

Name	Authors	Year	Age		Language	Description
The Carolina Curriculum for Infants and Toddlers with Special Needs, Third Edition	Johnson-Martin, Attermeier, and Hacker	2004	Birth–3 years	Yes	English, Spanish	Criterion-referenced assessment used with young children who have mild to severe developmental disabilities. Evaluates a child's progress through five areas: personal-social, cognition, communication, fine motor, and gross motor.
The Capute Scales: Cognitive Adaptive Test and Clinical Linguistic and Auditory Milestone Scale (CAT/CLAMS)	Accardo and Capute	2005	1–36 months	No	English, Spanish, Russian	Norm-referenced screening assessment that aids in identifying developmental delays in children. The CAT evaluates visual-motor functioning, while the CLAMS evaluates expressive and receptive language development.
Child Development Review–Parent Questionnaire	Ireton	1990	18 months–5 years	Yes	English, Spanish	Parent questionnaire provides information about a child's health and development. Contains a development chart that addresses five developmental areas: social, self-help, gross motor skills, fine motor skills, and language.
Communication and Symbolic Behavior Scales–Developmental Profile (CSBS DP)	Wetherby and Prizant	2002a	6–24 months (up to 72 months, if delayed)	Yes	English	Norm-referenced screening and evaluation tool that assesses a child's communicative competence. Includes assessment of symbolic play, nonverbal communication, and expressive and receptive language. Includes the Infant/Toddler checklist, a caregiver questionnaire, and a behavior sample.
Early Language Milestones Scale, Second Edition (ELM-2)	Coplan	1993	Birth–3 years	No	English	Assesses speech and language development in infancy and early childhood. Assesses the following areas: auditory expressive, auditory receptive, and visual.
Early Learning Accomplishment Profile (E-LAP)	Glover, Preminger, and Sanford	1995	Birth–3 years	No	English, Spanish	Criterion-referenced tool that provides a picture of a child's development in six domains: gross motor, fine motor, cognitive, language, self-help, and social/emotional abilities.
Early Screening Profile (ESP)	Harrison et al.	1990	2–6:11	No	English	Screening tool used to identify children who may be at risk for later learning problems. Areas assessed include cognition, language, motor, self-help/social, articulation, and home environment.

(continued)

TABLE 4-6
(Continued)

Instrument Title	Author(s) and Year of Publication	Year	Age Range	Parent Report	Languages	Description
Expressive One Word Picture Vocabulary Test, Fourth Edition (EOWPVT-4)	Brownell	2000	2:0–80+	No	English, Spanish	Standardized assessment of expressive vocabulary. Examinee is instructed to make word–picture associations.
Hawaii Early Learning Profile (HELP)	Furuno et al.	1988	Birth–36 months	No	English, Spanish	Family-centered curriculum-based assessment that assesses developmental skills and behaviors of children. Areas assessed include cognitive, language, gross motor, social-emotional, and self-help.
Infant/Toddler Checklist	Wetherby and Prizant	2002b	6–24 months	Yes	English, Chinese, Spanish, German, Slovenian, Swedish	Screening component of the *Communication and Symbolic Behavior Scales (CSBS)*. This tool provides for the early identification of children who are at risk for developing communication impairments. It is designed to measure seven language predictors: emotion and use of eye gaze, use of communication, use of gestures, use of sounds, use of words, understanding of words, and use of objects.
Infant-Toddler Developmental Assessment (IDA)	Provence, Erikson, Vater, and Palmeri	1995	Birth–3 years	Yes	English, Spanish Parent Report Form	Comprehensive, multidisciplinary assessment that provides for early identification of children who are developmentally at risk. Contains six phases: referral and pre-interview data gathering; initial parent interview; health review; developmental observation and assessment; integration and synthesis; and share findings, completion, and report.
Language Development Survey (LDS)	Rescorla	1989	18–35 months	Yes	English, Spanish	A vocabulary checklist designed as a screening tool for identification of language delays in young children. The checklist is completed by the parent, and a total vocabulary score is reported.

Measure	Author	Year	Age range	Available	Languages	Description
MacArthur-Bates Communicative Development Inventories, Second Edition	Fenson et al.	2007		Yes	Available in over 50 languages	Diagnostic tool that assesses expressive and receptive vocabulary and early grammatical production in young children. Includes two forms: Words and Gestures (for use with children 8–18 months) and Words and Sentences (for use with children 16–30 months).
Mullen Scales of Early Learning: AGS Edition	Mullen	1995	Birth–5:8	No	English	Standardized assessment that provides a measure of cognitive functioning in young children. Areas assessed include perceptual language, expressive language, gross motor, fine motor, and visual reception.
The Ounce Scale	Meisels, Dombro, Marsden, Weston, and Jewkes	2003	Birth–3:6	Yes	English, Spanish	Criterion-referenced assessment that evaluates a child's development and behavior. The scale is organized around six major developmental areas: personal connections, feelings about self, relationships with other children, understanding and communicating, exploration and problem solving, and movement and coordination.
Parents' Evaluation of Developmental Status	Glascoe	2006	Birth–8 years	Yes	English, Spanish, Vietnamese	Developmental screening tool that helps identify children with developmental and behavioral deficits. A parent questionnaire addresses concerns about a child's language, motor, self-help, early academic skills, behavior, and social/emotional/ mental health.
Peabody Picture Vocabulary Test, Fourth Edition	Dunn and Dunn	2007	2:6–90+	No	English, Spanish	Norm-referenced language assessment tool that evaluates the receptive vocabulary of adults and children.
Preschool Language Scale, Fifth Edition (PLS-5)	Zimmerman, Steiner, and Pond	2011	Birth–7:11	No	English, Spanish	Standardized comprehensive developmental assessment of language. This play-based assessment evaluates a range of receptive and expressive language skills. These language skills are presented in sequential, developmental order.

(continued)

TABLE 4-6
(Continued)

Instrument Title	Author(s) and Year of Publication	Year	Age Range	Parent Report	Languages	Description
Receptive One Word Picture Vocabulary Test, Fourth Edition (ROWPVT-4)	Brownell	2000	2–80+	No	English, Spanish	Norm-referenced tool that assesses an individual's receptive vocabulary development.
Receptive-Expressive Emergent Language Test, Third Edition (REEL-3)	Bzoch, League, and Brown	2003	Birth–3 years	Parent interview	English	Assessment tool used to identify infants and toddlers with developmental language impairments. Subtest areas include receptive language, expressive language, and a supplementary subtest (inventory of vocabulary words)
Reynell Developmental Language Scales, Fourth Edition	Edwards, Letts, and Sinka	2011	2–7:5 years	No	English	Assessment tool designed to identify speech and language delays and impairments in young children. Scales included in the assessment are comprehension scale and production scale.
Rosetti Infant and Toddler Language Scale	Rosetti	2006	Birth–3 years	Yes	English, Spanish	Criterion-referenced tool that evaluates preverbal and verbal aspects of communication and interaction in young children. Areas assessed include interaction-attachment, pragmatics, gesture, play, language comprehension, and language expression.
Sequenced Inventory of Communication Development, Revised Edition (SICD-R)	Prather and Tobin	1995	4–48 months	Yes	English	Diagnostic tool that assesses communication skills of young children. Assessment uses both parent report and observation of communication behaviors. Areas assessed include receptive language and expressive language.
Symbolic Play Test, Second Edition	Lowe and Costello	1988	1–3 years	No	English	Standardized assessment that identifies the early skills required for language development through play.

Assessment	Author(s)	Year	Age	Parent interview	Language	Description
Test of Early Communication and Emerging Language (TECEL)	Huer and Miller	2011	2 weeks–24 months	Parent interview	English Nonverbal AAC	Norm-referenced diagnostic tool that assesses the earliest communicative strengths and weaknesses, as well as emerging language abilities, in infants and toddlers.
Test of Early Language Development, Third Edition (TELD-3)	Hresko, Reid, and Hammill	1999	3:0–7:11	No	English, Spanish	Standardized assessment that assesses the language development of children. The assessment specifically focuses on the areas of semantics, syntax, and morphology, and its subtests include receptive language and expressive language.
Test of Pretend Play (ToPP)	Lewis and Boucher	1998	1–6 years	No	English	Designed to assess symbolic play, conceptual development, and the use of symbols in preschool children. Three types of symbolic play assessed are substituting one object for another object or person, attributing an imagined property to an object or person, and referencing an absent object or person.
Trandisciplinary Play-Based Assessment, Second edition	Linder	2008	Birth–6 years	Yes	English	Assessment that involves the child participating in structured and unstructured play situations to provide opportunities for developmental observations.
Vineland Adaptive Behavior Scales, Second Edition	Sparrow, Cicchetti, and Balla	2005	Birth–90 years	Yes	English, Spanish	Norm-referenced diagnostic tool designed to measure adaptive behavior. Consists of the survey interview form, the parent/caregiver form, an expanded interview form, and a teacher rating form. Four domains are assessed; communication, daily living skills, socialization, and motor skills.

cautions against selecting treatment targets from standardized tests and says not to measure treatment progress with these instruments. Thus, while formal tests are a part of assessment, they are a relatively minor part of the process.

Assessment of Structure and Function in Early Utterances

So far, we have briefly sketched the development of cognitive and social prerequisites to language. This section of the chapter deals with formation of the linguistic code in communicative development. Our discussion will consider two general phases: single-word and early multiword. These stages are based on length of utterance (Miller & Chapman, 1981) and linguistic attainment (Brown, 1973; Lund & Duchan, 1988). Each stage has certain acquisitions associated with it that may indicate that the child is ready for transition to the next stage.

Single-Word Utterances

After a period of using no real words and becoming more consistent with the use of vocalizations accompanied by gestures, the child begins to use single words to code objects and events. The words are not adult productions; they are typically CV or CVCV approximations of the correct production (Nelson, 1973). Nelson has found that children's early lexicons represent specific categories. Research has reported that subgroups of language-developing and language-disordered children are *referential* (word and object–oriented) or *expressive* (social and conversation–oriented). That is, the referential children use mostly nouns and refer to objects and events. They also like to play with objects and spend more time playing alone. The expressive children, on the other hand, enjoy talking to and being with people and use more personal-social words (Weiss et al., 1983). There are perhaps other ways to characterize early single-word productions, but the point is that children go through a period of talking, as Lois Bloom (1973) says, using "one word at a time." Toward the end of the single-word period, Nelson (1973) indicates that the child accrues an expressive lexicon of about 50 words and then begins to attempt word combinations.

Children in the single-word period can be examined for the number of words they use, the types of words they use, and the apparent reasons they use them. Parent report measures are indispensable in this age of working closely with families. O'Neill (2007) has developed the *Language Use Inventory (LUI)* to evaluate pragmatic skills of early preschool children on variables such as use of gestures, vocabulary, and use of longer utterances to serve a variety of communicative functions. Most of the items require parents to answer yes or no or to choose from options such as *never, rarely, sometimes*, or *often*. This inventory was found to discriminate between clinical populations and typically developing children with sensitivity and specificity ranges above 90%.

The form of single-word utterances has been viewed in different ways by various authorities. Nelson (1973), for instance, categorized single words as members of the classes in Table 4–7. Other researchers have found similar results (Benedict, 1975). Lahey (1988) provides a lengthy discussion and examples of a system for early-utterance analysis. Ideally, single words should be paired with functions such as those discussed earlier. Parent checklists are especially useful in obtaining data on lexicon size and content. Fenson et al. (2006) developed the *MacArthur-Bates Communicative Development Inventories* that provide normative data on children from 8 months to 30 months of age in terms of gestures, words, and multiword utterances. Heilmann, Weismer, Evans, and Hollar (2005) found significant correlations between the MacArthur-Bates CDI and direct language measures in 38 late talkers at 30 months of age. In a sample of 100 children (38 late talkers and 62 normal language children), they found that the CDI

TABLE 4–7

Percentage of First 50-Word Lexicon Accounted for by Grammatical Categories
in Two Major Studies

Category	Nelson (1973)	Benedict (1975)	Example
General nominal	50	51	*chair, kitty*
Specific nominal	11	14	*person's name*
Action word	19	14	*go, eat*
Modifier	10	9	*dirty, big*
Personal-social	10	9	*hi, no, please*
Function	0	4	*that, for*

identified children with low language skills up to the 11th percentile, and children with normal language were identified above the 49th percentile. Skarakis-Doyle, Campbell, and Dempsey (2009) found that the CDI total score coupled with chronological age effectively classified children studied into typically developing and language-impaired groups with 96% accuracy. The CDI has also been shown to have excellent validity for children with cochlear implants who are in the early stages of language development, albeit at a more advanced chronological age (Thal, DesJardin, & Eisenberg, 2007). Benchmarks are beginning to appear in the literature for various groups of children on standardized test performance. For instance, Nicholas and Geers (2008) provide benchmark scores for children with cochlear implants on the Preschool Language Scale, the Peabody Picture Vocabulary Test III, and the MacArthur-Bates Communicative Development Scale. The three measures were significantly correlated and the researchers indicate that while these do not constitute normative data, they can be used as benchmarks to compare other children with children with cochlear implants who have similar histories to the subjects studied in the research.

Rice, Sell, and Hadley (1990) provide a system for online coding of children's verbal initiations and responses in natural classroom settings as a function of environmental and play variables. Although the system does not examine types of single words used, it documents whether the child is using single-word, multiword, or gestural communications. Rescorla (1989) developed the *Language Development Survey* (LDS) to screen children at the single-word/early-multiword levels. The LDS is a checklist of communicative behaviors and lexical items to be completed by the parent. Rescorla has recommended the "Delay 3 cutoff" to determine which children should be recommended for a formal evaluation. Using this cutoff, a child who had less than 50 words or no word combinations at 26 months is effectively identified by the LDS as being at risk for language delay. Rescorla and Alley (2001) found the LDS to have excellent reliability, validity, and clinical utility as a screening instrument for expressive language delay in 2-year-old toddlers. Rescorla, Alley, and Christine (2001) also examined word frequencies in toddler lexicons using the LDS and extensive spontaneous samples. They found a high degree of consistency among vocabulary items reported on the LDS, words used in spontaneous samples, and words reported in diary studies of the first lexicon. Klee, Pearce, and Carson (2000) showed that supplementing the Delay 3 criterion with two additional questions (parental concerns about child's language ability and history of six or more ear infections) improved LDS specificity and predictive value while maintaining high sensitivity. Rescorla, Ratner, Jusczyk, and Jusczyk (2005) studied 239 children between 23 and 25 months of age and found that the LDS and CDI were highly correlated (>.90) and that both instruments can be used to rank-order toddlers on the variables of vocabulary size and length of phrases based on parental report.

Prior to the first word combinations, Dore et al. (1976) noted another transitional phenomenon known as the presyntactic device. Dore stated that a syntactic utterance is one in which two words that have a meaning relationship are combined under the same intonational pattern (e.g., "Mommy go"). A *presyntactic device (PSD)* is the combination of two elements under an intonation contour that do not have a meaning relation because one element is not a real word or because the word combination is reduplicated or a highly learned rote production. Thus, a child who says /WI KITI/ is combining a real word (KITI) with a nonword (WI) under an intonation contour. Other presyntactic transitional elements that have been reported are empty forms, which are consistently used productions that appear to be nonsense words (e.g., "wida," "gocking") (Bloom, 1973; Leonard, 1975). Bloom (1970) reports the use of two single words that have a meaning relationship, with a pause inserted between the two elements (e.g., "car . . . go"). All of the above presyntactic devices prepare a child to combine two meaningful language elements under an intonation pattern that is the essence of early multiword combinations. McEachern and Haynes (2004) conducted a longitudinal study of 10 normally developing children using single-word utterances. Children were sampled once a month from 15 months of age until they developed early multiword combinations. The study was designed to determine if certain types of gesture-speech combinations act as transitional phenomena preceding production of two-word utterances. Temporally synchronized gesture–speech combinations were analyzed over a 6-month period to describe whether they encoded one semantic element (pointing to a car and saying "car") or two semantic elements (pointing to a car and saying "big"). There was a significant increase in gesture–speech combinations encoding two semantic elements during the 6-month period, and the onset of these combinations preceded or co-occurred with the first productions of multiword utterances. Thus, the results support the notion that gesture–speech combinations encoding two elements may be a transitional period between single-word and the onset of early multiword combinations. Bain and Olswang (1995) point out the utility of using a dynamic assessment approach to examine readiness for learning early multiword utterances. This information would add a significant dimension to the assessment of a single-word communicator.

The Case of Late Talkers

Children who reach the age of 2 years with significant delays in expressive language despite normal cognitive, auditory, structural, and language comprehension abilities have been the subject of much research. These children usually have less than a 50-word lexicon and no evidence of multiword combinations at age 2. Some authorities suggest that as many as 50% of these children will be at risk for the language delay persisting beyond their third birthday, while the other 50% may catch up and exhibit near-normal communication at age 3. The children in the latter group have been called late bloomers or late talkers. One challenge of the diagnostician is to be able to distinguish children who will persist in their language impairment from those who are simply late talkers. A series of studies suggests that there are some potent variables to use in making this distinction (Paul & Jennings, 1992; Rescorla & Goossens, 1992; Thal & Tobias, 1992; Weismer, Branch, & Miller, 1994). Olswang, Rodriguez, and Timler (1998) provide a useful review of the literature in this area and a chart of prognostic variables related to late talkers. The following are signs that research has suggested may aid in discriminating late bloomers from those children whose language impairment will persist beyond age 3:

- Children whose disorders persist may have a family history of speech and language problems.
- Late talkers tend to have a higher frequency of communication acts.

- Children whose disorders persist tend to have less mature syllable structure, for example, fewer consonants in their phonetic inventories.
- Late talkers tend to have higher scores in language comprehension on measures such as the *MacArthur-Bates Communicative Development Inventories.*
- Late talkers have higher levels of symbolic play and more evidence of combinatorial play compared to children whose disorders persist.

Some recent research shows that there may be some caretaker and cultural variables that are predictive of children who do not resolve their language disorder. LaParo, Justice, Skibbe, and Pianta (2004) studied a national database of 73 children with preschool language impairment at age 3. Standardized assessment at age 4.5 revealed that 33 of the children had resolved their impairments, and 40 showed persistent language disorder. Maternal sensitivity and maternal depression contributed significantly to the prediction of group membership. Children who had greater comprehension deficits were also likely to be in the group that did not resolve their language problems. Caucasian children were over 13 times more likely to be in the resolved group compared to African American children whose mothers also scored lower on depression and sensitivity measures.

The clinician should look for *patterns* of such signs and should not base a decision on one indication alone. It is notable that the majority of these symptoms are not typically addressed in most of our standardized tests for early language; thus, nonstandardized tasks can provide critical information to the well-informed clinician.

Early Multiword Utterances

Perhaps the most researched and reported period of language acquisition is the time when children begin to combine lexical items to form meaning relationships (semantic relations). There has been a long history of interpreting these early utterances as traditional parts of speech (e.g., noun, verb), telegraphic speech (Brown & Fraser, 1963), pivot/open classes (Braine, 1963), and underlying structures of transformational grammar (McNeill, 1970). Currently, most authorities support a semantic view of early multiword utterances using a case grammar (Fillmore, 1968) and have rendered interpretations of early utterances using semantic relations (Bloom, 1970; Bloom & Lahey, 1978; Bowerman, 1974; Brown, 1973; Leonard, 1976; Schlesinger, 1974). Some of the basic early multiword constructions are composed of the semantic cases (Brown, 1973) in Table 4–8. Note that these basic semantic relations code aspects of the world that the child has learned about during the sensorimotor period of cognitive development, which is one reason that some authorities have indicated the strong cross-cultural similarities in early utterances (Brown, 1973). There are many more fine-grained analyses of children's early multiword utterances (Bloom, Lightbrown, & Hood, 1975; Braine, 1976; Leonard, 1976), and the basic relation types in Table 4–8 are included in these analyses, along with some other, more subtle distinctions.

Semantic relations must always be interpreted in light of the nonverbal context surrounding the utterance. The main point here is that children begin to use word combinations that code various common relationships in their environments; if we merely assign adult, syntactic categories (e.g., noun, verb) to the utterances, we miss some of the skill that children have in coding rather subtle relations that are cognitively understood in the sensorimotor period. This skill has been termed a "rich interpretation" by Brown (1973) and gives the child credit for being able to talk about various relationships that syntactic metrics do not. As in the single-word period, these semantic relations are used for various functions; that is, agent + action can be used as a comment/ label (e.g., "Mommy run"—when a child points to mother jogging) or as a regulatory

TABLE 4–8
Semantic Relations Reported by Brown (1973)

Nomination + X	"This ball"
Recurrence + X	"More milk"
Nonexistence + X	"All gone egg"
Agent + action	"Mommy run"
Action + object	"Hit ball"
Agent + object	"Mommy shoe"
Action + locative	"Go outside"
Entity + locative	"Ball kitchen"
Possessor + possession	"Mommy skirt"
Entity + attribute	"Ball red"
Agent + action + object	"Mommy hit ball"
Agent + action + locative	"Mommy run outside"

statement (e.g., "Mommy push"—when the child is trying to get mother to push the wagon). According to authorities, it is wise always to consider both the structure (form) and use (function) of early multiword utterances (Bloom & Lahey, 1978; McLean & Snyder-McLean, 1978). There is a more recent move toward not using a priori semantic relation categories and giving a child credit for a multiword relation only after he or she has demonstrated "productivity" of use (Howe 1976; Leonard, Steckol, & Panther 1983; Lund & Duchan 1988).

As mentioned previously, there are existing methods of viewing and analyzing early semantic relations in children's utterances (Bloom, 1973; Braine, 1976; Brown, 1973; Leonard, 1976; Retherford, 2000). As discussed, there are also a number of systems for examining communicative functions in children (Dore, 1975; Halliday, 1975). Few systems exist, however, that interactively analyze structure and function in early utterances. Lahey (1988) described an analysis system that takes into account structure and function. The system suggests that the clinician transcribe the child's utterances, the adult's utterances, and the nonverbal communicative contextual events that are relevant to the communication. Lahey (1988) prefers the use of video in recording a sample for use in the analysis because all linguistic and contextual information can be preserved and reviewed. Lahey recommends that the beginning clinician start by gaining practice with a particular coding taxonomy through carefully scoring video-recorded sessions. When speed and reliability are increased, then hand transcriptions may be easier and more accurate. Lee's (1966, 1974) method for analyzing developmental sentence types is another grammatically based system for analyzing speech samples that is appropriate for the early multiword stage of development.

At the very least, we recommend that the clinician video-record the child in an interaction with caretakers, teachers, or children so that the former can transcribe the child's utterances and note the context of communication. We feel that the following assumptions are important in a basic early multiword assessment:

1. Determine if there is a "basic" set of semantic relations or if the child uses just a few relations (Lahey, 1988; McLean & Snyder-McLean, 1978).

2. A child should be able verbally to code many relationships and aspects of the environment.

3. The clinician should obtain an inventory of communicative functions used by a child to determine if there is a "basic set" of uses of language (Wetherby et al., 1988).

4. Structure and function should be viewed interactively (Bloom & Lahey, 1978; Lahey, 1988; Muma, 1978).

5. The clinician may find it valuable to get a feeling for the percentage of time that a child initiates language versus the percentage of adult-initiated utterances (Bloom & Lahey, 1978; Wetherby et al., 1988).

6. The clinician must be able to analyze utterances from one to four words in length.

7. Early multiwords are analyzed in a way that is different from the analysis of later syntax (Bloom & Lahey, 1978; Bowerman, 1973; Brown, 1973; Leonard et al., 1983), typically by using semantic grammars.

8. The clinician should be sensitive to later developing forms present with the early multiwords (e.g., word endings, function words) to project development into later stages (Lahey, 1988; Miller, 1981).

Appendix D contains a suggested coding transcription sheet for use with the analysis. The clinician should first write down the child's utterance either phonetically or orthographically, then follow this transcription with the immediate interpretation of a semantic relation and function. Thus, the first three columns can be filled out at the time of each utterance. The video can be replayed for problematic utterances. This procedure could be used as a preliminary part of an assessment to find out basic semantic relations and functions in a child's communication. It can also be carried forward as a means of monitoring treatment progress. From the data, later analysis can determine the percentage of child-initiated versus adult-initiated utterances as well as the percentage of the use of each function and semantic relation in the sample. A summary sheet is presented in Appendix E. The remaining columns (4 to 6) of the transcription sheet can be filled out by the clinician subsequent to the evaluation session and can be used to complete the summary sheet. When a child is leaving the early multiword period, he or she has reached a mean length of utterance of over 2.25. At this point, the acquisition of a variety of syntactic conventions begins to emerge.

Assessment of Children's Early Language Comprehension

Confounding Factors: Nonlinguistic Context

Children's responses to language are determined by many factors. That is, a child's correct response could be primarily in reaction to nonverbal, contextual aspects of the situation. The following is a typical scenario:

> The mother says, "He can understand everything that we tell him. He just doesn't talk." The clinician leans forward and says, "Can you show me how you know he understands what you tell him?" The mother shifts uncomfortably in her chair and tells the child to "go turn off the light," as she points alternately between the light switch and the ceiling fixture. The child turns the light off and on several times. Later when the mother was told to provide only verbal stimuli, the child was not able to perform many one- and two-level commands if they were unaccompanied by gestures.

Thus, children and adults rely on the context in which language is used to aid in interpretation of what was said.

Confounding Factors: Comprehension Strategies

Chapman (1978) discussed the notion of "comprehension strategies" exhibited by children. According to Chapman, a *comprehension strategy* is "a short cut, heuristic or algorithm for arriving at sentence meaning without full marshaling of the information in the sentence and one's linguistic knowledge. Thus, it sometimes yields the correct answer, although it may more usually give the appearance of understanding" (p. 310). Clinicians who attempt to assess early language comprehension should be wary of correct responses by children that could have been generated by attention to contextual stimuli or comprehension strategies. An example would be that many children process the name of an object and then act on the object in a habitual manner. This behavior gives the appearance of knowing an entire sentence (e.g., "Throw the ball"), when in actuality the child may understand only the word "ball" and simply throws it as he usually would. Chapman gives many other comprehension strategies, and we encourage clinicians to become familiar with these patterns.

We have suggested that comprehension is difficult to test without contaminating influences from the context and comprehension strategies. Understanding of single words in young children appears to us to be the easiest to test. The clinician should make sure that objects are maximally separated in the evaluation room so that it will be clear which item the child turns toward when the examiner names it. If the child directs his or her attention to or retrieves the appropriate object when its name is uttered by an examiner (with appropriate controls for contextual cues), the child probably recognizes the lexical item. We begin to run into trouble when we try to test two-word utterances and larger sentences. Edmonston and Thane (1992) point out the difficulty in assessing relational words because of comprehension strategies. Some attempts have been made to remove the effects of context and comprehension strategies by using anomalous commands in the testing of children (Kramer, 1977). This technique involves giving to children commands that they are not likely to expect from their past experience. A child may be told to "Sit on the ball" or "Kiss the phone." If the child performs, he or she is said to have comprehended both elements in the command. If the child does not perform (and this is where we run into the problem again), is it that he or she has not understood? Perhaps anomalous commands are "silly" to children and are disregarded. There may be a cognitive mismatch between the command and the child's knowledge of the object's typical use. At any rate, failure to perform an anomalous command may not really mean lack of comprehension. The clinician should also not avoid more naturalistic assessment methods such as engaging the child in play or conversation and evaluating the appropriateness of verbal and nonverbal responses. Only a few standardized assessments have been designed to assess the receptive language of children under the age of 3. For example, the *Peabody Picture Vocabulary Test,* Fourth Edition (PPVT-IV; Dunn, & Dunn, 2007); *Receptive One-Word Picture Vocabulary Test,* Fourth Edition (ROWPVT-4; Martin & Brownell, 2010); and CSBS evaluate single-word receptive vocabulary. Several popular instruments rely on parental reports to gauge receptive lexicon size. For example, in *MacArthur-Bates Communicative Development Inventories* (Fenson et al., 1993), normative data are provided on lexical comprehension based on parental reports. However, parent checklists' for assessing receptive vocabulary have been found to be less reliable than those assessing expressive vocabulary, for reasons mentioned previously in this chapter (Dale, 1991; Thal, O'Hanlon, Clemmons, & Franklin, 1999).

Chapter 5 outlines some additional considerations in assessing language comprehension in older children.

Assessment of Utterances Using Length Measures

One of the most common measures recommended for use in a basic language evaluation is the *mean length of utterance (MLU)* (Miller, 1981). Length measures are not new in speech pathology and were used historically as a mainstay of our clinical repertoire. Early measurements included the mean length of response (MLR), in which the clinician segments the language sample into utterances, counts the number of words in each utterance, and divides by the number of utterances in the sample. This yields the average number of words per utterance. Later, clinicians began to use the MLU, which represents the average number of morphemes (free and bound) per utterance. The MLU gives the child credit for mastering bound morphemes such as plurals, possessives, progressives, and regular past tense, among many others.

There are several reasons that authorities have continued to recommend computing a length measure on utterances obtained in a language sample. First, there is a general correlation between the MLU and chronological age in many groups of children up to age 4 (Miller, 1981). Thus, the MLU may be used as a very gross indicator of language development in children up to age 4, but the clinician cannot simply rely on length measures alone in an analysis. A second important reason for computing MLU on a child is that Brown (1973) has used this length measure to demarcate his five stages of language development. Allegedly, MLU is a much better predictor of language development than is chronological age. Brown (1973) has postulated that if two children are matched on MLU, a clinician may predict that the constructional complexity of their language will be similar. Brown (1973) and Miller (1981) provide suggestions for the computation of MLU. Miller (1981) recommends a distributional analysis to ensure that the MLU has a relatively normal distribution around an average length. The analysis is simply a listing of the number of utterances at each morpheme level (e.g., 1, 2, 3, 4). If the distributional analysis reveals an MLU with a small variation, perhaps an organic condition or sampling error has played a role in the length of utterance. Johnston et al. (1993) found that children with language impairments tended to respond to questions with higher proportions of elliptical utterances compared to normal-language children. This finding certainly could affect MLU measures by increasing sampling error. Table 4–9 shows the general relations among Brown's stages, chronological age, and MLU data taken from Miller and Chapman (1981). One obvious point in these data is that the variability, as reflected in the standard deviations, generally increases with age. Research on temporal reliability for older children has also been published (Chabon, Udolf, & Egolf, 1982). These investigators report that MLU has weak temporal reliability in older children, and its use for prediction of language level may be less sensitive than previously thought.

The data from Miller and Chapman (1981) were gathered on a relatively small sample from the Madison, Wisconsin, area. It is axiomatic that any data we gather will reflect the characteristics of the sample of people tested. Thus, we would not expect every study on MLU to agree exactly with one another. There have been more recent attempts to provide MLU norms for clinical use. Much of the data on MLU that clinicians use in practice come from studies done over 30 years ago with relatively small samples. A more recent source of carefully gathered data comes from the Systematic Analysis of Language Transcripts (SALT) database (Miller & Chapman, 2008). This database has been developed since the 1980s and has been updated with each new version of the analysis software. The most recent MLU data come from Rice, Smolik, Perpich, Thompson, Rytting, and Blossom (2010) on 306 children, and the data are fairly evenly divided between children with language impairment and those who were typically developing. The data were very carefully gathered and the populations were meticulously described. The results for the typically developing children show, as in prior research, that MLU increases systematically with age, and that even the children with language impairment made gains as they got older, although they never caught up to the typically developing sample. Rice et al. (2010) show fairly reliable changes in MLU even in older age groups, which may be at odds with earlier research. These new data will be of great interest and utility to practicing clinicians.

TABLE 4–9
Relationships among Language Development, Chronological Age,
and Mean Length of Utterance

Brown's Stage	Chronological Age (±1 Month)	Predicted MLU and Standard Deviation (in Parentheses)
Stage I: relations or roles within the simple sentence (MLU 1.75)	18 months	1.31 (0.325)
	21 months	1.62 (0.386)
	24 months	1.92 (0.448)
Stage II: Modulations of meaning within the simple sentence (MLU 2.25)	27 months	2.23 (0.510)
	30 months	2.54 (0.571)
Stage III: Modalities of the simple sentence (MLU 2.75)	33 months	2.85 (0.633)
	36 months	3.16 (0.694)
Stage IV: Embedding of one sentence within another (MLU 3.50)	39 months	3.47 (0.756)
	42 months	3.78 (0.817)
Stage V: Coordination of simple sentences	45 months	4.09 (0.879)
	48 months	4.40 (0.940)
	51 months	4.71 (1.002)
	54 months	5.02 (1.064)
	57 months	5.32 (1.125)
	60 months	5.63 (1.187)

Source: Adapted from Brown (1973) and Miller and Chapman (1981).

We should always remember that MLU is not an objective measure such as height or weight. It is hopelessly entangled with the type of sample that is obtained by the clinician. Muma (1998) has shown that while the typical language sample size in our field is between 50 to 100 utterances, sampling error rates are very high until one analyzes samples of 200 to 400 utterances. Clearly, the larger the sample size, the better and probably more stable the grammatical and length measures that are calculated. The norms for MLU are presently reported on a rather narrow population, and further data gathering is necessary for different socioeconomic and cultural groups. The use of MLU may presently be in a state of transition, but until more conclusive data and viable alternatives are provided, we feel that MLU should be routinely calculated in a language evaluation of limited-language children. The rules for counting morphemes can be found in Table 4–10.

Infant, Toddler, and Family Assessment

The Individuals with Disabilities Education Act of 2004 (IDEA) mandates that the school speech-language pathologist assess and treat children between the ages of 3 and 5. Speech-language pathologists in many states are currently serving the birth-to-age-5 population, and this will no doubt become the norm. This section of the chapter provides some references for SLPs faced with the assessment of infants and toddlers.

TABLE 4–10
Rules for Assigning Morphemes to Utterances

1. Morphemes should be assigned to 100 consecutive utterances that represent the child's language abilities.
   a. Utterances should be consecutive and not selectively chosen because that could result in an inflated MLU.
   b. Avoid selecting utterances that include the child responding to high number of yes or no questions. Single-word responses to questions will artificially lower MLU.
2. Only assign morphemes to utterances that are intelligible.
   a. Do not assign morphemes to any repeated, partially intelligible, unintelligible, or interrupted utterances.
3. When stuttering or a false start occurs, assign morphemes to the complete form as if it were spoken fluently (e.g., "Her, her cat is black," count as "her cat is black").
   a. If a child repeats for emphasis or clarification, count all words (e.g., "her cat is really, really big").
4. Assign morphemes to short words like *hi* and *yes*.
   a Do not assign morphemes to fillers (e.g., *um, uh*).
5. Compound words (e.g. *mailman, baseball*) and related words (e.g., *good-bye)* should be counted as single words and assigned only one morpheme.
   a. Also, only one morpheme is assigned to indefinite and reflexive compound pronouns (e.g., *something, nobody, himself*).
6. Proper nouns (e.g. *the Statue of Liberty, Mr. Jones*) and ritualized reduplications (e.g., *choo-choo, night-night*) should be counted as single words.
7. Diminutive forms of words (e.g., *kitty, daddy, Willy*) should be counted as only one morpheme.
8. Auxiliary verbs (e.g., *will, have, may*) are assigned only one morpheme.
9. Catenative forms (e.g., *y'all = you all; wanna = want to*) are assigned only one morpheme.
10. Assign one additional morpheme to words that contain inflectional affixes (i.e., plural *–s*, singular and plural possessive *–s*, present third-person singular *–s*, regular past-tense *–ed*, past participle *–ed* and *–en*, present participle *–ing*, comparative *–er*, and superlative *–est).*
    a. If inflection is used incorrectly, it should not be counted as a separate morpheme (e.g., *wented*).
11. Assign only one morpheme to words that have inflections marked on gerunds and predicate adjectives (e.g., "*jumping* is hard"; "I am *tired*"). They are not counted as verb tense inflections.
12. Irregular past-tense and past-participle forms (e.g., *done, rung*) receive only one morpheme. Negative contractions are assigned two morphemes (e.g., *can't, isn't, haven't*) if the child uses both parts of the contraction independently within the transcript (e.g.,*can* and *not*).
    a. Only assign one morpheme if each part is not used independently.
13. Nonnegative contractions receive two morphemes (e.g., *I'm, we've, you'll*).
14. Derivational affixes are assigned their own morphemes (e.g., *re–, un–, –non, –ly, –ful, –ness*).

Source: Adapted from Brown (1973) and Retherford (2000).

Many categories of infants and children are at risk for communication disorders. There is a host of syndromes (e.g., Turner, 18Q, Down, Hurlers, Morquio, Goldenhar, Mohr, Treacher-Collins, etc.) with associated speech, language, and hearing problems (Clark, 1989). Also, communication disorders can result from a variety of other sources such as environmental toxins (mercury, lead, cadmium, fetal alcohol exposure), infections prior to birth (syphilis, rubella, congenital cytomegaloviris, toxoplasmosis), or postnatal acquired infections (herpes, otitis, streptococcus infections). Other groups such as premature infants and those suffering early respiratory distress or intracranial hemorrhages are also at high risk for communication disorders. In many cases, speech/

language problems are not necessarily the result of some insidious syndrome that directly attacks communication skills but more likely result from a condition that affects hearing or cognitive development (Paul, 2012). Children who have experienced maltreatment in the preschool years or prenatal alcohol exposure are especially vulnerable to manifold developmental delays across domains. Speech, language, and hearing are frequently affected, and communication disorders professionals will almost always be an important part of multidisciplinary teams working with these children and their families.

The good thing about early intervention is that children are being identified soon after birth, which allows the beginning of a dialogue between professionals and parents. Most states are now providing neonatal hearing screenings during the first weeks of life. Children who used to be identified as hearing impaired at 2 to 3 years of age when their speech/language development was delayed are now being found at birth. In many cases we can move to prevent or reduce the occurrence of secondary disorders such as speech/language problems if the early intervention is done effectively from the outset. The SLP is more frequently involved than ever before on evaluation and intervention teams working with high-risk infants and their families. Often, this population is intimidating to clinicians without experience serving infants and toddlers.

Assessment of infants and toddlers must involve several components: (1) assessment of the infant, (2) assessment of the family situation, (3) assessment of the primary caregiver, and (4) assessment of caregiver–child interaction patterns. Sparks (1989) provides some general guidelines for assessing the infant. First, the SLP should become intimately familiar with the child's prenatal and perinatal history. We must know the medical status of the child so that we can try to predict which types of communication disorders are likely to be associated with a particular syndrome or condition. This allows the SLP to take preventive measures against a variety of secondary impairments. Second, we should gain a general appreciation of the infant's ability to maintain homeostasis. This means learning how individual infants cope with handling, when they lose control, and how we need to help them to maintain respiration, thermal control, and proper nutrition (Sparks, 1989). Frequently used measures for this are the *Neonatal Behavioral Assessment Scale,* Fourth Edition (Brazelton & Nugent, 2011) and the *Assessment of Preterm Infant Behavior* (Als, Lester, Tronick, & Brazelton, 1982). Third, the child's oral-motor behavior is an important skill to evaluate. Often, these children have difficulty with feeding, and the speech-language pathologist is a primary participant in working with parents on evaluating and treating feeding disorders. Paul (2012) provides a useful overview of feeding assessment and intervention procedures for the SLP. Proctor (1989) provides an excellent description of vocal development and a detailed assessment protocol for use in evaluating infant oral/vocal skills. Developmental vocal assessment forms based on Proctor's protocol can be found in Paul (2012) or online though the American Speech-Language-Hearing Association (ASHA) website. Finally, the infant's hospital environment should be examined in terms of available stimulation and opportunities for communication. Often, these children are in neonatal intensive care units (NICUs) or in other hospital units, and these environments provide the child's only exposure to communication.

In terms of evaluating caregiver–infant interactions, numerous potential schemes are available (Cole & St. Clair-Stokes, 1984; Duchan & Weitzner-Lin, 1987; Klein & Briggs, 1987; Lifter, Edwards, Avery, Anderson, & Sulzer-Azaroff, 1988; McCollum & Stayton, 1985; Wetherby, Cain, Yonclas, & Walker, 1988). We are also interested in more basic issues, such as the availability of the caregiver and caregiver expectations about communication. The actual analysis of caregiver–child interaction embodies many behaviors discussed earlier in this chapter. Examine some of the references just listed for specific procedures.

Some team member, perhaps the SLP if he or she is the case manager, will participate in a family strengths and needs assessment. Bailey and Simeonsson (1988) provide procedures and suggestions for family assessment. With infants and toddlers, the assessments of family status and interaction patterns are as important as or even more significant than evaluation of the child. Without an intact family that functions adequately as a system, the planning and implementation of intervention cannot take place. Also, IDEA requires an individualized family service plan (IFSP), which specifies not only goals for the child but also objectives for the family as a unit. In most cases, the SLP will be an important part of a team of professionals who work with the family in assessing a child who is at risk for developmental delays. According to IDEA, and specifically Part C of this act, states must identify and provide early intervention services for children with established risks (e.g., hearing impairment), environmental risks (e.g., abuse, neglect), and biological risks (e.g., prematurity, respiratory distress) in the first 3 years of life. Working closely with the family, professionals must assist in developing an IFSP that documents information in several important areas: (1) the child's status in terms of present levels of functioning in areas that include physical, cognitive, communication, social, and emotional; (2) information on the family's strengths, needs, and concerns; (3) a list of measurable outcomes expected for the child and the family; (4) a detailed description of early intervention services, including frequency, intensity, methods, providers, and so on; (5) a description of any other services such as medical interventions; (6) a statement of projected duration of services; (7) a specification of who will be the service coordinator of the plan; and (8) a plan for transition from Part C services under the IFSP to IDEA services provided with an individualized education plan (IEP) in the school system. We bring up the IFSP here because it is clear that evaluation and assessment are an integral part of this process. It begins with an in-depth interview(s) with family members in which the SLP listens to concerns and preferred goals of the parents. To establish the child's present level of functioning in cognitive and communicative domains, the SLP must administer both standardized and nonstandardized assessments. The specification of measurable outcomes implies that assessment is ongoing and must continue through the intervention process to determine if progress is being made and if the goals need to be modified. Thus, it is not simply a clinician's arbitrary choice about what to do in early assessment/intervention; it is guided to a large extent by legal requirements.

Thus, assessing infants and toddlers typically involves a team approach, with the SLP working closely with social workers, psychologists, medical professionals, early childhood special educators, and others. As is typical for many other disorders, the SLP spends a large amount of time with families and is often placed in the role of counselor. Families of high-risk babies are faced with many challenges such as shock, grief, guilt, confusion, information overload, anger, fear, uncertainty, financial concerns, and the intrusion of too many professionals. Sometimes the SLP is a major source of support for the members of such families, who are going through perhaps the most difficult period of their lives.

One of the biggest challenges for the SLP is to train parents to recognize these various states in their child and to present communication stimulation at a time when it can do the most good. Stimulating language in a child who is too sleepy or too upset (e.g., crying) will only result in frustration for the parent and the child. Paul (2012) illustrates varying states of infant behavioral organization on a continuum ranging from (a) deep sleep, (b) light sleep, (c) drowsy, (d) quiet alert, (e) active alert, to (f) crying. It is important for parents and nursing staff to appreciate that the quiet alert state is optimal for language and communication and that infants can be moved from drowsy to quiet alert by gentle stimulation or from active alert to quiet alert by cuddling or consoling behaviors.

As a child matures, assessment must be continuous and ongoing because the goals during the first 6 months of life will differ from those in the following 6 months. As time goes on, the goals may shift from feeding to cognitive, to social, to linguistic. Therefore, the IFSP must be assessed and revised at regular intervals. Polmanteer and Turbiville (2000) and Paul (2012) provide examples of how IFSPs can be written in a family-responsive manner with language and goals that are not only relevant to the family but also intelligible to them.

Assessment of Special Populations

Communication Is the Major Focus

Because the nature of communication and language and the model to which we subscribe do not change with the client, the assessment of special populations should not be dramatically different from what we do with any child with a language disorder. That is, our business is still to assess the integrity of the communication system (cognitive, linguistic, social, pragmatic), and this process should be our focus, regardless of etiology. We feel, as do many others (Bloom & Lahey, 1978; Lahey, 1988; Paul, 2007), that the diagnostic group of which a child is a member contributes limited insight into his or her language impairment. Certainly, however, some characteristics are important to consider in evaluating specific populations. Paul (2012) and Nelson (2010) provide an excellent overview of the research on communication skills associated with intellectual disability, sensory deficits (blindness, hearing impairment), psychiatric disorders, specific language disorder, maternal substance abuse, attention deficit disorder/attention deficit hyperactivity disorder (ADD/ADHD), pervasive developmental disorders (PDDs), autism, traumatic brain injury, and acquired aphasia. The clinician should be familiar with this information because it helps in parent counseling as well as in knowing what to expect in an evaluation. Still, no matter what a child's etiology, the clinician's major tasks are to determine the child's linguistic capability and the status of cognitive/social/biological abilities, as well as to explore the child's use of language in the natural environment.

Increased Probability of Focusing Assessment on Precommunicative Areas

Working with special populations increases the probability of having to assess biological, social, and cognitive prerequisites to language. Some limited-language children are cognitively impaired (Cosby & Ruder, 1983; Kamhi & Johnston, 1982; Rogers, 1977; Weisz & Zigler, 1979). The clinician must be certain that the child possesses the cognitive abilities necessary for learning a particular symbol system in terms of being able to deal with its abstraction level (objects, pictures, words, gestures, etc.). Many children with autism have also been reported to have cognitive difficulties, and the clinician should attempt to gain insight into this area in the evaluation (Clune, Paolella, & Foley, 1979; Curcio, 1978; Rutter, 1978). Children with autism are frequently reported to be socially withdrawn, and their general nonverbal social interaction may have to be modified as part of a treatment program if they are expected to use functional communication (Baltaxe & Simmons, 1975; Opitz, 1982). One of the earlier indicators of autism is the absence or reduced production of protodeclarative gestures such as pointing to regulate adult attention. Current research suggests that a diagnosis of autism spectrum disorder (ASD) can be made reliably at 24 months (Woods & Wetherby, 2003). Many variables appear to be predictive: Impairments in social interaction and impairments in communication are early signs, and these are observable by 24 months. Use of restricted and repetitive activities/interests is usually not seen until closer to 36 months. Klinger and Dawson (1992) have found that children with ASD lacked the four following critical behaviors: pointing, showing objects, looking at the face of another, and orienting to their name. Woods and Wetherby (2003) suggested that failure to meet any of the following milestones should result in further evaluation: no babbling by 12 months, no gesturing by 12 months, no single words by 16 months, no spontaneous two-word combinations by 24 months, or any loss of any language or social skills at any age. These indicators are not just for ASD but for any developmental disorder. For children with autism, Prizant and Wetherby (1988) recommend assessment areas that are highly similar to those previously advocated for any child with a language impairment. Thus, one implication of special populations is that they may involve the clinician in a more broadly based analysis of both precommunicative as well as communicative behaviors presented by the child, coupled with a detailed analysis of the environment using the family as collaborators (Prelock, Beatson, Bitner, Broder, & Ducker, 2003).

Increased Possibility of Recommending Augmentative/Alternative Communication Modes

Another aspect involved in dealing with special populations is that the clinician has an increased probability of prescribing a nonverbal/nonvocal response mode or augmentative communication device. Research has shown that children with cognitive impairment or autism may benefit from training in nonverbal communication modes, and that using an augmentative and alternative communication (AAC) system may even increase communication attempts and speech production (Bondy & Frost 1998; Silverman, 1995). In a recent systematic review of research, however, Schlosser and Wendt (2008) found that while AAC speech treatments may result in more speech production, the gains were described as "modest," and we must be realistic in our expectations.

Thus, it may be incumbent on the diagnostician to determine the potential that a given client may have for learning a nonvocal system. Beukelman and Mirenda (1992) provide an excellent overview of the factors that should be considered in assessment and intervention with augmentative and alternative communication techniques. Clinicians who do formal evaluations in the area of augmentative communication should have specialized training and experience in this arena before prescribing a nonvocal mode for a client.

Prognostic Implications

Special populations, as a whole, generally have a poorer prognosis than do language-impaired children without complicating difficulties. The prognosis worsens in proportion to the number of ancillary problems that the child exhibits (hearing impairment, neuromotor involvement, intellectual disability, absent caretakers, etc.). Also, the existence of ancillary problems increases the likelihood that a larger multidisciplinary team will be involved in the evaluation. The assistance of special educators, audiologists, psychologists, and medical personnel is necessary and invaluable to the clinician in making treatment recommendations for children from special populations. As dictated by federal legislation, the SLP has the opportunity to collaborate in staff meetings with other professionals to discuss the assessment and treatment of language-disordered children. We have found this, in most cases, to be stimulating and in the best interest of all concerned, especially in early-language cases.

Noting Specific Characteristics

With certain types of children, the diagnostician should make an inventory of characteristic behaviors that may need to be modified in the treatment program. For instance, children with autism and/or cognitive impairments have been reported to engage in self-stimulatory behaviors (hand flapping, making vocal sounds, rocking, etc.). Some authorities believe that new learning cannot effectively take place while the child is in a self-stimulatory state. Thus, one goal of treatment might be to reduce the occurrence of self-stimulation, and these behaviors should be catalogued by the diagnostician. In these populations there have also been many reports of self-abusive behaviors. These should also be noted by the clinician as potential considerations in planning treatment. Bopp, Brown, and Mirenda (2004) describe the process of functional behavior assessment. This includes functional assessment interviews where the clinician asks for descriptions of problem behaviors, contextual and antecedent factors that predict behaviors, and consequences following occurrence of problem behaviors. A second component of functional assessment is direct observation. A final component involves functional analysis of the behavior to determine the effects of various consequences on the occurrence of the behavior. While functional behavior assessment was historically the province of psychologists and other professionals, current practice involves teachers, parents, and SLPs in the process.

Assessing Children from Culturally and Linguistically Different Backgrounds

Learning language in a bilingual environment does not negatively affect first-language learning in children with normal intelligence (Owens, 2012) or even children with Down syndrome (Bird, Cleave, Trudeau, Thordardottir, Sutton, & Thorpe, 2005). Speech-language pathologists are frequently called on to assess children who come to the United States through international adoption. These children represent many different languages and cultures, and arrive in the country as infants or toddlers. Although this kind of assessment is challenging, research has shown that assessing prelinguistic communication and vocabulary comprehension using measures such as the Communication and Symbolic Behavior Scales and the MacArthur-Bates Communicative development scales reliably predicted language outcomes at age 2 (Glennen, 2007). Research has shown that many children who are adopted from overseas ultimately perform well by school age. For example, Scott, Roberts, and Krakow (2008) found that a cohort of children adopted from China performed at the average or above-average level on tests of oral and written language in the early elementary grades.

Brown (1973) has noted striking similarities in children's early language acquisition cross culturally. That is, children from a variety of cultures tend to develop the same types of early word combinations, presumably because these semantic relations rest on concepts developed in the sensorimotor period of cognitive development. While we may not find differences in word combinations across cultures, there may certainly be variations in prelinguistic and single-word development in various groups. However, cross-cultural studies of caretaker–child interaction have demonstrated cultural differences in interaction style, play, speech register, use of objects in joint referencing, parenting, family values and beliefs, and general opportunities for interaction (Bornstein, Tal, & Tamis-Lemonda, 1991; Bornstein et al., 1991; Fogel, Toda, & Kawai, 1988; Heath, 1983, 1989; Saville-Troike, 1986; Schieffelin, 1985; Watson-Gegeo & Gegeo, 1986).

It is important for clinicians to be culturally and linguistically competent and to realize that all cultural groups have differences and similarities to one another. These potential cultural differences in caregiver–child interaction must be taken into account as the clinician examines parents and children in clinical settings. Social interactions and selection of activities for joint referencing may be very different in the home environment, and we should not expect everyone to interact in the same way when using mainstream toys and objects provided in clinical settings. Clinicians must endeavor to learn more about child rearing and interaction in different cultures and should not impose ethnocentric views on the families we serve.

When faced with the challenge of establishing whether there is a language difference or disorder, the dominant language or primary language needs to be determined. To meet the spirit of *least biased assessment* outlined in Part B of IDEA, testing should be provided in a manner that is consistent with the child's most proficient language. This can include both standardized and nonstandardized forms of assessment. Language dominance can be established through observation of communication behaviors in a variety of settings (e.g., home or preschool) or structured questionnaires (Kayser, 1995). If a majority of the language observed is in the child's home language or if gestures are significantly relied upon when English is required, then it would be appropriate to determine that English is not the dominant language. Numerous structured questionnaires can be used to establish language dominance. For example, the *Assessment Instrument for Multicultural Clients* (Adler, 1991) and *Bilingual Language Proficiency Questionnaire* (Mattes & Santiago, 1985) are available in addition to resources that can be found online through ASHA.

Under the most ideal circumstances, a child would be evaluated by a clinician who speaks the dominant language with standardized and nonstandardized measures that are designed for, and have normative or criterion-referenced information available in, the client's dominant language. In recent years we have begun to make large strides toward developing tests in language other than English, with the most common being Spanish. In Table 4–6 you will find a list of some the standardized and criterion-referenced assessments that are currently available in languages other than English. However, tests are not often available in a client's native language. Suggestions for modifying, adapting, or translating standardized assessments can be found in Brice (2002), Goldstein (2000), Kayser (1995), and Wyatt (2002). Clinicians need to be wary, however, of test equivalence issues that can develop when translating or modifying a test (Kwan, Gong, & Maestas, 2010).

Consolidating Data and Arriving at Treatment Recommendations

Even if the diagnostician adheres to an integrative model of language, the assessment process tends to fragment the child and the information obtained in the evaluation to a certain degree. Before arriving at treatment recommendations, suggestions for further testing, or referral decisions, the clinician should pause and take stock of what has been done in the assessment process. We have found it useful and insightful to summarize the following areas (see Appendix F).

Data Obtained in the Evaluation

This section refers to the actual behaviors observed and procedures administered to a child in the evaluation. It does not include the different analyses of the data. For instance, a spontaneous language sample can be subjected to a variety of analyses (MLU, form-function analysis, phonological analysis, etc.). At the end of an evaluation, a clinician will often be struck by the need for additional data that may be obtained in the initial phase of treatment. We sometimes wonder why we cannot make clinical judgments about certain aspects of a child's language, and then we find that we did not gather all of the data necessary to make these decisions. Appendix F provides a checklist for clinicians to use in summarizing the data collected.

Analyses Performed on the Data

This section of the model allows the clinician summarize the analysis procedures performed on the data collected. On the surface, this procedure may appear to be rather simplistic; because language has so many aspects that may be important to assess, however, it is easy to forget to gather certain data or perform certain analyses.

Areas of Concern and Strength

By examining the data and analyses of the communicative process and language development stages, the clinician will be impressed with areas of normality, strength, and concern. The clinician should look for patterns in the data that are revealed when a judgment must be made about the overall effectiveness of each area in the language model. For instance, a clinician may have concerns in the biological prerequisite area over poor motor coordination and remarkable birth and developmental histories. The same child may have performed poorly on cognitive tasks, and the clinician questions whether the child needs work on the conceptual bases for language development. Similarly, on social areas of the model, the child is not operating according to age level and is not exhibiting optimal social prerequisites for communication. Adaptive behavior scales show a delay in all areas of development. In the language development area, the child turns out to be nonverbal. When the clinician checks the areas of concern and strength, the child will get a minus (−) under biological prerequisites for neurological areas and minuses for social areas of play partner and reciprocity. The child would also earn minuses on the cognitive prerequisites of play level, sensorimotor substage, and symbolic play. Finally, the child would receive minuses for most categories in single-word, phonology, and early-multiword combination areas. By examining the summary statements, the clinician can develop a profile of areas of strength and concern for each case. If no clear-cut statement for concern or strength can be made, then the clinician should examine the data gathered and the analyses performed to determine if enough information has been accumulated. In most cases, an inability to make a general statement about areas of the model is due to insufficient information, poor-quality information, or insufficient analysis.

Recommendations

The areas that are covered in the recommendation section revolve around three topics. First, the child may require referral to other professionals to obtain further information. For instance, referral to a psychologist or special educator may be warranted to determine the child's cognitive ability and potential for learning. Audiometric referral may be another common need. Second, the clinician may have been unable to perform certain tests or analyses because of time constraints or lack of cooperation by the child. Before specific treatment recommendations can be made, more data may be required. By examining the sections on data obtained and analyses performed, the clinician can determine this need.

Third, if enough data were obtained and analyses performed, the clinician is in a position to make treatment recommendations. By examining the child's areas of strength and concern, the clinician can consider intervention avenues that are the most appropriate. For instance, if a child is biologically, cognitively, and socially ready for communicative development and the clinician has located the child in the language development process, an appropriate goal might be to begin concentrating on the language forms that develop next according to the acquisition literature and the child's need to communicate. If the child is normal in most respects and the major concern is intelligibility, then this carries with it a phonological treatment priority. If the child has cognitive and social problems in addition to language delay, then some of the treatment goals might include these areas (facilitating cognitive development, improving social nonverbal skills, etc.). The areas of concern and strength also carry with them prognostic implications. To date, we really have no certain method of computing a given child's prognosis for success in language treatment. So many variables relate to the child's capacities, skills, motivation, environment, caretaker participation, time in treatment, and so forth. One approach to prognosis that will probably reflect reality is to regard the child who elicits fewer concerns in the major areas of the model as having a more favorable prognosis than one who has many deficiencies.

CONCLUSION AND SELF-ASSESSMENT

We have attempted to show that assessment of limited-language children is no simple matter. It requires that the clinician learn a multitude of skills and read literature that covers wide-ranging topics in order to perform it competently. The diagnosis of language disorder requires more than just a single test or procedure. It demands that the clinician examine the communicative process differently for children of varying communicative levels and cultures.

After reading this chapter you should be able to answer the following questions:

1. How does a child progress through different stages of development to become an effective communicator?
2. What are the three general categories of children with limited language? What assessment parameters should be considered within each corresponding category?
3. What types of challenges and difficulties does an SLP encounter when engaging in the process of language assessment?
4. What are Muma's six diagnostic precepts that can inform an SLP's approach to language assessment?
5. Why is the preassessment portion of an evaluation important, and what types of information should be gathered during this portion of the assessment?
6. Why is evaluation of the caretaker–child interaction informative, and what parameters need to be considered during this observation?
7. How does a child's adaptive behavior inform our understanding of language development, and what parameters need to be considered when evaluating this domain?
8. What information can be gained from play assessment, and how could a clinician evaluate the parameters of play?
9. Why is it necessary to consider communicative intent and function? What factors are considered during this portion of an evaluation?
10. What assessment methods should be considered in the assessment of single-word utterances?
11. What assessment methods should be considered in the assessment of multiword utterances?
12. What are some confounding factors that should be considered when evaluating language comprehension?
13. When should measures of utterance length be incorporated into a language evaluation, and how are they used to understand language development?
14. What factors need to be considered when assessing the language of children from culturally and/or linguistically different backgrounds?

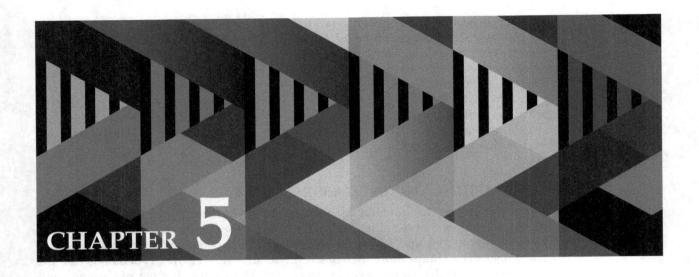

CHAPTER 5

Assessment of School-Age and Adolescent Language Disorders

LEARNING OUTCOMES

After reading this chapter you will be able to:

1. List and describe four groups of school-age students who have an increased likelihood of being diagnosed with a language disorder.

2. Describe the speech-language pathologist's role in screening school-age children.

3. Describe the purpose of the Common Core State Standards and implications for assessment.

4. Describe factors that require consideration when obtaining a language sample.

5. Describe the process of obtaining a language sample and the types of information that can be obtained from a language sample.

6. Describe measurements that require consideration when obtaining a language sample from a child who is later in her or his language development.

7. Outline factors that require consideration when assessing a child's language comprehension and where a breakdown in comprehension occurs.

8. Describe the four ways language comprehension is evaluated.

9. Outline some syntax analysis packages and the factors that require consideration when using a packaged analysis procedure.

10. Describe methods and factors that require consideration when conducting a pragmatic assessment.

11. Outline the process of obtaining a narrative sample and methods for analyzing narrative productions.

12. Describe the difference between analyzing the microstructure and macrostructure of narratives.

13. Outline what parameters can be evaluated when assessing conversational discourse.

14. Describe the impact that memory and executive functioning have on language assessment and diagnosis.

15. Describe the speech-language pathologist's role in evaluating reading disorders and areas that require assessment when a reading disorder is suspected.

16. Describe factors that require consideration when assessing written language.

The model by MacDonald and Carroll (1992) that was presented in Chapter 4 dealt with specific competencies required for communication development. Specifically, we talked about becoming *play partners, becoming turntaking partners,* and the beginning of developing a role as a *communicative partner* through the use of communicative intent, single-word, and early-multiword utterances. This chapter rounds out the last two components in the model by discussing the period when the child becomes a *language partner* through the use of semantic and grammatical rules. Finally, we will consider the child's becoming a *conversational partner* as pragmatic rules are developed to regulate the social use of language in a conversational context.

This chapter focuses on children who are speaking at the sentence level but may have difficulty with syntactic rules and who may also have deficiencies in semantics, pragmatics, metalinguistics, morphology, reading, writing, cognitive abilities, and general language processing. Thus, the assessment targets, tasks, and measurements we discuss in this chapter differ dramatically from those mentioned in Chapter 4. As Figure 5–1 indicates, however, the process of assessment remains the same. We are still interested in evaluating biological bases of communication, obtaining background information, performing standardized and nonstandardized testing, and evaluating the environments relevant to the child's communication. The areas of nonstandardized testing and evaluating relevant environments address pertinent aspects of the World Health Organization International Classification of Functioning, Disability and Health (ICF) model presented in Chapter 1.

Table 5–1 lists some common symptoms of language disorders in school-age and adolescent students. One can see that these symptoms span all areas of language and include comprehension as well as production impairments. There are also phonological disorders in this population that are addressed more fully in Chapter 6. When assessing morphosyntactic development, it is especially important to perform a careful evaluation of not only linguistic skills but also phonological abilities. The ability to produce final consonant clusters is certainly related to adding bound morphemes; however, it has been found that children with phonological disorder in addition to language impairment are at risk for morphosyntactic difficulties whether they can produce final consonant clusters or not (Haskill & Tyler, 2007).

Some of the symptoms in Table 5–1 are rather gross linguistic errors that would be easily detected in conversation (e.g., syntactic rule violations), whereas other errors are rather subtle and are discernible only with specialized communication sampling. Standardized tests may not reveal a subtle linguistic impairment in a school-age child (Plante & Vance, 1995). It is not unusual for an elementary-level student to pass many formal language tests and yet exhibit a significant linguistically based communication disorder. Many of these errors would only be seen in nonstandardized probing and conversational sampling. Similar difficulties have been found with some standardized language-screening instruments (Sturner, Heller, Funk, & Layton, 1993). Some surveys have indicated that the majority of public school speech-language pathologists (SLPs) routinely use a combination of formal (standardized) and informal (nonstandardized)

FIGURE 5–1
Critical Assessment Process in Later Language

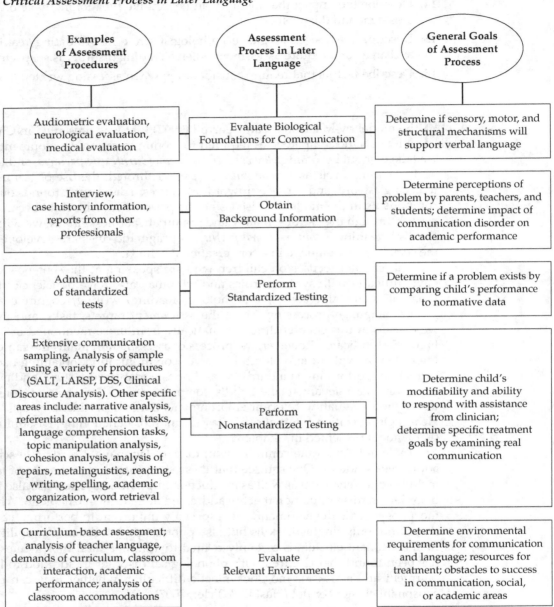

methods of assessment (Hux, Morris-Friehe, & Sanger, 1993; Wilson, Blackmon, Hall, & Elcholtz, 1991).

STUDENTS WITH LANGUAGE PROBLEMS: THE HIGH-RISK GROUPS

Several specific groups of school-age students have an increased likelihood of being diagnosed with a language disorder. We describe each group next.

TABLE 5–1
Common Symptoms of Language Disorders in Older Students

Semantics
- Word finding/retrieval deficits
- Use of a large number of words in an attempt to explain a concept because the name escapes them (circumlocutions)
- Overuse of limited vocabulary
- Difficulty recalling names of items in categories (e.g., animals, foods)
- Difficulty retrieving verbal opposites
- Small vocabulary
- Use of words lacking specificity (*thing, junk, stuff,* etc.)
- Inappropriate use of words (selection of wrong word)
- Difficulty defining words
- Less comprehension of complex words
- Failure to grasp double word meanings (e.g., *can, file*)
- Difficulty with figurative language

Syntax/Morphology
- Use of grammatically incorrect sentence structures
- Simple, as opposed to complex, sentences
- Less comprehension of complex grammatical structures
- Prolonged pauses while constructing sentences
- Semantically empty placeholders (e.g., filled pauses, use of *uh, er, um*)
- Use of many stereotyped phrases that do not require much language skill
- Use of "starters" (e.g., "You know . . .")

Pragmatics
- Use of redundant expressions and information the listener has already heard
- Use of nonspecific vocabulary (e.g., *thing, stuff*), and the listener cannot tell from prior conversation or physical context what is referred to
- Less skill in giving explanations clearly to a listener (lack of detail)
- Less skill in explaining something in a proper sequence
- Less conversational control in terms of introducing, maintaining, and changing topics (may get off track in conversation and introduce new topics awkwardly)
- Rare use of clarification questions (e.g., "I don't understand," "You did what?")
- Difficulty shifting conversational style in different social situations (e.g., peer versus teacher; child versus adult)
- Difficulty grasping the main idea of a story or lecture (preoccupation with irrelevant details)
- Trouble making inferences from material not explicitly stated (e.g., "Sally went outside. She had to put up her umbrella." Inference: It was raining.)

1. *History of language impairment as a preschooler.* Longitudinal studies of children who had language delays as preschoolers have shown a strong tendency for the emergence of academic and language problems as these youngsters get older (Aram & Nation, 1980; Bashir et al., 1983; Hall & Tomblin, 1978; King, Jones, & Lasky, 1982). Many of these studies suggest that over 50% of preschoolers with a history of language difficulties are at risk for academic and language problems. This is not just because of their "weakness" in the area of language but also because of increased academic difficulty and teacher language complexity as the child moves up the grade levels. Figure 5–2 shows the interaction of language ability, complexity of teacher language, and increased curricular demands as grade level increases. In the opinion of the authors of this text, the evidence suggests strongly that parents of preschoolers enrolled in language treatment, when they are dismissed from therapy, should be counseled about the possible

FIGURE 5–2
*Interactions of Language Ability, Teacher Language, and Curricular Demands
as Grade Level Increases*

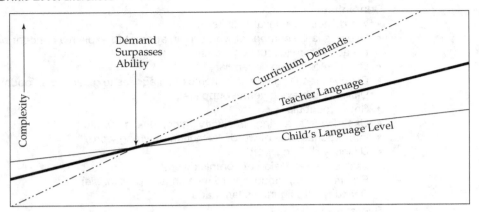

reemergence of language-based problems as the child is faced with increasing academic and linguistic complexity after entering school in the areas of English language arts, written language, reading, spelling, and mathematics.

More recently, Young et al. (2002) followed children with speech-only, speech and language, and language-only impairments into young adulthood to evaluate the academic outcomes associated with childhood language impairment. At the age of 19, they found that the children with speech-only difficulties had similar outcomes to the control group with no speech or language difficulties. However, the groups of children with language impairment were found to be behind the control group in several domains of academic achievement. The children with language impairment were found to be five times more likely than their non-language-impaired peers to experience academic difficulties that would merit classification as being learning disabled. Conti-Ramsden Durkin (2008) followed 118 typically developing children and 120 children with specific language impairment (SLI) into adolescence, taking data using parental and self-report measures related to independence of function in daily life. They found that, at age 16, the teenagers with a history of SLI were less independent than the typical group, and this was attributed to early language delay and poorer literacy skills in later years.

Johnson, Beitchman, and Brownlie (2010) followed a large sample of children identified as having language impairment at age 5 until they were 20 years old. They gathered data on family, education, occupation, and quality of life at four different time periods during the study. They found that the group with language impairments showed poorer outcomes at age 25 compared to a typically developing group in communication, cognitive, academic, educational attainment, and occupational status. The authors suggest that this information might be useful in planning treatment goals to target these issues and in counseling with clients and parents.

2. *Students with learning and/or reading disabilities.* The literature on learning disabilities has consistently supported the notion that the largest percentage of children diagnosed with reading and learning problems have either a history of language impairment or current linguistic difficulties (Beitchman, Wilson, Brownlie, Walters, & Lancee, 1996; Catts, Fey, Tomblin, & Zhang, 2002; Maxwell & Wallach, 1984). Publications have referred to this population as language-learning disabled,

emphasizing the pivotal role of language in their impairment. If a student is receiving services for reading problems or a learning disability, there is an increased risk that some form of language disorder may be present as well (Pennington & Bishop, 2009). Peterson, Pennington, Shriberg, and Boada (2009) conducted a longitudinal investigation that evaluated the impact of language skills and speech sound disorders on literacy outcomes in 123 children as they progressed from 5 to 6 years of age to 7 to 9 years of age. They found that language impairment was predictive of a later reading disability, with composite scores on the Test of Language Development Primary (TOLD–P:3) related to syntax being a greater predictor than composites scores in semantics. The current evidence suggests that children with comorbid speech sound disorders and language impairments (LIs) are most susceptible to developing a reading disability (see Pennington & Bishop, 2009).

3. *Students with behavioral, emotional, and social difficulties.* The literature on children with behavioral, emotional, and social difficulties (BESD) is growing and reflects a category of children who are being identified as having special education needs (Lindsay & Dockrell, 2013). Behavioral difficulties include externalizing kinds of behaviors such as attention deficit disorder (ADD), ADD with hyperactivity (ADHD), and conduct disorders. Emotional difficulties include internalizing types of behaviors such as anxiety and depression. Social difficulties include problems developing and maintaining peer relationships. There is emerging evidence that children with language impairments are more likely to experience or exhibit higher levels of BESD when compared to peer groups without language impairment (Conti-Ramsden, Mok, Pickles, & Durkin, 2013; Durkin & Conti-Ramsden, 2007; Goh & O'Kearney, 2012; St. Clair, Pickles, Durkin, & Conti-Ramsden, 2011).

4. *Students who are academically at risk.* Simon (1989) refers to a group of children who have "fallen between the cracks" of the educational system. These are students who have not been diagnosed as having a language problem but who are floundering academically on a consistent basis. Simon suggests that a significant percentage, maybe as many as 50%, of these students exhibit linguistic problems in addition to their academic difficulties. Simms-Hill and Haynes (1992) studied fourth-grade students who were rated as academically at risk by their teachers. These children consistently earned grades lower than C, were not receiving any remedial services in speech/language or in any other area, and had no history of language delay. Simms-Hill and Haynes (1992) found that over 50% of these students scored low enough on three different language tests to warrant clinical concern.

Thus, one mechanism of detecting school-age children with language disorders is to examine carefully students from the four high-risk groups just mentioned. This survey could be done through teacher referral, screening, or formal testing as part of a team evaluation of at-risk children.

SCREENING SCHOOL-AGE AND ADOLESCENT LANGUAGE DISORDERS

As indicated in Chapter 4, the purpose of a screening is to determine whether there is potentially a language problem and whether a child would benefit from a more in-depth language evaluation. Sturner et al. (1994) describe two different types of screening that take place within a school system: mass screenings and secondary screenings. Mass screening involves screening the general population, whereas a secondary screening occurs as a result of being referred for another problem such as speech. Therefore, the purpose of a secondary screening is to check out and determine whether there are any concomitant communication problems that might accompany an identified area of deficit. Some clinicians who are conducting a language screening will use locally developed or informal methods for screening school-age children and adolescents. While it is not particularly unusual to use these informal methods, it is not ideal, in our opinion. Screeners, just like any other assessment, should be tested for fairness and have robust psychometric properties. A screener's reliability, validity, sensitivity, and specificity, especially with regard to culturally and linguistically diverse populations, could be questionable and prove to be unfair when using informal or locally developed methods. Screenings conducted without norms and using solely clinical intuition or subjective criteria are inherently more likely to result in error.

Other clinicians use standardized methods or tests. *The Adolescent Language Screening Test* (ALST; Morgan & Guilford, 1984) provides a mechanism to screen children ages 11 to 17 years of age. It screens language use, content, and form through seven subtests that evaluate pragmatics, receptive vocabulary, concepts, expressive vocabulary, sentence formulation, morphology, and phonology. Also available is the *Screening Test of Adolescent Language- Revised* (STAL-R; Prather, Van Ausdal Breecher, Stafford, & Wallace, 1980). It identifies students between the ages of 11 and 18 with deficient language skills by measuring receptive and expressive vocabulary, auditory memory, language processing, and proverb explanation. And the *Clinical Evaluation of Language Fundamentals—Screening Test,* Fifth Edition (Semel, Wiig, & Secord, 2013) evaluates children 5 to 21 years of age in the areas of expressive morphology, syntax, receptive concepts, semantics, auditory comprehension, and pragmatics.

Regardless of the screener used, to be useful, it should be comprehensive enough to assess multiple domains of language to screen for language impairment. The efficiency with which this can be accomplished is another consideration. The feasibility of conducting a 15- to 20-minute screening on each child during a mass screening of, say, 750 children in an elementary school is questionable. While still unadvised, it is easy to see why some clinicians resort to locally developed and quick screening methods. With that said, teachers are an invaluable resource for screening. The teachers spend an enormous amount of time around the children in their classes and are usually pretty good at identifying when a child is struggling or experiencing deficits in a given area. Most schools also have their teachers administer curricular-based assessments, which are administered on a schoolwide basis, to track student progress. Poor performance on one of these assessments can serve as an initial red flag or trigger for more in-depth evaluation. For example, some schools use DIBELS (Dynamic Indicators of Basic Early Literacy) to evaluate the acquisition of literacy skills in kindergarten through sixth grade. This particular assessment includes multiple subtests and evaluates phonological awareness, alphabet knowledge, reading fluency, vocabulary, and reading comprehension. It is easy to see how failure to perform well on one or multiple parts of this assessment could be an indicator that a child needs to be evaluated for underlying language impairment. Comprehensive assessments used by the schools in an effort to assess requirements associated with the Common Core State Standards are also emerging and can serve as a guide for decisions about screening a child for a language disorder. These assessments are designed to assess and monitor student progress in the areas of language, reading, and writing, as well as other domains associated with the common core, like mathematics. The assessments adopted by a state could easily be used for screening and making decisions on whether a referral for a more in-depth language evaluation is warranted.

Most screenings have pass/fail criteria. If a child passes a general mass screening and there is no presenting concern from the parents or teachers, then the clinician can generally feel fairly confident in the favorable outcome. If a child passes the screening and there is documented concern about the child's language abilities, then the therapist should consider the following questions: (1) Did the screener evaluate the domain of language where the trouble exists? (2) Is a recommendation for a more in-depth evaluation justified? (3) Should it be recommended that the child be rescreened at a later time to monitor for improvement or decline? (4) Would a referral to another professional (e.g., psychologist, counselor, audiologist) be appropriate? If a child fails the screening and there was no presenting concern from parents or teachers, then the SLP should question whether there are any cultural or linguistic variables that could have contributed to the screening failure and recommend further evaluation to rule out a language disorder. If the child fails the screening and there were presenting concerns, then the child should be referred for a comprehensive language evaluation.

UNDERSTANDING COMMON CORE STATE STANDARDS

Due to concerns related to state-to-state rigor or differences in state-to-state criteria and test outcomes, national standards termed *Common Core State Standards* (CCSS, published in 2010) were developed. This effort, driven by the Council of Chief State School Officers and the National Governors Association, aims to provide learning objectives that would better prepare students for college and career expectations. Specifically, the CCSS standards were designed with a focus on promoting critical thinking, problem solving, and analytical thinking. The CCSS were published in 2010. In 2014, 45 states, the District of Columbia, and three U.S territories had adopted the two domains within the CCSS: *English Language Arts and Literacy in History/Social Studies, Science and Technical Subjects (2010a)*, and *Mathematics (2010b)*. Within each domain, the CCSS contain a hierarchy of knowledge and skills that a child should know when he or she finishes kindergarten through 12th grade. Information on the common core and the standards can be found at www.corestandards.org.

The CCSS standards have a few implications for assessment. First, the standards should guide assessment, and each state needs to have a mechanism in place that enables summative assessment and program evaluation for the two domains. K–12 grade-specific standards define end-of-year expectations and cumulative progression. Second, there is a clear focus on long-term outcomes at the end of each academic year and across grades K–12. Third, there must be established benchmarks that work toward the long-term outcomes and the summative assessment at the termination of each grade. Given that a student's success in the CCSS is dependent on communicative competence, the SLP has a distinct role in the implementation of CCSS. Ehren, Blosser, Roth, Paul, and Nelson (2012) describe how SLPs can become actively involved in implementing the CCSS:

- SLPs provide support for curriculum mastery by addressing linguistics and meta-linguistic foundations with children in general and special education.
- SLPs will be called upon to make sure that foundational language and emergent literacy skills are where they need to be for a child to meet the CCSS.
- SLPs will be called upon to assess and diagnose whether there is an underlying language deficit that is contributing to a child not being able to meet the CCSS.
- SLPs will be asked to assess and determine whether there are language skills or strategies that could help a child meet the CCSS.

USE OF STANDARDIZED TESTS WITH SYNTAX-LEVEL CHILDREN

As we indicated in Chapter 3, formal tests are best suited to comparing performance on a particular measure to the performance of same-age peers who took the test under similar conditions. Standardized tests address the issue of whether or not a problem exists. These measures are not particularly good at defining the nature of the problem or helping in the selection of treatment targets. We recommend that clinicians always use a standardized test to document the existence of a language disorder; most work settings require the use of such instruments as part of determining eligibility for services. Even if a child "passes" a standardized test, however, a language-based communication disorder may still exist. Many children's language disorders are not exposed until a conversational sample is elicited by the clinician or until the child's language abilities are challenged by increased difficulty on academic tasks, narratives, or other activities that stress the communication system. In general, the symptoms of language impairment become more subtle with age; therefore, our assessment techniques must be more subtle as well.

No area in communication disorders has as many standardized test instruments as syntax-level language disorders. As we stated in Chapter 4, it is not possible to summarize the hundreds of tests available for this population. Therefore we will focus on the process of assessment and provide a list of some commonly used assessments (see Table 5–2). Other sources that also provide general descriptions of many of these instruments include Nelson (2010) and Paul (2012).

Eickhoff, Betz, and Ristow (2010) conducted a nationwide survey of clinical procedures used by SLPs to diagnose SLI. Standardized tests and language samples were the most frequently reported measures used, with 50% of SLPs rating standardized tests as the most important measure in their diagnostic protocol and with almost 100% of SLPs rating standardized tests as one of the five most important assessment measures in their diagnostic protocol. Similarly, Wilson et al. (1991) surveyed clinicians in the state of California to determine which modes of assessment were used most in the public school systems. Almost all the clinicians used standardized measures, but like Eickhoff et al. (2010) most clinicians used a combination of standardized and nonstandardized methods to test both comprehension and production in the public school population. As we stated in Chapter 1, assessment embodies elements of both art and science. It makes sense that working clinicians find they must go beyond formal standardized testing and probe behaviors in more informal ways to gain adequate insight into a child's language system. For example, historically we have only examined semantic deficits by measuring receptive and expressive vocabulary size. There are many other areas of difficulty in children who have semantic deficits, such as (1) learning new words in indirect contexts, (2) using short-term memory to store phonological forms of new words, (3) creating/ storing elaborate lexical representations, and (4) using known lexical items in expressive language that involves word retrieval (Brackenbury & Pye, 2005). Most of these areas can be tapped by nonstandardized testing and using subtests of existing examinations.

Most existing instruments focus on structural aspects of language (syntax, semantics, literal meaning of sentences), although several deal with other areas as well (e.g., pragmatics, metalinguistics, concepts). Some of these tests may be used by the SLP to gain *preliminary* insights into selected aspects of language performance, and the tests certainly can fulfill institutional expectations for obtaining scores on formal instruments. An example of an instrument that has excellent psychometric attributes is the *Structured Photographic Expressive Language Test—Preschool*, Third Edition. The second edition of this examination was administered to groups of children with typical language development and those with language impairment, and the ability to discriminate the groups

TABLE 5-2
Commonly Used School-Age and Adolescent Language Test

Instrument Title	Author(s)	Year	Age Range	Languages	Description
Adolescent Language Screening Test (ALST)	Morgan and Guilford	1984	11:0–17:0 years	English	Screening tool that assesses the dimensions of adolescent language: form, content, and use. Subtests include pragmatics, receptive vocabulary, concepts, expressive vocabulary, sentence formulation, morphology, and phonology.
Assessment of Literacy and Language (ALL)	Lombardino, Lieberman, and Brown	2005	Preschool to grade 1	English	Diagnostic tool that assists in early detection of language disorders that may lead to reading deficits.
Auditory Discrimination and Lip Reading Skills Inventory (ALDR)	McFadin	2006	Pre-K to adult	English	Diagnostic tool that assesses skills needed to discern speech at the word and sentences levels. Includes six subtests: syllable structure, similar features, placement features, voicing, vowels, and sentences.
Auditory Processing Abilities Test (APAT)	Swain and Long	2004	5:0–12:11 years	English	Standardized assessment that identifies children with auditory processing disorder. Subtests include phonemic awareness, word sequences, semantic relationships, sentence memory, cued recall, content memory, complex sentences, sentence absurdities, following directions, and passage comprehension.
Bilingual Classroom Communication Profile	Roseberry-McKibbin	1994	4:0–11:0 years	English	Assessment questionnaire that helps teachers differentiate communication differences from communication disorders in bilingual children. Examines both structural and functional aspects of communication.
Boehm Test of Basic Concepts–Third Edition (Boehm-3)	Boehm	2000	5:0–7:11 years	English, Spanish	Norm-referenced assessment that assesses basic concepts necessary for success in school.
Clinical Evaluation of Language Fundamentals–Fifth Edition (CELF-5)	Semel, Wiig, and Secord	2013	5:0–21:0 years	English, Spanish CELF-4	Comprehensive language assessment that identifies the presence of language disorder. Subtests include sentence completion, linguistic concepts, word structure, word class, following directions, formulated sentences, recalling sentences, understanding spoken paragraphs, word definitions, sentence assembly, semantic relationships, reading comprehension, and structured writing. A pragmatics profile/checklist and an observational rating scale are also available.

(continued)

TABLE 5-2
(Continued)

146

Instrument Title	Author(s)	Year	Age Range	Languages	Description
Comprehensive Assessment of Spoken Language (CASL)	Carrow-Woolfolk	1999	3:0–21:11 years	English	Comprehensive oral language assessment that measures language processing skills and structural knowledge in four language structure categories: lexical/semantic, syntactic, supralinguistic, and pragmatic.
Comprehensive Receptive and Expressive Vocabulary Test–Third Edition (CREVT-3)	Wallace and Hammill	2013	5:0–89:0 years	English	Norm-referenced assessment that identifies students who are below their peers in oral vocabulary (expressive and receptive) proficiency.
Emerging Literacy & Language Assessment (ELLA)	Wiig and Secord	2006	4:6–9:11 years	English	Assessment that evaluates emerging literacy and language. Areas assessed include phonological awareness, sign and symbol recognition, rapid naming, word associations, and story recall.
Expressive One Word Picture Vocabulary Test-4 (EOWPVT-4)	Brownell	2000	2:0–80:0+ years	English, Spanish	Standardized assessment of expressive vocabulary. Child is instructed to make word–picture associations.
Language Processing Test 3: Elementary (LPT 3: Elementary)	Richard and Hanner	2005	5:0–11:11 years	English	Assessment used to diagnose language processing disorders. Assesses ability of children to connect meaning to information received and produce an expressive response. Subtests include associations, categorization, similarities and differences, multiple meanings, and attributes.
Montgomery Assessment of Vocabulary Acquisition (MAVA)	Montgomery	2008	3:0–12:11 years	English	Norm-referenced assessment that assesses receptive and expressive vocabulary. Evaluates a student's ability to recognize and identify three tiers of vocabulary words.
Oral and Written Language Scales–Second Edition (OWLS-2)	Carrow-Woolfolk	2011	3:0–21:11 (LC and OE), 5:0–21:11 (RC and WE)	English	Comprehensive evaluation of language and writing skills. Includes four separate scales: oral expression, listening comprehension, reading comprehension, and writing expression. Each of the scales assesses four linguistic structures: lexical/semantics, syntax, pragmatics, and supralinguistics.
Peabody Picture Vocabulary Test–Fourth Edition (PPVT-4)	Dunn and Dunn	2007	2:6–90:0+	English, Spanish	Norm-referenced language assessment tool that evaluates the receptive vocabulary of adults and children.
The Phonological Awareness Test	Robertson and Salter	1997	5:0–9:11 years	English	Standardized assessment that assesses prereading skills that are indicators of reading success, including phonological awareness, phoneme–grapheme correspondence, and phonetic decoding skills.

Test	Author	Year	Age range	Language	Description
Pragmatic Language Skills Inventory (PLSI)	Gilliam and Miller	2006	5:0–2:11 years	English	Norm-referenced rating scale that evaluates pragmatic language abilities. Three subscales include personal interaction skills, social interaction skills, and classroom interaction skills.
Rapid Automatized Naming and Rapid Alternating Stimulus Tests (RAN/RAS)	Wolf and Denckla	2005	5:0–18:11 years	English	Diagnostic tool used to assess the ability to perceive a visual symbol and name it accurately and rapidly. Identifies students who may be at risk for reading deficits.
Receptive One Word Picture Vocabulary Test-4 (ROWPVT4)	Brownell	2000	2:0–80:0 years	English, Spanish	Norm-referenced tool that assesses an individual's receptive vocabulary development.
Screening Test of Adolescent Language–Revised (STAL–R)	Prather, Breecher, Stafford, and Wallace	1980	11:0–18:0 years	English	Quick screening tool that identifies adolescent students at risk for a language disorder. Measures receptive and expressive language through vocabulary, auditory memory span, language processing, and proverb explanation.
Social Language Development Test Adolescent	Bowers, Huisingh, and LoGiudice	2010	12:0–17:11 years	English	Standardized assessment of social skills. Assesses students' responses in social situations and identifies atypical social language behaviors present. Subtests include making inferences, interpreting social language, problem solving, social interaction, and interpreting ironic statements.
Social Language Development Test Elementary	Bowers, Huisingh, and LoGiudice	2008	6:0–11:11 years	English	Standardized assessment of social skills. Assesses language-based skills of social interaction and identifies atypical social language behaviors present. Subtests include making inferences, interpersonal negotiations, multiple interpretations, and supporting peers.
Spelling Performance Evaluation for Language and Literacy (SPELL-2)	Masterson, Apel, and Wasowicz	2006	7 years to adult	English	Diagnostic tool that uses spelling error analysis to identify underlying language processes that interfere with a student's ability to read and spell.
The Strong Narrative Assessment Procedure (SNAP)	Strong	1998	7:0–12:0 years	English	Criterion-referenced assessment that evaluates narrative skills.
Structured Photographic Expressive Language Test–3 (SPELT-3)	Dawson, Stout, and Eyer	2005	4:0–9:11 years	English, Spanish	Norm-referenced assessment of specific language structures that may not transpire in spontaneous language samples. Test items assess use of morphology, verb form, pronoun usage, and syntax.
Test for Auditory Comprehension of Language–Third Edition (TACL-3)	Carrow-Woolfolk	1998	3:0–9:11 years	English	Standardized tool that assesses receptive spoken vocabulary, grammar, and syntax. Subtests include vocabulary, grammatical morphemes, and elaborated phrases and sentences.

(continued)

TABLE 5-2
(Continued)

Instrument Title	Author(s)	Year	Age Range	Languages	Description
Test of Adolescent and Adult Language–Third Edition (TOAL-3)	Hammill, Brown, Larsen, and Wiederholt	1994	12:0–24:11 years	English	Diagnostic tool designed to measure spoken and written language abilities. Subtests include word opposites, word derivations, spoken analogies, word similarities, sentence combining, and orthographic usage.
Test of Auditory Processing Skills–3 (TAPS-3)	Martin and Brownell	2005	4:0–18:11 years	English	Standardized assessment that identifies children and adolescents who have auditory processing deficits. Subtests include word discrimination, word memory, phonological segmentation, phonological blending, number memory forward, number memory reversed, sentence memory, auditory comprehension, auditory reasoning, and auditory figure-ground.
Test of Auditory Reasoning and Processing Skills–Third Edition (TARPS)	Martin, Brownell, and Novato	1993	5:0–13:11 years	English	Diagnostic tool that measures a child's ability to understand, interpret, draw conclusions, and make inferences from auditory stimuli.
Test of Early Written Language–2 (TWEL-2)	Herron, Hresko, and Peak	1996	3:0–11:0 years	English	Norm-referenced assessment that evaluates emerging writing skills. Subtests include basic writing, contextual writing, and overall writing.
Test of Language Competence–Expanded Edition (TLC-Expanded)	Wiig and Secord	1989	5:0–18:11 years	English	Diagnostic tool that evaluates metalinguistic advanced language functions. Subtests include ambiguous sentences, listening comprehension, making inferences, oral expression, re-creating speech acts, figurative language, and a supplemental memory subtest.
Test of Language Development–Primary, Fourth Edition (TOLD-P:4)	Newcomer and Hammill	2008	4:0–8:11 years	English	Standardized assessment that evaluates spoken language. Subtests include picture vocabulary, relational vocabulary, oral vocabulary, syntactic understanding, sentence imitation, morphological completion, word discrimination, word analysis, and word articulation.
Test of Language Development–Intermediate, Fourth Edition (TOLD-I:4)	Hammill and Newcomer	2008	8:0–17:11 years	English	Includes six subtests that measure semantic and grammar skills: sentence combining, picture vocabulary, word ordering, relational vocabulary, morphological comprehension, and multiple meanings.
Test of Narrative Language (TNL)	Gillam and Pearson	2004	5:0–11:11 years	English	Assessment that evaluates ability to use language in narrative dialogue. Utilizes three narrative formats: no picture cues, sequence picture cues, and single picture cues.
Test of Pragmatic Language–2 (TOPL-2)	Phelps-Terasaki, and Phelps-Gunn	2007	6:0–18:11 years	English	Diagnostic tool that provides a comprehensive analysis of social communication in context. Utilizes narratives and story contexts that involve natural communication and social interaction.

Test	Authors	Year	Age	Language	Description
Test of Problem Solving-3 Elementary (TOPS-3: Elementary)	Bowers, Barrett, Huisingh, Orman, and LoGiudice	2005	6:0–12:11 years	English	Norm-referenced assessment that evaluates how students respond to linguistically based critical thinking problems. Subtests include making inferences, sequencing, negative questions, problem solving, predicting, and determining causes.
Test of Problem Solving-2 Adolescent (TOPS-2)	Bowers, Barrett, Huisingh, Orman, and LoGiudice	2007	12:0–17:11 years	English	Diagnostic test of problem solving and critical thinking that evaluates language-based critical thinking skills through logic and experience. Subtests include making inferences, determining solutions, problem solving, interpreting perspectives, and transferring insights.
Test of Semantic Skills-Primary (TOSS-P)	Bowers, Huisingh, LoGiudice, and Orman	2002	4:0–8:11 years	English	Diagnostic tool that assesses the receptive and expressive semantic skills of children. Subtests include both identifying and stating: labels, categories, attributes, functions, and definitions.
Test of Semantic Skills-Intermediate (TOSS-I)	Huisingh, Bowers, LoGiudice, and Orman	2003	9:0–13:11 years	English	Diagnostic tool that assesses the receptive and expressive semantic skills of upper elementary school children. Subtests include identifying labels, identifying categories, identifying attributes, identifying functions, identifying definitions, stating labels, stating categories, stating attributes, stating function, and stating definitions.
Test of Word Knowledge	Wiig and Secord	1992	5:0–17:0 years	English	Diagnostic tool that assesses lexical skills, including: definitions, synonyms, antonyms, metalinguistics, and figurative language.
Test of Written Language-4 (TOWL-4)	Hammill and Larsen	2009	9:0–17:11 years	English	Norm-referenced assessment that measures structural elements in writing. Subtests include vocabulary, spelling, punctuation, logical sentences, sentence combining, contextual conversations, and story composition.
Token Test of Children-Second Edition (TTFC-2)	McGhee, Ehrler, and DiSimoni	2007	3:0–12:11 years	English	Norm-referenced assessment that assesses a child's receptive language skills using 20 tokens (that vary in size, shape, and color). Child manipulates tokens in response to directions.
Wiig Assessment of Basic Concepts (WABC)	Wiig	2004	2:6–7:11 years	English, Spanish	Norm-referenced assessment that assesses a child's receptive and expressive understanding of basic concepts.

was impressive, with a specificity of 100% and a sensitivity of 90.6% using a standard score cutoff of 87 (Greenslade, Plante, & Vance, 2009).

NONSTANDARDIZED TESTING

Sometimes clinicians are interested in eliciting particular syntactic structures from a child as opposed to administering an entire standardized test. This occasion would arise if the clinician wanted to probe the child's use of certain constructions, such as question forms in spontaneous speech. Mulac, Prutting, and Tomlinson (1978) suggest that a variety of tasks could be used to elicit a particular construction. They found that the most effective tasks for eliciting the "is interrogative" were those tasks that required intent, had contextual referents, and had some inherent structure to the activity. One example was a guessing game in which children had to guess what was in a bag (e.g., "Is it a ___?"). The notion of using several different informal elicitation tasks to evaluate certain syntactic structures has been supported by others as well (Eisenberg, 2005; Gazella & Stockman, 2003; Leonard et al., 1978; Lund & Duchan, 1993; Musselwhite & Barrie-Blackley, 1980; Paul, 2012).

The host of standardized tests available for examining the comprehension and production of language have more similarities than differences because there are only so many ways that expressive and receptive language can be sampled. Although many formal tests of language demarcate linguistic ability into expressive and receptive modalities, some question the notion of a purely "expressive" language impairment. For instance, Leonard (2009) points out that the research shows that expressive language impairments are usually accompanied by difficulties in the processing of language input. He recommends that clinicians use the expressive language disorder classification with caution.

It is instructive to move from thinking about *tests* toward thinking about *tasks* that these instruments use to sample language. For example, many tests involve asking a child to point at pictures when the clinician gives a verbal stimulus (e.g., "Show me airplane flying"). When all tests are examined from the perspective of the types of tasks they use in assessing comprehension and production of language, the tests appear highly similar. Decades ago, Leonard et al. (1978) studied formal tests and research protocols to determine which types of tasks were used to gain insight into child language. Table 5–3 illustrates some of the common threads they saw running through

TABLE 5–3
Elicitation Procedures Used in Nonstandardized Assessment

Comprehension	Production
Identification (pointing to, touching)	Elicited immediate imitation
Acting out (following directions)	Elicited delayed imitation
Judgment task (right, wrong, silly, polite)	
Conversation (requests for repair)	Cloze task (carrier phrase)
	Spontaneous evoked (naming, picture description, barrier)
	Story retelling (paraphrase)
	Narratives
	Conversation (legitimate)
	Free play

tests and research projects. Clinicians who want to probe language comprehension and production in children informally have a relatively finite number of ways to do it. This is both comforting and disturbing at the same time. When clinicians use nonstandardized methods to assess language, they must design stimuli and tasks that will give them information beyond that provided by standardized instruments. The tasks in both comprehension and production fall on a continuum of "naturalness." In production, for example, elicited imitation and cloze tasks are further removed from real communication than legitimate conversation and free play. There is nothing wrong with using a combination of tasks to probe a child's capabilities with specific linguistic forms. Use of less natural tasks can even give us insight into how much support a child requires in terms of context or cues presented by the clinician. As stated in Chapter 3, just because nonstandardized methods are used, the clinician is not absolved from having to be systematic in the way data are gathered.

LANGUAGE SAMPLING: A GENERAL LOOK AT THE PROCESS

A common thread that has woven its way through the text thus far has been the notion of ecological validity. When done appropriately, language sampling of a spontaneous conversation is perhaps the closest we come to evaluating real communication. As Miller (1981) says, we must broaden our definition of what we mean by sampling. Perhaps a better name for this process would be *communication sampling* rather than *language sampling* because a child can use flawless syntax and yet not communicate effectively if a pragmatic disorder is present. Spontaneous sampling is the only way to hold content, form, and use intact; thus, it is one of our most powerful tools.

Most SLPs have had the opportunity to sit in a small room with a child and attempt to record a representative sample of language. Most of us also have experienced the despair and humiliation (if we were being observed) of instead harvesting a string of one-word utterances and elliptical responses. Faced with this, we begin to put the pressure on the child for longer utterances and ask questions about the obvious. "What is in this picture?" we ask, when both the child and the clinician know the answer. "Tell me about what you did at school today," we cajole, and the child shrugs his or her shoulders, saying, "Nuthin." A very wise observation was made by Hubbell (1981) after he studied spontaneous talking in young children. When children feel they are being interrogated and there is a great deal of pressure for them to talk, they tend to clam up. Children need to feel at ease and not pressured to talk by the parent or clinician. Clinicians also should try to resist the very strong urge to "interrogate" school-age children and to question them about the obvious. As we mentioned earlier, all communication is affected by the context in which it occurs, and language sampling is no different. We have suggested that multiple samples in varied contexts provide a more realistic view of a student's communication, and even within a classroom situation there are different genres of communicative performance (e.g., peer play, group lesson, and sharing time). Because each sampling session is a product of an individual student, clinician, and communicative environment, it is impossible to provide guidelines that will work with all cases. All we can do is play the probabilities and provide some suggestions that may facilitate spontaneous talking in most cases.

For detailed treatments of language-sampling procedures, refer to the ample sources dealing with the topic (Barrie-Blackley, Musselwhite, & Rogister, 1978; Miller, 1981; Nippold, 2014). Some general factors to keep in mind follow.

1. *Always record the sample.* We tend to subjectively fill in utterances that are incomplete if we transcribe during the sample. Transcribing is distracting, and your attention

is inherently divided if you are attempting to carry on a legitimate conversation while scribbling on a tablet. Either we are engaging in a real conversation or we are not. We typically transcribe the communication sample after the session so that a permanent record is available for comparison at a later date. Paul (2012) has suggested that some analyses can be done with less time commitment if the clinician simply listens to the recorded sample while taking specific data on errors. This allows the clinician an opportunity to replay the recording in cases where the client's productions are less intelligible.

2. *Use a good digital recorder and position it for optimal recording.* This is one of the most often overlooked aspects of sampling language. It is a real disappointment when a clinician has done a masterful job of eliciting natural conversation from a child only to have the speech rendered unintelligible by a poor recording. The ideal recording device should have an appropriate sampling rate and quantization depth. Finan (2010) provides a nice overview of principles that require consideration when purchasing a digital recorder for clinical purposes.

3. *Minimize your use of yes or no questions.* As soon as you ask these questions, you know the answer will be yes, no, or "I don't know." Beginning clinicians typically bombard the child with yes or no questions, and the sample may be so loaded with single-word utterances that the child's mean length of utterance (MLU) is severely underestimated because of sampling error (see Miller, 1981).

4. *Minimize questions that can be answered with one word.* One example is "What color is your dog?" Although you have to ask some of these questions in the normal course of conversation, they do elicit single-word responses.

5. *Try to ask broad-based questions.* Examples include "What happened?," "What happened next?," "Can you tell me about . . .?," "Why?," "How?," and so forth.

6. *Do not be afraid to make contributions to the conversation.* One of the most common errors made by beginning clinicians is that they want the child to do all the talking. This is not a natural conversational situation. Furthermore, the child's utterances are typically in the role of responder. Think back to the last language sample you took and ask yourself if the child had opportunities to initiate conversation instead of merely respond to your interrogations. In addition, ask yourself if you were a legitimate conversational participant. Did you tell the child some of your feelings and experiences? Did you talk mostly about things that were obvious or trivial? It has been our experience that as soon as we stop the barrage of questions and begin to make some observations about what is going on in the session and what we think about things, the child begins to make some contributions to the conversation.

7. *As Miller (1981) says, try not to "play the fool" during a language sample, especially with an older child.* We have heard clinicians say, "I don't know what's in this picture; can you tell me?" Another example is a clinician who says, "Tell me how to make a sandwich. I don't know how." Give the child credit for knowing that you can easily describe pictures or that you know how to do simple, everyday tasks.

8. *Learn to tolerate periods of silence or pauses.* Beginning clinicians seem to feel that they have to fill up all the communicative space with verbalizations. Give the child an opportunity to initiate conversation. As a general rule, give the child approximately 5 seconds to respond before repeating or rephrasing the question.

9. *Stay on a topic long enough to converse about it.* Do not change topics after the child says one utterance on the issue or you will encourage a series of one-liners from children. The clinician will again be placed in the position of having to interrogate. It also interferes with the clinician's ability to gather a sample that is appropriate for analyzing conversational mechanisms, such as topic maintenance.

10. *Be aware of children's cognitive levels when you ask questions.* The clinician should be aware that children have differing conceptual frameworks from those of adults, as well as altered perceptions of time and space. We have heard clinicians ask 3-year-olds questions such as, "Why do you think the truck goes so fast?" Conversely, we do not want to ask questions that are cognitively too simple for older students.

There are variables that appear to affect the length and complexity of language samples obtained by researchers and examiners. First, the racial/cultural backgrounds of the participants could have a potential influence on a child's conversation. Several studies have suggested that some young African American children may engage in style shifting or code switching when confronted with a white, adult examiner (Cazden, 1970; Hester, 1996). Cazden has stated that African American children speak in a school register for teachers and administrators and a street register for peers and family. The school register is different in content, has a shorter MLU, is less complex, and is more disfluent than the street register. Of course, everyone style-shifts to some degree when conversing with another person from a different social, cultural, educational, or economic background. This certainly has implications for language sampling. Clinicians should realize that the samples they obtain from young children from a cultural group different from their own may underestimate linguistic abilities.

Verbalizations of the examiner also may affect language sampling. Lee (1974) suggests that the clinician attempt to speak with a variety of syntactic structures when sampling a child's language. Children are also sensitive to pragmatic aspects of a communicative situation. If they are placed in a play situation with younger children, their language will be simpler than it would be if they were talking to adults (Sachs & Devin, 1976). Presupposition may also play a role in the length and complexity of samples obtained from children. Like adults, children will elaborate linguistically about objects and events that are not present in the current communicative context (Strandberg & Griffith, 1969). If a child does not share visual access to the stimuli with the clinician, he or she will tend to elaborate linguistically to a greater degree (Haynes, Purcell, & Haynes, 1979).

Several studies have shown that children provide longer and more complex language samples if they are engaging in conversation as opposed to performing picture description tasks (Haynes, Purcell, & Haynes, 1979; Longhurst & File, 1977; Longhurst & Grubb, 1974). Picture description tends to lend itself to the naming of elements in a picture rather than elaborating linguistically about a topic unknown to the clinician. These are typically single-word responses or elliptical answers. Most important, if the clinician views the picture with the child, the task becomes not one of conversing but of naming aspects of pictures. Picture description, however, is a viable and sometimes necessary method of sampling language for some children. Certainly, some children will not readily engage in conversation, and picture description is needed to elicit some language for analysis (Atkins & Cartwright, 1982).

The topic of conversation may influence the productivity and syntactic complexity of a language sample. Nippold (2009) had school-age children who played the game of chess talk in three conditions: a general conversation, a conversation about the game of chess, and an explanation of chess. She found that the chess explanation task had significantly more length and complexity than the other tasks. This study highlights the possible effect of the interest and complexity of the conversational topic as it relates to the productivity and complexity of the language sample obtained.

Obtaining a language sample is a critical part of doing a language evaluation. A host of variables can affect the size and quality of the sample the examiner obtains. These variables, and their effect on sample size, may play a major role in the clinician's interpretation of the student's language sample and must be considered when analyzing the client's communicative ability. It would be nice if language samples had the reliability and validity of physical measures such as height and weight. Unfortunately, they do not. Many researchers have reported that the size of language samples has a critical effect on their sampling error rates. Specifically, sampling error rates found by Muma (1998) dropped from 55% in samples of 50 utterances to 15% in samples containing 400 utterances. Historically, a minimum of 50 intelligible utterances has been recommended, and the general thought has been the more utterances, the better. Heilmann, Nockerts, and Miller (2010) evaluated the stability of language sample measures for children between 2.8 and 13.3 years of age. They investigated whether differences in sample length (1-, 3-, and 7-minute samples), child age, or sampling contexts (narrative and conversation) would influence language sample measures. They found that the language sample measures were not affected by sample length or affected by the child's age or sample type. Casby (2011) also evaluated the effect of sample size on MLU in children with language impairment. Casby, like Heilman, Nockerts, and Miller, did not find significant differences in MLU across varying sample sizes. These findings indicate that there is some efficacy for using shorter samples in language sample analysis. However, as you might expect, more research on this topic will need to be conducted before a more definitive conclusion can be reached.

Eisenberg, Fersko, and Lundgren (2001) reviewed the MLU gathered from language samples. They caution against the use of MLU as a determiner of language impairment. First, it is not a measure of syntactic development; it is only one method of measuring utterance length or overall expressive language skill. A child can have an MLU that is within normal limits and still have structural or pragmatic language difficulties. Second, the normative data on MLU are presently limited, especially in older children; the measure may also suffer from poor test-retest reliability. Finally, as mentioned, there is considerable variability in the sampling of MLU, not only in the tasks and types of interactions but also in the sample sizes obtained. Eisenberg, Fersko, and Lundgren conclude that while a low MLU might be used as one piece of evidence for a language impairment, it should never be used as a sole measure.

Johnston (2001) found that MLU was affected by discourse variables such as answers to questions, imitation, and elliptical responding. Johnston studied differences between MLU calculated in the traditional manner and MLU computed without discourse variables, and found that certain children were affected more than others by discourse variables. Johnston reminds clinicians of the complex nature of MLU and cautions them on any MLU-based decisions related to children with relatively advanced language and severe impairments.

Balason and Dollaghan (2002) found significant variability in both the obligatory contexts and grammatical morpheme production in 100 4-year-old children. They took 15-minute language samples obtained in caregiver–child play. The variability brings into question the reliability of findings used to distinguish between normal and abnormal morphological development, especially when relatively small sample sizes are used. This may underscore the need for supplementary elicitation procedures to augment the spontaneous sample or the need to develop ways to make language sample analysis less time consuming. For example, Furey and Watkins (2002) sampled language from 22 preschoolers using a play-based sampling procedure that targeted 50 verbs. Target verbs were recorded by the examiner online and compared to a total language sample recorded. There were significant correlations between verb repertoires in the online recording and in the total language samples. This suggests that online sampling of specific grammatical forms may be an accurate method of evaluation. Although the sampling time is the same as in traditional language sampling, the time to transcribe a language sample is significantly reduced. Note that this method has not been validated on grammatical forms other than verbs.

LATER LANGUAGE DEVELOPMENT: EMERGING DATA

Structural analysis of a language sample can compare the child's production to the growing stockpile of normative data on youngsters between 9 and 18 years of age (Nippold, 2007). During the period from late elementary through high school, there are slow but systematic changes in measurements, such as sentence length (Klecan-Aker & Hedrick, 1985; Loban, 1976; Morris & Crump, 1982), use of subordinate clauses (Scott, 1988), understanding of cohesive devices (Nippold, Schwarz, & Undlin, 1992), and use of the literate lexicon and figurative language (Nippold, 1993).

Scott and Stokes (1995) talk about the need for more relevant grammatical measures for older students. The measures that are used on younger children are not appropriate for older children. Evaluating older children requires quantitative measures such as sentence length (oral and written); clause density (degree to which a student uses subordinate clauses); measures of word structure (derivational morphology); phrase and clause structures; use of complex sentences; and the use of higher-level connectives, conjuncts, and disjuncts (e.g., *therefore, however, in addition, for example,* etc.). The authors make the case for building a normative base for these more complex structures so that the SLP can have a basis for comparing students during an evaluation. Also, normative data on pragmatics are limited (Norris, 1995). Children and adolescents are expected to adapt their communication across varied modalities in classroom, home, and social environments, and little is known about normative performance in these areas. As children move to more decontextualized contexts and are called on to engage in more abstract discourse and semantic contexts, we know less about "normal" development. We also need to develop innovative methods of eliciting more complex sentence structures from students. For instance, Gummersall and Strong (1999) studied clinician support in the form of modeling specific complex language structures and the effect that practice with those structures had on children's production of complex language. They found that the assessment protocol was useful in eliciting a large and varied number of complex syntactic structures in a story context. Conversational samples may not be the best vehicle, however, to examine more complex syntactic development. Nippold, Mansfield, Billow, and Tomblin (2008) found that both typically developing and language-impaired adolescents produced more complex language in an expository task as measured by mean length of T-units, and use of clauses and subordination as compared to a conversational condition. We have maintained in the present text that gathering a narrative sample is an important part of any language assessment because narratives incorporate many complex aspects of linguistic ability. With older clients, we may want to include expository tasks as well to reveal use of linguistic complexity that may not be found in conversation alone. Nippold, Mansfield, Billow, and Tomblin (2009) studied groups of adolescents with typically developing language, specific language impairment, and nonspecific language impairment. They used a peer conflict resolution (PCR) task to sample language performance. This task involved solving a perceived conflict illustrated by a scenario presented by the researcher. The typically developing group had greater T-unit length and used more complex language than either group with language impairment. The PCR task seems well suited for use in gathering language samples from adolescent clients. Researchers are developing more databases on which we can compare performance on specific aspects of linguistic elaboration with development. For example, Eisenberg, Ukrainetz, Hsu, Kaderavek, Justice, and Gillam (2008) gathered data on 5-, 8-, and 11-year-old children to determine their ability to elaborate noun phrases in spoken narratives. They found a clear developmental progression that clinicians can use to determine expectations in typically developing children. At 5 years of age, children use simple designating noun phrases, 8-year-olds used simple descriptive noun phrases, and the oldest group used postmodification.

Earlier we illustrated the interaction that takes place among a student's language ability, teacher language, and the demands of the curriculum. Essentially, as the grade level increases, the student is asked to do progressively more abstract and complicated tasks with language as well as thought. Clearly, the syntactic complexity of language increases, as shown by progressively more use of conjunctions, subordinate clauses, and infinitives. The vocabulary becomes progressively more complex and technical with each grade level. The use of figurative language increases in lectures and in textbooks as grade level increases.

Most educators are familiar with Bloom's taxonomy, which is a progressively more demanding series of levels that require a student to use language and thought interactively to learn more complex material and demonstrate knowledge (Paul, 2012). The tasks in the hierarchy begin with listing and identifying on the simplest level. Then a student must demonstrate his or her grasp of a concept by explaining, describing, and restating relevant material. Later the student must show how he or she can apply the learned information to solve problems, analyze a novel situation, or debate/ defend a position using the information. Finally, a student must be able to compare and contrast and critically evaluate the information in relation to other perspectives. When we deal with students who have language impairment, we are often content to see them perform on the initial levels of Bloom's taxonomy (naming, listing, identifying). However, the classroom will stress their linguistic and cognitive systems much more using the higher levels of the hierarchy. Tests often ask students to compare and contrast, describe, explain, and apply learned information as the grade level increases. Thus, we must perform our language assessment on many levels to determine where the student has difficulty with using language in the service of cognition. If we find that a student cannot deal with higher levels of thought and language, these can be easily incorporated into the treatment program and result in communicative as well as academic payoffs. A good place to start is to determine what the classroom teachers expect of their students in terms of language and thought. This is part of what is sometimes called curriculum-based assessment.

TESTING LANGUAGE COMPREHENSION

Bransford and Nitsch (1978) point out that comprehension involves a situation plus an input. A human organism is not a static system but has a current state of excitation, a history, and background knowledge. A given input of language is placed in this situation along with the nonverbal context of communication. Many variables come to bear on the understanding of an input, not the least of which are the person's background, as well as the linguistic and nonlinguistic contexts. Rees and Shulman (1978) have written an article in which they indicate that most tests of language comprehension measure only the literal meanings of utterances. For example, if asked to point to a picture of a boy who is running, the child can choose the correct picture and not point to one of a boy who is standing. Thus, the child understands the notions of *boy* and *run* and can discriminate them from other literal meanings, such as *standing*. But comprehension involves so much more than the literal meaning of utterances. Miller and Paul (1995) provide several examples of other types of comprehension knowledge, as illustrated in Table 5–4. As another example, the skill of making inferences is used in almost every interaction and certainly many times during a school day. To comprehend fully an utterance such as "It's supposed to rain today, but I forgot my umbrella," one must infer that the person may get wet, although this is never specifically stated. Another broader notion of comprehension has to do with understanding the main point in a narrative, lecture, or conversation. If a child cannot comprehend the main point in a lecture, this is

TABLE 5–4
Selected Types of Comprehension Knowledge

- *Knowledge of literal meaning:* "Show me the picture of the monkey."
  A correct response would be to point to the monkey to show literal knowledge of the requested item.
- *Social knowledge:* "Do you want to be sent to your room without supper?"
  This is not a question from a mother to a child. It is actually a threat and requires knowledge of the situation to interpret appropriately.
- *Knowledge of sincerity conditions:* "Is the pope Catholic?"
  When someone produces this question, we know that this is just another way of saying yes in a conversation and is not a query about the religious affiliation of the pontiff.
- *Knowledge of cohesive devices:* "He fixed the car."
  One cannot comprehend this sentence correctly unless information from outside the utterance is considered. The listener must be able to figure out who "he" is and whose vehicle was repaired.
- *Knowledge of presupposition:* "They managed to sell their house."
  A listener must know not only that the people sold their home but also that it was done with some difficulty because of the word "managed."
- *General world knowledge:* "It's raining."
  Miller and Paul (1995) give an example of poll workers who know that rainy weather often results in low voter turnout, and thus the above utterance takes on special meaning beyond simply talking about the weather.
- *Specific background knowledge:* "I'm the Michael Jordan of soccer."
  Unless the listener knew about the prowess of this famous basketball player, it would be difficult to know that the utterance refers to playing soccer exceptionally well.

Source: Adapted from Miller, J., & Paul, R. (1995).*The clinical assessment of language comprehension.* Baltimore, MD: Brookes.

certainly as much of a comprehension problem as not understanding literal meanings. Comprehension of figurative language such as idioms and metaphors involves more than just literal meaning. If a teacher says, "This science project should really shine," the child should know that the teacher does not mean that the project requires lights (Simon, 1987).

We must go past the idea of assessing literal meanings when dealing with comprehension assessment. Most comprehension tests are quite artificial when compared to the richness of language comprehension in a natural situation. The typical comprehension assessment situation involves presenting a child with test plates containing pictures. The child is asked to point to the picture that best represents some verbal stimulus uttered by the examiner. The pictures are often line drawings, and the verbal stimuli are not discursively related to one another (in one case, the child is asked to point to a "monkey," and in the next plate the topic is "shopping"). In these tests, there is no temporal sequence of events that would allow a child to be able to predict what will be said, as in real language comprehension. Naturalistic situations also give the child the opportunity to ask for clarification or repetition in the face of information loss. The notion of comprehension monitoring implies that we are always scanning to determine if we understand someone's utterances; if we do not understand, we initiate repair sequences that can clarify information that we do not comprehend. Skarakis-Doyle and Dempsey (2008) found that children with language impairment performed significantly lower than typically developing children matched for receptive vocabulary on a comprehension monitoring task. We do not afford children this chance in comprehension testing. In fact, we are often forbidden by the examiner's manual from presenting a stimulus a second time, even if the child asks for a repetition! This discussion is meant only to reinforce the notion that real language comprehension is a highly complex phenomenon and cannot be assessed easily.

Millen and Prutting (1979) studied three language comprehension tests for consistency of response on specific grammatical features. They found that on the *Northwestern Syntax Screening Test* (NSST), *Assessment of Children's Language Comprehension* (ACLC), and *Bellugi Comprehension Test*, there was general agreement in the overall scores generated by the measures. There were significant differences among the tests, however, for more than half of the specific grammatical features evaluated. The investigators logically suggest that the tests are not equivalent and not clinically sound for generating specific remediation targets. Other stimulus, task, and subject variables have been studied in comprehension tests. Haynes and McCallion (1981) found that on the *Test of Auditory Comprehension of Language* (TACL), children with a reflective cognitive tempo, or long decision time, performed significantly better than impulsive children with a short decision time. These researchers reported that scores on the TACL improved significantly over standard administration when the subjects were given two stimulus presentations or if the test was administered imitatively. Skarakis-Doyle, Dempsey, and Lee (2008) investigated the individual and combined effects of three comprehension measurements on preschool-age children with typical and impaired language. The measurements (joint story retell, expectancy violation detection task, and comprehension questions) each classified children in their predetermined groups, but the combination of the three measures proved to be the most effective predictor (96%) of group membership. This study shows that comprehension impairments can be detected effectively in the preschool years using naturalistic tasks that take a total of about 20 minutes to administer.

Thus, it appears that variables other than language comprehension enter into test performance, and failure to do well on a comprehension test could be explained by other factors. Attentional set, hearing impairment, ambiguous pictures, test administration procedures (Shorr, 1983), cognitive style, and unrelated stimuli—all could account for poor performance on a standardized test of language comprehension. Gowie and Powers (1979) showed that a child's expectations about what a sentence was going to say significantly influenced his or her performance on a comprehension task. Gowie and Powers observed that "knowing a word involves a set of expectations about the referents and about the types of messages in which the word is likely to occur" (p. 40).

We have suggested that comprehension is difficult to test in limited-language cases without contaminating influences from the context and the child's use of comprehension strategies. We have said that failure to perform well on a test of comprehension does not necessarily indicate the presence of a comprehension disorder. Based on the current literature, about all we can say with some conviction is that adequate performance on a standardized test of language comprehension probably means that the child is capable of comprehending some language in a highly artificial situation. This does not necessarily represent comprehension ability in natural situations. Failure of a comprehension test, on the other hand, does not necessarily mean that the child is incapable of comprehending language either in the contrived testing situation or the natural environment.

Currently, language comprehension is tested in four ways by SLPs. First, there are a number of standardized tests of comprehension. Second, some researchers have tested comprehension by having children act out certain commands (Leonard et al., 1978). Third, several investigators have used a decision task in which the child makes judgments such as "good or bad" or engages in a preference task to say which of two sentences was the best. Finally, similar to the standardized tests, clinicians have used pictures or objects and have engaged children in an informal pointing task. Miller and Paul (1995) have developed an impressive series of nonstandardized comprehension assessment tasks for use with clients from under 12 months of age to those over 10 years old. Each task is directly related to a developmental level, and detailed instructions are provided for administration, scoring, and interpretation. Perhaps the "best" method of comprehension testing would be to examine it via several methods, both formal and informal. The clinician should utilize more naturalistic assessment methods such as engaging the child in play or conversation and evaluating the appropriateness of verbal and nonverbal responses. Observation in the classroom combined with teacher and parent interviews can provide valuable insight into comprehension in everyday situations. It also should be noted whether the child uses requests for clarification or repetition in conversation. Research has shown that these clarification/repetition requests can be elicited successfully by the clinician by using informal probes (Brinton & Fujiki, 1989). Gillam, Fargo, and Robertson (2009) illustrate the use of comprehension questions and think-aloud tasks to evaluate language comprehension beyond the typical tasks found on standardized tests. In their think-aloud tasks, expository stimuli are read by the clinician one sentence at a time, and the child is asked what he or she knows about the story so far. Comprehension questions are also asked about the story.

When a child does not comprehend an utterance, the clinician should systematically determine where the process of understanding begins to break down. Unfortunately, no single test is presently available to solve this dilemma; however, several researchers have made progress in this area (Miller & Paul, 1995). For older children, clinicians can experiment systematically with the variables listed in Table 5–5 to determine where the breakdown occurs.

TABLE 5–5
Selected Evaluation Areas to Determine Source of Comprehension Breakdown

Input Variables
- *Complexity of vocabulary (semantics).* Does comprehension break down when the vocabulary increases in complexity? Does the child lack knowledge of the literal meanings of words?
- *Syntactic complexity.* Does comprehension break down as sentences become more complex?
- *Sentence length.* Does comprehension break down as sentences become longer?
- *Context.* Does comprehension improve when there is a clear physical context to support the utterance? Does comprehension break down in decontextualized utterances?

Internal Variables
- *Auditory acuity.* Does comprehension break down because of hearing impairment?
- *Attentional abilities.* Does comprehension improve when a child is given a "set" to attend or when there is less distraction in the context?
- *Comprehension monitoring.* Does comprehension improve when a child is asked to judge continuously whether he or she understands utterances? When he or she is asked for repairs?

Specific Problems
- *Intersentence relations.* Does comprehension break down when meaning must be derived from analysis of multiple sentences?
- *Cohesion.* Does comprehension break down when the listener must derive the meaning of cohesive devices (e.g., pronouns) from prior discourse?
- *World or specific knowledge.* Does comprehension break down when the topic requires general types of knowledge? When it requires specific types of world knowledge?

ASSESSMENT OF SYNTAX USING ANALYSIS PACKAGES

After the SLP has obtained a language sample, judgments must be made regarding the syntactic development of the child. Analysis of syntax can be conceptualized on a continuum. On the left end of the continuum is the administration of formal tests. These measures can give the clinician some insight into general syntactic development. In the middle of the continuum, the clinician can analyze a language sample in accordance with specific packaged assessment procedures (Lee, 1974) and obtain more precise information than is available from standardized tests. Finally, on the right end, the clinician can analyze the sample by using knowledge of linguistics and language development and does not have to rely on a step-by-step package analysis procedure (Hubbell, 1988; Kahn & James, 1980; Lund & Duchan, 1993; Muma, 1973b; Retherford, 2000). The left end of the continuum requires less expertise than does the right end in terms of clinician experience and training. The left end of the continuum takes less time for the analysis than does the right, but it also provides less clinically relevant information. Thus, the clinician must make a decision about the time available for the analysis, training and expertise in linguistics, and the depth of information desired.

It is beyond the scope of this chapter to instruct clinicians in performing an analysis of a child's syntax. The best way to learn an analysis system is to obtain a sample and follow the guidelines provided by authors of complex analysis packages. Typically, the authors provide explicit instructions for obtaining a sample, segmentation, and analysis. Beginning clinicians should realize that any syntactic analysis method requires practice in order to be used effectively. The most widely known analysis procedures are listed in Table 5–6.

Muma (1978) points out that descriptive procedures have greater power than normative ones do because they help the clinician describe individual differences. Descriptive procedures, because they are based on spontaneous language samples, also provide the clinician with more relevant intervention targets because these procedures do not fracture the integrity of the content-form-use model the way that imitative and standardized tests do. Thus, there are advantages to performing a descriptive analysis, and package systems provide the clinician with guidelines for completing such an analysis. We should remember, however, that each analysis procedure reflects the author's bias regarding language, and that most systems look at a language sample in only limited ways.

Consumers who intend to use an analysis package should be aware that the procedures differ in important ways. These differences may determine whether or not a clinician finds it appropriate to use a particular package. We will use the Developmental Sentence Scoring (DSS) procedure in our examples because this methodology

TABLE 5–6
Selected Language Sample Analysis Procedures

- Assessing Children's Language in Naturalistic Contexts (Lund & Duchan, 1993)
- Assigning Structural Stage (Miller, 1981)
- Co-Occurring and Restricted Structures Analysis (Muma, 1973b)
- Developmental Sentences Analysis (Lee, 1974)
- Language Assessment, Remediation, and Screening Procedure (Crystal, Fletcher, & Garman, 1976)
- Language Sampling, Analysis, and Training (Tyack & Gottsleben, 1974)
- Linguistic Analysis of Speech Samples (Engler, Hannah, & Longhurst, 1973)
- Method for Assessing Use of Grammatical Structures (Kahn & James, 1980)

Source: Adapted from R. Owens (2014). *Language disorders: A functional approach to assessment and intervention.* Boston: Allyn & Bacon.

has been available for years (Lee, 1974), has been referred to in the literature as being a potentially useful procedure (Hughes, Fey, & Long, 1992), and is included in the computer-based language analysis programs (Long, Fey, & Channell, 2002). Using this procedure in our discussion is not meant to be a criticism or an endorsement of this particular approach.

1. Some package systems recommend obtaining a specific sample size before subjecting the language to analysis. For instance, Lee (1974) recommends using 50 subject-verb utterances for computation of the DSS. A later study stated, however, that a sample of 150 utterances may be more appropriate for reliable scoring. If the clinician does not have a large enough sample, perhaps a different procedure would be more appropriate.

2. The analysis packages vary considerably in the time required for completion. This may be due to several influences. First, some procedures are quite detailed and lengthy (Bloom & Lahey, 1978; Crystal, Fletcher, & Garman, 1976). Other procedures use very specific terminologies and vocabulary or have complicated scoring systems that require much time and practice in order for the clinician to use the procedure economically.

3. The procedures differ in terms of how they segment or separate utterances obtained in the sample. The DSS, for instance, analyzes only subject-verb utterances and does not score sentence fragments. However, some clinicians feel that there is much useful information in sentence fragments (e.g., elliptical responses) that may be important to analyze.

4. Some systems are recommended by their authors as ideal for use with particular treatment approaches. For example, Lee, Koenigsknecht, and Mulhern (1975) use the DSS as an input to their interactive language teaching strategy and continue to monitor progress by using the system.

5. Another way that evaluation systems differ is in terms of the structures they do or do not analyze. For example, the DSS does not specifically analyze certain forms (e.g., prepositions and articles) and accounts for their presence or absence by assigning a "sentence point" to an utterance if it is grammatical. Other systems specifically analyze most structural elements of English, even structures that may not be of interest to the clinician.

6. Analysis packages differ in their provision of normative data. The DSS has normative data, while some other packages are purely descriptive and make no attempt to gather numerical scores on normal and disordered children.

7. Finally, the analysis procedures are not uniform in applying the results to a normal language development progression. That is, some procedures are designed to examine linguistic elements without locating the child on a language development continuum. Others apply their results to the normal developmental progression (Crystal, Fletcher, & Garman, 1976; Lahey, 1988; Lee, 1974; Miller, 1981). Research has shown that many aspects of syntactic and morphological acquisition in children with language impairments develop in an order similar to that found in normally developing children (Paul & Alforde, 1993).

Several investigations have shown that some of the package analysis procedures appear to be capable of documenting language changes in children, at least in a general way (Hughes, Fey, & Long, 1992; Longhurst & Schrandt, 1973; Sharf, 1972). Any method that a clinician selects will require specific training and practice in order to use it effectively. Remember that any method used depends to a significant degree on the quality of the sample obtained and typically analyzes only the structural elements of language, independent of pragmatics. Thus, any analysis package procedure will take

TABLE 5–7
General Guidelines for Syntactic Analysis of Language Sample

- Obtain a conversation sample.
- Transcribe the sample orthographically (or in phonetics if the client has misarticulations).
- Locate errors in sample:
  Find sentences containing errors and highlight them.
  Mark specific errors within the highlighted sentences (circle them).
- Make a list of forms/structures the child uses correctly.
- Make a list of forms/structures the child misuses consistently (never correct).
- Make a list of forms/structures the child misuses inconsistently.
- For inconsistently misused forms/structures, make a list of contexts:
  List contexts where form/structure is correct.
  List contexts where form/structure is incorrect.
- Common variables to consider regarding contextual influence:
  Syntactic complexity of sentence
  Semantic complexity of lexical items used in sentence
  Type of sentence (e.g., question, declarative)
  Phonological complexity of sentence
  Pragmatic variables (e.g., listener uncertainty; narrative)
- Look for possible patterns using above variables that account for occasions when error occurs and does not occur.

the clinician time and practice to learn, and in the end will look at language only from a specific point of view (Miller, 1981).

The present authors believe that if clinicians are going to spend time learning about analysis of the structural aspects of language, their time would be better spent learning linguistics and language acquisition instead of one specific analysis package that probably would not be appropriate for all clients. An analysis package could always be learned later to supplement the clinician's linguistic knowledge and would probably be learned more easily owing to the experience with linguistics. Knowledge of linguistics would allow the clinician to analyze samples generally for structures that are present, absent, and inconsistent and to choose treatment targets that are relevant, instead of trying to find a package analysis procedure that is the "best fit" for the child. Several fine textbooks provide information on sentence structure (e.g., Hubbell, 1988). We feel that, ultimately, the clinician must determine (1) which structures the child appears to have acquired, (2) which structures are absent in obligatory contexts, (3) which structures are used inconsistently, and (4) which contexts seem to be associated with use and nonuse of the inconsistent structures. Muma (1973a) and Kahn and James (1980) have advocated such descriptive procedures that focus on determining present, absent, and inconsistent syntactic elements, and we view this as a commonsense approach to analysis that has direct clinical application. It also does not involve the clinician's commitment of time to learning one or two package procedures and their unique scoring systems. Tables 5–7 and 5–8 provide a hypothetical sample and analysis.

Recently, computer analyses of language samples have come to the fore. Software programs are available that provide detailed information about a language sample; however, the clinician must remember that some time is typically invested in coding the transcript into the program. In some cases, this may take more time than a paper-and-pencil analysis if the clinician merely wants to define treatment targets. In addition, the computer analyses may provide the clinician with more information than is really needed. The output from these programs is truly phenomenal.

TABLE 5–8
Transcript Analysis Example

1. Grant got one of them.	17. Him go to the hospital.
2. Him go flop flop.	18. Thats a hospital.
3. It go like that.	19. They are too big.
4. They have a wagon.	20. I running fast.
5. Jay is my brother.	21. They boys are driving a car.
6. Somebody drop a glass on the floor.	22. The cat is sleeping.
7. Him live at that house.	23. Her feed the baby.
8. Him the boy that live next door.	24. Her have a cold.
9. They are going to town.	25. We have to let him in car.
10. Him riding a bike.	26. We ride in car and go fast.
11. It is at home.	27. A boy on the rocker and one in house.
12. Her going fast.	28. They in parking lot while the boy sleep.
13. I don't know.	29. The cat is running up the drapes.
14. Smudge is a boy cat.	30. The girl is holding her ears.
15. I four years old and I live in Eufaula.	31. Him carrying a box of apples.
16. It brown and brick.	

Selected Forms Used

Proper noun	Uncontractible copula
Irregular verb	Personal pronoun ("my," "I")
Cardinal number	Prepositions
Plural pronoun	Definite article
Verbs	Auxillary ("are")
Demonstrative ("that")	Present progressive
Adverbial of manner	Auxillary ("do")
Indefinite pronoun ("somebody")	Adjective
Verb "have"	Conjunctions ("and," "while")
Nondefinite article	Plural ("boys")
Nouns	

Errors

"him"/"he" (objective for subjective
    pronominal case)
"go"/"goes"; "live"/"lives"; "feed"/"feeds";
"sleep"/"sleeps" (third person sing.)
"drop"/"dropped" (regular past "-ed")
Omitted copula "is"

Omitted auxiliary "is"

Omitted copula "am"

"have"/"has"

Omitted definite article

Omitted copula "are"

Errors Consistently Misused

"him"/"he"
Third person "-s"
Regular past "-ed" (1 instance)
Omitted copula "am"
"have"/"has"

Errors Inconsistently Misused

Omitted copula "is"
Omitted auxillary "is"
Omitted definite article
Omitted copula "are"

Context When Inconsistent Error Occurred

Copula "is":
   8: high complexity, embedding,
      "him"/"he" substitution
   16: complex, conjoining and deleting
   27: complex, conjoining
Auxillary "is":
   10: "him"/"he" substitution
   12: "her"/"she" substitution
   31: "him"/"he" substitution

(continued)

TABLE 5–8
(Continued)

	Copula "are":
	  28: complex, conjoining
	Definite article:
	  25: complex, embedding
	  26: complex, embedding
	  27: complex, embedding
	  28: complex, embedding

Context of Inconsistent Errors When
They Did Not Occur
Copula "is":
5: simple, "Jay is . . ."
11: simple, "It is . . ."
14: simple, "Smudge is . . ."
18: "That is . . ."
Auxiliary *is*
22: simple, "The cat is . . ."
29: simple, "The cat is . . ."
30: simple, "The girl is . . ."
Copula *are*:
9: simple, *They are . . .*
19: simple, *They are . . .*
21: simple, *The boys are . . .*
	Definite article:
	  6: simple
	  17: simple
	  21: simple
	  22: simple
	  23: simple
	  27: complex, conjoining
	  28: complex, conjoining
	  29: simple
	  30: simple

We would like to provide a very brief overview of two computer programs that are currently available and are particularly useful in language analysis. Both programs are impressive and are based on years of research and development. It would take many pages just to list the types of output from the programs. Thus, we cannot hope to do justice to either one in a couple of paragraphs. It is important, however, that clinicians move toward the use of computer analysis in language assessment. We have tried to make it clear in this text that conversational samples are the most valid target of a language assessment. Some clinicians have shied away from such analyses because of the time it takes to complete them and the expertise in linguistics required to make certain judgments. To some degree, these programs address both concerns and make language sample analysis more accessible to clinicians working in the field. Both programs have been developed with the cooperation of university faculty members and clinicians working in school systems and other settings. These two programs represent somewhat different approaches to the input of data and analysis of language samples. One program has been characterized as a data retrieval program; it requires the clinician to code utterances, boundaries, segmentation, errors, and so on, using codes specific to the software. Thus, the automatic part of the program is its summary of the data that has already been entered into the computer by the clinician. A second type of program uses a computer algorithm to parse the sentences and identify grammatical components for analysis, then summarizes the results. While the clinician still must type in a language transcript, certain decisions are made by the computer—such as the grammatical identities of sentence components, grammatical morphemes, and even the identification of phrases and clauses. Long and Channell (2001) analyzed 69 language samples using the grammatical analyses of MLU, LARSP, IPSyn, and DSS to determine if results using human coding and automatic computer analyses were in agreement. They found that "[r]esults for all four analyses produced automatically were comparable to published data on the manual interrater reliability of these procedures. Clinical decisions based on cutoff scores and productivity data were little affected by the use of automatic rather than human-generated analyses. These findings bode well for future clinical and research use of automatic language analysis software" (p. 180).

Both automatic analysis and data retrieval programs have significant value to the clinician attempting to analyze a language sample. We will give an example of each type of program. The first program, *Computerized Profiling* (Long, Fey, & Channell, 2002), which automatically parses utterances, can be downloaded from the Internet at no charge (www.computerizedprofiling.org) and thus is a resource available to all clinicians regardless of work setting. It has a variety of modules that are used to examine many linguistic areas. A module common to all analyses is the corpus module, which allows the user to create transcript files used by all other modules. In corpus mode, the clinician can input samples, edit, print, and even convert files for export to the SALT program (which we discuss next). Computerized Profiling's *PROPH module* analyzes a child's phonetic inventory, syllable shapes, phonological processes, and percentage of consonants correct using a traditional test or a conversational sample. The *Profile in Semantics (PRISM) module* examines the content of early and later vocabularies in children and provides a highly detailed lexical analysis based on semantic fields. It also has a submodule that analyzes semantic relations. There is a module for the *Language Assessment, Remediation, and Screening Procedure (LARSP)*, which provides an age- and stage-based system for profiling a child's syntactic development. A submodule in LARSP is Conversational Acts Profile (CAP), which examines a child's assertiveness and responsiveness in conversation. A prosody profile (PROP) is also included in Computerized Profiling for analyzing intonation patterns in grammatical structures. Finally, a module for Developmental Sentence Scoring (DSS) is included in the package. Channell (2003) found point-by-point agreement between computerized profiling using DSS and manual coding to be 78%, with a correlation of .97 between the two methods. Readers are encouraged to download the program, which is free of charge and has excellent help screens to guide new users in the analyses.

The second program we will consider is a data retrieval program called *Systematic Analyses of Language Transcripts* (SALT) (Miller & Chapman, 2008). Heilmann, Miller, and Nockerts (2010) provide an effective overview of the SALT database and how it might be used by clinicians. A long-standing use of these computer-based procedures has been to document clinical progress over time as measured by naturalistic language samples instead of formal tests. The above researchers have shown that language sample analysis using the SALT program can even discriminate between typically developing children and those with language impairment with a fair amount of sensitivity and specificity, with most values between 80% and 89%.

The SALT program allows the user either to type in a language transcript or to import a transcript from a word processing program. Once the transcript is entered, the clinician must segment it and enter certain codes in the form of slashes, asterisks, and other symbols to define certain conversational or grammatical categories (e.g., bound morphemes, abandoned utterances, etc.). After the codes are entered, the program summarizes a series of standard analyses at the word, morpheme, utterance, and discourse levels. A particularly useful measure of SALT is its in-depth analysis of mazing (use of repetitions, fillers, etc.) in conversational samples. Another aspect of SALT that is extremely useful is its reference database of normative data on nearly 350 subjects, representing children ages 3 to 13. There are norms for both conversation and narratives in the database. These norms are particularly useful because they indicate how many standard deviations away from the mean a child scores compared to the reference data-base. Because the norms are based on conversational samples, they represent a source of normative data for many variables that we might want to examine in connected speech. Miller and Chapman (2008) show how particular patterns on the SALT may relate to specific subtypes of language impairment.

The advantage of the computer would appear to lie in the multiple analyses that can be performed once the sample is input. That is, a clinician can take the same transcript and analyze it for insight into the child's semantic system, phonological system, syntactic system, and occurrence of speech acts (if appropriately coded). An important point to emphasize is that these programs are only as good as the coding of the language sample that they analyze. Some programs automatically classify lexical items or grammatical forms based on internal algorithms. Most programs allow the clinician to change these a priori classifications of transcript items if they are incorrect. That is, sometimes a program will not identify a word or grammatical construction correctly, and the clinician needs to check how the computer has classified transcript items. There is no substitute for close clinician monitoring when using these programs. The computer may pump out a profile or summary of a child's performance, but the clinician should at least spot-check the analysis for correctness. It is easy to be seduced into relying on complex summaries without checking on validity. Some excellent examples of how computer-aided language sample analysis can be used in clinical settings in initial assessment and measuring treatment progress are presented by Price, Hendricks, and Cook (2010).

No doubt we will learn much in the next decade from these procedures about patterns of error and subtypes of language disorder. No single procedure can tell a clinician all he or she needs to know about a child's language. Again, the clinician's judgment must be applied to a particular case, whether it is a decision to choose among several package analysis systems, rely on computer-assisted analysis, or simply to focus on a more specific, descriptive linguistic analysis.

ASSESSMENT OF CONVERSATIONAL PRAGMATICS

Many reports in the literature attest to pragmatic differences in children with language impairments. Some investigations report that these children have difficulty organizing narratives and staying on a topic (Johnston, 1982). Fey and Leonard (1983) have hypothesized that there may be subgroups of language-impaired children who exhibit a variety of pragmatic problems. There have been reports of children with language disorders who have difficulty taking listener perspective into account (Muma, 1975). Unfortunately, there are no tests that tap all relevant aspects of conversational pragmatics. Although some formal measures focus on limited facets of pragmatic ability (Blagden & McConnell, 1983; Shulman, 1986), it would be difficult to develop a broader assessment device because of the many aspects included under the rubric of pragmatics. Conversational abilities are also difficult to tap by using artificial tasks, limited samples, or contrived topics of discourse. If the clinician is interested in conversational abilities, there is no substitute for legitimate conversation. When the clinician focuses on conversation and discourse, it is necessary to obtain a sample of the child's conversational performance and to transcribe both the utterances of the child and of the interlocutor. This transcription is a time-consuming task; however, if the clinician is to obtain data on the child's conversational performance, the contributions of both participants cannot be ignored. The clinician might choose from several measures to analyze conversation, depending on which aspects of the discourse are of interest. Some of these measures may overlap to a certain degree. We recommend beginning at a general level and then progressing to more specific analyses.

Evaluation of General Pragmatic Parameters: Identification of a Potential Problem

Damico and Oller (1980) noted that classroom teachers find it easy to make appropriate referrals of pragmatic disorders to the speech-language pathologist. In fact, some pragmatic problems are even more noticeable than morphological/syntactic difficulties. Ask a teacher sometime if there are children in his or her class who consistently have trouble carrying on a conversation because of inadequate information, listener perspective problems, and significant mazing. They often remember these children more easily than one who omits a plural morpheme. Pragmatic difficulties are best observed in a natural context that allow for assessment of social, emotional, and communication behaviors.

The number of pragmatic assessments available is surprisingly limited. Most of the assessments available today are observational and involve having parents, teachers, or clinicians rate pragmatic behaviors through the use of checklists or questionnaires. For example, the *Children's Communication Checklist–2* (Bishop, 2006) is a caregiver assessment tool that evaluates pragmatic aspects of communication. Damico (1985) has advocated for the analysis of specific discourse errors in children with pragmatic language deficits. He provides a list of nine discourse errors that can be detected in conversation and computed into a percentage of utterances containing pragmatic difficulties. He recommends obtaining 180 utterances over two sessions in conversational interaction about home and school activities. The goal of the analysis is to describe specific discourse errors that exist in the interaction. Damico has gathered data on many typically developing children and those with language disorders, and proposes some error percentage ranges for determining very generally the existence and severity of a discourse problem.

Currently only two direct observational pragmatic assessments have published psychometric properties. First, is the *Pragmatic Protocol* developed by Prutting and Kirchner (1987), which gives an overall communicative index for children, adolescents, and adults. It includes 30 pragmatic aspects of language in the broad groupings of verbal, paralinguistic, and nonverbal skills. There are specific definitions for each parameter used in the system, and they provide preliminary data on both adults and children with normal and disordered language. This approach to evaluating a child's pragmatic abilities begins with a molar view of conversational performance to determine if certain types of errors are especially obvious to the clinician. Prutting and Kirchner (1987) rated children's conversation on the 30 parameters. The most inappropriate pragmatic parameters found in 42 children with language impairments involved turntaking, specificity/accuracy, cohesion, repair/revision, topic maintenance, and intelligibility. Another more recently developed measure is the *Pragmatics Observational Measure* (POM; Cordier, Munro, Wilkes-Gillan, Speyer, & Pearce, 2014). It was developed to assess pragmatic language of children between 5 and 11 years in a naturalistic context through evaluation of 27 items across five pragmatic domains: introduction of communication and responsiveness to social interactions, interpreting and using nonverbal communication, social-emotional understanding of peers intentions, executive functioning, and use of appropriate negotiation strategies when interacting with peers. Each of the items contained in the POM is rated on a 4-point scale, with 1 being rarely observed and 4 being almost always observed. Use of the protocols described above forces the clinician, at the very least, to consider the relevant parameters of pragmatics and to make a judgment regarding each. Then more concentrated evaluation tasks can be applied to the case that might define the nature of the conversational errors more specifically. Damico, Oller, and Tetnowski (1999) have developed another tool called the *Systematic Observation of Communicative Interaction* (SOCI) that can be used successfully to identifying children with pragmatic disorders. Another more detailed system is recommended by Bedrosian (1985). Again, this type of approach moves from general to more specific in terms of evaluating language in older students. More molecular analyses can be initiated after a student is identified by a general procedure.

Another general area intimately related to pragmatics is the child's social skills. Humans develop social relationships largely based on their ability to communicate with others in a relevant and efficient manner. Some studies show that children with language impairment have social difficulties compared to typically developing peers. Fujiki et al. (2001) studied the playground behavior of eight children with SLI and their age-matched peers and found that typically developing children spent more time interacting with peers on the playground compared to children with SLI. Conversely, children with SLI demonstrated more withdrawn behaviors compared to the typically developing children. The authors suggest that including social interaction behaviors in the treatment program for children with SLI might be appropriate. This again illustrates how the SLP should extend assessment beyond formal testing and determine environmental effects of the communication disorder and evaluate functional outcomes that extend beyond language. Fujiki, Brinton, and Todd (1996) studied 19 elementary school children with SLI and age-matched peers. They administered a number of measures to teachers and peers to determine a general measure of social skill and the quantity and quality of peer relationships. They found that the children with SLI had poorer social skills and fewer peer relationships than the age-matched controls. Also, the children with SLI were less satisfied with their peer relationships than were the typically developing children.

In a recent study, Conti-Ramsden et al. (2013) evaluated the BESD experienced by 139 adolescents with language impairment. The adolescents with a history of language impairment were found to report higher levels of BESD than were those in a typically developing (TD) control group. Social difficulties or difficulties with peer relationships were found to be the strongest differentiator. Specifically, they found that 25% of children with language impairment reported difficulties with peer relations by age 16; this is in marked contrast to the 2.4% who reported difficulties in the TD group. They also found that the lower the receptive language skills, the more likely the child with a language impairment would experience behavioral or emotional difficulties. Current evidence is highlighting the fact that we need to consider the relationship between reported mental BESD and the degree to which those children are influenced by an underlying language impairment. This again underscores the importance of evaluating the child's functioning in more than just language and of using teachers and peers as informants.

Narrowing the Focus: Assessment of Narrative Production

Narratives give an "account of happenings," as in telling a story, and adhere to some definable conventions or rules in the children's generation (Liles, 1993). Educational research has suggested that narratives are bridges between oral language and literacy because their structure resembles written text. Narrative skills have been shown to predict academic success reliably in children who are normally developing as well as those with learning disabilities and a specific language disorder (Paul, 2012). Narratives occur repeatedly in our daily discourse as we talk to others about weekend experiences, tell jokes, explain a process to a teacher, relate anecdotes, gossip, and describe our activities and possessions to impress our listeners. Thus, narratives are important academically as well as socially and communicatively. The narrative has been a topic of research interest over the past decade because it synthesizes a variety of abilities in order to be effective. For example, the ability to tell a story involves skill in sequencing events, creating cohesive text, use of precise vocabulary, nonreliance on contextual support, and understanding universal story grammar to structure the narrative production. According to Liles (1993):

> There is a consistency across investigators regarding the structural limitations of young children's narratives and the apparent acceleration in development around age 5. Researchers analyzing the structure of narratives in older children have generally agreed that by age 6 children can produce an ideal (e.g., adult) structure, but development continues in 9- and 10-year-old children. The development of narrative structure in older children is evidenced by both an increased number of episodes and the children's growing ability to link them together in complex ways (e.g., embedding one episode within another). More recent studies investigating narrative structure in older children . . . found that the number of complete episodes continued to increase in the narratives of children aged 8 to 16 years. (p. 875)

As narrative productions develop in children and become more complex, increasingly more elements of story grammar are incorporated into the narrative (Applebee, 1978; Johnston, 1982; Paul, 2012). For example, Johnson (1982) specifies that story grammar typically includes the following components:

- *Setting* This includes the social, physical, or environmental context as well as the main characters of the story.
- *Initiating event* It is some action, event, or change in the environment that affects the characters. This is often a "problem" of some sort (e.g., eruption of a volcano).
- *Internal response* The characters typically have an internal response to the initiating event, which may include emotions, goals, thoughts, and intentions.
- *Plan* The main character develops a plan of action.
- *Attempt* The plan of action leads to attempts or actions directed toward resolving the situation or attaining a goal.
- *Consequence* It is either the resolution of the problem or the attainment of the goal, or the failure to deal adequately with the situation.
- *Reaction* Finally, the character demonstrates a reaction that includes the character's internal states (e.g., feelings, thoughts) and response to the events that have occurred.

As narratives become more complex, the child includes more of the above elements in the production.

Studies of children with a specific language disorder have revealed narratives with some of the following characteristics (Merritt & Liles, 1989; Owens, 2004):

- Fewer total words
- Fewer different words
- Fewer story grammar components
- Fewer complete episodes
- Fewer protagonist plans and internal responses
- Fewer conventional story openings and closings
- Improper amounts of information (too much or too little)
- Fewer successful repairs
- Fewer accommodations to listeners
- Fewer complete cohesive ties and more incomplete and/or erroneous ties

Clinicians who wish to analyze narratives in children with language impairments might look for some of the differences just mentioned. As children become older, their language disorders often take on more subtle characteristics. The impairment may not be revealed in structural errors, but it may become obvious on a pragmatic-conversational level. Johnson (1995) points out that we need more information on the later development of narratives in school-age children and adolescents. Although we have information on early development, the establishment of norms on older children would be helpful to the diagnostician. Johnson also reviews information on situational variation and cultural diversity. Miller, Gillam, and Pena (2001) have developed a procedure for using principles of dynamic assessment to evaluate children's narrative production. An intervention program is coupled with this assessment procedure. Their assessment takes into account not only structural aspects of the narrative produced but also rating scales for clinician judgment about a child's response to dynamic assessment and his or her modifiability. The degree of modifiability during dynamic assessment seems to be a better indicator in classifying children with language impairment compared to pretest storytelling data (Pena, Gillam, Malek, Ruiz-Felter, Resendiz, Fiestas, & Sabel, 2006).

Paul (2007) talks about three major aspects of narratives that deserve assessment consideration. First, narratives include a basic plot and elements of story grammar that should be incorporated into the story; we briefly introduced story grammar elements earlier in this chapter. Applebee (1978) characterizes narrative development in part as the progressive inclusion of more elements of story grammar with age and the existence of a defined plot as the child becomes older. For example, Applebee proposes six stages of narrative development that involve increased use of story grammar components and plot. Looking for story grammar elements and basic plotting involves a general view of a child's narrative, so these components are often referred to as narrative macrostructure. See Table 5–9 for a description and example of the different stages.

A second assessment target for narratives according to Paul (2007) is evaluating cohesive ties in narratives. A section later in this chapter discusses cohesive adequacy, but for now it is enough to say that certain elements in an utterance gain meaning only by searching outside a particular sentence. For instance, in the sentence "John hit him," we do not know who was hit unless we look at the prior sentence, "John was pushed by Mark." Now we know that Mark was the one whom John hit. In narratives and conversation, we can use certain words only if we have introduced them in a prior utterance. If you have done a good job of cohesion, a person can find meaning in an utterance by referring to other parts of the narrative to derive meaning. This is called a *complete tie*, or the ability to tie an ambiguous part of an utterance effectively to some other part of the narrative. If you encounter a word such as *him* and you cannot figure out who "he" is, then the tie is incomplete. Paul suggests that kindergarten children have 85% complete ties in their narratives, and children with language impairment have a few as 60% complete ties. She recommends a cutoff of 70% complete ties as an indicator of concern.

A third aspect of narratives to consider in evaluation is what has become known as *sparkle* (Paul, 2007; Peterson & McCabe, 1983). Although sparkle is a bit artsy in its interpretation, several important elements are usually considered: richness of vocabulary, episode complexity, existence of a story climax, use of complex sentence structures, use of literate language style, and use of dialogue. The more these elements are included in the narrative, the more sparkle the narrative has. Newman and McGregor (2006) found that teachers and laypersons noted differences between children with SLI and typically developing children after hearing a short oral narrative. The narratives of the children with SLI were judged to be poorer in quality. In addition to some quantitative

TABLE 5–9
Applebee's Six Stages of Narrative Development

Stage	Age of Development	Description	Example
Heaps	2 years	Child provides a set of statements related to a story request, but the statements are not related to one another. There is no organizational pattern and the statements are predominately descriptive declarative sentences about events or actions. The common element is often the grammatical structure of the sentences.	A dog is barking. The cat is cute. Dad is cooking. Baby is sleeping. The end.
Sequences	3 years	Child provides a sequence that is linked by an event or attribute. There is no plot or temporal sequence and the components can often be moved around easily.	Mommy plays a game. Sissy plays a game too. Daddy plays a guitar. Doggy plays a toy. The end.
Primitive narratives	4 years	Story is organized around a central theme with events that relate to the central theme.	I went to the park. My sister wanted to swing. Mom pushed me on the swing. I went very high. I got scared. I cried. The end.
Unfocused chains	4–4.5 years	A string of events is linked but the attributes within the chain shift. There is no central theme.	I went to the pet store. I looked at fish and turtles. I fed the turtles. (shift) Turtles swim in the water. They like light. They climb on rocks. (shift) You get rocks outside. Some are big and some are small.
Focused temporal chains	5 years	A main character experiences a series of linked events.	A girl named Sarah found a penny. Her mom said "make a wish." And she did make a wish. And then she got a big surprise. A new puppy.
Narratives	Older than 5 years	The central theme of the story develops over the course of the narrative. The elements of the story compliment the theme. Elements and relationships may be concrete or abstract, and there is consistent movement toward the end of the story, where there is often a climax.	One day there was a princess named Lilly. She liked to play and sing music for all her animals. The animals liked to hear her music. One day, she got sick and could not sing. The animals were very sad. They went and found her a magic flower to make her feel better. When she held the flower her voice came back. Then they all singed and celebrated.

Source: Adapted from Applebee (1978)

variables such as utterance length and underdeveloped story themes, the laypersons also noted that sparkle was missing from the SLI narratives. A good place to start in a narrative analysis might be a standardized method of analysis, such as the *Test of Narrative Language* (Gillam & Pearson, 2004) or the Strong *Narrative Assessment Procedure* (Strong, 1998). These tests are two of the few measures that provide normative data on narrative production.

Narratives have been analyzed with regard to macrostructure and microstructure. *Macrostructure* has to do with inclusion of story grammar elements and the complexity of episode structure. One aspect of *microstructure* analysis is directed to the linguistic aspects of the narrative, including construction of noun phrases, use of conjunctions, and the inclusion of dependent clauses. Most authorities suggest that a thorough assessment of narratives includes both macro- and microstructural analyses. Justice, Bowles, Kaderavek, Ukrainetz, Eisenberg, and Gillam (2006) have developed the Index of Narrative Microstructure (INMIS) and provide preliminary normative data for 250 children between 5 and 12 years of age as they constructed narratives in response to a single picture stimulus. The authors found that microstructure analysis revealed two important factors of productivity (word output, lexical diversity, and number of T-units produced) and complexity (T-unit length, proportion of complex T-units). The procedure can be used in conjunction with macrostructural analyses to evaluate narrative development in children. Ukrainetz and Gillam (2009) studied 6- and 8-year-old children as they produced two imaginative narratives. They found that the younger, typically developing children and those with language impairment produced narratives with fewer orientations to the story, less evaluations, and fewer abstracts and codas compared to older, typically developing children. The type of narrative used in language sampling may be important in assessment. McCabe, Bliss, Barra, and Bennett (2008) gathered fictional (wordless picture book) and personal (experience-based) narratives from children with language impairment between the ages of 7 and 9. They found that the personal narratives included more components required in adequate narrative production compared to fictional narratives. Performance in one type of narrative did not appear to relate to the performance in the other genre. Heilmann, Miller, Nockerts, and Dunaway (2010) developed the Narrative Scoring Scheme (NSS), which deals with narrative macroscructure but goes beyond basic story grammar to include higher-level components such as cohesion, character development referencing, and conflict resolution (see Table 5–10). Each of the narrative components is scored using a 5-point scale ranging from minimal to proficient, and the clinician can obtain a total or composite score that represents a child's "overall narrative organization." The narrative can also be input into the SALT program and the child's results compared to NSS normative data. This is a relevant measure that can be used not only in diagnosis but also in monitoring treatment goals that focus on narrative production.

Narrative analysis is a valuable adjunct to our assessment repertoire and is regarded as an important diagnostic consideration by most current authorities (Owens, 2014; Paul, 2012; Swanson, Fey, Mills, & Hood, 2005). We must also remember that narrative production may vary according to a person's culture. Gutierrez-Clellen and Quinn (1993) indicate that narratives are influenced by a child's information and organization abilities, world knowledge/experience, the type of elicitation task, interactional style, and use of paralinguistic conventions. For certain disorder groups, the elicitation task may make a difference in gathering narrative samples. For instance, using pictures in eliciting narratives from children with Down syndrome resulted in longer utterances compared to an interview technique (Miles, Chapman, & Sindberg, 2006).

TABLE 5–10
Narrative Scoring Scheme from Heilman et al. (2010)

Characteristic	Proficient	Emerging	Minimal/immature
Introduction	Setting –Child states general place and provides some detail about the setting (e.g., reference to the time of the setting—daytime, bedtime, or season). –Setting elements are stated at appropriate place in story. Characters –Main characters are introduced with some description or detail provided.	Setting –Child states general setting but provides no detail. –Description or elements of story are given intermittently through story. –Child may provide description of specific element of setting (e.g., the frog is in the jar). OR Characters –Characters of story are mentioned with no detail or description.	–Child launches into story with no attempt to provide the setting.
Character development	–Main character(s) and *all* supporting character(s) are mentioned. –Throughout story it is clear that child can discriminate between main and supporting characters (e.g., more description of and emphasis on main character[s]). –Child narrates in first person using character voice (e.g., "You get out of my tree," said the owl).	–Both main and active supporting characters are mentioned. –Main characters are not clearly distinguished from supporting characters.	–Inconsistent mention is made of involved or active characters. –Characters necessary for advancing the plot are not present.
Mental states	–Mental states of main and supporting characters are expressed when necessary for plot development and advancement. –Various mental state words are used.	–Some mental state words are used to develop character(s). –A limited number of mental state words are used inconsistently throughout the story.	No use is made of mental state words to develop characters.
Referencing	–Child provides necessary antecedents to pronouns. –References are clear throughout story.	–Referents/antecedents are used inconsistently.	–Pronouns are used excessively. –No verbal clarifiers are used. –Child is unaware listener is confused.
Conflict resolution	–Child clearly states all conflicts and resolutions critical to advancing the plot of the story.	–Description of conflicts and resolutions critical to advancing the plot of the story is underdeveloped. OR –Not all conflicts and resolutions critical to advancing the plot are present.	–Random resolution is stated with no mention of cause or conflict. OR –Conflict is mentioned without resolution. OR –Many conflicts and resolutions critical to advancing the plot are not present.

(continued)

TABLE 5–10
(Continued)

Characteristic	Proficient	Emerging	Minimal/immature
Cohesion	–Events follow a logical order. –Critical events are included, while less emphasis is placed on minor events. –Smooth transitions are provided between events.	–Events follow a logical order. –Excessive detail or emphasis provided on minor events leads the listener astray. OR –Transitions to next event are unclear. OR –Minimal detail is given for critical events. OR –Equal emphasis is placed on all events.	–No use is made of smooth transitions.
Conclusion	–Story is clearly wrapped up using general concluding statements such as "and they were together again happy as could be."	–Specific event is concluded, but no general statement is made as to the conclusion of the whole story.	–Child stops narrating, and listener may need to ask if that is the end.

Scoring: Each characteristic receives a scaled score of 0–5. Proficient characteristics = 5; Emerging = 3; Minimal/immature = 1. Scores between (i.e., 2 and 4) are undefined; use judgment. Scores of zero and NA are defined below. A composite is scored by adding the total of the characteristic scores. Highest score = 35.

A score of zero is given for child errors (such as telling the wrong story, conversing with examiner, not completing/refusing task, using wrong language and creating inability of scorer to comprehend story in target language, abandoned utterances, unintelligibility, poor performance, or components of rubric are in imitation-only).

A score of NA (nonapplicable) is given for mechanical/examiner/operator errors (such as interference from background noise, issues with recording such as cutoffs or interruptions, examiner quitting before child does, examiner not following protocol, or examiner asking overly specific or leading questions rather than open-ended questions or prompts).

Source: Republished with permission of American Speech-Language-Hearing Association, from Properties of the narrative scoring scheme using narrative retells in young children. Heilman et al. (2009). *American Journal of Speech-Language Pathology*; permission conveyed through Copyright Clearance Center, Inc.

Assessment of Topic Manipulation in Clinical Discourse

Topic maintenance requires use of general knowledge shared by the conversational partners, information physically present in the context of the environment, or previously shared discourse. According to Keenan and Schieffelin (1976), much conversational space is taken up by communicators to establish a topic. Once the topic is established, an interactant can use a turn to either maintain the topic (*continuous discourse*) or change the topic (*discontinuous discourse*). When speakers continue a discourse topic by corroborating a previous utterance with a related statement, or incorporating information in a prior utterance into their statement, the topic is maintained. When a speaker discontinues a discourse topic, it is either by introducing a topic that is unrelated to previous utterances or by reintroducing a prior topic ("Getting back to what we said about . . ."). Thus, topic-maintaining utterances corroborate a prior statement or incorporate it into a new statement that is still on the topic. The length of continuous discourse increases with age. In assessment, we need to determine how a child is able to secure the attention of a listener in order to initiate a topic (by crying, yelling, gesturing, and tugging; or with loudness, prosody, or an introduction such as "Know what?"). We can measure the length of the topic unit in terms of number of turns taken per topic. We also can measure the topic-maintaining and -shifting utterances used by a child. It is important in assessment to examine a child's ability not only to continue topics but also to initiate them. In sampling, as mentioned previously, we may not often provide for this. Some of the most productive work on in-depth analysis of topic manipulation has been done by Brinton and Fujiki (1984, 1989), who provide detailed procedures for evaluating all relevant aspects of topic manipulation in clinical work. We need further research to define more specifically the normal development of topic manipulation in both children who are typically developing and those with language impairments. Some language-impaired children clearly have difficulty with these skills (Prutting & Kirchner, 1987), while other subgroups of children with linguistic impairment appear to manipulate topics normally (Edmonds & Haynes, 1988; Ehlers & Cirrin, 1983). Assessment of *contingency* (topic manipulation) may be important in documenting discourse problems in specific populations. For example, fragile X syndrome often co-occurs with autism spectrum disorders, and research has shown that boys with both of these disorders concurrently were significantly less contingent in discourse than those having only fragile X (Roberts, Martin, Moskowitz, Harris, Foreman, & Nelson, 2007). We also need to know more about topic manipulation throughout the lifespan to determine changes in these skills in aging normal subjects because there is some evidence that differences exist among age groups (Stover & Haynes, 1989).

Assessment of Repairs: The Contingent Query

Another major category of measurement of conversational competence is the *contingent query*. A number of studies (Garvey, 1977a, 1977b) show that contingent queries are used by adults and children to achieve cohesion in conversation. Children as young as 3 years use contingent queries. Basically, the queries serve multiple functions in conversation, many of which have to do with repair procedures that allow the conversation to continue. For instance, a contingent query can be used to request a general repetition ("Huh?"), a specific repetition ("A what?"), a request for confirmation ("A digital recorder?"), and elaboration ("We have to go where?"). There are more complex aspects of contingent queries that are explained in the above references. One can see, however, that these queries are important mechanisms of conversational competence and that a child who does not know how to ask for clarification, for instance, will have difficulty continuing a particular topic with an interactant. The term *conversational repair* has been used most often in association with contingent queries. Clinically, it would be important to determine if a child can both respond to and produce requests for conversational repair (Brinton & Fujiki, 1989). For example, we would like to see if a child can adjust an utterance to a listener's request for repetition, clarification, or elaboration. On the other hand, we would like to determine if a child would ask for clarification if a clinician asks for a *ferbis* or makes a statement violating truth constraints in a particular context. Brinton and Fujiki (1989) provide many helpful suggestions for both assessment and intervention with conversational repair mechanisms. Yont, Hewitt, and Miccio (2000) introduced a system for coding conversational breakdowns, called the *Breakdown Coding System* (BCS). This was piloted on typically developing preschoolers during natural interactions with caretakers. They found that the BCS had high interjudge reliability and was useful for profiling patterns of breakdowns in conversation. Further research on children with language impairment should be conducted.

Assessment of Cohesive Adequacy

Some children produce narratives or conversational turns that lack adequate *cohesion*, which refers to the relationships or ties between elements in discourse that are dependent upon one another (Halliday & Hasan, 1976). Stover and Haynes (1989) provide an example:

> Wash the *dirty dishes* that are in the sink. Dry *them* and then put *them* in the cabinet. In the second sentence *them* refers directly back to the *dirty dishes*, thus forming a cohesive tie. Of course, the cohesive marker may extend far beyond the immediately preceding sentence to an utterance produced earlier in the conversation. . . . In a *complete tie*, the referent to which a cohesive marker refers is easily found in a prior utterance with no ambiguity as in the above example. In an *incomplete tie*, a cohesive marker refers to something not mentioned in prior utterances (e.g., I like ice cream. *He* does too). In this example *he* cannot be associated with a particular person mentioned previously in the sentence. In an erroneous tie, there is ambiguity or error in interpreting who a referent is (e.g., Tom and Jerry live in the city. *He* likes it.). In this example, we do not know if *he* refers to Tom or Jerry. (p. 140)

Liles (1985) provides specific procedures for cohesion analysis. One can readily see that this type of analysis would be useful in cases that do not take into account the listener's perspective in discourse and that are not aware of the requirements of conversational rules (Grice, 1975). Some recent studies suggest that there may be subgroups of children with cohesion difficulties. For example, Craig and Evans (1993) found that children with both receptive and expressive language impairments produced significantly more incomplete, erroneous, and ambiguous cohesive ties compared to children with disorders exclusively in expressive language. It is easy to see that measurements such as percentage of complete, incomplete, and erroneous ties could be used as an index of progress in treatment.

ISSUES OF MEMORY, PROCESSING LOAD, AND EXECUTIVE LOADING

Over time it has been noted by clinicians and researchers that children with language impairments seem to have difficulty processing linguistic material effectively. This is especially true when the processing load becomes less manageable with the addition of semantic, syntactic, phonological, and/or cognitive complexity. This quite possibly accounts for the phenomenon we referred to earlier when the child with SLI finds it progressively more difficult to cope with the increasing linguistic and cognitive demands of the educational curriculum. This is easy to see in studies that have used a dual-task paradigm in which children are asked to complete two operations simultaneously. Johnston (2006) summarizes this eloquently:

> Other interpretations of dual-task findings stress the coordination of effort that is required, and argue that poor performance reflects inefficient deployment of knowledge, poor monitoring of performance, or difficulties in managing diverse responses. All of these interpretations rest on the assumption that the human mind functions as a limited capacity system. If there is a finite amount of mental energy available at any one moment, a task that requires great concentration or efficiency may use enough of this capacity that little remains for work on a second task. When the traffic is heavy, it's hard to talk and drive. (p. 54)

If children with SLI have a "weakness" in the area of language, they may use most of their processing capacity just to understand or produce an utterance, and few resources are left for more complex activities such as making inferences, selecting novel vocabulary, or constructing complex sentences. Thus, the more we can help a child learn about language through therapy, the more processing capacity is freed for use. Certain abilities, such as using working memory, are necessary in order to hold critical information in mind from the beginning of a sentence or a prior sentence while processing the rest of the utterance. Even in nonword repetition tasks (NRTs), children with SLI seem to run into processing difficulty as the stimuli become longer. We mention some specific examples here because clinicians may want to probe these abilities as part of a thorough language assessment. Montgomery and Evans (2009) found that children with language impairment performed lower than typically developing children on tasks designed to tap working memory. The memory task scores in the language-impaired group correlated with scores indicating comprehension of complex sentences. Scores on an NRT correlated with comprehension of simple sentences. There were no significant correlations found between memory tasks and language comprehension for the typically developing group.

Working memory has been found to be deficient in many studies of children with language impairment and is a skill that is required especially in a task requiring parsing of complex sentences. The processing load is significantly increased if a child is struggling to hold onto rapidly presented information while trying to make cognitive and linguistic judgments. Thus, compared to typically developing children, those with language impairment require more mental effort to process language, whether it is simple or more complex. A recent factor analytic investigation suggested that 14-year-old students with specific language impairment may experience processing limitations in speed and working memory (Leonard, Weismer, Miller, Frances, Tomblin, & Kail, 2007). Lum, Conti-Ramsden, Page, and Ullman (2012) evaluated and compared the working, declarative, and procedural memory of primary-school-age children with SLI and typically developing children. The children with SLI were found to experience impairments in visuospatial procedural memory, verbal short-term memory, and verbal working memory. No correlation was found between working memory and language, whereas declarative memory correlated with the lexical abilities of both groups of children. Grammatical abilities were also found to correlate with verbal declarative memory in the children with SLI. Overall, the results of their investigation suggest that children with SLI experience deficits in procedural memory and verbal working memory. Montgomery, Magimairaj, and Finney (2010) provide an excellent review of the research on working memory as it relates to language impairment and a list of sources for tests and measurements that can be used by the SLP to measure processing speed, executive function, working memory capacity, and short-term memory.

A recent meta-analysis of over 20 studies focusing on nonword repetition performance in children with language impairment found that this population exhibited significant impairments, performing an average of 1.27 standard deviations below typically developing children. The difficulties were on both short and long nonword stimuli; however, the problem became more significant on the longer stimuli. Also, the study found different effect sizes across studies that used different sets of nonword stimuli, suggesting that the specific tasks may not be equivalent. Another example of a nonword repetition task for preschool children was developed in Britain by Stokes and Klee (2009). They found, as most nonword repetition tests do, that the longer syllable tasks were more difficult for the children in the study and that the test could differentiate between late talkers and typically developing children with acceptable psychometric values for sensitivity and specificity. Chiat and Roy (2007) have developed a nonword repetition test for preschool children. They have found the typical result of increased difficulty with increased item length and more complex prosodic structure of the items. Children performed better with age between 2 and 4 years, and the performance was not affected by gender or socioeconomic level. They also found that the test could discriminate accurately between children referred to a clinic for evaluation and typically developing children with high interjudge and test-retest reliability.

Most tasks involving working memory and nonword repetition take little time to administer in an evaluation and may contribute one more piece to the picture of a child's total functioning in the area of language. NRTs have also been used with bilingual children or those who speak dialects of English because nonwords do not depend on the rules of a child's first language. Thus, these have been promising tasks for use in nonbiased assessment.

Executive functioning is a basket term that reflects cognitive abilities and goal-directed behavior that requires working memory, planning, flexibility in thought and action (switching), verbal and nonverbal fluency, and inhibition (Hughes, 2002; Miyake, Friedman, Emerson, Witzki, & Howerter, 2000). These skills have different developmental courses, with inhibition developing earlier than switching and working memory. Studies are emerging and documenting a relationship between language development and executive functioning ability (Carlson, Mandell, & Williams, 2004; Remine, Care, & Brown, 2008; Roebers & Schneider, 2005; Spaulding, 2010). Henry, Messer, and Nash (2012) used 10 measures of executive functioning to evaluate whether school-age children with SLI differ in executive abilities when compared to children with low language function and typically developing children with no language difficulties. They found that the children with SLI experienced more difficulty with 6 out of the 10 measures of executive function than the typically developing children. Specifically, they performed more poorly on tasks related to verbal and nonverbal working memory tasks, verbal and nonverbal fluency, nonverbal inhibition, and nonverbal planning. They also found that two-thirds of the children with SLI demonstrated executive functioning impairments in at least three of the areas of executive functioning evaluated. Significant differences were not observed between the children with SLI and the children with low language function, suggesting that even a low to moderate degrees of language impairment could influence executive functioning abilities.

EVALUATING LITERACY AND SCHOOL CURRICULUM

As we mentioned at the beginning of this chapter, several groups of youngsters are at high risk of developing a language disorder during the school years. First, children with a history of preschool language delay are likely to experience subtle language disturbances throughout their school years and be at risk for academic problems (Aram & Nation, 1980; Bashir et al., 1983; Hall & Tomblin, 1978; King, Jones, & Lasky, 1982; Strominger & Bashir, 1977). These children were often dismissed from language treatment and then later rediagnosed as having a reading or learning disability. Most of these children exhibited low academic achievement throughout school because the curricular demands increase significantly in terms of language and communicative expectations while the child's linguistic abilities may not improve to meet these challenges. A second group of children likely to demonstrate subtle language impairments consists of children diagnosed as having a reading or learning disability. The majority of students with learning disabilities have experienced language delays, and some of these problems continue into adulthood. Finally, children who are considered to be academically at risk because of poor school performance are also likely to have gaps in their ability to perform linguistic tasks (Simon, 1989). It is now clear that children with speech-language impairments tend to perform poorly on reading comprehension (Catts, 1993). Oral language skills are intimately related to reading achievement (Wise, Sevcik, Morris, Lovett, & Wolf, 2007). The SLP should carefully evaluate youngsters from the groups mentioned above, especially when they are referred by classroom teachers. Many of the specific language symptoms likely to be seen in these groups were listed in Table 5–1. One aspect that has not been emphasized, however, is specific examination of the types of language and communication abilities that are important for classroom success.

More than ever before, the speech-language pathologist is involved with literacy issues. This involvement may begin in preschool or early school age as early literacy screening programs are developed. Part of any thorough language assessment should address emerging literacy skills. If a child is lagging in literacy development, the SLP can incorporate literacy activities into treatment. Even in typically developing children, literacy issues can have a significant impact on learning. For instance, Foster and Miller (2007) studied groups of children from kindergarten to third grade who represented low, average, and high levels of literacy development on kindergarten entrance. These children came from a pool of over 12,000 youngsters who were part of the Early Childhood Longitudinal Study. Students in the middle and high groups achieved good scores on phonics (decoding) by the end of first grade. The low-level group did not meet such expectations until third grade. This group also manifested significant text comprehension difficulties. One can only speculate on the amount of information that these children had difficulty learning due to a struggle with literacy issues. Unfortunately, most children in the low-level performing group came from lower socioeconomic levels and had an overrepresentation of African American and Hispanic students. Justice and Ezell (2004) provide a good developmental sequence of written language awareness achievements and their associated print-referencing targets for assessment and treatment. Justice and Kaderavek (2004) and Kaderavek and Justice (2004) outline a developmental model for emergent literacy development, including phonological awareness, print concepts, alphabet knowledge, and literate language. Many literacy opportunities are available embedded in a child's natural environment and school setting, while other aspects may be approached explicitly by the SLP with small-group, classroom, and individual activities. It is helpful to know the developmental progression in choosing assessment targets and intervention goals. Boudreau (2005) determined that experimenter-administered measures of rhyme, environmental print knowledge, knowledge of print conventions, letter-name knowledge, letter-sound knowledge, and narrative ability were strongly related to a parent questionnaire that tapped similar areas and parent literacy practices. The implication here is that such a questionnaire might be combined with assessment tasks to gain a broader view of emergent literacy. Never underestimate the contribution that parents and teachers can make to evaluation. Some formal standardized measures commonly used to assess reading ability are the *Test of Early Reading Ability*, Third Edition (Reid, Hresko, & Hammill, 2001); *Gray Oral Reading Test*, Fifth Edition (Wiederholt & Bryant, 2012); *Gray Diagnostic Reading Test*, Second Edition (Bryant, Wiederholt, & Bryant, 2004); *Gray Silent Reading Tests* (Wiederholt & Blalock, 2000); and *Woodcock Reading Mastery Test*, Third Edition (Woodcock, 2011).

Many aspects of literacy (e.g., reading, writing, spelling, adequate narratives) are based on a child's oral language system, so it is not surprising that many of our clients with language disorder also have poor literacy skills. In the beginning of this chapter, we cited studies showing that children with language impairment are at high risk for reading problems and may have less academic success. Some more recent investigations address the relationships among language and metalinguistic abilities and reading. For example, Catts, Fey, Zhang, and Tomblin (2001) studied more than 600 children in kindergarten and tested them again in second grade for reading ability. They found that letter identification, sentence imitation, phonological awareness, rapid naming, and mother's educational level uniquely predicted reading outcome in second grade. Gilbertson and Bramlett (1998) studied informal phonological awareness measures to determine if they could predict reading ability in first grade. Participants were 91 former Head Start students. Gilbertson and Bramlett found that the phonological awareness tasks of invented spelling, categorization, and blending were the best predictors of standardized reading measures at the end of first grade. The three phonological awareness tasks correctly identified at-risk students with 92% accuracy. The authors suggest that the SLP can play a primary role in identifying and remediating children with language-based reading disorders.

Catts (1997) provides a checklist for SLPs and teachers to use for early identification of reading disabilities. The checklist provides a number of language deficits often associated with reading difficulties. It is designed to be used with children who are finishing kindergarten or entering the first grade. Children who demonstrate a large number of the characteristics listed within the checklist should be considered for further evaluation. The checklist contains seven sections, with each section containing five to seven items: speech-sound awareness, word retrieval, verbal memory, speech production/ perception, comprehension, expressive language, and other important factors. Boudreau and Hedberg (1999) studied 5-year-old children with SLI and normally developing language on a number of early literacy variables. The SLI children did not perform as well as normally developing children on tasks involving knowledge of rhyme, letter names, and print concepts. The SLI children also showed poorer performance on narrative measures of linguistic structure, recall of information, and total events included. Other research has examined literacy in terms of emergent readings in children with SLI. In emergent readings, a child who is not yet reading conventionally is asked to "read" from a familiar storybook, and the speech produced is analyzed for features of written language. Kaderavek and Sulzby (2000) studied SLI and normal-language children and found that children with SLI produced fewer language features associated with written language, and the SLI children had more difficulty with oral narratives. They suggest that emergent storybook reading may be useful as part of a language assessment protocol because it may provide insight into the relationship between language impairment and later reading difficulty.

Even in cases of late talkers who ultimately develop language in a relatively normal manner, some researchers have expressed concern. For example, Rescorla (2002) studied 34 children who were identified as late talkers as toddlers and followed them until the ages of 6 to 9 years. Most late talkers performed within the average range in most language skills by the time they entered school. Relatively few of the late talkers developed a reading disability, but the author regarded the early expressive language delay as a subclinical weakness in the skills that serve language and reading. Rescorla recommends providing extra exposure to activities for strengthening word retrieval, verbal memory, phonological discrimination, and grammatical processing. Thus, the speech-language pathologist should be involved in the early detection of literacy issues because these are likely to be present in children with language impairment. We are learning more and more about the long-term effects of language delay. Rescorla (2009) studied typically developing and late-talking children with normal comprehension between the ages of 2 and 17 years. At age 17, the children who were late talkers had significantly lower vocabulary, grammar, and verbal memory compared to the typically developing children. It is important to note that the scores of both groups were within normal limits, but the late talkers were significantly lower in this range. Justice, Invernizzi, and Meier (2002) developed a protocol for early detection of children with high risk for literacy difficulties. The protocol is designed for use by a team of professionals in a school district and focuses on written language awareness, phonological awareness, letter-name knowledge, grapheme–phoneme correspondence, literacy motivation, and home literacy. Guidelines are provided for designing and implementing an early literacy screening program and developing interpretive benchmarks for the protocol (passing scores, etc.).

As children get older, it should be the responsibility of the SLP to incorporate literacy issues into assessment as well as treatment activities. For example, Apel (1999) provides a rationale from the professional literature and ASHA-preferred practice patterns for assessing and treating reading and writing difficulties: ". . . [S]peech-language pathologists should assess and facilitate reading and writing skills, in addition to oral language skills, if they have been identified as areas of concern" (p. 229). This can be an important facet of diagnosis and treatment even in older cases. Speech-language pathologists may also participate in assessments involving other literacy areas such as spelling and writing. Masterson and Crede (1999) discuss the development of spelling and factors that influence spelling performance. They provide a case example of how a thorough assessment and intervention for spelling problems can show improvement in both formal and informal measures of spelling performance. There are three contexts that spelling is often assessed: dictation, connected writing, and recognition. For dictation, the therapist orally provides the word within the context of a sentence, and the student is asked to spell the word orthographically or aloud. In connected writing, the students spelling is evaluated from a writing sample; with a recognition task, the student is given multiple choices. Masterson and Apel (2000) indicate that students should be assessed in both dictation and connected writing. The *Test of Written Spelling–5* (Larsen, Hammill, & Moats, 2013) and *Test of Written Language,* Fourth Edition (Hammill & Larsen, 2009) are commonly used standardized methods for assessing spelling. Masterson and Apel (2010) developed the Spelling Sensitivity System (SSS) as a method for evaluating developmental changes in spelling accuracy and knowledge. Within this system words, are divided into elements, and the student's spelling is evaluated on a 4-point scale. Two scores are divided: SSS-Elements and SSS-Words. Guidelines are provided on how to score and evaluate the SSS-Elements and SSS-Words outcomes.

Graham and Harris (1999) illustrate how writing strategies can be assessed and explicitly taught in combination with procedures for regulating those strategies, working through the writing process, and eliminating undesirable behaviors that interfere with writing. As part of a comprehensive evaluation of the school-age student with a language disorder, we must remember that all modalities of language can provide important insights into the student's abilities and needs. A sample of the student reading several paragraphs aloud from one of his or her textbooks allows the SLP to note miscues, comprehension ability, and decoding strategies that may indicate difficulty processing written information. Similarly, writing samples of stories or narratives can usually be obtained in less than an hour, including time for planning. Obviously, the younger the student, the less writing can be accomplished in a sampling period. Nelson (2010) provides a nice overview of analysis of reading and writing, and additional Internet and written resources for the clinician. Puranik, Lombardino, and Altmann (2008) provide a method for SLPs to use in quantifying writing abilities. The procedure can be administered individually or in groups. Specific measurements to be computed on a writing sample are illustrated and data are provided for school-age children between grades 3 and 6. This procedure can also be of value in quantifying writing growth over time.

If a school-age child has some subtle language impairments and shows poor academic performance, part of a thorough evaluation should include the following:

1. Assessment of the child's knowledge of successful strategies to perform well in the school culture
2. Evaluation of the teacher's communication while instructing the child
3. Assessment of the curriculum and materials that the child is expected to learn
4. Assessment of literacy areas of reading and writing.

You may wonder why an SLP would be interested in assessing these factors when they are peripheral to the child's abilities. A school-age child is part of a complex system that is constantly changing its expectations for academic performance. The child may have to deal with differing types of educational content and a variety of teaching styles throughout the school day. The school-age child must use language in both comprehension and production for a variety of academic tasks that often involve complex metalinguistic ability and the learning of abstract concepts presented verbally by a teacher. Teachers and SLPs should remember that metalinguistic abilities appear to be acquired in a general developmental order (Wallach & Miller, 1988).

In addition, the child must be aware of the expectations of the school culture and must know how to study, memorize, and learn classroom material on which he or she will be thoroughly tested. If the child has no effective study skills or strategies for remembering and understanding information, failure results. Academic success requires self-discipline, prioritizing, organization, and time management, all of which are subsumed under the concept of executive function. *Self-regulation* involves self-monitoring, self-evaluation, and behavioral adjustment. Both executive function and self-regulation are intimately involved in learning and implementing strategies for oral language, writing, and reading comprehension. In Singer and Bashir (1999) they provide a case example that demonstrates how a client was taught to inhibit nonproductive responses and engage in systematic analysis of a situation, set goals for communication, and self-monitor. Executive functions and self-regulation are very important to evaluate and include in treatment programs.

The child's teacher could talk at a rapid rate during instruction or use figurative language and complex sentence types. The teacher could be quite adept at using audio and visual media as aids to instruction or could rely exclusively on the lecture modality. The reading curriculum could have a heavy emphasis on phonics or other metalinguistic tasks that may make the learning of reading extremely difficult or impossible for a child with metalinguistic problems. Conversely, the curriculum might emphasize a whole-language approach with little emphasis on phonics for a child whose phonological awareness is desperately in need of remedial work. In some cases, an alternative approach could help a child learn a particular skill. What we are saying here is that the diagnostician cannot fully understand the language-impaired child unless he or she is familiar with the child's learning environment. Sometimes, the most potent treatment recommendations include curricular, instructional, and learning strategy modifications. Without examining these areas in a thorough assessment, a clinician cannot hope to make effective suggestions for remediation. Obtaining input from teachers and the older child is an important factor in evaluation. Larson and McKinley (1995) and Paul (2012) provide examples of protocols to use in obtaining information from teachers and students with language impairments.

The rationale for using portfolios to evaluate students with language disorders is persuasive. It is important to examine these students from a variety of perspectives to determine the true impact of their communication disorders and abilities. First, portfolios provide a method of evaluation that is holistic and educationally relevant, as required by law. Second, traditional language testing is more related to labeling or placement issues and is not adapted to the development of treatment goals and strategies. Third, a portfolio represents a collection of a student's work across a variety of modalities and subject areas. Fourth, portfolios promote collaboration among team members in school settings. Finally, much of this information is readily available, and in school settings it is possible for the SLP to gather new information because he or she is working in the context. An important factor in using portfolios is that they should not simply be composed of random data but should be dictated by the clinician's questions and concerns. Kratcoski (1998) suggests that the clinician follow a four-step process: (1) define the student's problem, (2) form hypotheses about the causes and effects of the problem, (3) develop specific assessment questions, and (4) determine the specific items to be added to the portfolio that address the questions posed by the clinician. Kratcoski lists many potential items that could be included in a portfolio:

- Initial referral forms
- Language samples
- Story retell samples
- Referential communication sample
- Observational notes of class participation, work observation, and social interaction
- Work samples of tests, papers, assignments, speeches
- Teacher interviews
- Parent interviews
- Student interview
- Audio and video recordings
- Writing samples, journal entries
- Peer evaluations
- Testing data
- Conference notes

Portfolio assessment is a broad-based and invaluable source of information to be used in language assessment with school-age children.

Another area of interest for assessment is the child's ability to deal with the types of communication and linguistic tasks typically encountered in the classroom. Some useful measures that focus on classroom communication abilities or metalinguistics in older students (e.g., upper elementary through junior high) are *Evaluating Communicative Competence* (ECC) (Simon, 1994), *Classroom Communication Screening Procedure for Early Assessment* (CCSPEA) (Simon, 1989), and *Analysis of the Language of Learning* (ALL) (Blodgett & Cooper, 1987). These procedures will provide insight into a child's ability to perform classroom-like tasks and will pinpoint specific difficulties. The clinician can also experiment with any facilitating procedures that make difficult tasks easier to accomplish and can mention these in the examination report for teacher use.

CONCLUSION AND SELF-ASSESSMENT

One can easily see that the diagnosis and evaluation of school-age and adolescent clients is a complex activity. The SLP must work closely with teachers, parents, and other professionals in successfully dealing with these cases. The interplay among linguistic, metalinguistic, conversational, and academic areas is great, and the work of the SLP can potentially reap benefits in a child's educational performance.

After reading this chapter you should be able to answer the following questions:

1. What are the four groups of school-age students who have a greater likelihood of being diagnosed with a language disorder?
2. What is the SLP's role in screening school-age children?
3. What are the CCSS and what is their impact on assessment?
4. What parameters need to be considered when obtaining a representative language sample?
5. How does an SLP obtain and analyze a representative language sample?
6. What types of measurements can be performed on a language sample from a child who is delayed in his or her language development?
7. When evaluating a child's language comprehension, where can breakdowns in comprehension occur?
8. What are the four ways that language comprehension can be evaluated?
9. What are some available syntax analysis packages? What factors should be considered when using a packaged analysis procedure?
10. How can pragmatic language be assessed? What factors should be considered when evaluating pragmatics?
11. How can a narrative sample be obtained? What factors must be considered when analyzing narrative productions?
12. What factors must be considered when evaluating the microstructure and macrostructure of narratives? How do these structures differ?
13. What factors can be evaluated when assessing conversational discourse?
14. How can memory and executive functioning affect language assessment and diagnosis?
15. What role does the SLP play in evaluating reading disorders?
16. How are reading problems assessed and what areas require assessment when a reading disorder is suspected?
17. How is written language evaluated? What factors must be considered when assessing written language?

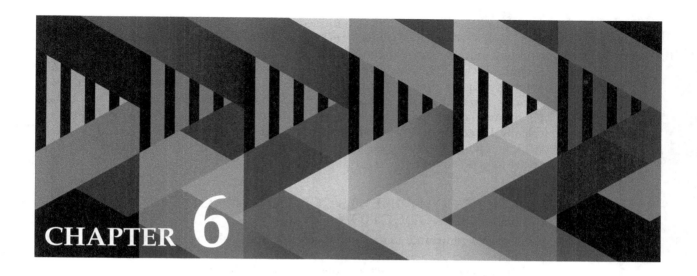

CHAPTER 6

Assessment of Speech-Sound Disorders

LEARNING OUTCOMES

After reading this chapter you will be able to:

1. Differentiate between articulation disorders and phonological processing disorders.
2. List at least four commonly heard phonological processes that may be awry in the speech-language production of children.
3. Cite general areas to assess when evaluating a young child with a speech-sound disorder.
4. Defend why it is important to assess (and treat) phonological processing disorders in children.

Historically, articulation was conceptualized by most researchers and clinicians as being primarily a motor act. This sensorimotor aspect of articulation was studied, and it was not uncommon for articulation treatment to emphasize almost exclusively the movements of the oral musculature through an emphasis on diagrams, models, and motoric drills. In these early years, the disorder was known as an articulation impairment, reflecting the importance of movements of the articulators in the vocal tract. Current views on the use of nonspeech oral motor exercises in treatment for speech-sound disorders suggest that such methods are not only controversial but unfounded.

In the mid-1970s speech-language pathologists (SLPs) became highly interested in the work of linguists who examined emerging sound production differences from the perspective of phonological theory. With the advent of greater attention to linguistics and the branch of phonology (the science and study of speech-sound usage) it was noted that articulation had more components than simply motoric activity. It is now well accepted that linguistic activity contributes significantly to the articulatory process. (See Kuhl [2004] for an overview of the evidence of children cracking the speech code.)

After linguistic theory was studied for decades, some articulation disorders began to be recognized as phonological processing disorders. Now that we are aware that both sensorimotor and linguistic factors can contribute to speech impairment, the encompassing terminology has changed to speech-sound disorder (though we will cover particular motor speech disorders in future chapters). Suffice it to say, our use of the term *speech-sound disorders* is inclusive of both articulation and phonological disorders, and indeed it is common for clinicians to use the terms denoting both linguistically based and motorically based disorders—despite their differences. Bernthal, Bankson, and Flipsen (2013) and Bauman-Waengler (2012) vary their terminologies in this manner, so we feel we are in good company.

MULTIPLE COMPONENTS CONTRIBUTING TO SOUND PRODUCTION

Many events contribute to the final motor act of articulating. First, the biological component provides the basic structures for articulation, such as the vocal tract and the articulators, as well as the intact nervous system, which allows us to perform the sensory (auditory, tactile, kinesthetic, proprioceptive) and motor functions necessary for controlled movement. Second, a cognitive-linguistic component allows the speaker to conceive of something to say. This thought then undergoes linguistic processing whereby semantic elements are selected, words are arranged in proper syntactic order, and the utterance is appropriately tailored to the communicative situation by the speaker, taking pragmatics into consideration. The selection of phonemic elements and their order is then accomplished by applying phonological rules of language. The details of linguistic processing of an utterance are not fully understood. It is enough to say, however, that linguistic processing involving semantic, syntactic, pragmatic, and phonological areas must occur at some point prior to expressing an utterance. Third, there is a sensorimotor-acoustic component that includes motor programming and motor learning of actual sequences of physical movement in a wide variety of phonetic contexts. The motor production in the vocal tract then gives rise to acoustic vibrations that travel through a medium of air and arrive at the ears of our listeners. This brief sketch of the processes that result in articulatory production is highly simplified.

This gross division of the articulatory process into biological, cognitive-linguistic, and sensorimotor components carries with it several important implications. First, the diagnostician must be prepared to assess and treat any or all aspects of the process in a given client. Bernthal, Bankson, and Flipsen (2013) indicate that speech-sound disorders can be motorically based errors (the ability to produce a target sound is not within the client's repertoire of motor skills) or that the sound disorder can be cognitively or linguistically based (the client can produce a sound but does not use the sound in appropriate contexts). Differentiating a motoric from a linguistically based disorder is not always easy. A disorder may be perceived as primarily motoric or linguistic, yet intervention typically involves elements of both. They point out that although it is convenient to dichotomize the motor/articulation and linguistic/phonologic aspects of most speech-sound disorders for organization purposes, normal sound usage involves both the production of sounds at a motor level and their use in accordance with the rules of the language.

Misarticulations can be categorized in several ways. Historically, speech pathologists have used the traditional classifications of (1) substitution of one sound for another ("thoup" for "soup"), (2) omission of a sound ("kool" for "school"), (3) distortion of a sound (nonstandard production of a sound), and (4) addition of a sound ("puhlease" for "please"). These historical classifications have persisted because they do describe most articulatory deviations. If there is any fault with the categories, it is that they are not specific enough. The diagnostician must say more than "the child has substitutions and omissions in his [or her] speech." We need to know which sounds are substituted for others, how often, and in what contexts. The same could be said for distortions, omissions, and additions. Another example of the superficiality of the historical categories is that they do not imply what part of the articulatory process is affected. That is, we cannot discern from the category of substitution whether the error is related to deficiencies in the client's sensorimotor or linguistic/phonological systems. The traditional classifications are, however, a good place to begin the assessment of speech-sound disorders. We can then assess further and attempt to determine the variability of performance in specific phonetic contexts as well as the ways in which misarticulation varies in utterances of different linguistic complexities.

Articulatory errors can also be divided into categories of *organic* (some physical cause for the misarticulation) and *functional* (no demonstrable organic cause). The latter term has come under criticism; the term *functional* is just a "diagnosis by default." The diagnosis of *organic* requires some positive proof of organicity, while the diagnosis of *functional* requires no positive evidence. The classification of *functional* is made only when a lack of evidence of organicity exists. The words most frequently associated with the *functional* classification are *learned* or *habit*. Although the classification of *functional* has been justifiably criticized, it is still widely held that the vast majority of articulation disorders have no significant, maintaining organic basis and that the treatment is behavioral in nature. Future research may yet uncover subtle organic or behavioral differences in these individuals. Assessment of organically based articulation disorders such as dysarthria and apraxia will be discussed in Chapter 9, on motor speech disorders. This current chapter focuses on speech-sound disorders that have no obvious organic component. As mentioned earlier, we will use the term *phonological disorder* to refer to functional cases that involve multiple phoneme errors presumably due to linguistic factors. The term *articulation disorder* will be reserved for clients who misarticulate only one or two phonemes, which may be more related to learned motor patterns habituated over a long time.

Another implication of a multicomponent conception of articulation is that no single measure is currently capable of adequately examining all parts of this complex process. It is naive to believe that administration of a traditional articulation test and an oral-peripheral examination are all that is necessary to perform a complete assessment of articulatory behavior. The articulatory process is just too complex and the disordered population too heterogeneous to rely on one or two standard tests. Independent and relational analyses should be done to provide complementary perspectives on a child's phonological system. Independent analysis simply describes a child's productions in terms of features, segments, and syllable shapes that actually occur in the speech sample. Relational analysis attempts to gloss a child's productions and compare them to standard, age-appropriate (or adult) models of "correct" speech-sound productions. Typically, the SLP dealing with infants and toddlers, who may not be using language for communication, will engage in independent analysis of vocal productions by the child. As children become older and develop a linguistic system, relational analyses are conducted to compare the child's productions to adult standards (Bernthal, Bankson, & Flipsen, 2013).

In this chapter, we emphasize the importance of knowing where to go and what to do to gain insight into aspects of articulation that are revealed to be problematic by the initial testing. As with any disorder area, no single chapter can possibly tell a student how to do everything well. Our goal is simply to make clinicians aware of the possibilities in the assessment of speech-sound disorders.

SEVEN IMPORTANT KNOWLEDGE AREAS FOR EVALUATION OF ARTICULATION AND PHONOLOGICAL DISORDERS

Before we discuss assessment of speech-sound disorders, we wish to introduce the clinician to some important bodies of literature. In actuality, there are more areas that could be considered, but these seven seem to us to be critical prerequisites to performing a diagnostic evaluation.

1. *Knowledge of the anatomy and physiology of the speech mechanism.* Before attempting to deal with an articulatory evaluation, the clinician should be completely familiar with the normal oral mechanism. Most students obtain this knowledge in their undergraduate training.

2. *Knowledge of phonetics.* It is one thing to know about the anatomy and physiology of the vocal mechanism, but it is quite another to be aware of how that apparatus actually produces the variety of consonant and vowel sounds in English (or any other language). Aside from knowing articulatory phonetics, the clinician must have well-developed skills in phonetic transcription. This expertise is important in order to record a client's productions accurately for later analysis. Reliable phonetic transcription abilities are especially important in order to accomplish phonological analyses. Among the clinical resources provided in Appendix B is a chart of English consonant and vowel symbols from the International Phonetic Alphabet, along with their place and manner of production.

3. *Knowledge of phonological development.* A major goal in diagnosis is to compare a child's articulatory performance to the behavior of other children in the same age range. In this way we can tell if a child's misarticulations are developmental in nature or they are clinically significant. The clinician should be familiar with at least three interpretations of articulatory development before doing an assessment.

The most abundant normative data available from the 20th century are traditionally oriented studies of children's phoneme production of words with the target sound in the initial, medial, and final positions. Although research design differences included what constituted sound acquisition, customary usage, or mastery, this body of work remains useful to parents, pediatricians, and SLPs. Figure 6–1 is an example of normative consonant development data. Most misarticulations in phonologically disordered children involve consonants, so only consonant development data are presented here. Vowels are typically developed by age 3 to 3½ (Bernthal, Bankson, & Flipsen, 2013; McGowan, McGowan, Denny, & Nittrouer, 2014). This does not mean that vowels are never involved in phonological disorder or that vowels are easily acquired.

Most preschool-and school-age children seen by the SLP will have difficulty primarily with consonants, and this is reflected by the content of most articulation tests. If the child is very young or exhibits a severe speech-sound disorder, however, clinicians will be interested in assessing the vowel system. Early intervention programs target infants between birth and 2 years, and these children are probably using more vowels than consonants in their productions. In such cases the clinician will want to perform a thorough assessment of vowels and diphthongs to determine the existence of vowel disorders (Ball & Gibbon, 2012).

In addition to data on the development of singleton consonants, there are some studies on the acquisition of consonant clusters. For example, McLeod, Van Doorn, and Reed (2001) review acquisition literature over the past 70-plus years and describe the acquisition of consonant clusters in childhood. The authors summarize this literature with 10 generalizations about the developmental progression, which may be useful to clinicians in assessment and treatment decisions.

FIGURE 6–1
Average Age Estimates and Upper Age Limits of Customary Consonant Production. The Solid Bar Corresponding to Each Sound Starts at the Median Age of Customary Articulation; It Stops at the Age Level at Which 90% of All Children Are Customarily Producing the Sound

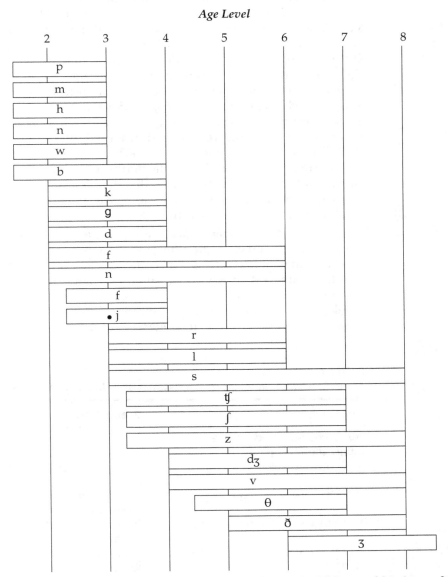

Source: Prather, Hedrick, & Kern, C. (1975). Articulation development in children aged 2 to 4 years. *Journal of Speech and Hearing Disorders,* 40, 179–191. Used with permission from the American Speech-Language-Hearing Association, Rockville, MD.

A second type of developmental data involves distinctive feature acquisition. According to linguists, speech sounds may be subdivided into unique binary attributes: If a given attribute is present in a speech sound, it is said to be positive (+) for it; if it is lacking, that attribute is coded negative (–). For example, most classification systems specify the distinctive feature of "nasal" and denote either its presence (+ nasal as in /m/) or absence (+ nasal as in /b/). The presence or absence of voicing is another distinctive feature; by examples /b/ is +voice while /p/ is −voice. The data from the analysis of a child's speech-sound disorder in terms of distinctive features that are present, absent, or confused might be used to devise a linguistically efficient treatment plan.

Finally, data are available regarding the occurrence of phonological reduction processes or patterns of error in typically developing children (Grunwell, 1988; Shriberg & Kwiatkowski, 1994; Singleton & Shulman, 2014; Stoel-Gammon & Dunn, 1985). These data provide some general age cutoffs for certain phonological processes and give the SLP a view of a child's error pattern not found in traditional norms. If a clinician sees a child who is deleting final consonants, for instance, the clinician cannot use traditional norms to determine when this tendency diminishes in normal children. Most studies have focused on children's phonological development between the ages of 3 and 8 years. Some investigations have concentrated on children age 1 to 3 years in response to the emphases on early intervention and increased interest in early development (Dyson, 1988; Grunwell, 1988; Kahn & Lewis, 2002; Stoel-Gammon, 1987). Table 6–1 provides an example of preschool developmental norms from a phonological process perspective. A major point we wish to make here is that the clinician can look at a speech sample from a variety of perspectives. Traditional as well as phonological norms provide a reference point to use in assessment and treatment.

4. *Knowledge of factors related to articulation disorders.* Whenever undertaking a speech-sound evaluation, the clinician can expect that parents will often ask questions regarding the etiology of the problem. The clinician must be familiar with the pertinent literature dealing with research on etiological factors, as well as skills and abilities of children with speech-sound disorders. Questions may be asked about language development, reading, spelling, educational performance, dentition, oral structures, gross and fine motor skills, intelligence, auditory abilities, and much more. Bernthal,

TABLE 6–1
Some Common Phonological Processes Typical in Early Development

Process	Description
Processes acquired but then suppressed by age 3	
Weak Syllable Deletion	The unstressed syllable is deleted in multisyllabic words (telephone → tephone).
Final Consonant Deletion	The final consonant in a word is omitted (/baet → bae/).
Doubling (also called reduplication)	Two-syllable words are produced by repeating the first syllable (bottle → baba).
Consonant Assimilation (also called harmony)	The manner or voice characteristics of one phoneme changes to be consistent with another (dog → gog).
Velar Fronting	Velar sounds such as /k/ and /g/ are replaced by alveolar sounds /t/ and /d/ (go → do).
Gliding	Liquids such as /r/ and /l/ become glides such as /w/ and /j/ (run → wun).
Processes that persist after age 3	
Cluster Reduction	Consonant clusters are simplified, often to a single phoneme (stop → top).
Stopping	Continuant sounds, often fricatives, are replaced by stops (see → tee).

Bankson, and Flipsen (2013) summarize this research handily, and this should assist clinicians in answering any questions.

5. *Knowledge of Dialectal Variation.* According to the American Speech-Language-Hearing Association and Battle (2012), the clinician performing an evaluation of speech sounds must be able to differentiate a communication disorder from a dialectal variation. In the last decade, much progress has been made regarding information helpful with diverse populations; for example, Spanish versions of assessment materials exist. Information on phonetic inventories for Arabic, Cantonese, English, Korean, Mandarin, Spanish, and Vietnamese can be found online at the website of the American Speech-Language-Hearing Association (www.asha.org/; search "templates & tools" for phonemic inventories across languages).

We recognize that cultures are not monolithic, and regional dialects certainly vary. Still, we offer a few "common" phonological characteristicss. For example, African American vernacular may exhibit final cluster reductions (as in "presen" for "presents"), deletion of "r" (as in "puhfessuh" for "professor"), and stopping of interdental fricatives in various positions (as in the initial position where "they" is spoken as "dey"). Examples of English spoken by native Spanish speakers may demonstrate confusion of "d" with the voiced "th" (as in "day" for "they"), devoicing of "z" (as in "lice" for "lies"), and affrication of "sh" (as in "chew" for "shoe") (Yavas & Goldstein, 1998). The clinician must become familiar with multicultural phonological characteristics and routinely consider them when evaluating misarticulations of diverse clients.

6. *Knowledge of Coarticulation.* For at least 40 years, researchers have known that speech is produced in a parallel fashion as opposed to a series of discrete events. This means that speech sounds are not isolated entities; they overlap motorically and acoustically in time. Put simply, sounds are influenced by other phonemes that surround them. This influence of one sound on another is called *coarticulation* and is one of the most basic facts about the articulatory process. The phonetic environment or phonetic context in which a sound is produced influences the production of that phoneme. Two major types of coarticulation can be described in terms of the direction of the influence of one sound on another. Left-to-right coarticulation refers to a preceding sound's having an effect on a following sound (the "t" in *boots* is produced with some lip rounding because of the rounding /u/ vowel that precedes it). This type of coarticulation is perceived by some to be a type of "overflow" of movement from the first sound to the second. Thus, the left-to-right coarticulation is thought to be primarily the result of mechanical-inertial factors. The other type of coarticulation is right to left. This means that a sound later in the speech sequence affects a sound earlier in the stream of speech. For example, the "t" sound in the word *tea* is produced differently from the "t" in the word *too*. The difference in the two situations is that in the word *tea*, the sound is followed by a vowel that is not produced with rounded lips. Thus, the "t" sound in *too* might be produced with lip rounding because the following vowel is rounded. In both cases, the sound that influences the "t" occurs after the "t" has been uttered. Researchers and theorists have suggested that the right-to-left influence is probably the result of articulatory preprogramming. That is, early sounds in a sequence are produced differently in anticipation of sounds that are yet to be said. This implies some sort of motor planning.

The implications of the existence of coarticulation for the assessment of speech sounds are significant. One implication is that testing sounds in isolation is an unrealistic and artificial enterprise. What a child can do with a sound in isolation may be totally different from the child's production in connected speech. Another implication has to do with testing in single words. When we speak, we typically do not put oral pauses or spaces between our words, as in the words you are reading right now. The speech stream essentially is an unsegmented whole, where the coarticulation effects of one sound on another can cross both word and syllable boundaries and where sounds located in two adjacent words can have an effect on one another. This means that testing sound production on the single-word level may not be representative of sound production in spontaneous speech because connected words may provide different coarticulatory effects compared to single words alone. We have known for some time that specific phonemes are misarticulated less often in consonant cluster contexts compared to consonant-vowel (CV) environments.

Yet another implication has to do with possible facilitating and sabotaging effects of phonemes surrounding a particular target sound. For instance, a misarticulated /r/ sound may be produced correctly by a child if it is preceded by a /k/ (e.g., /kræk/), perhaps because both sounds require grossly similar positioning of the tongue in the vocal tract. Conversely, an /r/ might be misarticulated as a /w/ if contexts surrounding the target sound contain a lip-rounded phoneme (e.g., /row/). Therefore, the effects of coarticulation can be positive or negative, facilitating or sabotaging, and this finding is especially important for the clinician to consider in assessment and treatment.

Perhaps the most important implication of coarticulation is in accounting for articulatory inconsistency. Most misarticulations are notoriously inconsistent, and if the clinician analyzes these productions, he or she can find that this "inconsistency" may actually be quite consistent indeed. Phonetic context is often the common denominator among errors that appear inconsistent on the surface. We need not only think of the notion of phonetic context as a purely motoric phenomenon. In performing linguistic phonological analyses, a consideration of context is critical. In evaluating assimilation processes (e.g., nasal assimilation), the clinician may note than nonnasal sounds in the initial word position are changed to nasals only when there is a nasal phoneme in the final or medial position of the words.

7. *Knowledge of the Linguistic-Articulatory Connection.* An important postulate in discussing articulatory assessment is the intimate relationship between language and articulation. This connection has been shown in several ways in the literature:

- Phonology is a component of language. Theoretically, phonology has been considered a classical component of language models.

- Syntactic complexity affects misarticulations. Several studies have shown that misarticulations are affected by linguistic complexity (Haynes, Haynes, & Jackson, 1982). That is, more misarticulations will occur as syntactic complexity increases. Here is a clear relationship between articulation and language.

- Semantic complexity affects misarticulations. Shriberg and Kwiatkowski (1994) have suggested that even the word's syntactic class may affect sound productions. For instance, blends may be reduced differently in verbs compared to the same blend in nouns. In early language development there appear to be more misarticulations on action words as opposed to object words in the first lexicon. This observation has been made with typically developing as well as phonologically delayed children.

- Pragmatics and communicative value affect misarticulations. When there is a greater chance of being misunderstood, the child may articulate more correctly.

- Language and phonological disorders typically co-occur. A relationship between language and articulation can be inferred from the high co-occurrence of the two disorders in children. Generally, children who have speech-sound problems are at high risk for language disorders, and vice versa (Shriberg & Kwiatkowski, 1994).

The implications of these connections between articulation and language are significant for assessment. First, routine assessment of articulation with an exclusively sensorimotor orientation is not appropriate. Language and articulation are hopelessly intertwined when a person speaks spontaneously. Second, when the speech pathologist is looking for sources of inconsistent phoneme production, he or she may find significant effects not only from phonetic context but also from semantic, syntactic, or pragmatic variables. Third, an evaluation that uses only single-word responses on which to base a clinical decision is incomplete because significant differences may exist between a client's performance on the single-word and connected-speech levels.

Gathering a spontaneous speech sample in a phonological evaluation has several advantages. First, the connected-speech sample keeps the actual process of producing utterances intact. Individual words are embedded within sentences, and thus the effects of stress, intonation, rate, and syllable structure can influence productions. Second, recall that, earlier in this chapter, we cited research that found the effects of syntax, semantics, and pragmatics can affect phonology. In conversation, all linguistic elements are present to allow such influences of language complexity on the sound system. Unfortunately, there are also disadvantages to conversational sampling. In cases where the client is unintelligible in connected speech, the clinician has little choice but to use shorter samples of single words or phrases in order to compare productions to an adult standard. Also, some children are reluctant to engage in conversation with an unfamiliar person. Finally, because a conversational sample is generated by the client, it may not include specific phonemes or syllable shapes of interest to the clinician. Single-word responses to picture-naming tasks offer a known target for the clinician to analyze. Many single-word tests suggest analyzing only one or two phonemes per word in accordance with their scoring sheets. We agree with Bernthal, Bankson, and Flipsen (2013) that much data are lost using this method. Clinicians should transcribe the entire word, including both consonants and vowels, in order to have a more robust set for analysis from single-word samples. One issue associated with single-word sampling is its fidelity to sound productions in continuous speech, with all of its attendant influences. It is well known that more errors occur in spontaneous connected speech; however, there are also reported instances in which more errors occurred on the single-word level. In general, most authorities recommend both single-word and connected-speech sampling in gathering data for a phonological evaluation (Bernthal, Bankson, & Flipsen, 2013).

We have made the point in this chapter that single-word tests may not reflect a child's productions in connected speech. Klein and Liu-Shea (2009) found that the substitutions and deletions that children exhibited in a continuous-speech sample were not predicted by their performance on a single-word articulation test. The authors suggest that in cases where a child may not qualify for remedial services based on single-word testing, a continuous-speech sample should be evaluated (and we add by well-developed data-gathering methods) to determine possible eligibility. They support the notion of including continuous-speech sampling in every thorough phonological assessment. The clinician can see that the most productive view would be to consider both sensorimotor and linguistic components in the assessment repertoire.

OVERVIEW OF THE ARTICULATION/PHONOLOGY ASSESSMENT PROCESS

Figure 6–2 presents the critical assessment mechanisms in articulation/phonology. Note that the same major areas of biological/linguistic foundations, background information, standardized testing, nonstandardized testing, and evaluation of the client's environment are relevant to a thorough evaluation. Note also that the figure covers all pertinent aspects of the World Health Organization International Classification of Functioning, Disability and Health (ICF) model presented in Chapter 1. The effects of the disorder are especially a focus when we perform nonstandardized testing and evaluate relevant environments.

FIGURE 6–2
Critical Assessment Process in Articulation and Phonology

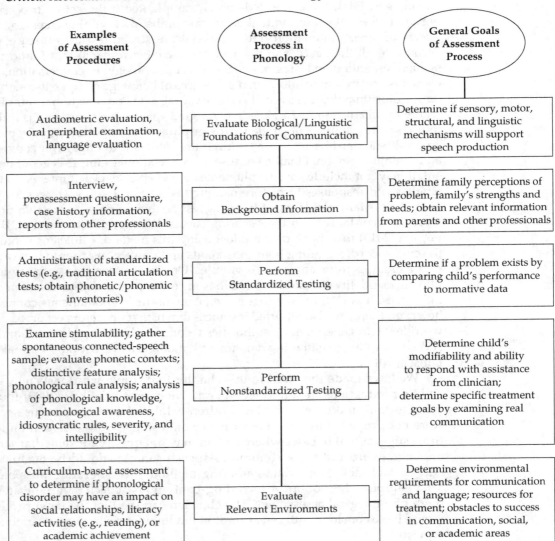

SCREENING FOR SPEECH-SOUND DISORDERS

One of the tasks performed by the SLP is screening for speech-sound disorders. The purpose of a screening is to determine if a person should be referred for a formal diagnostic evaluation in which the phonological system is analyzed in detail. Although screenings typically take a short time (less than 5 to 10 minutes), evaluations can take an hour or more. Usually, if a clinician has any doubt about the normality of a person's phonological system in a screening, the client is referred for a more thorough evaluation. Thus, if a child did not talk during a screening or a large enough sample could not be elicited, it is better to err on the side of caution and refer the child for an evaluation. According to Bernthal, Bankson, and Flipsen (2013), screening is appropriate for preschool children as part of early intervention programs. In some school settings the SLP will screen third-grade children for speech-sound errors because, at this age, most phonemes should be produced correctly. In older clients, a screening is sometimes done to ensure that the person meets certain speech standards required for admission to a degree program (e.g., broadcasting, teaching.) Of course, screening is performed when a person is referred to a clinic or school SLP with a suspected communication disorder. Screenings can be done informally with the use of clinician-constructed materials such as pictures, a conversational speech sample, or a reading passage. Often informal screenings involve counting, saying the days of the week, or describing pictures. One disadvantage to informal screening is the lack of normative data and identifiable cutoffs, indicating a passing or a failing performance. Often, school systems require a more formal method of screening to identify children for services. Some formal screening instruments that are available commercially include the following:

- Denver Articulation Screening Exam (DASE) (Frankenburg & Drumwright, 19731)
- Diagnostic Evaluation of Articulation and Phonology (screening part of DEAP) (Dodd, Hua, Crosbie, Holm, & Ozanne, 2006)
- Fluharty Preschool Speech and Language Screening Test (Fluharty-2) (Fluharty, 2000)
- Phonological Screening Assessment (PSA) (Stevens & Isles, 2001)
- Slosson Articulation, Language Test with Phonology (SALT-P, incorporates screening) (Tade & Slosson, 1986)
- Speech-Ease Screening Inventory (K–1) (Pigott, Barry, Hughes, Eastin, Titus, Stensil, Metcalf, & Porter, 1985)

Most of these instruments have standard scores or cutoff scores to use in making screening decisions. We also wish to point out that some full articulation/phonology tests can be efficiently administered in lieu of screening tools.

TRADITIONAL ASSESSMENT PROCEDURES

A variety of types of speech-sound assessments differ in their theoretical assumptions, method of sample elicitation, the type of information obtained, and their therapeutic implications. Perhaps the most common type of assessment is what we call traditional. The theoretical orientation of traditional testing is that each English consonant must be evaluated in the initial, medial, and final positions of words. These words are typically elicited from the client by means of pictures, word lists, sentences, or conversational sampling. Many studies examining articulation from a traditional perspective have shown that children tend to produce more singleton consonants correctly in single-word sampling contexts. On the other hand, when performance is examined from a phonological process perspective, some studies have shown no significant differences between single-word and connected-speech sampling conditions. Masterson, Bernhardt, and Hofheinz (2005) found few differences in the treatment ramifications between single-word and conversational speech samples. The conversational sample took three times longer to elicit and transcribe and still elicited less critical language targets compared to single-word sampling. The single-word targets were tailored to the child's phonological system based on limited sampling. While acknowledging single-word efficiencies and thoroughness, the researchers recommend conversational sampling to check on the representativeness of the single-word sample and for judging intelligibility and prosody.

Even though the data for the analysis might range from words to connected speech, the orientation of the clinician in these types of traditional tests is to determine omissions, substitutions, and distortions of phonemes in differing word positions. Many tests are available for use in traditional assessment and such inventories often include stimulus pictures for testing children and structured sentences for older clients to read. Tests often provide norms against which a child may be compared. Testing seeks to accrue a phonemic inventory of speech production performance.

Some of the readily available, traditional testing tools include the following:

- Arizona Articulation Proficiency Scale (Arizona-3) (Fundala, 2000)
- Fisher-Logemann Test of Articulation Competence (FLTOAC) (Fisher & Logemann, 1971)
- Goldman-Fristoe Test of Articulation (G-FTA-2) (Goldman & Fristoe, 2000)
- LinguaSystems Articulation Test (LAT) (Bowers & Huisingh, 2010)
- Photo Articulation Test (PAT-3) (Pendergast, Dickey, Selmar, & Soder, 1997)

Before we leave this topic, we wish to add that another traditional procedure is the testing of a client's stimulability, or response to stimulation, in which we evaluate the impact that the examiner's model has on the client's production. Is there some modification in the direction of normalcy? Or is there no change in the articulatory behavior? Testing for stimulability is extremely useful diagnostic procedure. If a client can produce the error correctly by imitating a standard model, either in isolation, in nonsense syllables, or in words, then there may be no serious organic obstacles that would prevent the eventual acquisition of the sound. Stimulability is also a useful prognostic sign; clients who can modify their articulation errors by imitating the examiner's standard production have a place to start the treatment process. Stimulability has also been implicated as a potential predictor of whether children will develop typical speech through maturation.

Stimulability is frequently given short shrift by practicing clinicians and students in training. Sometimes it is totally omitted. Often, we see students hurry through the stimulability testing, frequently giving inadequate instructions and rather imprecise models to the client. The real spirit of stimulability testing is to see how the client performs under maximal, multimodality stimulation. This is why most tests recommend that the model be presented two or three times after the client has been given a strong attentional set. Students sometimes indicate that the client was not stimulable for error phonemes after rather cursory testing. Subsequent stimulability trials, done more intensively, may reveal that the client, in fact, can produce the target sound. Prior to making negative stimulability statements in a clinical report, the clinician should be certain that the stimulation task was administered effectively. A good example of providing systematic information to a client during stimulability testing is presented by Glaspey and Stoel-Gammon (2005), in which various elicitation cues and phonetic contexts are altered.

It is our contention that traditional testing is a good starting point in assessing speech sounds. In many cases, a traditional assessment may be all that is needed, especially when the client has only a few articulatory errors and is stimulable. In cases like this, the clinician knows what the errors are and how often they occur in a test and in spontaneous speech if analyzed traditionally. The clinician also has a place to start production of the target sound because the client can make it correctly with stimulation. Probe tasks that focus on particular productions can also be used as a follow-up procedure. For example, specific probing techniques have been developed for use with consonant clusters (Powell, 1995). In the majority of cases, however, traditional testing does not go far enough. For instance, our discussion of coarticulation suggested that sounds will be produced differently in different phonetic environments. Most traditional tests examine only a limited number of these phonetic contexts. If a child or adult is not stimulable, the clinician may want to rely on experimentation with different coarticulatory transitions to determine if there is a facilitating context. Most traditional tests are not equipped to do this. Another example is that traditional testing procedures are not directed toward detecting patterns of error in a client's speech. To define patterns of error, a phonological analysis is the most efficient method to use. Traditional analyses do not systematically examine the effects of stress, syllable complexity, linguistic complexity, and pragmatics on misarticulation. Finally, traditional analyses do not focus on certain parameters that may be relevant to certain cases, such as distinctive feature acquisition and use. In short, no one method can do everything, and so it is with the traditional approach. The traditional test, however, is a viable instrument to use generically. If other analyses are required, they should be done when appropriate.

It is far easier to describe the testing of speech sounds than it is to administer an articulation test. A student's first attempt is generally a confusing situation that requires careful listening, attention to visual cues, recording the client's responses appropriately, and maintaining a positive client–clinician relationship. We recommend that the beginning clinician listen for only one sound at a time. When possible, have the child repeat the test words a number of times. Audio-record or, better yet, video-record the child's responses to assist in later scoring of the test. Experienced speech-language pathologists are able to save time by testing more than one sound simultaneously.

It is especially true with speech-sound assessment that the clinician is really the "test." Commercial articulation tests are nothing more than stacks of pictures bound together with metal or plastic. Articulatory responses are so transient and fleeting, so clinicians must listen carefully; practice frequently; and, above all, check their reliability. When judgments become more fine-grained, as in determining the nature of specific substitutions in certain word positions, our reliability tends to deteriorate. One can easily see that very complex analysis procedures such as those used in distinctive features and phonology are even more susceptible to misjudgments on the part of the clinician. The clinician must always strive to improve his or her reliability through practice and by rechecking results. A clinician's evaluation results are only as good as his or her ability to perceive the reality of the client's responses. No one, as an old professor said, has immaculate perception. Chapter 3 discussed interjudge reliability and provides a formula for its calculation.

TEST PROCEDURES THAT EVALUATE PHONETIC CONTEXT EFFECTS

After a traditional assessment, a client may be judged not stimulable. Procedures then need to be initiated to determine if a facilitating phonetic context can be found. As we mentioned in the section on coarticulation, phonemes are significantly influenced by other sounds that surround them. This phenomenon results in the existence of facilitating contexts that can encourage the correct production of a target consonant. The concept that certain phonetic environments can facilitate correct production is not new. Writers 50 years ago indicated there were key words in which a phoneme could be produced more effectively. If certain key words were discovered for a nonstimulable client, then treatment could commence in these contexts. Tests were developed using this notion that phonemes are produced differently depending on the sounds that precede and follow them. By systematically permuting a variety of consonants before and after a specific phoneme, the contexts in which correct production is observed can be noted by the clinician and can serve as a starting point for treatment.

Current tests that systematically evaluate phonetic context effects include the following:

- Context Probe of Articulation Competence (CPAC; available in English and Spanish) (Goldstein & Iglesias, 2006)
- Secord Contextual Articulation Tests (S-CAT) (Secord & Shine, 1997)
- Contextual Test of Articulation (Aase, Hovre, Krause, Schelfhout, Smith, & Carpenter, 2000)

Another way to examine phonetic context effects in children and adults is the use of sound-in-context sentences (Haynes, Haynes, & Jackson, 1982). Sentences can be read spontaneously by adults or imitated by children. Work with sentences has been done in research projects directed toward finding facilitating contexts for particular target consonants (mainly the /s/ and /r/ phonemes). The use of these sentence stimuli has shown that there are, in fact, facilitating contexts for /r/ and /s/ that occur for many clients. The essence of these sentences is that a clinician can ask the client to say any number of utterances that are constructed to determine phonetic context effects. For instance, if the clinician wants to evaluate the effects on /s/ production of a preceding /k/ sound and a following /p/ sound (e.g., /ksp/), a sentence can be constructed such as "The dress had a black spot." In addition, phrases may be used instead of sentences. The clinician can then use knowledge of coarticulation and devise stimuli to probe phonetic context effects on a given client's articulation.

ASSESSMENT OF SPEECH SOUNDS IN EARLY INTERVENTION

Historically, it has been a challenge to quantify the development of the sound system in children under the age of 3. Charts of consonant, vowel, and syllable development in the first years of life are instructive. These stages can be used to characterize a child's speech-sound development in the early years and track development. There are several methods by which phonetic and syllable shape data can be quantified in a single score that can be used to monitor development over time. Two such methods, Mean Babbling Level (MBL) and Syllable Structure Level (SSL), were reviewed by Morris (2010) in terms of their clinical usefulness. The MBL is a measure of vocal or nonlinguistic productions in which each vocalization is assigned from 1 to 3 points depending on the occurrence of phonetic elements and certain syllable structures. The more consonants included and the more complex the syllable structure, the higher the rating. Ultimately the ratings for individual vocalizations are averaged, and a score (e.g., 1.54) is obtained. You can see how an increase in the score suggests more complexity in the phonetic and syllable structure of a vocalization. The MBL was extended for use with productive lexical items and renamed the Syllable Structure Level (SSL) measure. Again, the SSL used a scoring system to quantify the phonetic and syllabic complexity of true words so that development could be monitored by a single value over time. After a review of the literature, Morris concluded that both the MBL and SSL provided clinically valuable and reliable information with which to characterize change in phonological development in the early years. We mentioned the notion of an independent analysis of phonology as being comprised of an inventory of consonants, vowels, and syllable structures. In the case of children who have not developed language for communication, such an analysis is all we have to work with regarding the phonological system. Samples of vocalizations can be obtained during normal caregiving activities and turntaking during play, and independent analysis can be conducted on the productions (Bernthal, Bankson, & Flipsen, 2013).

THE PHONETIC AND PHONEMIC INVENTORIES

A most important source of information about a phonologically disordered client is the phonetic inventory. After gathering a representative sample, one of the first operations a clinician should perform is to inventory the client's sound system in several ways. The phonetic inventory is a summary of sounds the client has produced either correctly or incorrectly in the sample and represents the sounds that can be physically produced by the client. That is, if the client produced a glottal stop, this sound is part of the phonetic inventory. If the client produces a /θ/s substitution and never produces the /θ/ correctly when it is required, the /θ/ is still included in the phonetic inventory. The phonemic inventory, on the other hand, includes sounds that are used contrastively and that are implemented to make a meaning difference in the client's language. Thus, although an /θ/ may be part of the child's phonetic repertoire, it may not be part of the phonemic system.

As we will discuss later, an examination of the phonetic and phonemic inventories is a critical part of assessing a child's possession and use of distinctive features of English phonemes. There are also some other ways to analyze data from a child's phonetic and phonemic inventories. Some authorities have recommended searching for various types of rules that may or may not be operating in a child's system, and the phonetic/phonemic inventories are an important part of these analyses. For instance, static rules (phonotactic constraints) may be operating to restrict the occurrence of certain sounds or phoneme combinations. Three types of phonotactic constraints have been reported. First, *positional constraints* are rules that allow the production of a sound in only certain contexts or word positions. Second, *inventory constraints* reduce the production of particular sounds because the phonemes are not included in the phonetic inventory. *Sequence constraints* are rules that may not permit the child to produce sounds in particular combinations (e.g., the child can produce the phoneme as a singleton but not in a cluster). One can see that examination of the phonetic and phonemic inventory is an important part of arriving at an appreciation of a client's phonotactic rule system.

There are a variety of systems for reporting a client's phonetic inventory. It would be most important for a phonetic inventory not only to reflect sensorimotor production of a sound but also to provide some indication of appropriate or phonemic use of the element. The phonetic inventory should also indicate failure to sample certain sounds so that the clinician does not assume the client cannot produce the sounds. The phonetic inventory in the Natural Process Analysis (Shriberg & Kwiatkowski, 1980) differentiates phones that are used correctly, appear in the sample, are glossed in the sample, and are never glossed. This analysis can tell the clinician if the phonetic element is phonemic (correct anywhere), whether it is used as a substitution for another sound (appears anywhere), whether it should have been in a word (glossed) but was not, or whether the sound was never expected to be produced in the sample. Other systems simply list the phones in the phonetic inventory from left to right in terms of place of articulation in the vocal tract (left = front, right = back). Another way to consider a child's phonetic/phonemic inventory might be to array the phonemes on the continuum of phonological knowledge, which we will discuss later.

However the clinician decides to examine a child's phonological system, a phonetic/phonemic inventory is a good starting point because it can give significant insights into phonotactic rules (e.g., inventory constraints) and the child's overall knowledge of the sound system.

DISTINCTIVE FEATURE ANALYSIS

As we mentioned previously, neither traditional analyses nor appraisals of phonetic context effects examine all pertinent aspects of a child's articulatory system. The most basic unit that speech can be reduced to is the distinctive feature, and the "reality" of features has been demonstrated both acoustically and physiologically. That is, as humans, we seem to pay attention to certain aspects of the speech signal both in perception and production. Phonemes are evidently made up of bundles of distinctive features that combine to produce a variety of different consonant and vowel sounds in a language. Children do not acquire phonemes one by one; rather, they acquire a feature (such as voicing presence/absence) that, when combined with other features, provides the basis for a number of phonemes in the language. Features, then, are a prerequisite to phonemes because without the knowledge of and ability to produce a given feature of language, certain sounds containing that feature will not be produced. For instance, if a child does not learn that the feature of voicelessness is important in differentiating certain sounds from each other, the phonemes with the − voice feature will not be produced (/s/, /f/, /p/, /k/, etc.). Distinctive feature theory attempts to specify the characteristics of phonemes according to the presence (+) or absence (−) of each feature that distinguishes or contrasts one speech sound from another.

The popularity of SLPs doing a distinctive feature analysis of a client's speech sample has waned in recent years. There are numerous linguistic systems of analyses, a lack of universality, and disparate bases (acoustic, articulatory, perceptual). One source of solace to the clinician is the fact that most systems have some characteristics in common. There are certain features that appear to be so significant and strong that they are included in the majority of systems. Specifically, the features of voice, nasality, some feature denoting duration, and a place feature are the most common for clinical use.

It has been suggested that there are at least two different types of feature problems exhibited by children: phonetic and phonemic. One type of distinctive feature difficulty is exemplified by a child who has not acquired the use of a feature at all. The child is not aware of the importance of the feature in differentiating English sounds and has difficulty producing the feature. The child might have one aspect or one-half of the feature (+ voicing), but does not have the other half (− voicing). Features are rather like light switches; they are only useful when you know about both turning them on and turning them off. Thus, a child has not really acquired the feature of voice until both voiced and voiceless sounds can be produced appropriately and contrastively. If a child's phonetic inventory does not include voiceless phonemes used correctly and incorrectly, the child does not have contrastive use of the voice feature. A second type of feature error is shown in a child who has acquired the feature but does not use it appropriately. Control of features, as with many things, is on a continuum. A child may be aware of the importance of a feature and be capable of producing both aspects (+ and −) of it, yet there are specific contexts in which the feature is not used appropriately. On the other hand, a child may not be able to produce the feature aspects without great difficulty in

TABLE 6–2
Example of Distinctive Feature Approach to Analyzing Articulation Errors

Error	Features Used Correctly	Features in Error	
Substitution/Target		**Target Phoneme**	**Substitution**
d/s	vocalic, consonantal, high, back, low, nasal	− voice + continuant + strident	+ voice − continuant − strident
d/z	vocalic, consonantal, high, back, low, nasal	+ continuant + strident	− continuant − strident
d/sh	vocalic, consonantal, high, back, low, nasal	− voice + continuant + strident	+ voice − continuant − strident
b/f	vocalic, consonantal, high, back, low, nasal	− voice + continuant + strident	+ voice − continuant − strident
b/v	vocalic, consonantal, high, back, low, nasal	+ continuant + strident	− continuant − strident
d/th (*th*ink)	vocalic, consonantal, high, back, low, nasal	− voice + continuant	+ voice − continuant
d/th (*th*at)	vocalic, consonantal, high, back, low, nasal	+ continuant	− continuant

Note: The features associated with phonemes are from the classic work of Chomsky and Halle (1968). Compare the feature bundles of the target and error phonemes to determine features misused. One can easily see that the most misused features are the voicing, continuancy, and stridency elements.

any context. Perhaps these two cases represent slightly different diagnostic groups. One child does not have the feature, and the other has it but misuses the feature in certain contexts.

Many authorities recommend the examination of distinctive features as part of the larger process of phonological analysis. That is, when we write phonological rules for a disordered child's system, we can use distinctive features to make our descriptions more specific and look for commonalities across different sound errors. Table 6–2 gives an example of how six individual sound errors can be construed as basically a problem with one distinctive feature (+ continuant). A phonological process analysis of the same errors would reveal a stopping rule, which is essentially a misuse of the + continuant. It would be important to determine if the child in the example ever produced the + continuant feature in the speech sample. One can easily see that using distinctive features is just another way to look at a client's misarticulations and can add some specificity to our descriptions as well as allow us to see relationships among individual sound errors.

It was mentioned earlier that a major decision we must make in a distinctive feature analysis is whether a child has not acquired a feature or whether he or she is a feature misuser. This decision is typically quite easy for a clinician to make after looking at the child's phonetic inventory to see if whole classes of sounds and features are missing. An experienced clinician can examine a child's speech sample and accurately predict which features are most in error. In many cases this may be enough to help the clinician to decide whether the treatment should be directed toward establishing a feature in a child's repertoire or altering the use of a feature that has already been acquired but is being used inconsistently in a child's system.

We see four advantages of considering distinctive features in our analysis of misarticulations:

1. They provide a model for understanding errors in many clients, as in an error on a give feature (e.g., voicing) that is shared by more than one misarticulated phoneme.
2. Considering distinctive features may provide one gauge of the severity of sound substitution in that the more feature differences between a target sound and its substitution, the more severe the problem.
3. They provide a basis for the selection of a target sound for therapy; the clinician can select the phoneme that shares features with many other misarticulated sounds.
4. They provide a basis for more efficient therapy by facilitating generalization to sounds not being directly treated.

Despite these advantages, some factors limit the application of distinctive feature theory to clinical practice. Nevertheless we believe that whatever method the clinician uses to analyze distinctive features in a given client, the following points are important:

The diagnostician should "think features" at some point in the analysis of a child with multiple articulation errors. In other words, one should at least be able to make a judgment about whether all features are present or if error patterns reflect consistent, repeated misuse of specific features in certain contexts.

The clinician should determine if a child (a) has not acquired a feature or (b) is a feature misuser. If the child does not produce a particular feature in his or her phonetic inventory, then treatment may best be directed toward basic introduction of the feature into the child's repertoire. If the child is a feature misuser, then further phonological analysis (which implies feature use) is indicated, and the clinician must determine the extent and loci of feature misuse. Phonological analysis techniques are more suitable for this purpose. More recent nonlinear phonological analyses include a feature level in their hierarchy.

Substitution errors especially should undergo a distinctive feature substitution analysis in which the feature bundles of the target and substituted sounds are compared and features that are misused are noted by the examiner, as in Table 6–1.

PHONOLOGICAL ANALYSIS

Another approach to analyzing a child's articulatory behavior is to perform a phonological process analysis. A landmark book by David Ingram (1976) entitled *Phonological Disability in Children* sparked an interest in a more linguistic approach to misarticulation analysis. Ingram cited linguists and others about the existence of common patterns of articulatory simplification in children's speech. That is, most children develop the ability to articulate gradually, and before perfecting an adult production, they reduce the complexity of words in characteristic ways. Space in this chapter does not permit us to provide examples of each phonological pattern reported in the existing literature, and most training programs now include extensive exposure to phonological processes in coursework.

A phonological approach rests on certain assumptions. First, phonologists assume that there is a structure to every child's sound system and that even in the most unintelligible child there is a pattern of phonemic production. In other words, sounds do not occur in random combinations. Second, a phonological approach assumes an underlying system that gives rise to the observable sound combinations that we hear from children. The implication is that a phonological error may be a product of the underlying system that organizes the overt sound combinations.

Earlier in this chapter, we indicated that there can be both linguistically based and sensorimotor-based misarticulations. The linguistically generated errors could be construed as products of rules generated by the child's underlying phonological linguistic system. Rules, to a certain degree, imply patterns of performance, and phonological rules can be written to describe these patterns simply. Phonological rules, then, are descriptive of the way in which a child uses classes of phonemes. Many investigators have reported that, in development, it is commonly observed that children tend to simplify their word productions in comparison to adult models. The simplifications are typically in the direction of producing physiologically easier sounds for more difficult ones. For reasons not presently known, some children appear to persist in using these simplification strategies, and if enough of these strategies are retained, the child is likely to be quite unintelligible. Most authorities report that many of the patterns of error found in disordered children's speech are those observed in typically developing youngsters at earlier ages. Also, deviant rules not usually found in typically developing children may appear in youngsters with phonological disorders. Phonological rules can describe these simplification techniques, and each rule implies a change in the use of distinctive features. That is, a child who substitutes stops for continuants is altering an important distinctive feature of the target phonemes.

+ continuant		− continuant
s		t
ʃ	⟶	t
f		p
θ		t

The clinician wishing to gain insight into phonological processes generally administers a commercially available test to the client and is guided by the manual through the analysis. A nonexhaustive list of such instruments includes the following:

- Bankston-Bernthal Test of Phonology (BBTOP) (Bankson & Bernthal, 1990)
- Comprehensive Test of Phonological Processes (CTOPP) (Wagner, Torgeson, & Rashotte, 1990)
- Hodson Assessment of Phonological Patterns (HAPP-3; Computerized Analysis also available as HCAPP) (Hodson, 2004)
- Khan-Lewis Phonological Analysis (KLPA-2) (Khan & Lewis, 2002)
- Spanish Articulation Measures (SAM) (Mattes, 1994)

These measures provide picture or object stimuli and ask the child to give a single-word or connected-speech response. Responses are analyzed by the clinician for particular phonological simplifications. We add here that it also has been suggested that traditional test stimuli can be used to aid the clinician in a gross analysis of phonological process use.

The measures mentioned above can be administered in a reasonable time period (under 1 hour); the scoring time will vary with the clinician's experience in using the test and the severity of the phonological disorder under evaluation. Most of the measures do not evaluate spontaneous connected speech, however; therefore, the phonological rules obtained may only approximate those typically used by the child in conversation. Some research suggests more similarities than differences, however, between single-word and connected-speech productions. Clinicians need to be aware of the importance of sampling when attempting to complete an in-depth phonological analysis. A given sample must adequately examine a variety of word shapes (e.g., CVC, CCV, CVCVC, etc.) and a variety of sequences of phonemes and features. That is, phonemes and features (e.g., place, manner) must have the opportunity to occur adjacent to one another and in more distant relationships. Clearly, it is difficult to predict if a spontaneous sample will provide many word shapes, phonemes, and sequences, so the case is made for supplemental sampling to determine the true nature of phonological errors. It is only with detailed and strategic sampling that we can effectively describe a child's phonological system and know the appropriate contexts to target in treatment.

Bernhardt and Holdgrafer (2001) provide a nice overview of the advantages of both single-word sampling and connected-speech sampling for the analysis of phonology. Thy offer a conceptual summary of nonlinear phonology and state that both single-word and connected-speech samples are necessary to examine word/syllable structure, segments, distinctive features, and phrasal aspects of phonology.

Another level of phonological analysis is to gather a spontaneous speech sample, transcribe it in the International Phonetic Alphabet, and attempt to discern patterns of error (processes) in the data. This is obviously more time consuming than the measures just mentioned, but it may also be more valid because the clinician is examining actual utterances that were generated by the client's cognitive-linguistic system. The analysis of a spontaneous speech sample is recommended by Shriberg and Kwiatkowski (1994) in the Natural Process Analysis (NPA). This procedure specifically targets eight processes for analysis and provides a unique and useful phonetic inventory. The Natural Process Analysis can provide valuable information for the practitioner and represents a well-planned procedure.

The earlier Procedures for the Phonological Analysis of Children's Language (PPACL; Ingram, 1981) includes a phonetic analysis, homonym analysis, substitution analysis, and phonological process analysis. Twenty-seven specific processes are targeted. However, Ingram stated that the analysis is open ended and can continue until all the substitutions in a child's speech have been explained.

There appears to be some agreement that certain processes are high risk in phonologically disordered children. Specific phonological processes may be more important than others in terms of focusing on them for assessment targets. Although there is considerable variation among the assessment techniques in the number of processes examined, there is also a high degree of agreement regarding processes that seem to be most at risk in unintelligible children. The actual number of processes targeted in an evaluation seems to be related to the clinician's goals in the analysis. If the clinician wants to write a relatively complete generative phonology for a client, it would obviously focus on a larger number of rules than if the clinician's goal were to determine which major processes interfered most with intelligibility. In the latter case, the clinician may find that six phonological processes account for more than 80% of the child's misarticulations, and treatment targets might be selected from the processes having the most impact on intelligibility. For instance, if a child is exhibiting unstressed syllable deletion, final consonant deletion, and stopping, these three will be initial treatment targets; rules such as epenthesis, vocalization, gliding, and so forth, which may have less effect on intelligibility, will not be of immediate concern. It should be noted that most of the evaluation techniques discussed allow for the assessment of other processes as discovered by the examiner, even though the processes may not be specifically evaluated.

Work in the area of nonlinear phonology points out the importance and utility of considering hierarchical relationships in child utterances. The relationships among words, syllables, segments, and features are illustrated in Figure 6–3. The initial

FIGURE 6–3
Hierarchical Levels Described in Nonlinear Phonology

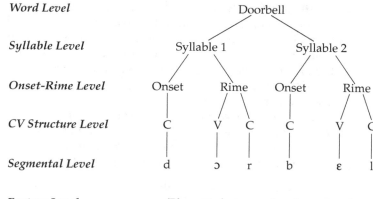

consonant(s) in a syllable is(are) called *onsets,* and *rimes* are a vowel and any consonants following the onset. All English syllables require a rime, but the onset is optional, as in the vowel-initiated first syllable in the example *outside.* Segments in this model are similar to phonemes, and features can be viewed from a variety of perspectives as simple as place-manner voicing and as complex as other distinctive feature systems mentioned earlier in this chapter. The elegance of hierarchical models is that they allow analysis of syllable, onset-rhyme, CV structure, and segmental and feature levels and may account for misarticulations in a way not possible with traditional or phonological process modes of analysis. Analysis of onset and rhyme usage currently is popular in the area of literacy development and disorders. Stoel-Gammon (1996) provides excellent examples of using nonlinear phonology in the analysis of disordered phonology.

The Intersection between Phonology and the Lexicon

Barlow (2002) discusses the interaction between phonology and the lexicon, including relationships to morphosyntax and the use of morphophonemic alternations in assessment (e.g., *pig/piggy*). It is clear that theoretical and clinical approaches to phonological analysis are not segment-oriented but rather word-oriented. That is, it is not reasonable to separate phonemes from lexical items in a child's phonological system.

Velleman and Vihman (2002) cite evidence that children enter language acquisition first from a word or phrase point of view. For example, children produce word approximations or primitive word combinations (e.g., "more juice") as formulaic structures. They state that only later, and construction by construction, the child begins to decompose and creatively re-create such units and do so very slowly. This view is that phonological development begins with whole-word learning. As such, children learn phonology through explicit learning (intentionally trying to replicate adult patterns), whereas implicit learning is incidental, unintentional, and the product of mere exposure to the language.

Ingram and Ingram (2001) advocate a whole-word approach because children acquire words, not individual phonemes. Early on, children have little awareness of segments, and they differ in their acquisition patterns and phonological learning strategies. Whole words have been assessment targets for some time. But rather than a simple tally of words used, they compute the percentage of whole words correct (PWW) in a child's utterances. As children learn language, the complexity of their words increases in terms of syllable structure, number of phonemes, and complexity of sounds produced, and so work by the Ingrams was refined. They developed a measure called phonological mean length of utterance (PMLU), which focuses on the number of segments in words and the number of correct consonants in those words. The PMLU is calculated by counting each segment (consonant and vowel) in the child's word and giving each segment a single point. Next, each correct consonant earns an additional point. The clinician then adds the total number of points for the words analyzed and divides by the number of words.

Other calculations were critical to Ingram and Ingram's (2001) assessment approach. Their four components included *whole-word analysis, word shape analysis* (syllables), *segmental analysis* (matches and substitutions of phonemes), and *phonological analysis* (determination of mastery of contrasts based on the acquisition of distinctive features).

If a clinician wishes to write phonological rules from a child's conversational sample, certain basic issues are common to most procedures:

1. *Glossing and segmentation.* The clinician must interpret the child's utterances and provide adult interpretations, or glosses, of what the child was trying to say. One cannot arrive at a phonological rule system unless the intended utterance is known. Several methods of segmenting or arranging the data have been reported. One method is to arrange correct and incorrect child productions and glosses word by word in phonetic transcription:

Child's Production	Adult Gloss
/ki/	/ki/
/bækI/	/bæskIt/
/pæ/	/fæn/
/go/	/go/

This allows the clinician the opportunity to compare productions with the adult model and hypothesize a phonological reduction pattern (e.g., final consonant deletion in the words *basket* and *fan*). Another method of segmentation is to keep spontaneous connected speech intact and divide the sample into utterances:

Child's Production	Adult Gloss
/tidəgɔgi/	/siðədɔgi/

This method of segmentation can sometimes help the clinician account for certain phonological reductions in a word that are influenced by sounds in previous words. There are a variety of methods for organizing segments once they have been glossed: alphabetically, by syllable shape, by consonant, and so on. The purpose of these varied organizational schemes is to aid in the retrieval and comparison of individual words and sounds when the clinician is attempting to prove the existence of a phonological rule.

2. *Hypothesizing a natural process.* After arranging the data from a sample, the clinician attempts to account for errors by hypothesizing a phonological reduction pattern. For instance, when comparing a child's production of a word to the adult gloss, a deletion of the final consonant may be noted. The clinician may hypothesize the process of final consonant deletion. The high-risk processes listed in Table 6–1 should be ruled out before any deviant processes are suspected.

3. *Finding support for hypothesized rules.* It is not enough simply to postulate that final consonant deletion has occurred in a child's sample. Evidence must be obtained from the utterances to determine whether the process has, in fact, occurred. For instance, the child may have deleted the final consonant in a CVC word. The clinician

should examine all other words in the sample that end in singleton consonants to determine the frequency of occurrence of the hypothesized phonological reduction. If there is widespread support for the occurrence of final consonant deletion, then the clinician may write the rule. If only certain final consonants are deleted consistently while others are produced normally, then the clinician must change the hypothesis to a rule that specifies particular kinds of final consonant deletion (e.g., stop and nasal deletion). This is where the use of distinctive features is helpful.

4. *Specification of frequency of occurrence.* Authorities differ in their methods of specifying the frequency of occurrence of certain phonological rules. Some processes appear to be obligatory (occur almost all the time), and others seem to be optional. In specifying optionality of a phonological rule, some authors recommend the three-stage system of "always," "sometimes," and "never" (Shriberg & Kwiatkowski, 1994). Other authorities (Ingram, 1981) recommend the use of percentage ranges such as 0–20, 21–40, 41–60, 61–80, and 81–100. Whatever method is used, the important point is to indicate how often the process is occurring.

5. *Writing the rule.* After the clinician has gathered support for a rule from the transcript, the rule is written, specifying the target phonemes, how they are changed, what context they are changed in, and how often the rule occurs. A phonological rule for final stop consonant deletion may look like this:

p

b

t → Ø/ CV-# 80–100%

d

k

g

This rule says that the consonants *p, b, t, d, k,* and *g* are deleted in the context of the CVC word when the target sound is at the end. The slash stands for "in the context of," the blank represents the location of the target sound, and the # refers to a word boundary. Note that the percentage of occurrence is indicated after the rule.

6. *Recycling of steps 1–4.* As each rule is written and proof is gathered for each phonological reduction, the clinician repeats the process of examining the errors, hypothesizing a phonological process, looking for data to support the rule, and writing the rule. Soon, the clinician can account for the majority of the errors in the child's transcript, with the exception of a small number of words that the rules do not describe. At this point, the clinician may wish to hypothesize a phonological rule that is typically seen in children's articulatory development. For instance, the child may delete initial consonants of certain types; however the procedure is still the same. The clinician must hypothesize the rule and find support for it before it can be written.

The detection of phonological simplification patterns can be a powerful tool in the hands of the well-trained clinician. A sample of speech that appears to have many unrelated misarticulations can be reduced to only a few phonological reduction patterns. The clinical implication of these processes is that the child does not need to work on a single sound but may need to focus on the pattern of error. The assumption is that the observable error pattern is generated by an underlying rule; if the rule is to be altered, then many of the segments that it affects should be targeted. Again, the only way to discover these patterns of misarticulation is to search for them through a phonological analysis technique. The commercially available traditional tests listed previously are not constructed for this purpose, although they certainly could be suggestive for further analyses and could provide hints for the clinician as to error patterns. We find the SPAT-DII by Dawson and Tattersall (2001) flexible in this regard.

We might several cautions regarding phonological analysis of a child's misarticulations. First, a phonological approach requires that a clinician transcribe words and/or sentences of spontaneous speech. Although most speech clinicians have completed courses in phonetics during their undergraduate education, many of these courses did not offer students the opportunity to transcribe disordered speech from a variety of male, female, adult, and child speakers. Some clinicians may not have adequate experience to transcribe connected speech reliably. Unfortunately, some clinicians only use their phonetics training to fill in the little blocks on the Goldman-Fristoe score sheet! It may be quite a leap, then, for some clinicians to transcribe words or connected speech in practice. Second, if our reliability is low in scoring phoneme errors, then we can only assume that reliability is even more of an issue in phonological transcription and analysis because we must construct rules from the data. Interjudge reliability is important, but test-retest reliability should be considered as well. Earlier we mentioned the notion of independent analysis in evaluating the vocal productions of children. Recall that, in such analyses, we are not judging the accuracy of production, just the presence of phonetic elements and syllabic complexity. As we discussed in Chapter 3, reliability is an important variable in any type of measurement we use in clinical assessment. Morris (2009) studied the test-retest reliability of independent measures of toddlers' speech and found syllable structure level and index of phonetic complexity achieved to have high test-retest reliability, while word-final phonetic inventory and word shape analyses had moderate but not significant reliability. Word-initial phonetic inventory was not reliable in their study.

A third concern is the compelling and captivating nature of phonological analysis. It makes an articulatory assessment rather like an interesting puzzle. When the clinician reaches the "solution" and divines the phonological rules, it is tempting to view the child's problem from a linguistic-phonological perspective only and apply this type of treatment. Be cautious about calling an observed pattern a phonological rule or process because the analysis is only a descriptive exercise based on a limited sample of speech.

Children of various etiological groups will demonstrate phonological regularities in their speech. Even if the disorder has a sensorimotor basis, phonological rules can be written and the child perceived as a phonological-linguistic case. Shriberg and Kwiatkowski (1994) suggest that the clinician must examine linguistic, sensorimotor, and psychosocial aspects of a child's behavior and select appropriate treatment goals. Clinicians should not assume a linguistically oriented treatment simply because the child exhibits a systematic phonology. The treatment of choice for each child may require different emphases, which could include focusing on sensorimotor aspects of articulation. There is no doubt that phonological analyses are useful and constitute a major innovation in articulatory assessment, but the clinician must be careful to check reliability and should not apply a phonological linguistic interpretation to all errors without examining sensorimotor and social aspects as well.

Computer-Assisted Analysis of Phonology

Much of the work in phonological analysis is laborious and repetitive. Some of the major difficulties are keeping track of the data on a host of different worksheets, tallying percentages and frequency counts, and cross-checking a variety of relationships found in different portions of the client's transcript. The nature of these tasks is ideally suited to computer analysis. The computer can take several examples of language and the gloss of each utterance and produce more information than even the most zealous clinician would like to know about a child's phonological system. In some cases, computer analyses of human behavior are rather superficial, and the programs available are just in the early stages of development. In the case of phonological analysis, however, the computer programs are detailed, user friendly, and here to stay. An analysis that might take a clinician several hours to accomplish can be completed in a matter of minutes by most programs. Some commercially available tests of phonology with computerized analysis include:

- Computerized Analysis of Phonology Patterns (HCAAP) (Hodson, 2003)
- Computerized Articulation and Phonology Evaluation Systems (CAPES) (Masterson & Bernhardt, 2001)

On the Web, one can find various types of speech analysis software; some can be downloaded for free. In general, the software is compatible with most types of hardware in the majority of school systems, universities, and households of prospective users. Programs differ in their scope, ranging from those designed to analyze the responses from a particular test of phonology to those focusing on the assessment of connected speech-language samples.

Computerized Profiling is a set of wide-ranging programs for language analysis. It is free and can be downloaded from www.computerizedprofiling.org/. Of particular relevance here is the Profile of Phonology (PROPH) phonological analysis module, which include various statistical analyses, analyses of word attributes (such as shape, stress, prosody, phoneme types), phonological process analysis, percent consonant correct (PCC), phonological mean length of tterance (PMLU), proportion of whole word proximity (PWP), and other usuful clinical components. By now, you should be aware that thorough clinical speech analyses almost certainly include both phonological process analysis as well as features of the child's syllable shape.

SIL International provides downloadable platforms for linguistic analysis; phonetics; and, of importance here, the Phonology Assistant. Its website (www.sil.org/) provides a wide range of training assistance as well as phonology task analyses.

While computer-assisted phonological analyses have advanced the clinical process, we would like to dispel some misconceptions about them. It would be ideal if the client simply talked into a microphone that was plugged into a computer, and in a few seconds a miraculous printout appeared that revealed the secrets of the phonological system. Unfortunately, this is not the case. The clinician must still obtain the sample; transcribe the sample; input the sample into the computer through the keyboard; and in many cases do some other work, responding to menus and prompts produced on the screen. The tasks just described constitute a lot of painstaking work on the part of the clinician. Just transcribing a sample of connected speech can take hours of careful listening. The beauty of computer-assisted analysis is that the clinician does not have to spend several *more* hours organizing data, scanning the transcript again and again, and performing mathematical operations. The computer also provides elegant summaries of the data, such as phonetic inventories, canonical shape analyses, positional inventories, phonological process analysis, and measures of severity (such as the widely used percentage of consonants correct, PCC). Some computer analysis programs even suggested treatment targets.

Thus, one misconception that some people might have is that computer analysis takes away all of the clinician's tedious work. The truth is, it takes away much of this work but not all of it. A second misconception some people may have is that the computer will always come up with the "right answer" with regard to a client's phonology. Although the algorithms in most phonology programs are quite sophisticated, they have difficulty dealing with idiosyncratic processes and certain types of analyses. The one thing the clinician can expect, however, is output; it may not always be correct, but it *is* output. A clinician should be aware of the limitations of phonological analysis programs and practice by running phonological samples that have been done by hand to see if there is general agreement between the two methods.

Assessment of Phonological Knowledge

Simply put, phonological processing is the use of sounds in a language system with phonological knowledge as a foundation for receptive understanding and expressive output, both verbally and later written language. There has been an explosion of research, with educational and clinical applications bringing phonological knowledge and awareness to the forefront. How and when does a typical toddler develop phonological knowledge and awareness? How can SLPs (and other educators) assess and address atypical processes? As part of the linguistic system, we know that phonological awareness is fundamental to speech-sound production, which in turn is related to manipulating syllables and words. And this sets the stage for future abilities in reading and spelling. In essence there is a direct line between early phonological knowledge and literacy. SLPs in many work settings are heavily involved in these issues among children.

Bauman-Waengler (2012) says that phonological awareness is a subdivision of phonological processing. Awareness is a skill that allows the person to break down words into smaller units. Three smaller levels of skill have been described in the literature along with measures to asses a child's ability for each, and there is a presumed developmental progression of tasks with each of the three levels.

First is the skill level of *syllable awareness*, in which a child understands that words can be divided into syllables. Bauman-Waengler (2012) provides four syllable awareness subskills and assessment examples:

1. Syllable segmentation: Can the child segment a multisyllabic word into the component beats (such as "ba-by")?

2. Syllable completion: Can the child supply the missing syllable when cued with a picture of a rainbow and the examiner says "Rain__"?

3. Syllable identification: Can the child indicate what part of *rainbow* and *raincoat* sound the same?

4. Syllable deletion: Can the child say "rabbit" and then be instructed to repeat it again, but without the "ra"?

The second type of phonological skill level awareness is known as *onset-rime awareness*, in which there is a recognition that syllables are structured into two parts: the onset of the syllable and the rime. The syllable onset includes all sound prior to the vowel nucleus, and the rime is the rest of the syllable. Onset-rime awareness is often assessed via rhyming tasks. To rhyme, a child must be able to separate the onset and the rime portions of syllables (and hence words). The words *cat, bat,* and *hat* rhyme because the rime ("at") stays the same even though the onset changes. Bauman-Waengler (2012) provides four assessment types for onset-rime awareness as well:

1. Spoken rhyme recognition is typified in this example: "Do these words rhyme: *hop* and *top*?"

2. Recognition that words do not rhyme can be demonstrated by having a child select from a string of choices, such as *cat, sat, car.*

3. Spoken rhyme production asks the child to say a word that rhymes with *dog.*

4. Onset-rime blending asks the child to merge two components into one, as in this example: Blend "c" and "at" to make "cat."

The third skill level related to phonological awareness is *phonemic awareness*. The ability to manipulate sounds can be assessed in a variety of ways. Bauman-Waengler (2012) provides 10 skills and sample tasks to assess; we highlight three in the following list:

1. In phoneme detection, the child can be asked, "Which one of these words has a different first sound—*rose, red, bike, rabbit*?"

2. In phoneme matching, the child can be asked, "Which word begins with the same sound as *rose*?"

3. In phoneme isolation, the child can be asked, "Which sound do you hear at the beginning of *toad*?

The other seven phonemic awareness skills listed by Bauman-Waengler (2012) are phonemic completion, phonemic blending, phonemic deletion, phonemic segmentation, phonemic reversal, phonemic manipulation, and spoonerisms. We leave these for your further investigation.

With the relationship among phonological awareness, developmental literacy, speech disorders, and even language impairments, it is logical for SLPs working with young children to be involved in assessing phonological knowledge. A nonexhaustive list of some commercially available tests for phonological awareness includes the following:

- HearBuilder Phonological Awareness Test (Wiig & Secord, 2011)
- Test of Phonological Awareness in Spanish (TPAS) (Riccio, Imhoff, Hasbrouck, & Davis, 2004)
- Test of Phonological Awareness Plus (TOPA-2+) (Torgensen & Bryant, 2004)
- Test of Phonological Awareness Skills (TOPAS) (Newcomer & Barenbaum, 2003)
- The Phonological Awareness Test 2 (PAT2) (Robertson, 2007)

We wish to close this section on phonological knowledge with the following information on clinically targeting sounds because it is still useful for clinicians today. Gierut, Elbert, and Dinnsen (1987) state that children acquire and exhibit various sets of phonological knowledge along a continuum of simple to more complex and also that some rules are more generalizable than others. They also contend that the phonological knowledge continuum may relate to the amount of generalization to be expected in treatment. Basically, training of sounds with least phonological knowledge resulted in generalization across the entire phonological system, whereas training of sounds with most knowledge resulted in generalization to only the specific class of phoneme trained. Thus, the implication is that greater effects may be obtained by training phonemes for which the child has least knowledge. Gierut (2007) suggested that selection of more complex treatment targets may result in more progress and generalization. This suggestion, of course, goes against the traditional view that treatment should begin on the earlier developing, simpler segments rather than those that are more complex. The research on this issue appears to be mixed. For instance, Rvachew and Bernhardt (2010) found that children who received treatment for simple targets made more progress toward the acquisition of the target sounds and demonstrated emergence of complex untreated segments and feature contrasts. This was relative to children who received treatment for complex targets and made little measurable gain in phonological development. These researchers did not suggest that complex targets should be avoided in treatment; rather, they espoused both horizontal and cyclical goals and strategies, with no need to limit treatment targets to simple or complex structures exclusively.

OTHER TESTING

We now return our focus in this chapter to issues of assessment and consolidation of areas to assess. We have already covered many approaches to assessing the speech-sound disorder per se, but seven additional areas of examination relate significantly to a competent and thorough evaluation of a client. While the importance of each of these areas may fluctuate, depending on the type of case and its severity, the clinician should be prepared to assess each one as appropriate.

1. *Case history.* As in any evaluation, a complete assessment of speech-sound disorders must include a thorough case history and interview with the parent and/or client. Bernthal, Bankson, and Flipsen (2013) recommend the following important areas of information: (1) possible etiological factors; (2) the family's or client's perception of the problem; (3) the academic, work, home, and social environment of the client; and (4) medical, developmental, and social information about the client. When interviewing the parent of a young child, the SLP may find the clinical resources in Appendix B useful, in particular information on developmental milestones and also some hearing-related questions to ask.

2. *Language Assessment.* The clinician examining a child's articulatory system should expect the bulk of these cases to exhibit some language deviations as well. Many authorities report the high co-occurrence of articulation and language disorders.

In several chapters of the present text we have cited research on nonword repetition tasks as a means for screening children with language disorders. In most cases, children with language disorders also have some phonological involvement. One can see the dilemma of attempting to use a nonword repetition task when the child cannot produce certain phonemes or syllable structures. Shriberg et al. (2009) developed a syllable repetition task (SRT) for use with children who have speech-sound disorders. The SRT includes one early developing vowel and four early developing consonants. Preliminary research shows that the task is valid and psychometrically sound for use with children who misarticulate.

The clinician should routinely gather a spontaneous language sample and administer standardized language tests for each client with a speech-sound disorder.

3. *Hearing Screening.* A second diagnostic procedure that should be administered routinely is a pure tone hearing screening. It is critical that the possibility of hearing impairment be eliminated prior to beginning treatment. This becomes especially important if the parents report suspected auditory problems or if the child has a history of ear infections. Appendix B provides guidelines for administering a hearing screening test.

4. *The Oral Peripheral Examination.* This examination is an integral part of the articulation examination (see Appendix A for guidelines in conducting this procedure). Oral peripheral examination results may be important in distinguishing a sensorimotor from a linguistic disorder of articulation. Assessing the motoric speed and coordination of the oral musculature may be particularly insightful in clients with speech-sound disorders. Norms exists for children and adults in tasks called either diadochokinetic testing or alternating motion rate assessment (see Appendix A).

5. *Articulation in Connected Speech.* In situations where neuromotor deficits are apparent to the diagnostician (e.g., head/neck cancer, dysarthrias, and other conditions in upcoming chapters), the SLP should judge speech-sound articulation not only at the single-word testing level but also in conversational speech, reading aloud, and/or in elicited sentences. Appendix B provides reading passages for various age levels.

6. *Auditory Discrimination.* This area has been a classical component of assessment because it is not uncommon for children with speech-sound disorders to perform poorly on auditory discrimination tasks. Consequently, early treatment programs incorporated an obligatory module of auditory discrimination training. Criticisms emerged regarding clinicians' methods of auditory discrimination testing and the efficacy of auditory discrimination training in treatment. Currently, the most defensible position appears to be assessing the auditory discrimination of misarticulated sounds only (Bernthal, Bankson & Flipsen, 2013) rather than all phonemes and to evaluate in a way that avoids the use of paired comparisons (mass-math). It is not clear if auditory discrimination testing needs to be part of routine articulatory evaluations or if it should be embarked upon only when some suspicion of a discrimination problem is demonstrated in trial therapy. The present authors favor the latter option.

7. *Phonological Awareness.* Many children with phonological disorders have been shown to exhibit decreased levels of phonological awareness that relate to academic and literacy skills (Bernthal, Bankson & Flipsen, 2013; Bird, Bishop, & Freeman, 1995). Clinicians can examine these abilities with a variety of techniques, as mentioned previously. It is often recommended that preschool children with speech-sound disorders be evaluated for phonological awareness skills prior to entering elementary school, and their articulation, phonological awareness, and literacy skills should receive ongoing monitoring (Rvachew, Chiang, & Evans, 2007). Others suggest that the SLP consider the assessment of phonological awareness as well as incorporate phonological awareness goals and development of sound–letter correspondence into an overall treatment program.

Preston and Edwards (2010) studied preschool children with speech-sound disorders and found that lower scores in phonological awareness were associated with more atypical articulation errors and lower scores on a measure of receptive vocabulary. They note that while phonological awareness assessments are not routinely performed on children with speech-sound errors, such evaluations should be recommended for children with such difficulties, especially in cases where the articulation errors are atypical in nature. Schuele and Boudreau (2008) provide an excellent tutorial on incorporating phonological awareness into an intervention program.

INTEGRATING DATA FROM THE ASSESSMENT

One issue of the *American Journal of Speech-Language Pathology* (Volume 11, Number 3, August 2002) was devoted to several clinicians outlining how they would orchestrate a 90-minute evaluation of a preschool child with a phonological disorder. Thus, each approach was constrained by time, ostensibly to mirror real-world time limitations. Most of the clinicians spent time doing a parent interview, language testing, hearing screening, oral peripheral exam, and taking a case history that consumed a large portion of the available time. Many of the clinicians administered a traditional articulation test or one of the phonological process instruments, and most also took a small language sample. At the end of the series of suggested phonological assessments, three reviews were presented: All pointed out limitations in the approaches suggested. Of course, it was not the purpose of the forum to outline the "ideal" phonological assessment, just one that could be done in 90 minutes. First, let us state that we are not of the opinion that time constraints should be a major determining factor in the assessment of a severe disorder. Certainly, some cases can be served well by applying a Band-Aid; however, others require major surgery. As speech-language pathologists, we should be prepared to do more in-depth analyses spanning several diagnostic sessions for cases that require such attention. All children with phonological disorders will not require an intensive evaluation; in fact, the majority of children with articulation problems present relatively straightforward difficulties that are easily understood by traditional testing procedures. For children with severe problems and poor intelligibility, however, the speech-language pathologist possesses expertise that no other professional has to offer for an in-depth analysis of the child's phonological system and principled selection of treatment targets based on this detailed analysis. After all, the state of knowledge about phonological disorders in our profession is also part of the real world and should not be ignored. With all that we know about the significant co-occurrence of severe phonological disorders with language, social, reading, and academic difficulties, it is important for us to spend all the time necessary to understand the child's problem fully, without arbitrary time constraints degrading the process. Overby et al. (2012) found links between speech-sound disorders and reading risks in children. Children whose speech-sound errors were atypical (nondevelopmental) scored more severe in speech (lowest 75% percentile) and had coexisting language disorders, deficits in phonemic awareness, and persistence of speech-sound disorders into early academic years that showed later as reading disorders.

Skahan, Watson, and Lof (2007) conducted a national survey to determine methods used by SLPs in assessing speech-sound disorders. They found that most clinicians administered a standardized articulation test, estimated intelligibility, engaged in stimulability, and performed a hearing screening. Most SLPs also used nonstandardized procedures in addition to these measures. The authors conclude that while these measurements may be adequate to qualify children for entrance into a caseload to receive services, they may not contain sufficient information to develop a comprehensive treatment program.

It is reasonable that after an articulation evaluation, the clinician should, at the very least, be able to make statements about the following areas: (1) biological prerequisites (hearing, structure/function of the speech mechanism); (2) linguistic ability; (3) phonetic and phonemic inventories; (4) distinctive features acquired, used correctly, absent, or misused; (5) response to stimulation by sounds that the child should have acquired, according to normative data; (6) phonological processes evident in the sample; (7) an indication of facilitating phonetic contexts, if any, in cases where stimulability is unproductive; (8) a judgment of intelligibility; and (9) a judgment of severity/prognosis.

Articulatory ability can be assessed in a variety of ways. The broader the view taken by the clinician, the more realistic the picture obtained of the client. For instance, if only the results of a traditional articulation test are considered, the clinician may be able to summarize a phonetic inventory and make some preliminary judgments about distinctive feature acquisition (but perhaps an inventory of phonological processes may not be possible because of limited sampling). Furthermore, traditional norms that might be used in comparing the child's phonetic inventory to other children are not applicable to phonological processes. The nine areas mentioned above are simply different ways of looking at the child's articulatory system and should at least be examined in every case to the extent that the clinician can make a statement about each area. Then further exploration might be undertaken in areas of concern, such as writing a phonology from a spontaneous speech sample if problems are indicated on single-word measures. If a child is noted to be missing entire classes of phonemes, then a more intensive distinctive feature analysis might be indicated. The point is that results from a variety of areas need to be considered and used as indicators for further analyses.

Some have suggested that clinicians consider possible causal correlates of articulation disorders, and gathering data on each client in the areas of cognition/language, speech mechanism integrity, and psychological/social parameters may be undertaken. Gathering specific data on children from different etiological groups could add additional insight into differences in speech-sound disorders and ways to assess them. For example, Barnes et al. (2009) found that children with fragile X syndrome, both with and without autism spectrum disorder, used similar phonological processes compared to typically developing children but were less intelligible in connected speech. This suggests that further evaluation of other factors such as motor speech ability, prosody, rate, and fluency of connected speech may be important to include in assessing these populations.

Consideration of these areas helps to keep the clinician from becoming too narrowly focused in the conception of articulation assessment and treatment. It also forces the clinician at least to consider the possibility of a variety of single or interactive maintaining factors in the articulation disorder. If a clinician is enamored of phonology and a linguistic interpretation of most articulation problems, such an approach forces the clinician to gather at least some information on psychosocial and speech mechanism variables. Conversely, if a clinician has a sensorimotor orientation, the approach forces the evaluation of more linguistic aspects. The findings of such a broad-based analysis may provide the clinician with important information on prognosis and a treatment goal that otherwise would not have been considered. Gathering this type of information allows construction of short- and long-term outcome data on children with phonological disorders and to begin to define subgroups of this population.

SEVERITY AND INTELLIGIBILITY

Although traditional articulation tests can easily identify children with phonological disorders, the tests have difficulty clearly defining different levels of severity. Several investigators have considered the problem of assigning a severity rating to children's misarticulations. We often hear clinicians rate a child's difficulty as mild or moderate; when asked how this rating was determined, the clinicians sometimes have no empirical basis. Flipsen, Hammer, and Yost (2005) asked 10 highly experienced SLPs to rate 17 phonologically disordered children on the severity of their disorder. Severity ratings were correlated with common objective measurements, such as percentage of consonants correct (PCC) and whole word accuracy (WWA), and it was found that the severity ratings by the "experts" were highly variable. They concluded that "impressionistic rating scales" used even by highly experienced clinicians were so inconsistent that it raises questions regarding their usefulness.

Shriberg and Kwiatkowski (1982a) suggest that use of the percentage of consonants correct (PCC) in a spontaneous sample is a reliable predictor of severity ratings. They had judges rank-order variables that were thought to contribute to severity, and intelligibility was ranked first as an influencing factor. They also had clinicians rate recordings of spontaneous speech on severity (mild, mild–moderate, moderate–severe, severe). Statistical analyses showed that the measure most predictive of severity rating was the PCC. Basically, the PCC is a calculation of the number of correct consonants divided by the numbers of correct plus incorrect consonants. The resulting number is multiplied by 100 to arrive at the PCC. Shriberg and Kwiatkowski (1982b) outline specific procedures and a worksheet for use in computation of the PCC. The point here is that the percentage of consonants that are correctly articulated relates to severity and severity relates to intelligibility. The number of errors a child has obviously affects the PCC.

Johnson, Weston, and Bain (2004) compared imitative sentence production with a conversational sample in computing the PCC to determine if severity ratings differed in the two elicitation methods. They found the PCC computed on imitated sentences was comparable to the PCC obtained from a conversational sample in children between the ages of 4 and 6 years. The imitative method took considerably less time to administer and complete.

Hodson and Paden (1991) offered the Composite Phonological Deviancy Score (CPDS) as a measure of severity. The system considers age in the calculation as well as a number of phonological processes occurring in the analysis of phonological processes. Edwards (1992) suggests the Process Density Index, which calculates the number of process applications per word, as a measure of severity and reports good reliability with listener judgments of severity. Shriberg (1993) developed the Articulation Competence Index for use in genetic research. This index takes into account distorted productions that were not included in the original development of the PCC.

Gordon-Brannan and Hodson (2000) studied 48 prekindergarten children to measure intelligibility and severity. The measure used was the percentage of words understood by an unfamiliar listener and correctly transcribed orthographically from a continuous-speech sample. They found four groups of children, based on the percentage of words correctly understood. Children with adult-like speech had percentages between 91% and 100%. Children in the mild category had 83% to 90% understood. A third group, the children in the moderate category, had 68% to 81% of their words understood, and children in the severe category group had between 16% and 63% understood. The range of the top three groups was 68% to 100%, with a mean of 85%. According to the authors, if a child 4 years of age and older falls below 66% (2 standard deviations [SD] below the mean), it could be an indicator of a phonological disorder. Recall also that Ingram and Ingram (2001) proposed the proportion of whole-word proximity (PWP) as a measure that might logically correlate with intelligibility ratings. Although the above methods may have their critics, they are at least attempts to objectify severity in cases of articulation disorders and are available for use by practicing clinicians.

Another gauge of severity might be to have independent judges rate the severity of speech samples based on their perceptual judgments. Although this is not a quantitative measure, it certainly is an indication of society's reaction to a person's phonological disorder. Garrett and Moran (1992) compared the ratings of experienced listeners (speech-language pathology majors) and inexperienced listeners (elementary education majors) to more objective measures such as the PCC and CPDS. They found all measures to be highly intercorrelated. The two objective measures appeared to be useful as clinical indicators of severity. This is especially interesting because the CPDS is derived from a single-word sample and the PCC from connected speech.

Of course, a clinician assessing the overall severity of a child's problem also has to consider other variables in addition to phonology. For instance, if a child has a concomitant language disorder or hearing impairment, the severity level increases. Reliability is an important issue in making judgments of severity, and SLPs should become familiar with normative data, especially for younger children. Rafaat, Rvachew, and Russell (1995) found that phonological severity judgments by SLPs for preschool children were not adequate (40% agreement) for children under 3.5 years of age, but they were adequate for older preschool children.

No matter how a child performs on an articulation test, a major concern of both the clinician and the parent is intelligibility in spontaneous speech. How understandable is the child in his or her daily interactions? Intelligibility is difficult to measure because it is affected by many variables. For instance, variables such as utterance length, fluency, word position, intelligibility of adjacent words, phonological complexity, grammatical form, and syllabic structure may have an effect on intelligibility judgments for a particular word (Weston & Shriberg, 1992). Kent, Miolo, and Bloedel (1994) summarized 19 different intelligibility evaluation procedures and discussed the issues to be considered in testing intelligibility. They concluded that no single method would be adequate for assessing intelligibility and that a clinician should use some combination of assessment devices. Selection of a measurement should consider the child's age, language abilities, other disabilities, time available for assessment and analysis, and the purpose of intelligibility testing.

There are few data relating intelligibility to age, although we know that children become more intelligible as they get older. A child of age 3 should be generally intelligible to strangers; an inability to understand a child of this age is reason for clinical intervention. Bernthal, Bankson, and Flipsen (2013) reviewed the literature on childhood intelligibility and said that commonly accepted standards for intelligibility are as follows: 3 years, 75% intelligible; 4 years, 85% intelligible; and 5 years, 95% intelligible.

A child will be more intelligible to those who know him or her well because the latter have unconsciously decoded the child's "system" of substitutions and omissions. Kwiatkowski and Shriberg (1992) found, however, that caregivers evidenced more difficulty than was anticipated in glossing their children's speech and overestimated their children's syntactic development. Another variable affecting intelligibility is the sound that the child misarticulates. Some sounds occur more frequently in the language than others; if the child's error is on a sound that occurs frequently, intelligibility will be affected to a greater degree than when errors are on infrequently occurring phonemes. An obvious factor that could logically affect intelligibility is the number of phonemes that a child misarticulates. Another variable affecting intelligibility may be the consistency of the error in the child's speech, which would also affect the PCC calculation. A final factor that can affect intelligibility could be the type of error (omissions, substitutions) that the child exhibits.

At the very least, a clinician can rate the client according to a rating scale. Fudala and Reynolds (1993) recommend using a continuum similar to the following for rating intelligibility:

1. Speech is not intelligible.
2. Speech is usually not intelligible.
3. Speech is difficult to understand.
4. Speech is intelligible with careful listening.
5. Speech is intelligible, although noticeably in error.
6. Speech is intelligible with occasional error.
7. Speech is totally intelligible.

Every assessment of articulatory ability should contain some judgment regarding intelligibility. This factor can be an important deciding variable in making treatment recommendations.

CONCLUSION AND SELF-ASSESSMENT

Speech-sound disorders may stem from sensorimotor problems (a disorder of articulation) or from linguistic impairments (especially in the phonological processing area), or they may exhibit a blend of both issues. Speech-sound disorders may affect both children and adults (though discussion of motor speech disorders is reserved for a later chapter). In this chapter, we reviewed the theoretical underpinnings of assessing disorders of speech sounds, from brief speech screenings to traditional testing, phonetic inventories, distinctive feature analysis, phonological processing analysis (assisted or not by computerized programs), and phonological awareness. Information garnered from the type of misarticulations and assessment guides the clinician in treatment planning. Ancillary areas to assess for a thorough diagnostic and evaluation of a client were discussed as well.

Long-Term Impacts

Phonological processing analysis has become the gold standard when a young child presents with a speech-sound disorder that is marked in character (affects multiple phonemes, is moderate to severe, and/or demonstrates low intelligibility). It is widely accepted that many individuals with speech-sound impairments, whether or not they receive treatment, experience academic difficulties. This, of course, could be related to the co-occurrence of phonological and language disorders in the majority of cases. Lewis and Freebairn (1992) found that subjects with a history of preschool phonological disorders performed more poorly than matched controls on measures of phonology, reading, and spelling for age groups from preschool to adult. Subjects with a history of language disorder, in addition to the phonological problem, performed even lower on the measures.

In a 28-year longitudinal study, Felsenfeld, Broen, and McGue (1994) followed a group of children who had phonological disorders as preschoolers that persisted through first grade. When they interviewed these subjects in adulthood, the phonological history group, when compared to matched controls, reported lower grades earned throughout school, more academic remedial services required, fewer years of formal education completed, and tendency to choose semiskilled or unskilled occupations. The long-lasting effects of speech-sound disorder can even be seen in parents who were treated for articulation problems as children. Lewis et al. (2007) found that such adults scored lower on multisyllabic word repetition, nonword repetition, reading, spelling, and language tasks when compared to parents without a history of speech-sound disorder. Although these abilities did not affect educational or occupational outcomes, they do suggest that residual effects are seen in adults with a history of speech-sound disorder. In view of the relation between phonological disorders and academic performance, clinicians should not underestimate the importance of early assessment, intervention, and counseling.

After reading this chapter you should be able to answer the following questions:

1. What is an articulation disorder?
2. What is a phonological processing disorder?
3. Give an example of traditional testing of the speech sound /s/ in the initial, medial and final positions in words.
4. Describe at least four phonological processes seen in speech-language development.
5. Explain why it is important to assess (and treat) young children with speech-sound disorders.

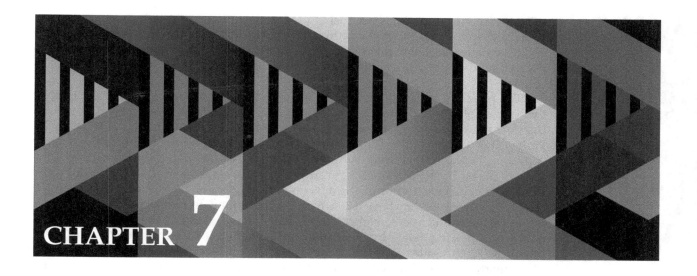

Disorders of Fluency

LEARNING OUTCOMES

After reading this chapter you will be able to:

1. Define stuttering and its salient features.
2. Describe and distinguish among different types of fluency disorders.
3. List and describe the types of disfluencies observed in the speech of people who do and do not stutter.
4. Differentiate stuttering from nonstuttering-like disfluencies.
5. Describe the overt features of stuttering that can be assessed during a fluency evaluation.
6. Provide criteria for distinguishing a normally disfluent child from a child with incipient stuttering.
7. Describe procedures that can be used for determining stuttering frequency and rate of speech.
8. Describe information that should be obtained during the case history portion of a fluency evaluation.
9. Provide some examples of commonly used tests for the evaluation of stuttering severity and covert features of stuttering.
10. Describe factors that should be considered when making a prognosis with a fluency client.
11. Describe factors that require consideration when assessing a person with a fluency disorder from a different culture.

*S*tuttering is a sometimes astonishing, curious, and complicated disorder that certainly represents a difficult way to talk. Why is the flow of speech, seemingly so easy and automatic for others, marred by tense interruptions? Unfortunately, the answer to that question continues to elude both clinicians and researchers—stuttering remains an enigma.

The puzzling nature of stuttering creates a dilemma for students who are looking for simple solutions. Confronted with a voluminous literature and a large number of treatment possibilities—each with its own advocates—it is easy to give up in despair. Perhaps the negative attitude toward working with people who stutter held by so many clinicians, in part, stems from the overwhelming confusion about the disorder and the paucity of solid academic training (Yaruss, 1999; Yaruss & Quesal, 2002). Yet for some beginning clinicians, the dramatic and ominous nature of the disorder and even the confusion among experts have a fascinating appeal; they present a challenge.

We will assume in this chapter that the reader has a good foundation concerning the nature of stuttering. Books by Bloodstein and Ratner (2008), Conture and Curlee (2008), Manning (2009), Guitar (2013), and Yairi and Seery (2014) provide excellent discussions of the many aspects of stuttering. We present the following list of "facts" about stuttering that have diagnostic implications and have been gleaned from the literature. For purposes of exposition, we have eschewed lengthy lists of references. Each item can be documented, however, even though some might disagree with our particular selection or interpretation.

1. The basic speech characteristics of stuttering consist of relatively brief repetitions, prolongations, and blocks on sounds or syllables. These oscillations and fixations may be audible or silent, and they tend to occur more frequently at the beginning of an utterance and on words and phrases that are more motorically complex (such as long words and less frequently used words).

2. Stuttering is a disorder of childhood, generally having its onset in the preschool years (especially between 2 and 5 years); rarely does it begin in older persons, and when it does, it may be a distinct subtype of the disorder (such as psychogenic and neurogenic stuttering).

3. Stuttering (also known as developmental stuttering and, in parts of the world, stammering) is found more frequently among males.

4. Stuttering tends to run in families.

5. Multiple etiologies may account for stuttering: genetics, child development, neurophysiology, and environmental factors.

6. Stuttering may be precipitated (and perpetuated) by certain environmental factors, particularly the critical, demanding behaviors of others, and a fast-paced lifestyle.

7. Stuttering tends to appear more frequently in children described as sensitive, who may be vulnerable or susceptible to stress. People who stutter may have a low threshold for autonomic arousal.

8. Stuttering tends to appear more frequently in children who were slow in acquiring speech or who manifest certain inadequacies of oral communication (articulation errors, language disturbances) other than fluency breakdowns.

9. Stuttering is variable and tends to exhibit cycles of frequency and severity in a given individual.

10. A significant number of individuals (perhaps 80%) recover from stuttering, while others continue to stutter.

11. Stuttering tends to change in form and severity as the individual matures.

12. Stuttering is eliminated or markedly reduced in a variety of conditions: speaking while alone, choral speaking, singing, prolonged or slow speaking, talking in time to rhythm, or under masking conditions.

13. Stuttering, in its developed form, can include a variety of escape and avoidance behaviors. That is, stuttering becomes as much about what the individual does in an attempt to cope with stuttering as it does with the emission of the speech disfluency.

14. Stuttering is also characterized by speech and voice abnormalities other than disfluency (such as narrow pitch range, vocal tension, lack of vocal expression, muscular lags, and asynchronies) that can be detected in nonstuttered speech. These anomalies *may* reflect a basic impairment of phonation (difficulty in initiating phonation, making consonant-vowel transitions), respiration (abnormal reflex activity), neuromotor coordination, or cortical integration; they *may*, however, simply be *effects* of stuttering.

15. Stuttering, in its developed form, is often associated with an expectancy or anticipation of its occurrence.

16. Stuttering becomes personal; individuals who stutter report fear, frustration, social penalties, dissatisfaction with themselves, lower level of aspiration, and a felt loss of social esteem. There is a tendency for problems common to all human beings to become associated with the speech disturbance. However, there is no particular "stuttering personality," nor is the disorder a manifestation of psychoneurosis.

Even though the fluency disorder of stuttering remains a tantalizing mystery, there is much that we can do to help persons who seek our services.

DIFFERENTIAL DIAGNOSIS

Speech is *fluent* when words are produced easily, effortlessly, smoothly, quickly, and in a forward flow. Speech is *disfluent* when one word does not flow smoothly and quickly into the next. Obviously, then, all speakers are, at times, disfluent and these so-called normal disfluencies should be of no consequence. The speech-language pathologist (SLP) needs to be able to differentiate typical from atypical disfluencies; often this proves to be no easy feat with young children. If the clinician does identify a speaker's disfluencies as atypical or clinically significant, the next decision is to distinguish the problem of stuttering from other conditions in which speech fluency is disrupted. A final aspect of the differential diagnosis process may be to identify subtypes within the stuttering population and thus select the most appropriate form of treatment. Let us discuss these three aspects of differential diagnosis.

Sorting out the Types of Fluency Disorders

Assuming that the clinician has already identified a speaker as having abnormal amounts or types of disfluencies, the diagnostic task is one of deciding *which* disorder of fluency is exhibited. Along with a behavioral analysis of the disfluencies, the case history information will go far in suggesting the disorder type. We will provide an overview of some of the fluency breakdowns that can be confused with the common variety of stuttering, called developmental stuttering (or, simply, stuttering).

Episodic Stress Reaction

It is well known that all speakers exhibit some degree of disfluency—revisions, interjections, word and phrase repetitions, and occasionally even part-word repetitions and prolongations. Speech fluency is often considered a sensitive barometer of a person's psychological state because stress tends to increase a speaker's disfluency. Fluency breakdowns that result from episodic stress show a number of consistent identifying features: an acknowledged source of intense or prolonged stimulation; tension overflow throughout the body (including the oral area), which may also produce a tremulous voice; an exacerbation of "normal" disfluency, including broken words, incomplete phrases, interjections, and repetitions of whole and parts of words; and no avoidance but feelings of fear. Finally, the most crucial characteristic is that the disfluency decreases markedly or stops when (or shortly after) the stress terminates. These acute, or episodic, periods of disfluency are usually not clinically significant.

Psychogenic Stuttering

Most persons who stutter, particularly confirmed adult cases, acquire negative feelings about their speech. A few clients, however, show symptoms of a primary neurosis. For these individuals, stuttering is a maladaptive solution to an acute psychological problem. *Psychogenic stuttering* has also been known as neurotic or hysterical stuttering. Referral to or a team approach with other healthcare professionals may be in order. The SLP is well equipped to diagnose and provide treatment for the overt symptoms. Following is a scenario the depicts how a case of psychogenic stuttering could present itself:

> Colleen, an eighth-grade parochial school pupil, began to stutter suddenly following the death of her parents in an automobile accident. She collapsed upon hearing the tragic news and remained mute, almost transfixed and catatonic, for several hours. During the planning for the funeral and extended period of the wake, she started to stutter—a monotonous repetition of the initial syllable of words. She showed no struggle, no avoidance behavior. She looked directly at the listener when she spoke and smiled bravely. We followed this case closely until the remission of stuttering 2 months later, and her disfluency was always the same; it never varied in form or severity from situation to situation. When she read a passage several times, she did not show the typical reduction (adaptation) in stuttering. School documents, as well as interviews with several relatives, indicated that Colleen had no prior speech difficulty. One maternal aunt whom we interviewed did recall, however, that the girl had several "spells" of uncontrolled weeping and laughing during her first menses the year before. The child had received an incredible amount of attention and solace after her parents' death, perhaps even more so because of her "stuttering," from sympathetic adults.

Psychogenic stuttering is a rare fluency disorder that is characterized by a sudden onset of rather stereotypical stuttering behavior. The onset may occur at any age, including adulthood, yet usually happens in an older child. Some severe (and lasting rather than episodic) psychological trauma, emotional upheaval, or stress seems to precipitate the occurrence of stuttering. When a formal diagnosis of psychopathology is present, it usually takes the form of a conversion reaction, anxiety, or depression (Baumgartner & Duffy, 1997; Mahr & Leith, 1992). However, other problems such as having a personality disorder, substance abuse problem, or a post-traumatic neurosis are also possible. In contrast to the exacerbation of "normal" disfluencies seen in episodic stress, Deal (1982) indicates that psychogenic stuttering is often characterized by a stuttering-like pattern that typically takes the form of lengthy repetitions of initial or stressed syllables, although prolongations and laryngeal blocks are also possible. There is often little change in the form and frequency of stuttering behaviors observed and little to no spans of fluent speech. The speech pattern observed is generally not affected by fluency-facilitating activities like choral reading, singing, and delayed auditory feedback. The adaptation effect that is commonly observed during repeated reading of a passage with developmental stuttering is also often absent (Baumgartner & Duffy, 1997). Although highly aware of these suddenly developed disfluencies, the person may or may not be frustrated by them or express interest in their occurrence. Therefore, no secondary or avoidance behaviors are generally observed (Deal, 1982). The level of concern and motivation to change are important elements for the SLP to assess because they may shape the prognosis for change and the direction of intervention.

Neurogenic Stuttering

Stuttering behaviors, or a stuttering-like subset of fluency disorders, may occur following nervous system damage in adolescents or adults. *Neurogenic stuttering* has not been correlated with a lesion in any particular part of the brain. In fact, neurogenic stuttering has been associated with lesions in both hemispheres, all lobes of the brain, the cerebellum, thalamus, and brainstem. Most cases may occur as a result of stroke, traumatic brain injury, infection, anoxia, or tumor. Nervous system disorders like Parkinson disease or Tourette syndrome are frequently affiliated with disfluencies and tic-like movements. The designation of neurogenic stuttering establishes these as fluency disorders. We also have observed disfluency in clients suffering from some types of cerebral palsy, apraxia of speech, and other neurological impairments. There are also reports of fluency disruptions in alcoholics, drug addicts, and patients afflicted with AIDS and with dialysis dementia. Palilalia, perhaps a subtype of neurogenic stuttering, may be caused by bilateral subcortical brain damage. Individuals with palilalia repeat words and entire phrases, typically not sounds or syllables, and they do so with increasing speed and diminishing loudness.

Several patients with aphasia with whom we have worked, particularly those clients who show good progress in word finding but who have residual syntactic difficulty, exhibited fluency breakdowns superficially similar to stuttering.

> Ms. Horn had suffered an aneurysm in the circle of Willis, leaving her hemiplegic, apraxic, and with mild expressive aphasia. When we examined her almost a year after the cerebral vascular episode, her speech pattern resembled clonic stuttering. She would begin a word, repeat a phoneme or syllable several times, back up, and try again; if blocked once more, a repetition might reverberate almost endlessly. She frequently pounded on the table as if to time her utterances. We could discern no evidence of fear or avoidance, just severe frustration. Interestingly, when she spoke or read swiftly her fluency increased dramatically; she also talked freely when distracted from closely monitoring the acts of speaking. Here is a sample of her speech taken from a tape recording during a group session: "I can't-I can't (sigh) . . . I-I-I-I have tr-trouble with my, ah, with my speech . . . and, ah, my leg is, is, you know is, stiff."

The disfluencies noted are rather typical: whole-word repetitions, revisions, interjections, broken words, and gaps in the flow of speech. This client had difficulty formulating messages and then programming the proper motor sequences to utter the thought. Unlike stuttering, where the difficulty is often associated with the beginning of an utterance, Ms. Horn's fluency breakdowns occurred at any point in a sentence.

Helm-Estabrooks (1999) provides six characteristics that can be considered when trying to distinguish neurogenic stuttering from developmental stuttering:

1. Disfluencies result on function as well content words with equal rate of occurrence, whereas in developmental stuttering, they are typically observed on content words.

2. Disfluencies such as repetitions, prolongations, and blocks are seen in all word posi-tions, whereas in developmental stuttering, they are typically observed in the initial position.

3. Stuttering-like behaviors are observed to be consistent across speech tasks and lack the variability commonly observed in developmental stuttering.

4. The speaker may be frustrated but is not anxious about the stuttering behavior.

5. Secondary coping behaviors (i.e., fist clenching, eye blinking, etc.) commonly ob-served with developmental stuttering are rarely associated with the stuttering be-haviors observed in neurogenic stuttering.

6. The adaptation effect generally observed with repeated readings of a passage is absent.

While individuals with neurogenic stuttering may have some fluency characteristics that are unique to their speech, like those listed above, clinical symptoms by themselves are not sufficient for distinguishing neurogenic from developmental stuttering (De Nil, Jokel, & Rochon, 2007; Jokel, De Nil, & Sharpe, 2007; Van Borsal, 1997). Clinicians can't depend solely on the characteristics listed above because contradictory evidence and cases that do not conform to the characteristics listed above have been documented in the literature. Hence, they should be considered more as a rule of thumb rather than distinctively characteristics of neurogenic stuttering. The Stuttering Foundation (www.stutteringhelp.org) provides brochures on neurogenic stuttering that are useful with clients and families.

Cluttering

Cluttering is sometimes confused with stuttering, but it encompasses more than just a disorder of fluency. Cluttering has varied symptomatology and co-occurs with other speech, language, and behavioral disorders. Cluttering symptoms may include part- and whole-word repetitions (including repetitions of multisyllabic words), *mazing disfluen-cies* (too frequent to be within normal limits for false starts, revisions, and fillers or inter-jections), omissions of syllables and small words (*telegraphic speech*), excess speech rates (*tachylalia*), *speech disrhythmia* (spurts of speech), misarticulations, lack of awareness of how the speech sounds and poor monitoring of it, syntactic disorganization, short atten-tion span, perceptual issues, poorly organized thinking, and possible motor disabilities (wise to assess diadochokinetic rate). Other academic difficulties, noted by clinicians, teachers, and researchers, include reading and writing disorders, difficulty with many language-dependent skills (because of subtle language disorders), lack of rhythm and musical ability, and restlessness and hyperactivity (Daly, 1996). Of course, not all these symptoms need to be present in a child or adult for a diagnosis of cluttering. Excessive rate of speech and language formulation problems seem to be the hallmark features of cluttering, along with poor intelligibility because of some of the speech-language symptoms just cited. In addition to Daly, the Myers (1996), Myers and St. Louis (1996), and Ward and Scott (2011) publications are particularly useful in understanding this fluency disorder and in making a differential diagnosis apart from that of stuttering. The Stuttering Foundation (www.stutteringhelp.org) offers a DVD and brochure on cluttering that may be useful to clients and clinicians alike. Information, resources, and support are also available through the International Cluttering Association (ICA) at http://associations.missouristate.edu/ica. Following is an example of how a case of cluttering might present itself:

Ralph was referred to us as a person who stutters by his supervisor during his semester of student teaching. When we evaluated him, he revealed no fears or avoidances, exhibited only a few short part-word repetitions, and had no fixations; he said that he enjoyed talking, did a lot of it, and that he was asked frequently to repeat himself, "especially when I talk fast." Ralph's difficulty seemed to take place on the phrase or sentence level; his interruptions broke the integrity of a thought rather than a word. In addition, he frequently omitted syllables and transposed words and phrases; he said "plobably," "posed," and "pacific" for *probably, supposed,* and *specific.* Ralph's speech was sprinkled with spoonerisms (he said "betadase" for *database*) and malapropisms (he described getting lost while hunting because the road he was following "dissipated" and told us he had a good "dialect" going with his roommate). His speech was swift and jumbled; it emerged in rapid torrents until he jammed up, and then he surged on again in another staccato outburst. In spontaneous talking, his message was characterized by disorganized sentences and poor phrasing. He gave the overall impression of being in great haste. When we asked him to slow down and speak carefully, there was a drastic improvement, but he soon forgot our recommendation and reverted back to his hurried, disorganized style. By and large, Ralph was unaware of and indifferent to his fluency problem. He was an impatient, impulsive young man, always on the go. His coursework was characteristically done in a great, almost compulsive rush; he had difficulty reading, and his handwriting was a scrawl.

Frequently used tools that clinicians can use to make differential diagnostic discriminations between stuttering and cluttering as well as measure cluttering severity are the *Predictive Cluttering Inventory* (PCI; Daly, 2006) and the *Cluttering Severity Instrument* (CSI; Bakker & Meyers, 2011).

Distinguishing among Subtypes of Stuttering

Are there different kinds of developmental stuttering? Although there is no conclusive answer to that question, clinical opinion is that there must be—if only to explain the wide variety of clients, symptomatologies, and responses to intervention programs. Possibilities that come to mind include interiorized and exteriorized speaker characteristics, *predominantly clonic* (repetitive disfluencies) and *predominantly tonic* (with tension, prolongations, and blockages) persons who stutter, clients who feature escape techniques, those who are addicted to avoidance, and those who can predict an occurrence of stuttering and those who cannot. Perhaps there are even variations in stuttering that stem from cultural influences.

Differentiating Stuttering from Nonstuttering Disfluencies

We saved this aspect of the differential diagnosis for last in this section, although the clinician must determine it first. It is a vast topic. The literature shows good agreement regarding the general principles for distinguishing between stuttering and nonstuttering types of disfluency. All speakers are disfluent from time to time. Where to draw the line between typical and atypical types and amounts of disfluency is still a matter of clinical debate and philosophy. In the past it was thought that persons who stutter and persons who do not stutter commit the same sorts of disfluencies initially, but that both parents and others in the immediate environment react negatively and cause the child's speech to spiral unacceptably—with more fragmentation and tension being the by-product in speech. In contrast, and based on considerable research evidence, the current philosophy holds that young nonstuttering and stuttering children's disfluencies are categorically divergent. Let us begin our discussion with the various types of speech disfluencies. A nonexhaustive list of some types of disfluencies includes the following and, as we will see, some types pose more concern than other, innocuous types:

1. Whole-word repetition: "My, my ball went under the car."
2. Part-word repetition (either easy or with tense, fleeting, or multiple iterations): "My i-i-ice cream is melting."
3. Phrase repetition: "I want, I want some ice cream."
4. Sentence revision: "It went—My ball went under the car."
5. Filled pause/interjections (fillers include *uhm, ah, uh*): "I want some . . . uhm . . . ice cream."
6. Unfilled pause (either relaxed hesitation or tense silence/inaudible block): "Daddy, I want (relaxed pause before next word) some ice cream." "Daddy, I (lips in posture for /w/ but blocked and unable to flow forward in audible speech) want some ice cream."
7. Sound prolongations: "SSSSSally took my ball."
8. Broken word: "I w-ant some ice cream."

Some of these types of disfluency overlap by definition, and frankly, some types of disfluency are of more concern than others. Keeping track of so many types of disfluency can be clinically cumbersome and imprecise.

The often-cited works by Yairi's research team at the University of Illinois segmented *stuttering-like disfluencies (SLDs)* from *other disfluencies (ODs)* (Ambrose & Yairi, 1994; Ambrose & Yairi, 1999; Yairi & Ambrose, 1992, 2005; Yairi, Ambrose, & Niermann, 1993; Yairi & Lewis, 1984). The types of disfluencies that characterize SLDs and ODs are shown in Table 7–1. By describing only three types of stuttering-like disfluencies, Yairi simplifies the multitude of descriptors that have been used. *Disrhythmic phonations* include events such as within-word disruptions of air flow, sound prolongations, blocks (whether audible or inaudible), instances of noticeable stress, as well as unusual patterns of intonation.

What types of disfluencies and other factors represent early signs of concern for the onset of stuttering? How should a speech-language pathologist proceed? There are many opinions in answer to these questions. There also are many tools available to the SLP for appraising developmental stuttering near onset in the preschool years as well as for adolescents and adults with persistent stuttering. Gordon and Luper (1992) reviewed six often-used protocols for identifying beginning stuttering. Two of these will be mentioned here. Adams (1977) provides a clinical strategy for differentiating the child with typical disfluencies from one beginning to stutter; his criteria and guidelines for clinical interpretation are summarized in Table 7–2. Also useful is the *Protocol for Differentiating the Incipient Stutterer* (Pindzola, 1988; Pindzola & White, 1986).

In making decisions about typical disfluency versus stuttering disfluency, the clinician should be guided by information available in the literature. The clinician then

TABLE 7–1
Stuttering-Like Disfluencies (SLDs) Compared to Other Disfluencies (ODs)

Three SLDs	Example ODs
Part-word repetitions	Interjections
Single-syllable word repetitions	Polysyllabic word repetitions
Dysrhythmic phonations	Phrase repetitions
	Revisions

TABLE 7–2

Adams's Guidelines for Distinguishing between the Normally Disfluent Child and the Incipient Stutterer

Criterion	Nonstuttering Disfluent	Incipient Stutterer
Total frequency (all types)	Nine or fewer disfluencies per 100 words	Ten or more disfluencies per 100 words
Predominant type	Whole-word and phrase repetitions, interjections, and revisions	Part-word repetitions, audible and silent prolongations, and broken words
Unit repetitions	No more than 2 unit repetitions ("b-b-ball")	At least 3 repetitions ("b-b-b-ball")
Voicing and air flow	Little or no difficulty starting or sustaining voicing or air flow; continuous phonation during part-word repetitions	Frequent difficulty in starting or sustaining voicing or air flow; heard in association with part-word repetitions, prolongations, and broken words; more effortful disfluencies
Intrusion of the schwa	Schwa not perceived ("ba-ba-baby")	Schwa often perceived ("buh-buh-buh-baby")

pulls together a vast array of information collected on and about the client to arrive at a diagnosis. We admit this is a judgment call on the part of the clinician, but if the evaluation is done thoroughly, it is an informed judgment call. Overt features we like to assess include:

- Predominant type of disfluency (SLDs versus ODs)
- Frequency of disfluency
- Duration of the disfluencies
- Presence of struggle or tension
- Speech rhythm and rate
- Presence of any learned behaviors and physical involvement

We have discussed various types of disfluencies, but now a few words about how to get a representative frequency count because it is an important diagnostic measure. The frequency of stuttering is provided as a percentage, with either the word (% Words Stuttered) or syllable (% Syllables Stuttered) serving as the unit of measurement. The ideal number of syllables or words to collect is an item of debate among professionals in the field. As a rule of thumb, it is best to collect a minimum of two different speech samples spanning different situations and tasks that contain a minimum of 300 syllables or words in each sample (Conture, 2001). Assessing the child's speech across different situations will give you a better understanding of how the child's speech varies across different contexts in response to differing demands. Factors that should be considered across the samples include the setting or location, the task, the linguistic complexity, number of conversational partners and their familiarity with them, degree of familiarity or comfort with the topic being discussed, and emotional state or stressors present during the speech sample. Obviously, the larger the samples and the more situations sampled, the more representative your overall sample is likely to be. We highly encourage clinicians to obtain at least one sample outside the speech clinic.

The clinician must also determine what behaviors to count, meaning that the SLP must adopt an acceptable system for evaluating disfluency types observed in a speech sample. See Table 7–3 for some guidelines for counting disfluencies. Reardon and Ya-russ (2004) described a real-time analysis method of counting fluent and disfluent syllables (or words) from a speech sample. The choice of whether to use syllables or words is one of personal preference. We prefer to use syllables because clients can stutter on more than one syllable in a multisyllabic word and because it is often easier to do an online tally with the rhythm of syllable beats than words. After deciding on the unit of measurement, a piece of graph paper or a page marked with small blocks for marking syllables (or words) spoken can be used to keep track of moments of disfluency. On this chart, instances of disfluent syllables (or words) are coded as Rs for sound or syllable repetitions, P for prolongations, B for blocks, Rw for word repetitions, Rp for phrase repetitions, Rv for revisions, and I for interjections or filler/starters. Fluent syllables are often coded with a dot or dash. A percentage of disfluency can then be calculated as follows:

$$\text{Percentage disfluency} = \frac{\text{number disfluent syllables(or words)}}{\text{total number of syllables(or words)}} \times 100$$

For example, a clinician obtains a 200-syllable sample of a child's conversational speech. In the sample, she observes 30 disfluent syllables. For this child, the frequency of disfluency is calculated as follows (and is equal to 15% SS):

$$\text{Percentage disfluency} = \frac{30 \text{ syllables}}{200 \text{ syllables}} = .15 \times 100 = 15\%$$

Totals per type of disfluency can also be analyzed for pattern trends and to determine the percentage of SLDs and ODs. The disfluency types are determined by evaluating the occurrence of each disfluency type in comparison to the overall percentage of disfluency. Percentage for each disfluency type can be calculated as follows:

$$\text{Percentage type disfluency} = \frac{\text{number disfluent syllable for a given type (or words)}}{\text{total number of disfluent syllables (or words)}} \times 100$$

TABLE 7–3
Guildlines for Counting Disfluencies

When counting the number of syllables or words in an utterance, count them as if the utterance were spoken fluently.
Repetitions are counted as one moment of disfluency regardless of the number of iterations.
When counting the number of itertations in a repetition, count the ones preceding the release of the word (e.g., p-p-pet = two-unit repetition)
Prolongation of a sound counts as one disfluency regardless of duration.
A block is counted as one disfluency regardless of its duration.
A pause is counted as one disfluency if it is unnatural or long enough to call attention to itself.
A revision is counted as one disfluency regardless of the number of syllables or words included in the revisions
Filler words are counted as one disfluency. When multiple filler words are used in succesion, they are counted as one disfluency (e.g., uh, well, uh what kind of car do you drive?)
In cases where one syllable or word has more than one type of disfluency, it is counted as only one moment of disfluency. (e.g., wwwwell-well-well)
When in doubt, count the syllable or word in question as fluent.

Source: Adapted from Bloom and Cooperman, 1999.

Using our previous example, the clinician documented 30 disfluencies in a 200-syllable sample. For the 30 observed disfluencies, let's assume that 21 were part-word repetitions and 9 were sound prolongations. The percentage for each disfluency type is calculated as follows and results in 70% part-word repetitions and 30% prolongations:

$$\text{Percentage part-word repetitions} = \frac{21 \text{ syllables}}{30 \text{ syllables}} = .70 \times 100 = 70\%$$

$$\text{Percentage prolongations} = \frac{9 \text{ syllables}}{30 \text{ syllables}} = .30 \times 100 = 30\%$$

When a speech sample is evaluated, it is also often marked for duration analysis. This is often expressed as an average number of reiterations of the repetition or as an average amount of time stuck in an audible or silent disrhythmic phonation. The following excerpts from a sample are provided:

"Mmmmake a snake" (1 P/1s)

"Sitting on the the the the couch" (1 Rw with 2 units)

"Lllllike th-th-th-th-that" (1 P/1s, 1 Rs with 4 units)

"Mmmmmmmay I have more, p-p-please" (1P/2s, 1 Rs with 2 units)

In this example from a 100-syllable speech sample, the client demonstrated a total of 6 SLDs. The percentage syllables stuttered, then, is 6% (total of 6 divided by 100 syllables) with 1- to 2-second prolongations and two- to four-unit repetitions.

In addition to using a paper tally, several handheld devices, online tools, or apps are available for conducting fluency tallies. Handheld devices include both mechanical and electronic tally counters. Online counters and apps can also be easily located and downloaded. Several of these applications allow for an analysis of syllables spoken by calculating the percentage of syllables stuttered, the percentage of fluent syllables, the average duration of disfluencies, and the rate of speech. Some allow for an analysis disfluency type.

It should be obvious to the reader by now that the type of disfluency that predominates in a client's speech and the size of the speech unit affected by the breakdown influence society's judgment of normal fluency. For example, repetitions of whole phrases are quite common in all speakers; whole-word repetitions are disfluencies typical of both persons who do and persons who do not stutter. Yet a predominance of part-word repetitions and prolongations distinguishes stuttered from nonstuttered speech (especially if done frequently), and this is true in preschool children and adults. Hesitations or pauses before phrases or before words may likewise be less worrisome than blocks or gaps within words (i.e., preceding syllables or sounds) or when disfluencies are accompanied with tension. The rule of thumb is that the smaller the speech unit affected, the more atypical the disfluency.

The frequency with which disfluent behaviors occur has long been recognized as important in the diagnosis of stuttering. As we have shown, there are various types of disfluencies and ways to measure them for use clinically. A host of normative data is also available for the different systems. A clinician needs to be careful in applying similar systems and interpretative data. Dissimilar information is not interchangeable. Norms reported by Yairi and Seery (2011) comparing the popular and straightforward stuttering-like disfluencies (SLDs) to other disfluencies (ODs) are summarized in Table 7–4.

As part of the assessment, the clinician gauges the duration of the client's disfluency. If the typical duration of prolongations exceeds 1 second, or if repetitions involve

TABLE 7–4
Percentage of Syllables Disfluent in Preschool Children Who Do and Do Not Stutter

Disfluency Type	Mean Percentage Disfluent for Children Who Stutter	Mean Percentage Disfluent for Children Who Do Not Stutter
SLDs (part-word repetitions, single-syllable repetitions, dysrhymic phonations)	Over 11%	Under 2%
Other disfluencies (ODs)	Over 5%	Under 5%

numerous reiterations—say, three to five or more—then these behaviors may be interpreted as signs of concern, perhaps stuttering. Audible effort while speaking is not typical and therefore, when noticed, may be indicative of stuttering. There are many signs of audible effort; some examples include disrupted air flow, hard contacts (explosive, crisp articulation), effort or tension heard in the voice, and a pitch rise during a moment of stuttering.

An audible insight into differentiating stuttering from nonstuttering may be the overall impression and speech naturalness. When adults or children who do not stutter have speech repetitions, those disfluencies preserve the normal rhythm and rate of speech. Not until the tempo of the multiple reiterations speeds up or the rhythm becomes irregular and choppy is there substantial reason for concern. The SLP, then, should subjectively judge the client's rhythm, tempo, and speed of disfluencies when trying to make a differential diagnosis.

The presence of learned behaviors, also called *secondary characteristics*, is strongly suggestive of stuttering rather than other innocuous disfluencies. In this case, the clinician should determine whether the client uses concealment devices (such as word substitutions or talking around a word, which is called a circumlocution), postponement devices, starting tricks, and so forth. Visually, the clinician may note physical involvement of the face, head, and body. Frequently observed contortions are eye blinks, wrinkling of the forehead, distortions of the mouth, overt mandibular tension, head jerks, and the more subtle head turnings to divert eye contact.

Once the SLP has made a differential diagnosis and determined that the client is stuttering, the next issue to be resolved is the developmental progression or severity of the disorder. In actuality, the information gathered to differentiate typical from atypical speech disfluencies speech is part of the same kind of information needed to determine the level of severity. Assessment instruments guide the SLP in determining the severity level (mild, moderate, and severe). The next decision confronting the clinician is the recommended course of action. Is treatment warranted? If so, the assessment information should help the SLP decide on the direction of intervention and treatment goals.

THE APPRAISAL OF STUTTERING

In our discussion about making a differential diagnosis, we glossed over the details of how to obtain the information necessary to make such a decision. What information is necessary? What published appraisal instruments are available to help collect and make sense of this information? What less tangible factors need to be judged, albeit subjectively, by the clinician? We will now try to answer these questions. Bear in mind, however, that the answers may differ for different clients depending on their age, intelligence, reading abilities, and so forth.

Case History Information and Parent Materials

We will discuss two forms of the case history intake: one done with the parents of a child who stutters or is beginning to stutter and one done with a teenager or adult who stutters.

Initial Interview with the Parents

The initial interview with the parents of a child beginning to stutter is of critical importance. We must establish our professional competence, demonstrate our genuine interest, and convince the parents that we can be trusted. In short, our primary task in this initial contact is to build a relationship for subsequent counseling sessions. We also listen carefully to the parents' presenting story: How do they see the child's problem? In their view, what might have caused it? What do they identify as their role in the onset of the child's stuttering? What expectations and apprehensions do they have regarding the nature and the outcome of treatment?

We like to regard the initial interaction between parents and clinician as a time for information gathering and information sharing. As we said, we first want to hear the presenting complaint—and encourage the telling of their child's speech story. We may opt to be more or less directive in our style with the parents; it does not matter, as long as we can obtain the information we need. A parent's careful review of the many factors involved in the child's problem tends to foster objectivity. It also shifts the focus away from a general impression of "trouble" to the observation of specific behaviors. Here are some questions we use as guides in assembling information from parents:

1. When did the child begin exhibiting disfluencies?
2. What were the circumstances under which the disfluencies were noted?
3. How long has the child been exhibiting the disfluencies?
4. Was anything special going on in the child's life when the disfluency started?
5. What changes have been noted in the frequency or form of the disfluencies?
6. What factors seem to increase or decrease the child's disfluency?
7. In what ways has the family tried to help the child?
8. What is the child's reaction to the family's efforts to help?

Additional items to assess in obtaining a case history include (1) a specific review of the familial incidence of stuttering; (2) the impact, if any, of siblings, relatives, teachers, or babysitters on the child; (3) a description of how the child spends a typical day; and (4) a description of any prior professional treatment.

The case history interview can be done either before or after the child has been seen and evaluated by the clinician. Consequently, this initial meeting may, in fact, involve several points of interaction or separate sessions. We try to refrain from being influenced by the parents' push for us to provide too much information prematurely; naturally, parents want to know what caused their child's disfluency and what can be done (quickly) about it. We do enlist the parents' help in collecting observations of the child's behavior in the home environment.

What factors at home seem to promote fluency and what seems to promote disfluency? Is it all right for the parents to remind the child to slow down (as advocated by Cooper & Cooper, 2004; Yairi & Ambrose, 2005), or is that counterproductive and something to be considered taboo (owing to earlier philosophies)? We do not know the answers to these questions for a *particular* child; the parents must find out. Parents' recording of home behaviors is a clinically useful assignment.

We often find that simply asking parents to monitor the antecedents and consequences of their child's speech disfluencies is sufficiently motivating to engender change. Environmental events that disrupt a child's flow of speech typically become obvious when parents begin to chart. The reader is encouraged to read the work of Ratner (2004) because she dispels some commonly held beliefs on caregiver–child interactions that have clear implications for counseling and treatment.

Even though there is much information that we simply cannot give the parents early in the clinical process (often because we do not yet know the information), clinicians have a responsibility to help educate the parents. That is, clinicians need to provide a good understanding of stuttering and its many ramifications. In addition, clinicians like to provide the parents with reading materials; some are of their own preparation, while others are brochures and booklets from published sources such as the Stuttering Foundation (www.stutteringhelp.org), the National Stuttering Association (www.westutter.org), and the American Speech-Language-Hearing Association (www.asha.org). Videos and printed matter available from these sources are invaluable in helping parents understand how they can help their children.

The clinician may wish to have one or both parents complete a checklist or questionnaire that may prove useful in identifying parental perceptions, attitudes, and topics in need of exploration at subsequent counseling sessions. Most texts on stuttering guide the clinician in such areas, as does the *Parent Attitudes toward Stuttering Checklist* in the program by Cooper and Cooper (2004).

It is important that parents obtain some closure from these initial interviews. Let us demonstrate a typical conversation, showing how we relate our diagnostic findings to the parents of a client named Stephen.

> Stephen does indeed have some breaks in speech, more than normal for a child of his age. He is doing some stuttering, but it is still the "less troublesome kind." He is not struggling or avoiding and, most important, he doesn't seem to be very aware that talking is tough. (We drew a rough sketch of the stuttering gauge depicted in Figure 7–1 and showed them that Stephen exhibited only the first three early danger signs of stuttering.) We want to prevent the problem from developing further and cannot do anything without your help. We need to find out why he is having speech breaks; we need to know when he does it and under what circumstances. In short, we have to start looking at behaviors, at what he *does*, not a condition he *has*. In many cases like this, if we identify and alter certain environmental situations or the demands placed on the child, the child stops stuttering or can become markedly more fluent. You were very wise to bring him in now, before the fear and frustration have a chance to develop. Let's plan on meeting again tomorrow, and together we can begin to review Stephen's background and then decide how to gather information on what is happening now.

Case History Interview with Older Clients

The case history and initial interview with older clients who stutter are obviously different from those we just described. Prior to undertaking formal observation and testing, clinicians like to perform an intake interview. This brief preliminary discussion is designed to accomplish four objectives: (1) to inform the client what to expect in the diagnostic session, (2) to determine why the client is coming for treatment at this particular time, (3) to assemble historical information, and (4) to establish a working relationship.

Because the clinician wants the client to be a partner in the exploration of the problem, it is important for the client to know *what* the clinician intends to do and *why* the

FIGURE 7–1
Signs of Concern Depicted Vertically

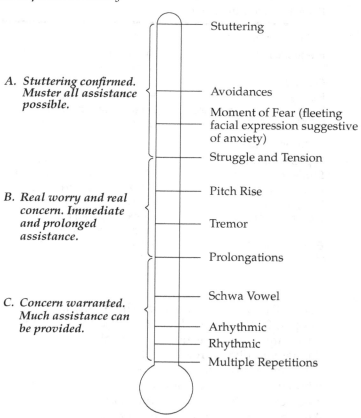

A. *Stuttering confirmed.*
   Muster all assistance
   possible.

B. *Real worry and real*
   concern. Immediate
   and prolonged
   assistance.

C. *Concern warranted.*
   Much assistance can
   be provided.

Stuttering

Avoidances

Moment of Fear (fleeting
facial expression suggestive
of anxiety)

Struggle and Tension

Pitch Rise

Tremor

Prolongations

Schwa Vowel

Arhythmic

Rhythmic

Multiple Repetitions

clinician proposes to do it. The clinician also likes to determine why the client is coming (or being sent) to an SLP at this particular point in time. Has the individual undergone a bottoming-out experience, a severe crisis in his or her social, occupational, or educational life? What does he or she expect from treatment? What do others expect? Answers to these questions are useful in determining the client's motivation and in making a prognosis. All in all, the initial contact with a client is of inestimable importance in establishing a working relationship and communicating your belief in the client's capacity for self-help.

Differentiating and Predictive Scales

As we discussed earlier in this chapter, one of the clinician's major responsibilities is differentiating speakers having typical disfluencies from persons who are stuttering. This may be obvious in the evaluation of some clients, but it may be quite difficult with others—particularly young children.

Complicating the issue further with young children is the notion of spontaneous recovery. Estimates are that as many as 80% of the children who begin to stutter recover after a transient period of stuttering. The transient period is believed to conclude within the first 18 to 36 months after onset for reasons that are not well understood (Mansson, 2000; Yairi et al., 1996; Yairi & Seery, 2011). Although clinicians are far from being able to differentiate precisely children who will recover from stuttering from those who will

TABLE 7–5
Child Risk Factors Believed to Be Important in Predicting Recovery versus Persistence of Stuttering

Of Top Importance	
Frequency of disfluency	Stable or increasing amounts over time, which is suggestive of persistence.
Gender	Boys are at higher risk.
Family history	Persistent stuttering is more likely when relatives stutter.
Time elapsed since onset	After 3 years of stuttering, the chance of natural recovery diminishes to about 15%.
Of Importance	
Types of disfluencies	SLDs rather than ODs.
Stuttering severity	More severe stuttering may or may not be more persistent.
Phonological skills	Coexisting disorder is a complicating factor.
Language skills	Coexisting disorder is complicating factor.
Motor coordination	Coexisting oral motor difficulties (diadochokinesis) may be complicating factors.
Environmental	Parental/society assistance, not ridicule, may aid recovery.

not, SLPs do have some help. The *Stuttering Chronicity Prediction Checklist* (Cooper & Cooper, 2004) and the *Stuttering Prediction Instrument for Young Children* (Riley, 1981) are examples of published and available prediction instruments, though with poor predictive validity, as reviewed by Biddle et al. (2002). In the hands of an experienced clinician, all assessment indexes provide information useful in predicting who will and who will not recover from stuttering. Table 7–5 summarizes important symptoms and risk factors helpful in predicting stuttering recovery as opposed to persistence (Yairi & Ambrose, 2005). Those who do not recover—with or without intervention—may be said to have persistent stuttering that can be managed or improved in therapy but not likely eliminated.

Clinicians have at their disposal, either commercially or in research publications, an assortment of tools that guide the assessment and interpretative process. The assessment of overt, observable features of stuttering is more straightforward than covert features, which, of course, tend to be less observable, hidden, and subjective. Tables 7–6 and 7–7 list many of the available assessment instruments, useful for a variety of purposes.

Severity Scales

The clinician's primary mission in the evaluation of a person who stutters is to perform a careful analysis of the individual's speech disfluency behavior. This is necessary not only for differential diagnosis but also for the appraisal of the severity of the disorder. With regard to treatment, the disfluency assessment also accomplishes two basic purposes: It delineates the behaviors to be altered, and it provides a base measure to which the clinician can refer when monitoring the impact of treatment. The majority of published assessment instruments help the clinician determine the extent of the speech problem. We will call these instruments *severity scales* whether or not the score from the test yields a severity modifier, such as mild to very severe.

Table 7–6 lists some of the available instruments that assess the overt features of stuttering. By using a variety of these instruments, many aspects of the stuttering

TABLE 7-6
Some Available Instruments for the Assessment of Overt Features of Stuttering, Including Diagnostic, Severity, and Predictive Scales

Instrument Title	Author(s) and Year of Publication	Year	Age Range	Description
A Protocol for Differentiating the Incipient Stutterer	Pindzola and White	1986	Children	Protocol that helps clinicians differentiate between children who experience normal disfluencies from incipient stutterers. It is arranged into four sections: auditory behaviors, visual behaviors, covert psychological feelings, and summarizing evidence.
A Stuttering Chronicity Prediction Checklist	Cooper and Cooper	2004	Children	Checklist that is used to differentiate between chronic and episodic stutterers. It is divided into three sections: historical indicators of chronicity, attitudinal indicators of chronicity, and behavioral indicators of chronicity.
Assessment Form: Systematic Fluency Training for Young Children–Third edition	Shine	1988	Preschool to third grade	Criterion-referenced assessment used to identify children who stutter. Assessment consists of six subsections: parent interview, rate of stuttering instrument, stuttering severity instrument, comprehensive stuttering analysis, physiological speaking process, and description of struggle behaviors.
Assessment of Stuttering Behaviors	Tanner	1990	3–6 years	Diagnostic tool that is used to evaluate a child's speech fluency in various environments. Instrument includes the Parental Diagnostic Questionnaire and the Classroom Fluency Checklist.
Cooper Chronicity Prediction Checklist	Cooper	1973	Children	Checklist that helps to determine the likelihood a child's stuttering will persist. It is scored based on the number of yes responses concerning the historical, attitudinal, and behavioral aspects of stuttering in children.
Pragmatic Stuttering Intervention for Adolescents and Adults	Tanner, Belliveau, and Siebert	1995	13–21 years	Assessment that evaluates pragmatic components of stuttering and identifies specific sound error patterns. Includes assessment protocols, stuttering history record forms, and methods for documenting disfluency.
Scale of Stuttering Severity	Williams, Darley, and Spriesterbach	1978	School-age children	Scale that uses a seven-point rating scale to assess overall level of stuttering severity. Evaluates a variety of behavioral characteristics, including frequency counts, facial grimacing, and associated movements.
Stocker Probe for Fluency and Language– Third Edition	Stocker and Goldfarb	1995	Preschool children	Diagnostic tool used for assessment of fluency and language. Consists of five levels of probes used to elicit different types of responses.
Stuttering Prediction Instrument for Young Children	Riley	1981	3–8 years	Diagnostic tool that measures a child's stuttering severity. Identifies part-word repetitions, prolongations, frequently stuttered words, and any negative reactions a child displays.
Stuttering Severity Instrument for Children and Adults (SSI-4)	Riley	2009	2:10+ years	Norm-referenced assessment that evaluates a child's stuttering severity in four areas of speech behavior: frequency, duration, physical concomitants, and naturalness of speech.
Stuttering Severity Scale	Lanyon	1967	Adolescents and adults	A 64-item true/false statement inventory that discriminates between stutterers and nonstutterers, as well as supplies severity levels of stuttering.
Test of Childhood Stuttering (TOCS)	Gillam, Logan, and Pearson	2009	4–12 years	Norm-referenced tool that assesses a child's stuttering severity through four tasks. These four tasks are rapid picture naming, modeled sentences, structured conversation, and narration. Observational rating scales and a supplemental clinical assessment are also available for use by clinicians.

TABLE 7-7
Some Available Instruments for the Assessment of Covert Features of Stuttering, Including Situation/Avoidance Checklists, Perception/Attitude Scales, and Quality of Life Impact Scales

Instrument Title	Author(s) and Year of Pulication	Year	Age Range	Description
A19 Scale	Guitar and Grims	1977	Kindergarten to fourth grade	Scale that includes 19 questions to determine whether a child has developed negative attitudes toward communication. The higher a child's score, the more likely he or she has developed negative attitudes toward communication.
Behavior Assessment Battery (BAB)	Brutten and Vanryckeghm	2003	children	Assessment battery includes three subscales: a Speech Situation Checklist for emotional reactions, a Speech Situation Checklist for speech disruption, and a behavior checklist.
Communication Attitudes Test (CAT)	Brutten and Dunham	1989	7.0+ years	Diagnostic tool that evaluates children's attitudes toward their own communication. Consists of 35 true/false questions that individuals complete.
Communication Attitude Test of Preschool and Kindergarten Children Who Stutter (KiddyCat)	Vanryckeghem and Brutten	2007	3–6 years	Assessment tool that evaluates a child's awareness and attitudes toward speech. Includes 12 yes or no questions that children respond to from their own perspective.
Culture-Free Self-Esteem Inventory–Second Edition	Battle	1992	6:0–18:11	Self-report inventories used to determine the level of self-esteem in students. Three forms are developed: primary, intermediate, and adolescent.
Inventory of Communication Attitudes	Watson	1988	Adolescents and adults	Self-report instrument that includes 39 statements of common speaking situations. An individual's score reflects her or his attitudes in general conversational situations. They are measured on four response scales (affective, behavioral, cognitive-A, and cognitive-b) and a frequency scale (1- to 7-point rating system).
Iowa Scale of Attitude Toward Stuttering	Ammons and Johnson	1944	Children	Scale that samples an individual's general attitude toward stuttering.
Modified Erickson Scale of Communication Attitudes (S-24)	Andrews and Cutler	1974	Adults	Measures interpersonal communication attitudes about stuttering
Overall Assessment of the Speaker's Experience of Stuttering (OASES)	Yaruss, Quesal, and Coleman	2010	7.0+	Comprehensive self-report that measures the impact of stuttering on a person's life.

Tool	Author	Year	Age	Description
Pragmatic Stuttering Intervention for Adolescents and Adults	Tanner	1995	13–21 years	Assessment that evaluates pragmatic components of stuttering and identifies any specific sound-error patterns in individuals who stutter. Includes assessment protocols, stuttering history record forms, and many ways to document disfluencies.
Pragmatic Stuttering Intervention for Children–Second Edition	Tanner	1994	7–11 years	Assessment that helps to identify social issues that may arise from a student's disfluencies. Includes assessment protocols, stuttering history record forms, and many ways to document disfluencies.
Perceptions of Stuttering Inventory	Woolf	1967	Adolescents and adults	Measures perceptions of the presence of struggle, avoidance, and expectancy of stuttering.
Revised Communication Attitude Inventory (S-24)	Andrews and Cutler	1974	Adolescents and adults	Clients respond to a series of 24 true/false statements according to whether or not the statements are characteristic of themselves. Higher scores indicated a negative attitude about communication.
Self Efficacy for Adolescents (SEA-Scale)	Manning	1994	9–19 years	Assessment tool that shows the individual's degree of confidence in approaching certain speaking situations. The individual answers 100 questions on a 10-point scale, according to his or her confidence level in that speaking situation.
Self Efficacy for Adults Who Stutter Scale (SESAS)	Ornstein and Manning	1985	19 + years	Assessment tool that shows the individual's degree of confidence in approaching and maintaining fluent speech in varied speaking situations.
Stutterer's Self-Ratings of Reactions to Speech Situations (SSRSS Scale)	Guitar	2006	Adolescents and adults	This tool presents 40 different speaking situations. Each column has a 1 to 5 rating scale, and a person responds to each question to reflect the degree to which she or he engages in each particular experience.
Stuttering Attitudes Checklist	Cooper and Cooper	2003	Adolescents and adults	Checklist is completed by individuals to determine their attitudes toward stuttering. They complete the form by placing a + or a – next to each statement.
Subjective Units of Distress Scale (SUDS)	Marks	1987	Adolescents and adults	Rating scale that reflects the level of fear and anxiety felt by an individual at a given time. Ratings are made on a scale from 0 to 100 or from 0 to 10.
The Wright and Ayre Stuttering Self-Rating Profile (WASSP)	Wright and Ayre	2000	Adolescents and adults	Comprehensive tool that identifies behavioral and attitudinal features of stuttering for adolescents and adults. Individuals respond to 24 items that are grouped into five sections: stuttering behaviors, thoughts about stuttering, feelings about stuttering, avoidance due to stuttering, and disadvantage due to stuttering.

problem can be tapped, including the frequency of disfluency, the duration of the disfluency, the physical behaviors that accompany speech attempts, and so forth. Judging from the length of this (nonexhaustive) list, there are many stuttering evaluation and severity scales from which to choose. We will highlight a commonly used scale of severity: the *Stuttering Severity Instrument*, which is in wide use and now in its fourth edition (SSI-4; Riley, 2009). The SSI-4 is useful with both children and adults and has provisions for testing those who can and cannot read. The number of syllables stuttered and the number of total syllables spoken are computed by the SLP as the client reads or is engaged in conversation. Frequency, expressed as a percentage of stuttered syllables, is then computed. The clinician also monitors the duration of the longest stuttering events and rates the presence and conspicuousness of physical behaviors concomitant with the speech attempts.

Frequency, duration, and physical concomitant task scores are then combined for a total score. The fourth edition also includes an assessment of the individual's speech naturalness, although this does not contribute to the severity score. The severity of the client's stuttering can be ascertained by comparing the total score to the normative data provided in the test manual. Stuttering severity may be described as very mild, mild, moderate, severe, or very severe in this manner. The SSI-4 kit includes optional computerized software for assistance in scoring. This recent edition also addresses its reliability and validity, a weakness that was previously raised (Biddle et al., 2002).

The *Test of Childhood Stuttering* (TOCS) is another test that has grown in popularity and is being used more widely in the assessment of children ages 4 to 12 (Gillam, Logan, & Pearson, 2009). The TOCS uses four speech tasks to identify stuttering-related behaviors and determine stuttering severity: rapid naming, modeled sentences, structured conversation, and narration. Through these tasks you assess how fluently the client can produce single words in a time-stressed context, utterances with varying linguistic complexity, utterances in the context of dialogue, and utterances in the context of monologue. The test includes observational rating forms that provide a means for evaluating stuttering and its related behaviors from the perspective of parents, teachers, and others with whom the child might interact. The TOCS kit also includes a means for conducting supplemental clinical assessment and provides guidance for those clinicians who wish to do a detailed analysis of the disfluency data obtained.

The appraisal of the overt symptoms of stuttering need not require administration of a commercial test. The clinician's analysis, whether using a formal published test or an informal look at a speech sample, should include a thorough description of the stuttering pattern (topography) and measures of the relative frequency with which various features of the pattern occur. Several authorities also recommend assessing the client's rate of speech during speaking and reading tasks (Guitar, 2013; Shapiro, 2011), but others do not (Ingham, 2005). Speech rate is a basic element of fluency and therefore, in our opinion, warrants assessment. The rate at which parents talk may also merit observation and sometimes assessment. If a client's speaking rate is too fast or too slow, it will often often communicative effectiveness, the perceived fluency, and sometimes the intelligibility of the client's spoken message. Some clinicians prefer to measure speech rate at the word level; others measure at the syllable level. Rate of speech can be easily derived by counting the number of syllables (or words) spoken and dividing that number by the talk time in minutes. For example, if a client produces 300 syllables in 2 minutes and 30 seconds, the rate of speech would be calculated as follows:

$$\text{Rate of speech} = \frac{300 \text{ syllables}}{2.5 \text{ syllables}} = 120 \text{ syllables per minute}$$

The average conversational rate of typically speaking adult males is 168 words per minute (wpm) and 221 syllables per minute (spm). Adult females tend to speak slower and use longer but fewer words. Their conversational speech rates average 151 wpm or 204 spm (Lutz & Mallard, 1986). Clinicians often assume that it is possible to convert between word and syllable counts for basic clinician measures, but be cautious. The existing conversion factor of approximately 1.5 syllables per word is derived from adult speech samples. Slower speaking rates of 3- to 5-year-old children generally range between 119 and 183 syllables per minute (Pindzola, Jenkins, & Lokken, 1989). If you are counting words, be aware that young children produce fewer multisyllabic words than do adults. Yaruss (2000) demonstrated that a conversion factor of 1.15 syllables per word is more accurate and stable for children ages 3 to 5.

The Assessment Process

We will now walk you through our assessment process, which is shown in Figure 7–2 in a stylized form. We often begin with the discussion of the presenting complaint and with nonstandardized testing to obtain a disfluency analysis of a representative sample of the client's speech. The operative word here is *representative*; stuttering is an intermittent disorder, and the amount of difficulty an individual has depends on the speaking task, the situation, and other variables. If it is possible to do so, collecting samples of the client's "real" communication in naturalistic settings—the playground, informal group situations, the family dinner table—has obvious advantages. Generally, however, clinicians rely on data obtained from speaking tasks, such as reading aloud a standard passage, giving a monologue, or conversing. Be sure to audio-record or, even better, video-record the session and note the time elapsed for each segment of the total sample: It will then be easier to specify rather precise frequency and severity values. We always ask the client to discuss both neutral topics (hobbies, sports, vacations) and challenging topics (family, school, dating) to ensure that we obtain a range of speaking difficulty. It is important to know what produces stress and how the individual responds to it; we experiment in the session with factors like hurrying the client, feigning listener loss, and asking the client to repeat.

An Overall Description

We begin the analysis with a global description of the individual's speech behavior. What is his or her typical speech like in terms of rate, rhythm, degree of tension, articulation, and voice? What are the salient features of the stuttering pattern?

Core Behaviors

The lowest common denominators of the problem of stuttering seem to be repetitions (*oscillative phenomena*), prolongations (*fixative phenomena*), and blocks. Although other overt disfluencies and related behaviors are part of stuttering, most individuals have either predominately repetitive or predominately tense disfluency patterns—with a dose of variability thrown in. A key feature of the disfluency analysis, therefore, is a precise description of the observed core stuttering behaviors. The methods of counting, presented earlier, need to be decided upon for a thorough description and comparison to norms.

With respect to *repetitions,* the clinician should identify the size of the unit (phrase, whole-word, syllable), the duration or number of oscillations per unit (e.g., b-boy versus b-b-b-b-boy), clients' tempo (fast or slow), degree of tension involved, and how units are terminated. Are there silent oscillations or articulatory postures? Does the client have difficulty finding the proper vowel during the course of the repetitions?

FIGURE 7–2
Critical Assessment Process in Disorders of Fluency

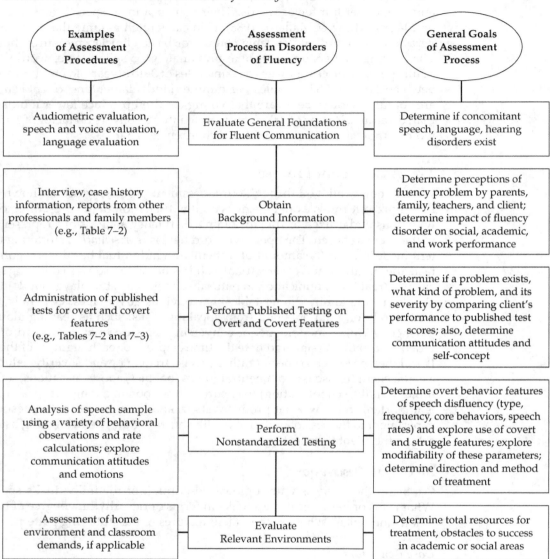

In terms of *prolongations,* the clinician is interested in the anatomical site of the fixations, whether they are silent or audible, how long they last, the degree of tension involved, and how they are terminated. *Disrhythmic phonation* is an umbrella term for a collection of SLDs such as within-word disruptions of air flow, sound prolongations, blocks (whether audible or inaudible), instances of noticeable stress, and unusual patterns of intonation.

Struggle-Tension Features

Very rarely does a client exhibit *only* a pattern that includes repetitions, prolongations, and blocks. Anyone who has observed persons who stutter knows that they can experience tension and often make extraneous sounds and movements while attempting to speak. Persons who stutter display a wide variety of these physical mannerisms, which may vary in frequency of occurrence and degree of involvement in particular clients; some individuals manifest an astounding array of eye blinking, head jerking, postponement rituals, and other behaviors, whereas others appear relatively quiescent, at least overtly. The clinician should take note of these accessory features. Several scales listed in Table 7–5 can be used as well.

Covert Measures

In developed stuttering, the overt symptoms may be only the tip of the problem. After years of difficulty in speaking, and especially because the amount of difficulty varies with the speaking situation, it is only natural that the person would develop hidden feelings and attitudes about speech. Vanryckeghem et al. (2001) show evidence that mal-attitudes and negative emotions are evident in even young children who stutter. Yairi and Ambrose (2005) have similar evidence. The negative feelings may be generalized but are often directed toward particular speaking situations, conversational partners, and even particular word and phoneme combinations. Following on the heels of apprehension, dislike, and fear of these events comes the avoidance of them. Therefore, measuring the covert side of a client's stuttering problem is often part of the diagnostic process. This approach is consistent with the World Health Organization's Classification of Functioning, Disability and Health (World Health Organization, 2002) as depicted in Figure 7–3. It is also consistent with the recent shift in treatment from behavioral fluency approaches to cognitive, comprehensive lifestyle integration approaches (Blood & Conture, 1998). The impact of stuttering can affect one's quality of life, regardless of age. Early on, perhaps in the initial session, we attempt to discuss with the client his or her feelings, attitudes, fears, and experiences. This helps us get to know the client and better understand the depth of the disorder. Counseling may need to be part of the treatment program for some clients. Manning (2010) is a good resource for counseling strategies and techniques. In addition to discussions of feelings, the clinician can utilize published instruments. Several of these instruments are listed in Table 7–6; some of the dated items are now classics and are still in use.

We would be remiss if we did not acknowledge that some behavioral clinicians opt not to measure, or clinically deal with, covert feelings and attitudes. The focus of intervention may, indeed, be to train fluency and let the covert aspects drop out of the client's repertoire on their own, in due time. Likewise, the clinician may use an attitude scale as a baseline measure, proceed with a behavioral approach that focuses only on the overt side of stuttering, and then probe for attitudinal change as a consequence of successful fluency. Evidence-based practice often uses such an approach.

The clinician *is* interested in avoidance behaviors that the client exhibits. We feel that, clinically, avoidance behavior is an important feature to deal with because it tends to reinforce and compound the speaker's difficulty. Rather than diminish, fears tend to incubate and grow when a person recoils from them; avoidances cause apprehension to increase and the problem to expand.

Avoidance is characterized by reduction or cessation of communication: The person who stutters retreats from the act of talking. The clinician can discern the types of speaking situations and listeners who increase or decrease the client's stuttering. This evaluation can be accomplished by interviewing the client or by having her or him fill out a checklist. The clinician can devise a form for recording data (simply listing different speaking situations, topics of conversation, and so forth) or use a published inventory. Table 7–7 lists assessment instruments useful with the covert side of stuttering. We admit that most of the measures lack reliability and validity; still, they remain classics.

FIGURE 7–3
Assessment of Stuttering Using the World Health Organization's International Classification of Functioning, Disability and Health (ICF)

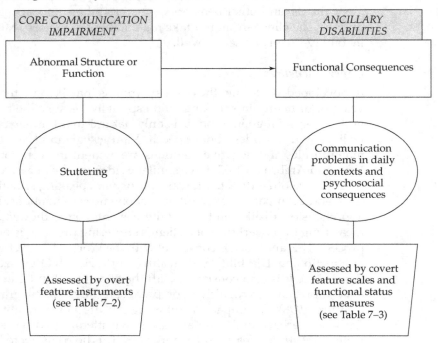

The *Speech Situation Checklist* (Brutten & Shoemaker, 1974) is still in use clinically and in research (Ezrati-Vinacour & Levin, 2004). The checklist has the client rate his or her degree of emotional response and severity of speech disruption in 51 life situations. Although no formal instrument is supplied, various circumstances (audience size, specific people, different talking situations) may be useful in sampling actual speech. In addition to listing the conditions under which stuttering is increased or reduced, the clinician may ask the client to rank-order the items in terms of speech difficulty and emotional impact. The *Communication Attitudes Test* (CAT) is another self-report tool that has stood the test of time and is still used as a research and clinical attitude scale, even with grade-school children (Brutten & Dunham, 1989; Vanryckeghem et al., 2001).

In addition to situation fears, many who stutter report that they have particular difficulty with certain words and speech sounds. We make a list of these items and then examine the speech sample to determine if, in fact, there is more stuttering on some sounds or words. During attempts at trial treatment, we like to show the client ways of ameliorating the stuttering and often use his or her most feared words as stimuli.

Any assessment of stuttering should also include the client's own perceptions of the magnitude and impact of her or his stuttering. This includes both severity self-assessment and quality of life impact measures; both are useful as pre- and post-treatment measures to document change. The clinician can obtain such information from many of the instruments listed in Tables 7–5 and 7–6. In particular, we like to administer the *Perceptions of Stuttering Inventory* (PSI) (Woolf, 1967); it is available free online. The PSI is devised to assess three dimensions of stuttering behavior: struggle, avoidance, and expectancy, as perceived by the person who stutters. It yields a profile that the clinician can then compare to scores obtained by a reference group of stutterers. With renewed clinical research emphasis into daily functioning and disability impacts by the World

Health Organization (World Health Organization, 2002), this area of assessment has again become popular.

The *Overall Assessment of the Speaker's Experience of Stuttering* (OASES) is a quality of life measure we like to give to clients who are over the age of 7 (Yaruss & Quesal, 2010). This measure is based on the theoretical framework provided by the World Health Organization and contains four different sections designed to evaluate a client's experience of stuttering: general information, reactions, communication in daily situations, and quality of life. These sections evaluate the client's perceptions of and knowledge of stuttering in general; affective, behavioral, and cognitive reactions; speaking difficulty across different communicative contexts; and speaker satisfaction and well-being, respectively. For each section of the OASES, impact scores are derived; higher scores indicate a greater degree of negative impact. In addition to impact scores, impact ratings are provided and indicate degree of stuttering impact (i.e., mild through severe), much like a severity rating does.

Having now discussed the predictive instruments, severity scales, and a myriad of covert measures typically used in the evaluation of stuttering, let us turn our attention to some general evaluation principles and special considerations for clients of various ages.

EVALUATION AT THE ONSET OF STUTTERING

Experienced clinicians agree that the problem of stuttering is much easier to prevent or manage in children than to treat in chronic adult clients. Indeed, early detection and management of children beginning to stutter is one of the most significant contributions a speech clinician can make. The SLP must seek answers for a great many questions: Is the child stuttering? If so, how likely is it that it will persist? When did it begin? What factors were associated with the onset of the problem? How aware is the child of the speech disturbance? How do listeners attempt to help, and how does this affect the child's efforts? How can the SLP alter the child's environment to prevent the problem from getting worse?

Throughout this text, we have repeatedly suggested that diagnosis and treatment are not separate undertakings. The careful assessment of a client's speech-language is often therapeutic; only by working with an individual (and his or her parents) for a period of time does the clinician truly come to know the dimensions of the disorder. This is particularly true in the management of children beginning to stutter. In planning for the evaluation, we delineate several objectives that guide the clinician's efforts:

1. Determine if the child is stuttering (problem/no problem determination).
2. If the child is stuttering, identify to what developmental extent the disorder has progressed (factors include overt and covert severity).
3. Obtain the parent's perception of the onset and current status of the disorder.
4. Sample the child's general level of functioning in regard to auditory, motor, social, articulatory, and cognitive-linguistic abilities.
5. Commence the development of a counseling relationship with the parents.

We have already discussed most of these objectives. Various assessment instruments are available to help the clinician make a differential diagnosis, determine the severity of the speech difficulties, appraise the home situation and parental attitudes, and begin a healthy dialogue with the parents of the child who is beginning to stutter. What remains to be discussed are the ancillary areas that need to be assessed in the young child.

Speed and coordination of repetitive oral movements may be tested using norms for *diadochokinesis*, which, among other places, can be found in the *Oral Speech Mechanism Examination* (St. Louis & Ruscello, 2000). Recent literature suggests the need to assess and monitor lexical and word retrieval skills (Hall, 2004; Silverman & Ratner, 2002); pragmatic competencies (Weiss, 2004); linguistic utterance length and complexity, especially as related to fluency breakdowns (Ryan, 1974; Weiss, 2004); and in general to assess language skills and phonology. Phonological disorders seem to co-occur frequently with stuttering (about 16% of the time), as do language disorders (about 10% of the time). Some 7% have concomitant learning disabilities, and about 6% have reading disabilities (Arndt & Healey, 2001; Blood et al., 2009; Conture, 2001; Yairi & Seery, 2011).

Various articulation and language tests should be used as part of a thorough fluency evaluation. Information and evaluation procedures described in Chapters 4, 5, and 6 are certainly relevant. The presence of speech and language disorders concomitant with stuttering may affect the planning of an appropriate treatment program. Along with these areas of assessment, we routinely screen the oral mechanism, voice, and hearing. We advocate referral for additional testing of cognitive, motoric, and psychological status, as needed, with particular clients.

Prognosis with Young Children

We are very impressed with the efficacy of treatment for young children who are beginning to stutter. When the clinician can intervene before the child develops fear and avoidance reactions, and if the parents are amenable to counseling, the prognosis for recovery is excellent—remember the 80% recovery rate discussed earlier. The reader is also encouraged to review the recovery factors presented in Table 7–5. It is worth reiterating these and other intuitive factors that the clinician must consider when estimating a client's prospects for recovery:

1. How long has the child been stuttering? Time is an enemy of recovery.

2. What is the frequency of disfluency?

3. What are gender and familial factors that may shade the prognosis?

4. What types of disfluency are exhibited and what is their severity?

5. What co-existing speech-language and other disorders exist?

6. What type and intensity of environmental reactions has the child been exposed to?

7. Is the child aware of speaking difficulties? Decreased awareness and a positive appraisal of communicative behaviors are more suggestive of a favorable prognosis.

8. How amenable are the parents to counseling? An all-out concerted effort on the home front is ideal, perhaps essential, for amelioration (see Reitzes, 2014).

9. What is the child's level of intelligence? We have had more limited success with cognitively or intellectually delayed children.

10. Are there organic or psychological factors that figure in the onset of stuttering? Chances for recovery are more limited if either is present.

Our clinical success or failure with children who are beginning to stutter is also related to the characteristic pattern of factors present at the onset of stuttering. We find these areas important to synthesizing diagnostic information and making a prognosis about a young disfluent child. The many variables that may be involved in the onset of stuttering are organized into three major categories: physiological, psycholinguistic, and psychosocial (Figure 7–4). Note how the three categories overlap. For example, a child

FIGURE 7–4
Factors Influencing Early Childhood Stuttering

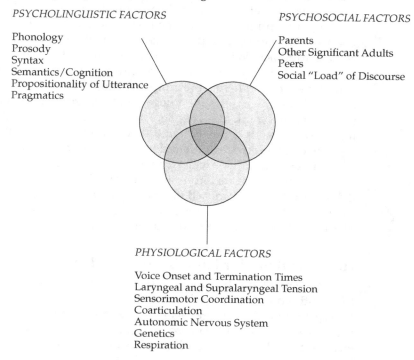

PSYCHOLINGUISTIC FACTORS

Phonology
Prosody
Syntax
Semantics/Cognition
Propositionality of Utterance
Pragmatics

PSYCHOSOCIAL FACTORS

Parents
Other Significant Adults
Peers
Social "Load" of Discourse

PHYSIOLOGICAL FACTORS

Voice Onset and Termination Times
Laryngeal and Supralaryngeal Tension
Sensorimotor Coordination
Coarticulation
Autonomic Nervous System
Genetics
Respiration

delayed in language development and deficient in motor skills could be particularly susceptible to high parental standards or communication competition with siblings.

One question continues to nag clinicians who work with young children: Would the children have gotten better without the clinicians' help simply because of the passage of time and some internal recovery potential in the child? Although we cannot answer that question with any authority, we do see that, in most instances, the child's recovery from stuttering occurred too swiftly after the initiation of treatment (2 weeks to several months) to be attributed to spontaneous recovery.

EVALUATION OF THE SCHOOL-AGE STUDENT
Elementary Students

Appraising and treating elementary school students who stutter is particularly challenging. These children, approximately 7 to 12 years old, are no longer beginning stutterers; they are not simply repeating and hesitating. They struggle noticeably when speaking and attempt to avoid or disguise their difficulty; they are frustrated, and it is now necessary to deal directly with the stuttering.

The clinician is faced with several thorny problems when planning an examination of a young person who stutters: (1) Young children frequently lack the insight and cooperation necessary to analyze their problem objectively and rationally; (2) children are often reluctant or unable to verbalize their internal feelings freely; (3) the speech clinician is associated in the child's mind with the teaching personnel, who may in some cases be penalizing or disturbing listeners, and the clinician may be identified with authority figures, which tends to undermine a trusting relationship; and (4) last, and perhaps most significant, the child usually has no choice about entering treatment because it is most likely that the student is brought for evaluation by the parents, referred by a teacher, or identified in a screening by a speech clinician.

The clinician may find that these students respond to an honest, straightforward clinical approach. With early elementary school children, we use descriptive language, such as *tensing* or *getting stuck*, to inquire about their speaking difficulty, not out of any fear of the word *stuttering* but simply because the term either doesn't mean much to the child or, in some cases, is too negatively charged. With older elementary school children, we use a frank, direct style. Establish trust and confidence by showing the client that the clinician is competent and *knows* about the problem of stuttering.

The evaluation of a student does not differ greatly in substance from an assessment of an older individual except that with young children, environmental, parental, and school factors are more important. Figure 7–5 outlines an assessment plan prepared by a diagnostic team composed of a faculty member and graduate students; it also reveals the range of information generally sought. The plan was compiled for the evaluation of a 10-year-old child referred to a university speech clinic by a public school clinician.

Junior and Senior High School Students

The assessment and treatment of stuttering in older students is even more challenging than with youngsters. Denial of the problem, lack of cooperation, and lack of motivation seem typical in the teenagers we have seen. The assessment outline does not differ much from the example shown in Figure 7–5. The process, however, is very adult-like; environmental and parental factors are downplayed.

Prognosis

What factors are crucial for improvement with students? What variables should the clinician consider when making a prognosis? We believe that the most significant improvement in treatment is noted in cases with the following operative factors:

1. No prior record of unsuccessful treatment. An absence of treatment seems more conducive to success than a history of therapeutic failure.
2. Cooperative and knowledgeable parents who are willing to participate meaningfully in a program of counseling and understand the nature of the disorder.
3. More severe stuttering pattern. Stuttering patterns characterized as mild typically show little improvement.
4. A predominantly clonic stuttering pattern featuring struggle and escape: Students adept at avoidance generally have more difficulty.
5. Cooperative teachers and other school personnel.
6. No other significant problems (reading difficulty, a scholastic problem independent of stuttering, and so on).
7. Other available resources (expertise in scouting, athletics, music).
8. A schedule of intensive therapy (at least three, preferably four, contacts a week).

ASSESSMENT OF THE ADULT WHO STUTTERS

The disorder is fully developed in the adult client: Speech interruptions are more complex and characteristically compulsive; fears and apprehensions become chronic; avoidance, disguise, and negative attitudes hamper and distort the individual's relationships

FIGURE 7–5
Assessment Plan for School-Age Child

I. *Identifying Information*

Obtain all the usual information regarding address, grade level, and so on. This can be obtained from Mrs. Hronkin, the referral source, or in the parent interview. Be sure to inquire about living arrangements: Ms. Hronkin mentioned that a parental grandfather may reside with the family, and apparently he is a dominant force in the family (reportedly, he is against Alan receiving speech therapy and insists he overcame stuttering by eating mashed potatoes!).

II. *Description of Stuttering*

A. *Global description.* What are the salient descriptive features of Alan's stuttering behavior? Is it basically fixative or oscillative? Are there long silent periods of internal struggle, or does he exhibit a more overt pattern?

B. *Core behaviors.* Make an analysis of the repetitions and prolongations observed—the number of oscillations per unit, tempo, duration, and so forth.

C. *Tension-struggle features.* Note the occurence and location of any ancillary behaviors.

D. *Frequency.* This analysis will serve as our baseline for reevaluation of Alan, so we need to be especially precise. Collect data (count repetitions, prolongations, other salient features of his moments of stuttering) on at least three types of speech samples—reading, paraphrasing, and spontaneous speech. We can compute the relative frequency of stutterings per minute, or per total syllables uttered, by analyzing the videotape later.

E. *Severity.* We will use the Stuttering Severity Instrument-4 (Riley 2009); this instrument employs the three dimensions of frequency, duration, and physical concomitants and yields a score that can be converted to a percentile. A severity measure like this (particularly when it allows the examiner to score a client on a common scale of 0 to 100) is useful when communicating the results of the evaluation to the parents, teacher, even the child himself.

F. *Variations in frequency/severity.* Explore with the child and his parents whether his stuttering comes and goes in cycles, which situations or listeners provoke variations in his speech, and whether there are any words or sounds that are particularly difficult. Determine what impact delayed auditory feedback and masking noise have on his speech, and the impact of a rhythmic metronome. Probe fluency changes as a function of linguistic length and complexity, while both answering and asking questions, and while following a model of easy-onset speech and stretched (slow, prolonged) speech.

G. How does the child try to control his stuttering? What techniques has he devised for coping with speech interruptions? How effective are they? Additionally, we need to identify which speech-altering strategies—slowing, easy onset, and so forth—induce fluency. Use Cooper and Cooper's (2004) Disfluency Descriptor Digest as a checklist to record observations.

H. Can the child predict when he is about to stutter? Ask him if he can; but also have him underline words he thinks he might stutter on as he reads silently a simple passage. Have him read it aloud and determine the degree to which he can accurately predict his stuttering.

I. What is the client's poststuttering behavior? Does he continue talking, give up, become angry, or cry? Does he appear indifferent?

III. *Attitude Dimension*

This is the most difficult and least reliable aspect of the evaluation. Some information can be obtained through observation of Alan and his parents and by what they say about the problem. We can also administer several self-inventory scales such as the A-19 Scale (Guitar, 2006). What is the child's attitude toward treatment? How much does he know about stuttering? Has he been teased at school or home because of his problem?

IV. *Case History*

We will want to obtain background information with respect to four basic areas: history of general development (motor, language, social), onset and development of stuttering, medical history, and family history. These areas can be explored in the parent interview.

V. *Present Functioning*

A. *Personality.* Describe the child's personality in general terms (shy, aggressive, and so on) and identify any special features (fears, tics, nail-biting, and the like) that may apply to him. Ascertain his special interests or hobbies.

B. *School.* Obtain information relevant to his academic and social adjustment in school.

C. *Related testing.* Is a psychological or medical referral indicated? Perform screening evaluations on the child's motor behavior, hearing, voice, phonology, and language ability. The latter two are particularly important, as we have discussed in this chapter. Select tests accordingly.

D. *Diagnostic session.* How did the child behave during the diagnostic session? What could be discerned about his level of motivation? How did he respond when put under communicative stress? How did he respond to trial therapy?

with others. At this stage, a speech breakdown is not simply a response; it is also a stimulus—the problem has become cyclic and self-reinforcing. Clinicians agree that the treatment of stuttering at this advanced stage is complicated—but far from impossible. There is a bewildering array of treatment approaches (and indexes of their successes); we will not attempt to summarize them here, however, but refer the reader to works by Bothe (2004); Bothe, Davidow, Bramlett, and Ingham (2006); Guitar (2013); Prins and Ingham (2009); Manning (2010); and Onslow (1996).

Prognosis

Making a prognosis about success and failure in stuttering is an inexact science. As noted earlier, recent research efforts have tried to delineate some factors that may be involved in determining successful outcomes. We present an incomplete and heuristic list of factors that help in making prognoses. The items are presented in random order because, at present, we have no data that would allow us to assign weight to them.

1. *Severity.* Paradoxically, persons with more severe stuttering, other factors being equal, seem to make better progress or gains than do clients with milder cases.

2. *Motivation and attitude.* Motivation to change is, of course, a most significant variable in all intervention programs. The better the client's pretreatment attitude, the more successful the outcome of treatment is likely to be.

3. *Timing.* A client's motivation for treatment is often related to crucial life experiences. Persons who have reached a critical stage and feel blocked by their disordered speech; barred from job advancement, education, or marriage; and who voluntarily seek treatment have a more favorable prognosis.

4. *Age.* Adolescents, particularly between the ages of 13 and 16, are especially resistant to treatment. Similarly, clients over 40 tend to do poorly in treatment.

5. *Sex.* Women seem to be more difficult to treat than men.

6. *Nonstuttered Speech.* The more well integrated the client's nonstuttered speech is, in terms of prosody, the better the prognosis.

7. *Type of stuttering.* Those with predominantly repetitive stuttering make more rapid progress than do those with predominantly fixative disfluencies; clients who feature escape reactions are easier to work with than persons who engage in chronic avoidance. Interiorized stutterers—especially those manifesting laryngeal blocking—are very resistant to treatment.

8. *Concomitant problems.* Clients presenting with organic complications (e.g., sensory, intellectual, or motor impairments) or psychological symptoms require more prolonged treatment and do less well than clients without concomitant problems.

9. *Prior Treatment and Intensive Treatment.* Clients with a history of therapeutic failure have a poor prognosis. Token treatment may be worse than no treatment at all. When intensive treatment (minimum daily contact of at least 1 hour) is available and the client can participate in a comprehensive program, the prospects for recovery are more favorable.

Multicultural Considerations in Fluency Disorders

Given that we live in such an ethnically diverse society, we are only beginning to appreciate how cultural values might affect the incidence, development, and ultimately the treatment of communication disorders such as stuttering. Multicultural sensitivity on the part of the SLP is necessary. Early examinations of stuttering within cultures and

TABLE 7–8
Cultural Variables and Stuttering

Gender/Sex
There is unequivocal evidence that more males than females stutter, regardless of the society or national origin.

Family and Societal Issues
Early research suggested that discipline, humiliation, and indulgence affect the occurrence of stuttering.
Parents of children who stutter display temperament and attitude differences (Yairi, 1997).
Persons who stutter, on the whole, though research is equivocal, show sensitive temperaments and inhibitions (as reviewed by Yasiri & Ambrose, 2005).
Living in a volatile society, such as Israel, may also affect stuttering (Amir & Ezrati-Vinacour, 2002).

Demographics
Equivocal research suggests that stuttering is more prevalent in urban rather than rural areas (Brady & Hall, 1976). Yet Dykes (1995) found that rural areas had a greater prevalence of stuttering (0.49%) than urban areas did (0.34%).

Bilingualism
It is generally accepted that bilingual children are more likely to stutter than monolingual speakers. Borsel, Maes, and Foulon (2001) cites a prevalence rate of 2.8% among bilinguals versus nearly 1% in the general population. In contrast, Montes and Erickson (1990) found no significant differences in the occurrence of stuttered speech behaviors in English and Spanish bilingual children. They also noted that the types of disfluencies associated with second-language learning are often misidentified as stuttering.

Race and Ethnicity
There is a long history of research comparing stuttering among different cultures, including Eskimos and various tribes of Native Americans; however, recent investigations are lacking. Also, little is known about stuttering in the Asian American community. Prevalence of stuttering among Puerto Ricans living in New York City was reported by Leavitt (1974) to be 0.84%, a value similar to that of whites; by comparison, the prevalence among Puerto Ricans living in San Juan was 1.5%. Proctor et al. (2001) examined over 3,400 preschoolers and found stuttering prevalence overall was 2.46%, with no group differences among African Americans, European Americans, and other minorities.

across nations were motivated by theorists espousing environmental etiologies of stuttering. Stuttering has no geographic boundaries; it is observed around the globe and no evidence exists to suggests that there is a culture in which stuttering does not exist. Table 7–8 cites information regarding culture and stuttering as presently understood. Robinson (2012) describes several factors that should be kept in mind when evaluating a person from a different culture who stutters:

- Need to gather information on the degree of cultural assimilation or the extent to which a client identifies with a particular culture.
- Need to consider the perceptions or attitudes a given culture has toward communication disorders and stuttering in particular.
- Are there any existing myths or beliefs regarding stuttering etiology and treatment?
- To what degree does a client's religious practice, or lack thereof, influence acceptance and treatment decisions?
- Need to be cognizant of nonverbal behaviors associated with a given culture because they could be misconstrued as avoidance or secondary behaviors (e.g., silence or lack of eye contact).
- Need to develop an appreciation for events or stressors associated with a given culture (e.g., holidays, family activities, or ceremonies).

The likelihood that you will encounter bilingual clients is increasing. There is some evidence to suggest that bilingual clients have an increased risk for developing stuttering behaviors (Van Borsel, Maes, & Foulon, 2001). The challenge to working with these clients is determining the extent to which stuttering occurs in both languages and also determining whether the observed disfluency is the result of increased linguistic demand or limited proficiency with the non-native language. Vigilant evaluation of both languages and observation of cognitive and affective reactions can aid in this determination. It is also important to keep in mind that some clients coming from another culture may speak a different language than your own. In these cases, an interpreter can be helpful with not only translating but also in providing relevant cultural information that will aid in the translation of both verbal and nonverbal information obtained during the course of the evaluation.

CONCLUSION AND SELF-ASSESSMENT

We wish to echo the preferred practice patterns of the American Speech-Language-Hearing Association (2004) with regard to expected outcomes of a fluency assessment, which include identification and description of the person's:

- Type of fluency disorder (the diagnosis)
- Characteristic fluent, disfluent, and covert behaviors
- Fluency impairments and their effects on the individual's daily activities
- Contextual factors that act as barriers to or facilitators of communication
- Co-occurring communication disorders, if any
- Prognosis for change
- Recommendations for intervention and support

The diagnosis of a fluency disorder requires a lot more than just a single test or procedure. It necessitates a current understanding of the nature of fluency disorders and the impact it can have on clients' decision-making processes and lives. Stuttering is a heterogeneous disorder marked by significant interspeaker and intraspeaker variability, and is affected by a variety of cognitive and affective factors as well as self-imposed and/or environmental demands. Compassion, warmth, a sincere interest in the client's story, and a tolerance for ambiguity are a few of the prerequisite factors for conducting an effective evaluation.

After reading this chapter you should be able to answer the following questions:

1. What behavioral and nonbehavioral details characterize stuttering?
2. How can developmental stuttering be distinguished from other fluency disorders, such as neurogenic, psychogenic, and cluttering?
3. What types of speech disfluencies are commonly observed in the speech of fluent and disfluent speakers?
4. What types of overt behavioral characteristics can be observed and documented during a fluency assessment?
5. What types of covert behaviors and attitudes should be considered and documented during a fluency assessment?
6. What types of questions would you ask a fluency client during the interview portion of an assessment? What types of questions would you ask of a parent, child, or adult?
7. What factors should you consider when deriving a prognosis for a fluency client?

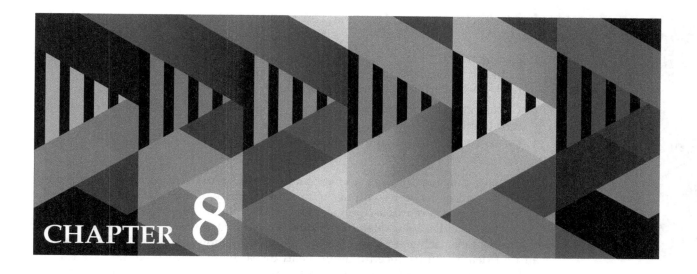

CHAPTER 8

Assessment of Aphasia and Adult Language Disorders

LEARNING OUTCOMES

After reading this chapter you will be able to:

1. Define *aphasia* and cite common causes.
2. Cite types of aphasia and common speech-language symptoms of each type.
3. Differentiate aphasia from other types of adult language disorders.
4. Explain subtle deficits often seen after a right (nondominant) hemisphere stroke.
5. Discuss cognitive-communicative aspects of the dementias.

When an adult suddenly loses the easy use of language, it is a devastating experience for the individual and for her or his family. Aphasia and other adult language disorders affect that which makes us uniquely human—our ability to communicate with each other via a system of language symbols.

THE NATURE OF APHASIA

Aphasia is the most common disorder of communication resulting from brain injury. Damage occurs in the hemisphere of the brain that is dominant for language; for most of us, this is the left hemisphere. An adult (or post-language-acquisition child or adolescent) with aphasia has a basic interference with *comprehension* and *use* of language in its many forms. More specifically, aphasia is a syndrome of language deficits resulting from destruction of cortical tissue and is characterized by one or more of the following symptoms:

1. Disturbance in receiving and decoding symbolic materials via auditory, visual, or tactile channels. Although the individual can still hear and see, he or she has difficulty deciphering the learned associations of messages.
2. Disturbance in central processes of meaning, word selection, and message formulation.
3. Disturbance in expressing symbolic materials by means of speech, writing, or gesture.

Aphasia may result from traumatic brain injury, brain tumor, certain inflammatory processes, and degenerative disease. The vast majority of aphasias, however, are the consequence of a cerebrovascular accident (CVA), commonly called stroke. The cerebrovascular accident is a relatively common illness that affects approximately a half million persons each year. In the United States, CVA now stands as the third leading cause of death (outdistanced only by heart disease and cancer). No one knows precisely how many surviving stroke victims are left with language impairment; estimates suggest that at least one-quarter of victims present some degree of aphasia that warrants treatment.

It is an exciting time to be an aphasiologist—a speech-language pathologist (SLP) who specializes in the diagnosis and rehabilitation of adult language disorders. There is an explosion of new technologies to aid in understanding the brain's biology. New and promising pharmacologic approaches are now available to aid the brain's recovery immediately following CVA. And medicines are becoming more effective in aiding cognition.

Etiology can influence the onset, progress, and type of aphasia symptoms. The onset of symptoms is likely to be insidious when caused by tumor and to be abrupt when due to CVA. Improvement is more likely if the aphasia is caused by a CVA than by a tumor, and patients with tumors may have wide differences in abilities across modalities (reading, writing, listening, speaking). Such large differences are less likely from a CVA. Aphasia resulting from trauma is often accompanied by a greater variety of cognitive deficits, but it shows a faster recovery than does aphasia resulting from CVA.

A host of other disorders may resemble aphasia and have brain damage as their basis. These include the language of confusion, language of intellectual deterioration (the dementias), communication deficit subsequent to a nondominant lesion (usually right hemisphere damage), language associated with psychosis, and motor speech disorders. These other language disorders will be discussed later in this chapter as part of the differential diagnosis process.

The severity of aphasia can vary greatly, from minimal, temporary language dysfunction to almost total and permanent inability to use and comprehend language. It is important to remember that the impoverishment of language observed in aphasia is *not* due to loss of mental capacity, impairment of sensory organs, or paralysis of the speech apparatus. These problems, however, can co-occur with aphasia, making differential diagnosis important. Current research is starting to acknowledge cognitive aspects within aphasia (Chapey, 2014; Helm-Estabrooks, Albert, & Nicholas, 2014; Hinckley & Nash, 2007).

Classifying a patient as to the *type* of aphasia displayed can be an important feature of diagnosis and treatment planning. Many labels and classification systems have been put forth through the years for this purpose. Three methods are currently in wide use: (1) fluent–nonfluent dichotomy, which is based on the patient's length of utterance; (2)

TABLE 8–1
Neurolinguistic Features of the Major Types of Aphasia

Broca's Aphasia
Impaired fluency; limited verbal output
Relatively good auditory comprehension
Impaired articulatory agility
Stereotyped grammar
Telegraphic and agrammatic (especially reduced use of articles, prepositions, auxiliaries, copulas, and derivational endings)
Prosodic alterations

Transcortical Motor Aphasia
Preserved ability to repeat
Nonfluent
Some auditory comprehension impairment, similar to Broca's aphasia
Superior naming ability compared to spontaneous speech

Global Aphasia
Severe loss of all receptive modalities
Severe loss of all expressive modalities
Almost totally absent speech
Stereotypic utterances (perhaps with normal melody and intonation)

Wernicke's Aphasia
Fluent; copious verbal output
Impaired auditory comprehension (often severe)
Frequent paraphasias (especially semantic types)
Neologisms and jargon, if severe
Normal articulatory agility

Normal prosody
Normal or supranormal phrase length
Full range of grammatical forms
Preserved syntax
Impaired naming and repetition abilities

Transcortical Sensory Aphasia
Preserved ability to repeat
Conversation resembles symptoms of Wernicke's aphasia
Extreme difficulty with nouns
Excessive paraphasias
Impaired auditory comprehension, resembling Wernicke's

Conduction Aphasia
Poor repetition ability
Fluent speech; good articulation and phrase length
Frequent paraphasias (especially literal types)
Some auditory comprehension impairment
Acute awareness of errors

Anomic Aphasia
Severe word-finding deficits
Frequent circumlocutions
Minimal paraphasic errors
Fluent speech; good articulation and phrase length
Appropriate grammatical forms
Good auditory comprehension

the "Boston" classification system by Goodglass, Kaplan, and Barresi (2000); and (3) the Western Aphasia Battery (WAB) taxonomy by Kertesz (2006). The Boston and WAB systems are quite similar and use fluency, auditory comprehension, repetition, and naming abilities for arriving at a diagnostic label. Table 8–1 lists characteristics of each of the major types of aphasia.

Although there is some controversy as to our ability to localize language functions in the brain, there is fairly good agreement with site of lesion information and the language characteristics seen in individual patients. Lobes of the brain and primary language areas of the left (dominant) hemisphere associated with various types of aphasia are shown in Figure 8–1. Anterior lesions generally produce nonfluent aphasia, such as Broca's and transcortical motor aphasias. Posterior lesions are associated with the fluent aphasias, such as Wernicke's, conduction, and transcortical sensory aphasias.

Site of lesion (anatomical areas affected) and type of lesion (tumor, CVA, and so forth) can usually be determined by modern methods of brain imaging such as computerized tomography (CT), positron emission tomography (PET), and magnetic resonance

FIGURE 8–1
Lobes of the Brain (Left Figure) and Areas of the Left Hemisphere Associated with Some of the Types of Aphasia (Right Figure)

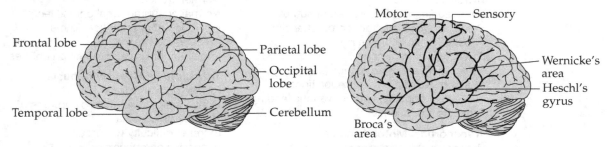

Source: Justice, (2010). *Communication science and disorders: A contemporary perspective.* Pearson Allyn & Bacon.

imaging (MRI). These methods have contributed greatly to aphasiology. The emerging role of single photon emission computed tomography (SPECT) might aid in the prediction of recovery (Mimura et al., 1998). Although anatomical evidence supplied by the neuroradiologist is diagnostically valuable, the speech-language pathologist may be wise to focus on carefully describing what the individual can and cannot do with respect to language. The clinician must, first and foremost, delineate the patient's ability to talk, listen, read, and write. In our zeal to identify the neurolinguistic dimensions of aphasia, it is possible to forget that brain injury is a grave health problem. The individual has suffered a major life crisis that has profound medical, psychological, and social consequences. In addition to the language impairment, the patient may present paralysis or paresis of the extremities (generally the right side, sometimes including the face), sensory abnormalities, and behavioral disturbances. There seems to be little, if any, relationship between these difficulties and the extent of the language impairment. Above all, the clinician must remember that aphasia is both a personal catastrophe and a family crisis.

CASE HISTORY

It is wise for SLPs to remember that they work with *persons* who have aphasia, not aphasia. Language treatment for an adult with aphasia has to be very personalized. Therefore, SLPs need to know as much as possible about their clients when planning a rehabilitation program. What sort of people were the clients before the strokes? How did they meet their problems? What educational levels were achieved? What were their occupations? Their avocations? What changes in behaviors, if any, have occurred following the brain injuries? The style, pace, and content of treatment will be based on the answers to these and many other questions.

Unfortunately, the aphasic patient is often in no position to provide the kind of detailed information we seek. In some instances, official records (educational tests, military records) and personal documents (diaries, letters) are helpful. Usually, however, we must rely on the accuracy and veracity of informants who are familiar with the patient. The most common method of assembling information about the language-impaired individual is a case history form that is filled out by a spouse or other close relative. Sample questions from a typical case history form are listed in Table 8–2. Another style of template (see Appendix B) is the Demographic and History Form from the American Speech-Language-Hearing Association (ASHA); search its website at www.asha.org/.

TABLE 8–2
Sample Questionnaire Topics for a Case History

Personal
Marital status
Name and occupation of spouse
Names and locations of children
Information about grandchildren
Amount of education
Occupation
Current employment status (retired?)
Hobbies and special interests
Preferences in reading material, television entertainment, and use of writing
Preferred hand
Native language, knowledge of other languages
Description of personality
Description of involvement in group activities (e.g., bowling leagues, church fellowships)
Description of any changes since the injury in mood, personality, ability to care for self, and the like

Medical
Date of injury
Cause of injury (accident, stroke, disease)
Length of unconsciousness, if any
Description of paralysis, if any
Complaints of dizziness, faintness, headaches, if any
Description of any visual or hearing problems
Description of any other problems, illnesses, or injuries

Communicative
Description of the patient's speech at the onset of the problem
Description of how the speech has changed
Check the appropriate column as it applies to the patient *now:*

Can	Cannot	
_____	_____	indicate meaning by gesture
_____	_____	repeat words spoken by others
_____	_____	use one or a few words over and over
_____	_____	use swear words (often)
_____	_____	use some words spontaneously
_____	_____	say short phrases
_____	_____	say short sentences
_____	_____	follow requests and understand directions
_____	_____	follow radio or television speech
_____	_____	read signs with understanding
_____	_____	read newspapers and/or magazines
_____	_____	tell time
_____	_____	write name without assistance
_____	_____	write sentences, letters
_____	_____	do simple arithmetic
_____	_____	handle money, make change

Ideally, the clinician also interviews the respondent to clarify any ambiguities in the written information and to permit additional questioning. Keep in mind, however, that a long-term marriage partner typically sees the patient as less impaired than objective language testing may show. On the other hand, acontextual tests of language do not measure communication; thus, the client may, in fact, perform better in a "real" setting. Health history of the patient is ascertained, in part, during the case history interview (recall Table 8–2), but medical records provide greater specificity. Information concerning the current medical episode is particularly useful in differential diagnosis and treatment planning. At a minimum, the following medical data should be collected:

1. Major and secondary medical diagnoses (e.g., thrombosis of left middle cerebral artery, organic brain syndrome, diabetes, CVA with right hemiparesis, and the like)
2. Date of onset with regard to etiology of communication disorder
3. Localization of brain damage (hemisphere and lobes affected) and source of data (e.g., CT, MRI, and other techniques)
4. Previous central nervous system (CNS) involvement (type and date of onset)
5. Brainstem signs (e.g., facial weakness, extraocular movement, dysphagia, other bulbar signs)
6. Limb involvement
7. Vision (acuity, corrective lens, visual field deficits, etc.)
8. Hearing (acuity, discrimination, amplification, etc.)

Access to the patient's medical chart is therefore essential to the SLP. In addition to the physician/neurologist report, entries by the neuroradiologist, social worker, nurse, and other healthcare professionals are enlightening. Important information can be gained from this telegraphic chart note entered by a neurologist:

> This alert, oriented adult male suffered a CVA on 3-19-14. Expressive-receptive aphasia. Right hemiplegia. Babinski sign on the right. Gross motor functioning of involved leg is returning; arm and hand are doubtful. CT scan revealed a focal lesion in the left parietal-temporal region. Right side astereognosis. Right homonomous hemianopsia.

This brief report told us several important details about the patient: The neurologist observed that the brain damage was apparently localized and was not widespread. He also observed that the aphasia was probably not transitory because lesions in the region cited generally result in more persistent language impairment, the patient could not identify objects by touch when they were placed in his right hand, and he could not see in the right field of vision. This last anomaly would require that we present testing materials from the patient's left side. Information assembled by the neurologist is, of course, very useful to the SLP. In addition to the size and locale of the lesion, the nature of the injury may be pertinent diagnostically. (For example, patients incurring traumatic brain injury often experience a different course of recovery from persons suffering vascular episodes.) The chart note also underscores the importance of being familiar with pertinent medical terminology.

After garnering case history information, the SLP should have a rather detailed description of the salient aspects of the patient's premorbid personality, health history and current status, and social orientation. But what impact would this sudden illness have? How much change could be expected, and in what areas? Would the patient's responses to the language impairment and physical disabilities merely be an exaggeration of earlier behavior patterns?

There are only limited answers to these questions. We suspect, however, that the nature of the illness, the treatment the patient receives, and premorbid factors are all crucial in determining the impact of the problem on the individual. Impact measure and quality-of-life scales may be done at a later point in intervention. In summary, any and all information about the individual that can be pulled together is important and may shape our course of assessment and treatment.

DIAGNOSIS AND FORMAL TESTING

A comprehensive evaluation of an adult with aphasia includes several clinical tasks: (1) a review of pertinent medical information and the sequence of events leading up to the referral; (2) a preliminary interview with the patient's spouse or other close relatives; (3) a case history, including information about the impact of brain injury on the patient and how much natural or spontaneous recovery has taken place; (4) an inventory of the client's language/communication performance; (5) observation and related testing (including informal assessments, oral peripheral examination, hearing test, and the like); and (6) a diagnostic determination with recommendations about the nature of treatment and a judgment about the individual's prospects for recovery. This process is shown in Figure 8–2. In arriving at a diagnosis, the clinician first determines whether a communication problem exists and, if it does, what kind of problem. This involves sorting out among various possible conditions and among subtypes within specific conditions.

Having discussed the first three tasks in the list, let us now turn our attention to the fourth and see how the evaluation process leads to a diagnosis. The SLP may need a quick idea of the client's language abilities and disabilities in order to determine the need for further testing and to better choose the most appropriate standardized tests to employ. Therefore, a screening test may be administered. The SLP will need to collect diagnostic and evaluation performance data but also organize and make sense of the information.

Screening for Aphasia

When a patient is referred in a medical setting, the SLP may begin with a *bedside consultation,* the term that reimbursement agencies prefer to use (rather than *screening*). A screening instrument is designed to evaluate a patient's language abilities swiftly before the administration of a more thorough (and lengthy) examination. One reason for using a screening instrument is that it allows the SLP to advise relatives and health-care professionals quickly about the best means of communicating with the patient. In addition, patients' symptoms change rapidly during the first days and months following brain injury; screenings allow for frequent reassessments to document the patient's progress (or lack of progress) and to modify suggestions about how best to communicate with the patient. Frequent readministrations of formal, standardized tests—many lasting 1 to 6 hours—would not be practical. Table 8–3 lists some of the available screening tests for aphasia. Salter et al. (2006) compared six of these screening tools (the Acute Aphasia Screening Protocol, Frenchay Aphasia Screening Test, Mississippi Aphasia Screening Test, Reitan-Indiana Aphasia Screening Examination, ScreeLink, and Ullevaal Aphasia Screening Test) on the basis of reliability, validity, classification sensitivity, and practical utility. While measurement properties and clinical utility appeared limited in all the tests, they reported that the Frenchay Aphasia Screening Test is the most thorough and, based on a literature review, the most widely used.

Some experienced clinicians design their own screening device—usually one that is more cursory than published tests. In some work settings, for example, the SLP must

FIGURE 8–2
Critical Assessment Process in Aphasia and Adult Language Disorders

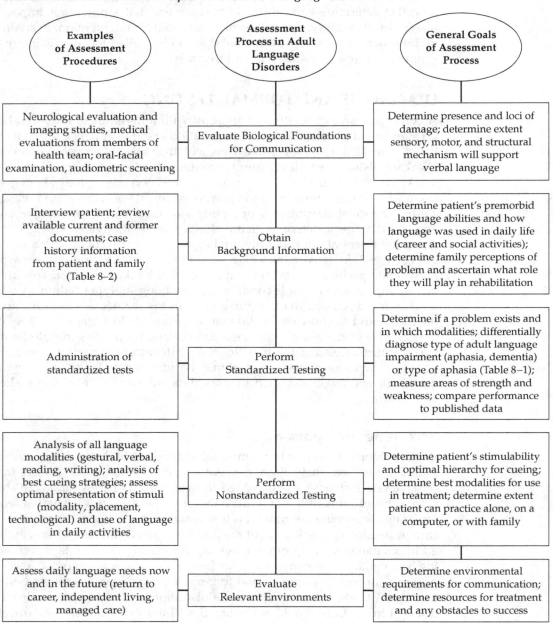

quickly (in 5 minutes or so) interview and screen all newly admitted patients to determine if a communication problem exists and to decide whether to suggest that the physician order a speech-language consult. This is done because third-party reimbursement agencies require that evaluations be medically necessary and physician ordered. Typically, the SLP elicits spontaneous conversation and judges it for contextual accuracy, topic maintenance, length of utterance, syntactic variety, facility with word selection,

TABLE 8–3
Some Screening or Bedside Tests for Aphasia

Acute Aphasia Screening Protocol (AASP)
　(Crary, Haak, & Malinsky, 1989)
Aphasia Language Performance Scales (ALPS)
　(Keenan & Brassell, 1975)
Aphasia Screening Test (AST-3)
　(Whurr, 2011)
Bedside Evaluation and Screening Test of Aphasia, Second Edition (BEST-2)
　(West, Sands, & Ross-Swain, 1998)
Bedside Western Aphasia Battery-R
　(Kertesz, 2006)
Children's Acquired Aphasia Screening Test (CAAST)
　(Whurr, 1999)
Frenchay Aphasia Screening Test (FAST)
　(Enderby, Wood, & Wade, 2006)
Language Screening Test (LAST)
　(Flamand-Roze et al., 2011)
Mississippi Aphasia Screening Test
　(Nakase-Thompson et al., 2005)
Multimodal Communication Screening Test for Persons with Aphasia
　(MCST-A) (Garrett & Lasker, 2007)
Quick Assessment for Aphasia
　(Tanner & Culbertson, 1999)
Reitan-Indiana Aphasia Screening Examination
　(Reitan & Wolfson, 1985)
ScreeLing (Doesborgh et al., 2003)
Sheffield Screening Test for Acquired Language Disorders
　(Syder et al., 1993)
Sklar Aphasia Scale (SAS)
　(Sklar, 1983) (also available in German)
Ullevaal Aphasia Screening Test (UAS)
　(Thommessen et al., 1999)

and fluency. Limited or absent conversation may lead the SLP to assess more basic skills quickly, such as naming and pointing to objects in the room, repeating, following commands (nonverbally), and responding to yes or no questions (verbally or gesturally). Such a quick, albeit incomplete, screening permits the clinician to judge (1) whether a communication problem exists on a gross level, (2) the need for further testing (and hence the need for a physician-ordered consult), and (3) which formal tests would be best suited to the patient's level of functioning.

Standardized Testing

To devise a plan of treatment, as well as to predict the probable course and outcome of treatment, the SLP needs a comprehensive appraisal of the patient's present language abilities. Where is the patient having difficulty? Which modalities are working best? How are errors made, and are there discernable patterns to the errors? To answer these and other questions, we inventory the patient's language.

　The SLP has many published tests from which to choose; Table 8–4 lists some of the more commonly used tests of aphasia. Only a cursory discussion of the more popular—and different—tests will be presented here. Beginning clinicians often ask which aphasia

TABLE 8–4
Commonly Used Tests for Aphasia and for Measures of Treatment Outcomes

Aphasia Diagnostic Profiles (ADP)
  (Helm-Estabrooks, 1992)
Assessment of Communicative Effectiveness in Severe Aphasia (ACESA)
  (Cunningham et al., 1995)
Assessment of Language-Related Functional Activities (ALFA)
  (Baines, Heeringa, & Martin, 1999)
Bilingual Aphasia Test (BAT)
  (Paradis, 2011)
Bilingual Verbal Ability Test (BVAT)
  (Munoz-Sandoval et al., 2005)
Boston Diagnostic Aphasia Examination, Third Edition (BDAE-3)
  (Goodglass, Kaplan, & Barresi, 2000)
Boston Assessment of Severe Aphasia (BASA)
  (Helm-Estabrooks et al., 1989)
Communicative Abilities in Daily Living, (CADL-2)
  (Holland, Frattali, & Fromm, 1999)
Examining for Aphasia: Assessment of Aphasia and Related Impairments (EFA-4)
  (LaPointe & Eisenson, 2008)
Functional Assessment of Communication Skills for Adults (ASHA FACS)
  (Frattali et al., 1997)
Functional Communication Profile, Revised (FCP-R)
  (Kleiman, 2003)
Minnesota Test for Differential Diagnosis of Aphasia (MTDDA)
  (Schuell, 1973)
Multilingual Aphasia Examination (MAE-3)
  (Benton, Hamsher, & Sivan, 1994)
Multilingual Aphasia Examination, Spanish (MAE-S)
  (Rey, Sivan, & Benton, 1994)
Porch Index of Communicative Ability—Revised (PICA-R)
  (Porch, 2001)
Western Aphasia Battery—Revised (WAB-R)
  (Kertesz, 2006)

test they should select for examining patients. We prefer not to advocate any particular instrument but instead ask the clinicians to specify their purposes in testing. What do they want the test to show? If prediction of the course of the patient's recovery is important, the PICA-R (Porch, 2001) or the Western Aphasia Battery–Revised (WAB-R) (Kertesz, 2006) are the instruments of choice. If the clinician is more interested in the site of lesion, the Boston Diagnostic Aphasia Examination (BDAE-3) (Goodglass, Kaplan & Barresi, 2000) or the WAB-R are indicated. If the clinician wants to know how the patient performs on basic to complicated language functions, then the classic Minnesota Test for Differential Diagnosis of Aphasia (Schuell, 1973) is a good choice, although it is dated and in limited supply. To sample a patient's communication ability in natural settings, the Functional Assessment of Communication Skills for Adults (Frattali et al., 1997) or the Communicative Abilities in Daily Living (Holland, Frattali, & Fromm, 1999) would be the instrument of choice. For use with diverse populations, the SLP may consider the Spanish version of the Multilinguistic Aphasia Examination (MAE-S; listed in Table 8–4); the Bilingual Verbal Ability Test (BVAT), which is available online from the publisher in Arabic, Chinese, English, French, German, Haitian-Creole, Hindi, Hmong, Italian, Japanese, Korean, Navajo, Polish, Portuguese, Russian, Spanish, Turkish, and

Vietnamese; or the Bilingual Aphasia Test (BAT), which is available free online in more than 60 languages (www.mcgill.ca/linguistics/research/bat/). A good tutorial on multicultural aphasia testing was provided by Ivanova and Hallowell (2013).

In the hands of a skilled and perceptive clinician who is thoroughly familiar with the materials, *any* of the published tests will provide a detailed description of an aphasic patient's language disturbance. As we pointed out earlier in this text, a test is only a tool, a way to help the clinician make relatively precise observations of a particular individual. With this in mind, let us comment further on a few popular, even classic, tests with regard to assessment philosophy and content coverage.

The Porch Index of Communicative Ability–Revised

Better known as the PICA-R (Porch, 2001), this is a psychometrically well-constructed test that assesses verbal, gestural, and graphic responses to common objects. Although now infrequently used as an aphasia test, the PICA-R features a multidimensional scoring system that is necessary in the administration of other instruments, such as the still popular Revised Token Test (McNeil & Prescott, 1978), which is good for subtle auditory comprehension issues, particularly in patients with traumatic brain injury. The multidimensional scoring system uses 1 to 16 categories that allow the clinician to make precise observations of the patient's responses. Scores with percentile norms, performance plots, and recovery curves are generated through data manipulation. Speech-language pathologists have found the overall score (as a single index of communication ability) and the recovery predictions extremely useful information to share with physicians.

On the other hand, we find that administration of the PICA-R is time consuming and that starting the examination with the most difficult task often overwhelms the aphasic person and disturbs his or her subsequent performance. The PICA-R offers only limited information about a patient's verbal ability: Only 4 of the 18 subtests elicit verbal behavior; only one of the four, "describing how objects are used," affords any insight into how the patient talks.

The Boston Diagnostic Aphasia Examination

The BDAE-3 (Goodglass, Kaplan, & Barresi, 2000) operates on the localization premise that test scores and profiles correspond to specific types of aphasia. We particularly recognize as a strength the conversational and expository speech section that rates six features: melodic line, phrase length, articulatory agility, grammatical form, paraphasia, and word finding. Subtests cover a wide variety of skills and modalities, making it a well-rounded examination. Supplementary tests are included for use with related disorders. However, we do find that the BDAE-3 is a lengthy test and one that may frustrate low-level patients.

Western Aphasia Battery–Revised

The WAB-R (Kertesz, 2006) is based on neurolinguistic and neuroanatomic models of language. With an efficient administration time of 1 hour, the Western Aphasia Battery assesses various language abilities through subtests such as information content, fluency, auditory comprehension, repetition, and naming; it taps the auditory modality but also the communicative modalities of reading, writing, and calculation. Analysis of the patient's performance yields an Aphasia Quotient that enables the clinician to classify the patient's type and severity of aphasia. The test battery provides data on language functioning that are useful in establishing a prognosis, designing treatment, and tracking progress.

Communicative Abilities in Daily Living, Second Edition

Holland, Frattali, and Fromm (1999) designed the CADL-2 to sample the patient's functional communication skills in naturalistic situations. It supplements traditional tests of aphasia; it does not replace them. As such, it does not lend itself to differential diagnosis. The content of the CADL-2 is unique; it includes categories such as role playing, utilizing nonverbal context, and analyzing speech acts. All in all, it is a test that measures what it purports—communication in daily activities.

Regardless of the test used, the evaluation process permits the clinician to identify islands of communication ability retained by the patient. In many instances, however, the SLP will want to do additional, more extensive testing in particular areas. Discussion of some specialized tests follows.

1. *Auditory comprehension.* Almost every comprehensive aphasia battery has at least one section that evaluates auditory comprehension. Because the integrity of the auditory modality is so crucial in predicting recovery, we urge thorough, standardized testing. We acknowledge that some focused auditory comprehension tests were published in the 1970s and that some current audiology tests can be adapted for nonstandardized explorations.

2. *Expressive abilities.* Early aphasia batteries have been criticized for not evaluating the spontaneous speech of patients. The Boston Diagnostic Aphasia Examination–3 is a well-known exception. Discourse analysis with adult patients has shown clinical promise, albeit time-consuming, with contextual, syntactic, and semantic assessments of expressive output. On a syntactic level, the Sentence Completion Test, available in journal form (Goodglass et al., 1972), is useful in assessing sentence construction abilities and the patient's use of derivations. The many psychology-based sentence completion tests are less useful.

3. *Word-finding abilities.* Word fluency and naming difficulties (*anomia*) are a common sequela of adolescent and adult brain damage, such as from stroke or traumatic brain injury. Specialized testing might include the Boston Naming Test (BNT-2) (Kaplan, Goodglass, & Weintraub, 2001), the Test of Adolescent and Adult Word Finding (TAWF) (German, 1990), and the neuropsychological Test of Verbal Conceptualization and Fluency (Reynolds & Horton, 2007). Some SLPs test the patient's vocabulary abilities as a rough indicator of single-word recall and verbal IQ. The popular Peabody Picture Vocabulary Test (PPVT-4) is an example, with a patient age range of 2 to 90+ years of age (Dunn & Dunn, 2007). Also we mention the Expressive Vocabulary Test (EVT-2) (Williams, 2007) with the same patient age range.

4. *Reading ability.* While subtests of comprehensive aphasia batteries measure reading ability, the SLP may wish to assess more in depth. The Reading Comprehension Battery for Aphasia (RCBA-2) (LaPointe & Horner, 1998) is appropriate but other, more general reading tests for child to adult are also available.

5. *Neuropsychological/neurolinguistic analysis.* Batteries that assess aphasia from this different perspective include the Psycholinguistic Assessments of Language Processing in Aphasia (PALPA) (Kay, Lesser, & Coltheart, 1997).

6. *Caregiver rating and daily living impact.* The SLP may wish to ascertain how the spouse or caregiver perceives the communicative functioning of the patient with aphasia. The Communicative Effectiveness Index (CETI) (Lomas et al., 1989) covers 16 common activities of daily living and includes speech, language and nonverbal communication behaviors. The Stroke and Aphasia Quality of Life Scale–39 (SAQOL-39) (Hilari et al., 2003) uses self-reporting on 53 items to ascertain impacts and adjustments to daily life, particularly in long-term survivors.

7. *Others.* Additional special testing almost surely includes an oral-peripheral and motor examination (see Appendix A), a hearing screening (see Appendix B), as well as others deemed necessary for particular patients (such as cognitive assessment, single-word/sentence production tasks, intelligibility testing, and so forth). In this vein, we also want to mention that the American Speech-Language-Hearing Association (ASHA) offers an adult language and cognition assessment template that guides the SLP through various areas of informal testing and/or use of formal subtests (search the ASHA website at www.asha.org/). Finally, we do not feel that a clinician should abrogate his or her personal clinical responsibility for judgment by deferring to a test or the numerical scores it generates. A combination of clinical intuition, patient observations, lesion information, and test scores and performances should shape our diagnoses and predictions.

DIFFERENTIAL DIAGNOSIS AND OTHER LANGUAGE DISORDERS

The SLP must often distinguish among aphasia, language changes associated with typical aging (as covered in the definitive text by Toner, Shadden, and Gluth [2011]), and a number of other conditions involving abnormality in speech-language or cognition. A variety of special tests may be needed to replace or supplement standard aphasia batteries in order to facilitate differential diagnosing. Table 8–5 lists some tests useful in differentiating aphasia from other language disorders seen in adults (or adolescents and children post–language acquisition). Special tests delineate a patient's strengths and weaknesses beyond the realm of language; areas such as intelligence, cognition, memory, perception, mood, and behavior need to be tapped. Various functional levels, spanning simple orientation to executive language functions (linguistic-cognitive skills such as anticipation, planning, execution, self-monitoring; Purdy, 2011), are listed in Table 8–5 so the clinician has a resource from which to select to meet the needs of the patient.

We present the following brief discussion of some disorders that might be confused with aphasia. Keep in mind, however, that impairment of symbolic functioning can coexist with any of these conditions. Often the patient's case history, medical referral information, and brain imaging studies clarify the nature of the patient's communication disorder.

Motor Speech Disorders

Motor speech disorders often coexist with language disorders, particularly aphasia. The presence of a speech disorder certainly affects the language treatment goals and procedures. For example, facilitative articulation techniques must often be incorporated into the total management program. Therefore, the evaluation of a patient with brain damage should include tasks to determine the existence of either *apraxia of speech* or one of the *dysarthrias.* We will discuss these disorders, and the process of differential diagnosis, in Chapter 9.

Right Hemisphere Damage

Most individuals are left hemisphere dominant for language, yet injury to the right hemisphere (such as from stroke or other insult) can cause communication and other deficits. Typically patients with right hemisphere damage (RHD) exhibit deficits in visual perception, attention, cognition, and complex communicative forms (both verbal and nonverbal). These communicative inefficiencies are often higher-level executive

TABLE 8–5
Useful Tests for Cognitive-Communicative Assessments and in Tracking Outcomes

Arizona Battery for Communication Disorders of Dementia (ABCD)
   (Bayles & Tomoeda, 1993)
Behavioral Assessment of Dysexecutive Syndrome (BADS)
   (Wilson et al., 1996)
Boston Naming Test, Second Edition
   (Kaplan, Goodglass, & Weintraub, 2001)
Brief Test of Head Injury (BTHI)
   (Helm-Estabrooks & Hotz, 1991)
Burns Brief Inventory of Communication and Cognition
   (Burns, 1997)
Butt Non-Verbal Reasoning Test (BNVR)
   (Butt & Bucks, 2004)
Cognitive Linguistic Quick Test (CLQT)
   (Helm-Estabrook, 2001)
Delis-Kaplan Executive Function System
   (Delis, Kaplan, & Kramer, 2001)
Dementia Rating Scale–2 (DRS-2) (Mattis, 2001)
Functional Independence Measure and *Functional Assessment Measure* (FIM + FAM system)
   (Hall, 1992)
Functional Assessment of Verbal Reasoning and Executive Strategies (adult FAVRES)
   (MacDonald, 2005)
Functional Assessment Staging Tool (FAST)
   (Sclan & Reisberg, 1992)
Functional Linguistic Communication Inventory (FLCI)
   (Bayles & Tomoeda, 1994)
Galveston Orientation and Amnesia Test (GOAT)
   (Levin, O'Donnell, & Grossman, 1979)
Global Deterioration Scale of Primary Degenerative Dementia (GDS)
   (Reisberg, Ferris, & Crook, 1982)
Mini-Cog (Borson et al., 2003)
Mini-Mental State Examination (MMSE-2)
   (Folstein & Folstein, 2010)
Monterey Cognitive Assessment (MoCA)
   (Nasreddine, 2003)
Revised Token Test
   (McNeil & Prescott, 1978)
Ross Information Processing Assessment–Geriatric (RIPA-G:2)
   (Ross-Swain & Fogle, 2011)
Scales for Cognitive Ability for Traumatic Brain Injury (SCATBI)
   (Adamovich & Henderson, 1992)
Test of Nonverbal Intelligence, Fourth Edition (TONI-4)
   (Brown, Sherbenou, & Johnsen, 2010)

functions that can be subtle. In essence, these issues do not resemble aphasic symptoms. Table 8–6 summarizes deficits typically seen in patients with right nondominant hemisphere impairment. The interested reader is referred to works on right hemisphere communication disorders (Blake, 2011; Myers, 2008; Thompkins, 1995; Thompkins & Lehman, 1998).

Only in recent years have tests of right hemisphere communication impairment been marketed. Typically, SLPs and neuropsychologists form a test battery using selected subtests from standard tests of aphasia, learning aptitude tests, perceptual tests,

TABLE 8–6
Sequelae of Right Hemisphere Damage

General Symptoms
Denial of illness
Impaired judgment
Impaired self-monitoring
Poor motivation
Memory problems
Disorganization
Problem-solving deficits

Visuospatial Deficits
Visual field deficits (especially neglect of left half of space)
Visual memory and imagery problems
Facial recognition difficulties (disorientation to person)
Geographic and spatial disorientation (to place)
Visual hallucinations
Visuoconstructive deficits (constructional apraxia)

Deficits in Affect and Prosody
Indifference reaction
Reduced sensitivity to emotional tone
Impaired prosodic production and comprehension

Linguistic Deficits
Problems with figurative language (interprets literally)
Impaired sense of humor
Impaired comprehension of complex auditory material
Word fluency difficulties
Word recognition and word–picture matching deficits
Paragraph comprehension difficulties
Higher-order (executive function) deficits in organizing information
Tendency to produce impulsive answers with unnecessary detail
Insensitivity to contextual cues and pragmatic aspects of communication

and others (recall Table 8–5). Informal test items are also often part of the assessment battery. Of particular importance are the patient's abilities and disabilities with visuospatial perception, prosody, judgment, and high-level communication. Nevertheless, some of the cohesive tests in clinical use are presented.

The Right Hemisphere Language Battery (RHLB-2) (Bryan, 1995) consists of subtests such as metaphor–picture matching, written metaphor choice, inferred meaning comprehension, humor appreciation, lexical semantic recognition, emphatic stress production, and discourse production. Rating scales for scoring the discourse sample along 11 parameters are used.

The Mini Inventory of Right Brain Injury (MIRBI-2) (Pimental & Knight, 2000) is a 27-item screening tool that assesses visual scanning, integrity of gnosis, body image/ body schema and praxis, visuoverbal processing, visuosymbolic processing, affective language, higher-level language skills, emotion and affect processing, and general behavior/psychic integrity.

The Rehabilitation Institute of Chicago Evaluation of Communication Problems in Right Hemisphere Dysfunction-3 (RICE-3) (Halper, Cherney, & Burns, 2010) has sections focusing on assorted aspects of this disorder. Included are general behavioral patterns, visual scanning and tracking, assessment and analysis of writing errors, assessment of pragmatic communication violations, and metaphorical language.

Psychosis

Although it is rather easy for the professional to distinguish *aphasia* from *psychosis,* it is understandable why laypeople are often confused. The person with aphasia may say yes when he or she means no, use obscenities and other antisocial language or gestures freely, laugh or cry often, lapse into euphoria, deny his or her symptoms, or withdraw into severe depression and despair. The distinguishing features of psychosis are rather obvious, however: severe personality decomposition—not just frustration or emotional overflow when trying to comprehend or speak—and distortion of, or loss of contact with, reality. The vast majority of patients with aphasia do not show evidence of mental deterioration or gross disturbances in processing reality. In addition, the person with aphasia will generally try hard to communicate with others; for the psychotic, interpersonal contact is irrelevant.

Considering all the frustrations that persons with aphasia encounter, we have often wondered why they do not behave in a more abnormal manner than they do. Indeed, their demeanor and social interaction, aside from the language impairment, are remarkably normal. Nevertheless, some individuals with aphasia do experience psychotic episodes and periods of severe depression.

Language of Confusion

The straightforward, sometimes short-lived *language of confusion* describes patients with irrelevant and confabulatory language, cognitive confusion and unclear thinking, reduced recognition of the environment and other perceptual issues, faulty memory, and disorientation to time and place. Syntax, word retrieval, auditory comprehension, and ability to repeat are usually not impaired. The patient's relatively good language is, therefore, unlike aphasia.

The onset of confusion typically is sudden because of a traumatic injury. In persons who exhibit the language of confusion, the injury to the brain is widespread and perhaps affects the hemispheres bilaterally. The following case example illustrates the irrelevance and confusion:

> Tom Snively, a 20-year-old college junior, suffered a closed head injury in a skiing accident. He was in a coma for 2 weeks. Now, 2 months post-onset, he is an inpatient in the Marquette Rehabilitation Center. When evaluated with a standard test of aphasia, Tom showed no disturbance of vocabulary or syntax; he did have some limited word-finding difficulty. The examiner noted, however, that the young man had trouble attending and staying in touch with the test situation. The patient tended to give responses that, although syntactically correct, were often irrelevant. Additionally, Tom was disoriented and, particularly in response to open-ended questions, gave rambling, fabricated answers. Here is a portion of an interview conducted by a medical social worker that reveals the patient's disorientation and tendency to confabulate:

> Worker: Where are you?
>
> Tom: Ah, in training camp. Colorado Springs. And tomorrow we do time trials for the giant slalom.
>
> Worker: But what is this place?
>
> Tom: A training center. I had a hamstring pull and need whirlpool treatments.

Sequela of Traumatic Brain Injury

Young and old alike may experience a traumatic injury to the brain. Youth and young adults are particularly susceptible due to causative activities in which they are involved: bike and trampoline falls, car accidents, gunshot or explosive head wounds, factory accidents, and so on. Traumatic brain injury (TBI), of course, is not a language diagnosis but may be an underlying cause of a host of cognitive-communicative deficits, and so we mention it in this chapter. TBI often triggers a multitude of deficits that the SLP may need to assess. These include, but are not limited to, aphasia (especially auditory comprehension of complex multistage instructions but also of repetition, reading, writing, and math), oral motor/speaking difficulties, attention deficits, cognitive changes (including reasoning, logical thinking, and memory), impulsivity and emotional control issues plus various visual-perceptual deficits.

The type of trauma to the head (closed impact or open wound) as well as the location and extent of brain trauma (ranging from frontal lobe to the brainstem) affect the patient's circumstance both early on and later. Kimbarow (2011) provides a good overview on the subject of TBI and its early sequel that may run the gamut from coma to post-traumatic amnesia, to environmental disorientation, to higher level cognitive-communicative issues. Table 8–5 includes various assessment instruments suitable for patients with TBI at various levels of ability. For example, the Galveston Orientation and Amnesia Test (GOAT) by Levin, O'Donnell, and Grossman (1979) is in wide use for early or low-functioning patients. At the other extreme would be test batteries appraising executive cognitive-linguistic functioning (including skills of anticipating, planning, executing, and self-monitoring). This testing sometimes parallels that done with right hemisphere damage patients.

The SLP working with school-age patients will certainly assess these various areas, collectively lumped together under the rubric of cognitive-communicative deficits. Again, collection of the patient's case history, medical documentation, and patient interview questions (also of parents and teachers, if appropriate), as presented earlier in this chapter, will go a long way in pointing out areas and levels to assess. Findings, in turn, shape the intervention goals. The following might be some insightful interview queries. What do you think has changed since your TBI? Give examples of areas you have found hard to do or understand. What do you do when you do not understand the teacher's directions?

While Table 8–5 includes various cognitive-communicative instruments useful with this clinical population, we wish to highlight two that were designed for TBI patients: the Brief Test of Head Injury (Helm-Estabrooks & Hotz, 1991) and the Scale for Cognitive Ability for Traumatic Brain Injury (Adamovich & Henderson, 1992). The American Speech-Language-Hearing Association has a practice portal on traumatic brain injury in adults that can be searched at www.asha.com/.

Mild Cognitive Impairment

Adults with mild cognitive impairment (MCI) may present with memory loss and some subtle declines in cognitive-communicative abilities. This may go undetected unless it is tested with challenging tasks, although family members have a nagging sense that something is now not quite right with dad. Petersen et al. (1999) purport that the individual with MCI has memory deficits well beyond what might be typical for the person's age and also to a degree worse than that seen in the mild or moderate dementia but with less cognitive impairment than that seen in dementia. This memory-impaired population of MCI patients may or may not deteriorate further in cognitive abilities. Devolution examples might be in cases of primary progressive aphasia or one of the dementias, but longitudinal research is needed in this area. Currently, multidisciplinary investigations are hoping to refine early identification and targeted management strategies to optimize outcomes. Given the increasing incidence of dementia and related disorders, this research is important.

A growing body of healthcare information suggests that early signs of MCI might include changes in executive functions as much or more so than significant memory issues. Executive functions are higher-order cognitive-communicative processes such as awareness of action-reaction consequences in thinking, sequencing abilities, logic, and so forth. While aphasia batteries cited in Table 8–4 and cognitive instruments in Table 8–5 may be used, those with challenging subtests may prove more fruitful for the SLP in detecting MCI. In particular we cite the following as some informal and formal starting points:

1. Memory—such as informal assessment recalling strings of numbers or words, especially after a time delay and having the patient perform other tasks before recalling the items; the Revised Token Test (McNeil & Prescott, 1978) also challenges linguistic memory.

2. Word Fluency—such as naming as many animals that start with a certain letter in a time period; published versions of these subtests were cited earlier.

3. Picture Description—a speech-language sample analyzed for linguistic details and sequential logic can be insightful; the Cookie Theft picture is a well-known example from the BDAE-3 (Goodglass et al., 2000).

4. Explaining the meaning of complex statements or of proverbs—allows for judgment of the patient's clarity of thought and logic; instrument cited in Table 8–6 on right hemisphere strokes might be useful.

5. Discourse analysis—provides the SLP with various cognitive-linguistic information, including the use of high-level thought processes (or lack thereof); discourse analysis to assess executive functioning in suspected cases of MCI is advocated by Fleming (2014).

With early identification of MCI the healthcare team unfortunately is faced with our limited pharmaceutical and behavioral interventions. In progressive disorder types, however, the SLP can do much to educate the patient and family, help build and store current memories (through paper or online scrapbooks for future use), and assist with communicative strategies that evolve with changing needs over time. Assessments and re-assessments not only advance our scientific knowledge of this disorder, they also appraise the patient's changing cognitive-linguistic abilities for optimizing patient and caregiver interaction strategies.

The Dementias and Cognitive Assessment

The *dementias* are a group of disorders that feature generalized cognitive declines; speech-language declines figure prominently in the dementias, but there can be a host of other symptoms. Depending on the type of dementia, causes may include infectious diseases, tumor, and multiple strokes. The area of the brain affected is diffuse and may be cortical, subcortical, or both. While Alzheimer's disease is a well-known type of dementia, other examples include Parkinson diseases, advanced Down syndrome, and vascular dementia stemming from repeated strokes, to name but a few (Bayles & Tomoeda, 2007). There also is evidence that dementia may be associated with motor neuron disease (such as amyotrophic lateral sclerosis [ALS]); it was previously thought to be limited to motor or motor-sensory functions. The dementias often have a gradual, insidious onset.

The physician and entire healthcare team, including the SLP, are involved in the diagnosis and evaluation of a patient with suspected dementia (and in determining the cause and type of dementia). While cognitive deterioration is the hallmark of dementia, there are related changes. Before a clinical diagnosis of dementia can be confirmed, several key features must be present:

1. A sustained deterioration of *memory,* plus a disturbance in at least three of the following areas: (a) orientation in time and place, (b) judgment and problem solving (dealing with everyday situations), (c) community affairs (shopping, handling finances), (d) home and avocations, and (e) personal care
2. A gradual onset and progression
3. A duration of at least 6 months or longer

While cognitive decline can co-occur in patients with the language-based disorder of aphasia, aphasia and dementia are different entities. Cognitive dysfunction (in many forms) is the cardinal indicator of dementia, which may be evident in both linguistic and nonlinguistic performance. Table 8–7 highlights differences between dementia and aphasia for the SLP.

Like a square is a rectangle but a rectangle is not necessarily a square, it is important to remember that the well-known disease of Alzheimer is but one type of dementia.

TABLE 8–7
Cognitive and Communicative Differences between Aphasia and Dementia

Variable	Aphasia	Dementia
Progression	Rapid onset; improvement is typical.	Slow onset and progressive deterioration.
Cognition	Cognition is generally intact.	Cognition is mildly to profoundly impaired; it worsens with the condition; problem solving is poor.
Memory	Memory is generally intact.	Memory ranges from mildly forgetful to profoundly impaired or amnesic; it worsens with the condition.
Emotionality	Mood is typically appropriate with occasional periods of depression or frustration.	Person is typically labile, is apathetic and withdrawn, intermittently shows agitation, and can exhibit depression or mania.
Pragmatics	Socially appropriate skills are evident despite some comprehension failures; communication efforts typically show relevance.	Social skills are mildly to severely affected; inappropriate behaviors and irrelevant comments are typical; thought processes are disorganized.
Repetition ability	Slightly to severely impaired.	Generally intact unless the condition is severe.
Semantics	Word-retrieval difficulties can be mild to severe; semantic and literal paraphasias may be used.	Impairment ranges from mild word-retrieval difficulties to visual misrecognitions, to severe vocabulary reductions.
Syntax	Syntax is affected to varying degrees; it can be classified as fluent or nonfluent based on length of utterance.	Syntax is intact when disorder is mild; there is reduction of syntactic complexity as the disorder progresses.
Phonology	Phonology is impaired in nonfluent aphasia; it may be present as literal paraphasia in fluent aphasia.	Phonology is generally intact unless the condition is severe; dysarthria is possible.

The Alzheimer's Association offers useful resources for professionals, patients, and their families; in particular we suggest that the SLP access the information on cognitive assessment from its website at www.alz.org/. Search for a video demonstration of a physician screening a patient's mental status, immediate and delayed memory recall of words, and the often-used test to draw a clock face of a specified time. Their Cognitive Assessment Toolkit is provided "as a guide to detecting cognitive impairment quickly and efficiently during the Medicare Annual Wellness Visit"; this toolkit includes assorted tests that the SLP may find useful for screening purposes.

To illustrate the salient behavioral and cognitive-communicative symptoms observed in dementia, we include a portion of a diagnostic report on a patient in the second phase of Alzheimer disease (Powell & Courtice, 1983):

> This 64-year-old patient manifested the following behaviors: lowered drive and energy level, memory loss, slow reaction time, and difficulty making decisions. Her personality has changed in the past year so that now she typically is dull, bland, and unresponsive socially.
>
> Mrs. Davis's language abilities are only mildly impaired at this time. She can match objects; point to and name pictures; and repeat words, phrases, and short sentences. Phonologically and syntactically, her speech is within normal limits. She does have limited output, however, and restricted usage. The patient's speech performance is slow and often, after trying to respond to a task, she will say, "I don't know."
>
> The patient's language disturbance was more evident on tasks requiring greater intellectual effort and abstraction. For example, Mrs. Davis was unable to find and correct semantic errors in sentences ("My sister is an only child") or discern the ambiguity in sentences ("Visiting relatives can be a nuisance").

As mentioned, the SLP has many dementia instruments available (e.g., Table 8–5); here we provide an overview of but a few. The Arizona Battery for Communication Disorders of Dementia (ABCD) (Bayles & Tomoeda, 1993) profiles patient performance along the subtests of mental status, linguistic expression, visuospatial construction, episodic memory, and linguistic comprehension. The ABCD is a popular test and can be used to document disease effects over time.

Dementia scales are useful summary tools to categorizing progression of the disease. The revised Dementia Rating Scale (DRS-2) (Mattis, 2001) is one example; the Functional Assessment Staging Tool (FAST) (Sclan & Reisberg, 1992) is another. The FAST uses the following seven stages to express the severity and progression of Alzheimer disease in terms of functionality (each will be discussed briefly here):

- Stage 1—no impairment (including normal memory exhibited in the interview and/or test session).
- Stage 2—very mild cognitive decline; person has memory lapses, for example, keys and/or glasses misplaced (may be typical age-related changes or early signs of Alzheimer).
- Stage 3—mild cognitive decline; early-stage Alzheimer can be diagnosed in some but not all individuals (family aware of memory or concentration problems); difficulties noted with word-finding, reading comprehension, performance issues at work or social settings, losing valuable objects, decline in planning/organizing.
- Stage 4—moderate cognitive decline; early-stage or mild Alzheimer; detailed assessment reveals decreased knowledge of current events, impaired mental arithmetic (for example, counting backward from 75), decreased capacity to perform

complex tasks (for example, paying bills or planning a dinner), reduced memory of personal history, and social, withdrawal.

- Stage 5—moderately severe cognitive decline; mid-stage Alzheimer; major gaps in memory and in cognitive function (for example, unable to recall address and/or phone number, unclear where they are or the date, naming family members and/or spouse), but needs no assistance eating or toileting.
- Stage 6—severe cognitive decline; further loss of abilities and awareness; needs help with customary daily activities; tends to wander and become lost.
- Stage 7—very severe cognitive decline; late-stage Alzheimer; loss of recognizable speech; needs help eating, dressing, toileting; may be incontinent; lost walking and sitting.

In summary, with dementia patients at any level, whichever test is selected, the SLP assesses cognitive and communicative aspects including memory, orientation, associative thought, intelligence, reasoning (both verbal and nonverbal), story retelling, object descriptions, explanations, and vocabulary. The American Speech-Language-Hearing Association offers a practice portal on dementia, its assessment, and evidence-based guidelines (search for the practice portal on dementia at www.asha.org/).

Cautionary Thoughts on Formal Diagnostic Testing

Defining aphasia remains controversial, even among the experts. Many definitions of aphasia exist—some broad and all-encompassing; others quite specific and limiting. Speech-language pathologists will be wise to keep this in mind as they seek to differentiate aphasia from other speech and language disorders. In the final analysis, labels we use reflect speech-language diagnoses, not medical diagnoses. The evaluation process is likened to taking an inventory of the patient's communicative strengths and weaknesses; this can be done informally as well.

THE ART OF INFORMAL ASSESSMENT

Regardless of which standardized test the clinician administers, it is important for treatment planning to examine *how* the patient made the errors. Did the patient seem to perseverate? At what level of complexity did responses break down? Did the patient give synonyms or associations for words when asked to name pictures or objects? For example, when asked to name a picture of a dollar bill, a patient who says, "Put it . . . pocket . . . wallet . . ." is making a "better error" than a response of "soup" or "don't know." Was the patient attempting to correct the errors? Are responses significantly delayed? How did the patient respond to various cueing techniques? What strategies, if any, were used to assist in word retrieval. Examples of self-cueing strategies include using a functional gesture, writing the word in the air or on paper, saying the phonetic start of the word, or uttering a semantically similar word. Answers to these questions are based more on clinician observations during the testing process than on test scores. Informal assessment with activities that probe treatment levels and cueing needs may be most insightful.

In evaluating a patient, it is not *necessary* to use a test at all, although tests do lend scores some degree of statistical validity and reliability that are important for evidenced-based practice. Functional communication skills exhibited by the patient are relevant to designing treatment. Questions that should come to the mind of the clinician include the following: Which of the patient's strategies should be capitalized on and reinforced? Which can be made more effective? Which strategies are counterproductive and interfering? Should alternative modes of communication be employed to develop functional responding? The evaluation provides an excellent time to observe *patient-generated facilitation strategies,* such as gesturing an action to aid in word retrieval, finger tapping to pace speech production, requesting repetitions or using a delay to gain extra processing time, and the like. In addition, before designing a management program, the SLP must consider *characteristics of the stimulus* and which *cues and prompts* may be presented to the patient to increase the likelihood of response accuracy. Treatment probes to determine these details may be initiated during the evaluation stage but should continue to be used throughout the management program to maintain efficiency. (Patient progress is often uneven, and "steps" in the program may be skipped from time to time.)

Characteristics of the stimulus affect the patient's ability to respond. The prevailing clinical assumption is that parameters of the stimulus can be hierarchically arranged to produce a level of responding that is not only continual but also correct (appropriate) more than half the time. Some general guidelines can be summarized here; the clinician may want to probe the patient's needs regarding the following stimulus characteristics:

1. Presentation of a stimulus through more than one modality increases the likelihood of a correct response. This also provides more contextual information.

2. Salient and nonambiguous stimuli affect performance positively—for example, large pictures without distracting backgrounds, or intense auditory stimuli with a favorable signal-to-noise ratio.

3. Reduced length and complexity of presentation, such as using short words or short and grammatically simple sentences, improves comprehension and production accuracy.

4. Presentation of stimuli at reduced rates for longer periods of time and with an imposed response delay affects performance favorably.

Various cues and prompts may be presented to increase the likelihood of response accuracy. These may be provided by the clinician initially and later, through training, may be faded from use or become self-generated cues, thus helping the patient become a self-sufficient, functional communicator. Cueing can also be part of computer software programs (Katz, 2001). Cueing characteristics and optimal hierarchies are an often-researched area in aphasiology. Table 8–8 lists a 10-level cueing hierarchy, which

TABLE 8–8
A Hierarchy for Word Retrieval

Step 1	Tell patient, "Say [word]." (Patient imitates.)
Step 2	Ask patient to complete a sentence with the first and second phonemes supplied (e.g., "You sleep in a be _____.").
Step 3	Ask patient to complete a sentence with the first phoneme supplied (e.g., "You sleep in a b _____.").
Step 4	Ask patient to complete a sentence with first the phoneme silently articulated (e.g., "You sleep in a [form /b/ on lips]").
Step 5	Ask patient to complete a sentence (e.g., "You sleep in a _____.").
Step 6	State function, demonstrate function, and supply a carrier phrase (e.g., "You sleep on it [motion sleep]. It's a _____.").
Step 7	State function and supply a carrier phrase (e.g., "You sleep on it; it's a _____.").
Step 8	Direct the patient to demonstrate the function (e.g., "Show me what you do with it.").
Step 9	Direct the patient to state the function (e.g., "What do you do with this?").
Step 10	Request the name (e.g., "What is this?").

TABLE 8–9
Compensatory Strategies for Aphasia

Comprehension Strategies
- Repeat the utterance for the patient; later ask the patient to assume the responsibility of requesting repeats.
- Augment verbal material with the same information in writing; patient eventually should ask for material to be written if this modality aids comprehension.

Stop-and-Go Strategies
These stop strategies are useful with patients who have fluent aphasia and assist in controlling fluency and monitoring empty speech or paraphasic errors.

- If desired, model a slow rate of speech and monitor the patient's pace, stopping to correct when needed.
- Encourage the patient to listen to him- or herself. Frequent verbal reminders to "listen" may be employed.
- Actively stop the patient's speech output, if necessary. This can be done by touching the lips, saying "Stop," using a gesture signal (such as hand up), or any combination of these that successfully terminates the jargon. Fading of the stop cue should be incorporated into the treatment plan.
- Encourage self-correction in the patient. Direction to use another strategy, such as a word-retrieval technique, may be helpful.

These go strategies are useful with patients who have nonfluent aphasia and encourage the patient to keep communication going by using telegraphic speech, gestures, or graphics on which to expand.

- Get the patient started; you can suggest a gesture or key word to initiate a telegraphic response.
- Keep the patient going; you can replay or feed back to the patient what was said initially and encourage expansion or elaboration.

is useful in assisting patients with word-retrieval problems. Cue the patient at the highest step possible to initially aid in word recall and back down the steps, supplying more assistance as needed. Table 8–9 explains strategies that might prove helpful during the informal assessment and that later can be integrated into treatment. We have often used such stop-and-go strategies to elicit optimal, elaborate, on-target responses from our patients in both assessment and treatment situations.

SUMMARY FINDINGS AND PROGNOSTIC INDICATORS

Information on patient abilities and disabilities obtained through the formal and informal evaluation process permits the SLP to diagnose the type of aphasia (or other communication disorder), if any. The diagnostic label is useful as a summary statement. The information collected is used in determining the patient's prognosis for recovery. It also shapes the direction that treatment will take. Of course, the ultimate goal of evaluation and diagnosis is to ensure that the patient's symptoms are managed appropriately.

Prognosis

Selecting patients for treatment who have the best chance of recovery from aphasia is an unsettling task. Rather than abandon anyone, the clinician's impulse is to attempt to work with every person, even though prospects for improvement in cases of severe language impairment are dim. When there is little real progress, the patient's labors are like those of Sisyphus.

How, then, can the SLP identify patients with the best potential? A list of inter-related factors that we have found helpful for making a prognosis is presented here; however, we trust the reader's forecasting will be guided by four important maxims: (1) Do not make a final prognosis on the basis of a single evaluation session—a period of trial therapy is always highly informative, (2) do not make a prognosis solely on the basis of a single measure of behavior (such as one test), (3) do make evidence-based decisions (such as knowing the poor relationship between a patient's motivation and improvement potential), and (4) be sure you understand the value of predictors—they can be potent self-fulfilling prophecies.

1. *Initial severity.* Initial severity of aphasia is the single best predictor of recovery. The more severe the patient's language impairment at the time of assessment, the poorer the prognosis. The following three aspects of language functioning are particularly im-portant in predicting recovery:

- *Auditory recognition.* Patients who make errors (even a few errors—2 or 3 out of 10 items—are significant) when identifying pictures or common objects named by the examiner have an unfavorable prognosis; an impairment at this level is apparently irreversible.

- *Comprehension.* Patients who have marked difficulty in comprehending ver-bal messages make poor candidates for treatment. In fact, a reliable index of the severity of language impairment in aphasia is the degree of disturbance in comprehension.

- *Speech fluency.* Patients who speak more fluently seem to make better recoveries. But the presence of jargon, especially when it is coupled with a lack of self-monitoring, euphoria, or denial, is a poor clinical sign.

2. *Time elapsed since onset.* Many studies have concluded that patients who receive language treatment before 6 months has elapsed since the cerebral insult show the most significant gains in treatment. The longer the time elapsed since the onset of aphasia and the beginning of treatment, the poorer the prognosis. Habits of dependence, with-drawal, and possible secondary gains accruing from a nonverbal role tend to defeat therapeutic intervention.

3. *Type of aphasia.* Recovery of aphasia seems to follow a pattern of evolution. Prog-ress in global aphasia is often poor, but when improvement occurs, it is toward the symptoms of Broca's aphasia. Broca's aphasia typically shows fair to good recovery; when symptoms diminish, the patient usually retains word-retrieval difficulty and dys-fluency. Wernicke's aphasia carries a split prognosis, with some patients doing fairly well and others poorly. Although the symptoms of Wernicke's aphasia often persist, recovery can occur, with symptoms evolving toward conduction or anomic types of aphasia. Conduction aphasia improves toward symptoms of anomic aphasia or may re-cover completely. Anomic aphasia also shows complete recovery or recovery with only the persistence of mild word-retrieval difficulties.

4. *Etiology.* Depending on the location and extent of the lesion, patients who have suffered traumatic brain injury tend to make better recoveries than do individuals who have had thrombotic or other vascular episodes and tumors.

5. *Age.* The importance of age as a prognostic variable is not clear because it often overlaps with factors such as etiology. For example, trauma patients tend to be younger

than CVA patients. However, it can generally be said that younger patients recover faster and more adequately than do older patients. Presumably this is because younger brains show more plasticity, and older patients may have more widespread cerebral damage due to arteriosclerosis. In addition, aphasic patients in or near retirement may lack the energy and motivation to persist in a treatment program.

6. *Presence of other health problems.* In our clinical experience, aphasic patients presenting health problems in addition to the brain injury (such as diabetes, systemic vascular disease, or kidney disease) often do poorly in treatment.

7. *Family response.* Patients whose families provide supportive understanding and appropriate stimulation and who permit the individual to regain his or her role within the family unit have a more favorable prognosis. Said another way, patients who are discharged to their homes have a better language outcome than do those discharged to long-term institutional care.

8. *Extent of the lesion.* The more extensive the brain injury, the poorer the prospects for recovery. However, there is evidence that CT scan data per se are not predictive of patient outcome.

9. *Location of the lesion.* This variable overlaps with the type of aphasia. In general, damage occurring posterior to the fissure of Rolando, especially at the junction of the parietal and temporal lobes, tends to result in more persistent aphasia.

10. *Premorbid personality.* The more outgoing, flexible individual generally responds better to treatment than does an inhibited, introverted person. Personality and temperament are often said to have altered as a result of brain damage. Behavior patterns seen in some aphasic patients have been labeled egocentricity, catastrophic response, concretism, and the like. Despite the tremendous frustration and alteration in self-concept that aphasia produces, most of our clients have not exhibited much change in their basic personality traits.

11. *Intelligence and education.* The more intelligent, better-educated patients make better candidates for treatment. Although this is generally true, a few of our most highly educated patients were so vividly aware of the discrepancy between their premorbid abilities and their present condition that they simply withdrew in futility.

12. *Self-monitoring.* Patients who are aware of their errors and attempt to correct them have a more favorable prognosis than those who do not. Patients who are attentive and cooperative during initial testing tend to be those whose outcome includes independent daily living.

13. *Handedness.* Left-handed patients have better prognoses than right-handed ones. However, it may be that left-handed individuals are more likely to become aphasic regardless of which hemisphere of the brain is damaged, suggesting that left-handers show bilateral language representation.

As we near the end of this chapter, let us remember that aphasia and other adult language disorders affect the daily lives of our patients. It behooves us as clinicians to assess such functional impact at the beginning, middle, and end of our intervention. Only in this manner can we objectively collect functional status measures and track the communicative impacts and improvements in daily living—or lack thereof. The World Health Organization's International Classification of Functioning, Disability and Health (ICF) (see Figure 8–3) focuses attention on the patient's functioning and disability rather than on the disorder per se, and so it is a useful schema for thinking about health outcomes (World Health Organization, 2002).

FIGURE 8–3
Assessment of Aphasia and Adult Language Disorders Using the World Health Organization's International Classification of Functioning, Disability and Health (ICF)

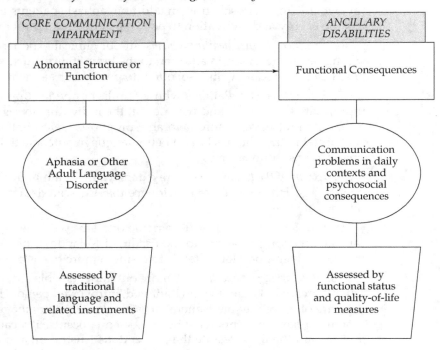

CONCLUSION AND SELF-ASSESSMENT

Throughout the chapter and its many tables we have mentioned various instruments for the functional assessment of communication. One's level of communication competence and the ability to participate in social activities are inextricably linked. In general, there is a direct relationship between a person's quality of life and the severity of the persisting aphasia or other adult language disorder. One to 3 years after a stroke or brain episode, the person's quality of communication is related to the presence or severity of depression: the more severe the communication disorder, the more severe the depression. Holland and Thompson (1998) reviewed the literature on aphasia and concluded that treatment indeed improves both the quality and quantity of language as compared to if no treatment was received. The knowledge and skill of the SLP, however, are the foundation on which diagnosis, ongoing evaluation, and treatment are built. Information presented in this chapter therefore is consistent with ASHA's preferred practice patterns (American Speech-Language-Hearing Association, 2004b) wherein the SLP is expected to:

- Assess the individual's underlying strengths and deficits related to spoken and written language factors.
- Appraise the effects of the language disorder on the individual's activities and participation in ideal settings and in everyday contexts.
- Explore contextual factors that serve as barriers to or facilitators of successful communication and participation.

After reading this chapter you should be able to answer the following questions:

1. What is aphasia? Differentiate some of the various types by name and by presenting features.

2. What is anomia (a common problem in various adult language disorders)? How might an SLP assess the utility of facilitating strategies?

3. Explain some of the subtle communication issues following a right (nondominant) hemisphere stroke.

4. Explain how an SLP might assist a patient with dementia at various stages of cognitive decline.

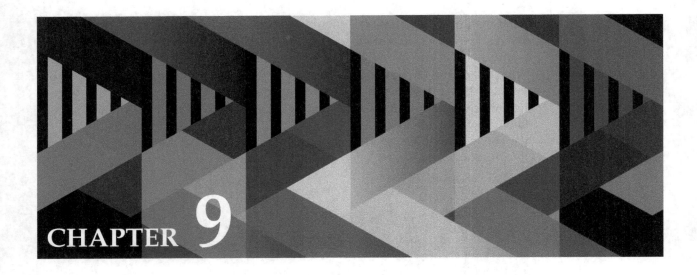

CHAPTER 9

Motor Speech Disorders

LEARNING OUTCOMES

After reading this chapter you will be able to:

1. Cite typical causes of motor speech disorders (dysarthrias and apraxias).
2. Name and describe the types of dysarthria.
3. Differentiate symptoms of adult dysarthria and apraxia of speech.
4. Describe characteristics of childhood apraxia of speech as distinct from articulation disorders.
5. Explain important motor speech characteristics to assess in a patient for both differential diagnosis and for setting intervention goals.

Motor speech disorders is an umbrella term that includes many diverse, neurologically based problems. Those that may come to mind first are the many adult dysarthrias. The cerebral palsies originate in infancy, and the speech impairment that may coexist with the movement disorder is also considered dysarthria. (Neuromuscular difficulties also may result in feeding and swallowing disorders; these will be covered in Chapter 10.) Then there are the apraxias that may affect various parts of the body, in particular the control of oral muscles, leading to oral (nonverbal) apraxia or apraxia of speech (verbal apraxia). All in all, we have our work cut out for us in this chapter.

APRAXIA OF SPEECH IN ADULTS

The Greek word *praxis* means "action." The performance of action can go awry with damage to the central nervous system, and the resulting disruption of movement control can affect various body parts and abilities. Limb apraxia, constructional apraxia, and a myriad of apraxic conditions have been reported; we will focus our discussion on apraxia of speech in adults, with brief mention of its close cousin, oral (nonverbal) apraxia.

Cortical damage to the inferior-posterior region of the frontal lobe in the left (dominant) hemisphere can impair oral movements and speech production. This condition has been called by many names, but it is generally known as *apraxia of speech* (AOS). Prevailing opinion, though not without controversy, and the perspective of this chapter is that apraxia is a nonlinguistic speech disorder. It can coexist with other disorders, and it is frequently observed in concert with aphasia and/or dysarthria. The differential diagnosis of a patient's motor speech deficit is important in shaping the appropriate management program. This view of AOS as a motor planning and control disorder is reflected in its definition provided by McNeil, Robin, and Schmidt (2009):

> Apraxia of speech is a phonetic-motor disorder of speech production caused by inefficiencies in the translation of a well-formed and filled phonological frame to previously learned kinematic parameters assembled for carrying out the intended movement, resulting in intra- and interarticulatory temporal and spatial segmental and prosodic distortions. (p. 264)

The Characteristics of Adult Apraxia of Speech

The hallmark of AOS in a patient is articulatory groping and searching for articulator placements. Speech output may sound struggled, even stuttering-like, or speech may mimic errored word selection (saying something sounding like "chicken" when intending to say "kitchen"). Individual symptoms vary. The motor speech output may well be a distortion rather than a pure articulatory substitution. This needs to be remembered, even when most writings about apraxia of speech differentially diagnose it from dysarthria on the basis of articulatory distortion. Our overview suffers this fate as well, but it is an acceptable way to learn about both of these motor speech disorders. Another hallmark of apraxia of speech is the impact on volitional productions of articulation and prosody. These articulation and prosodic disturbances do not result from muscle weakness or slowness (as in dysarthria) but from inhibition or impairment of the central nervous system's programming of oral movements. Auditory comprehension, in pure cases of apraxia, is relatively unaffected. Probably for this reason, most individuals with apraxia of speech have good monitoring skills and are aware of, even frustrated by, their motor speech attempts. The most frequent speech symptoms associated with acquired apraxia of speech in adults are (in no particular order):

1. Perceived substitutions and distortions
2. Perceived omissions and additions
3. Effortful articulation
4. Trial-and-error groping
5. Slow speech
6. Difficulty imitating
7. Excess and equal stress; aberrant prosody
8. Part-word repetitions
9. More errors on polysyllabic words
10. Inconsistent errors
11. Islands of error-free speech
12. Nonverbal in severe cases

This consensus list is a prelude of assessment indicators for the speech-language pathologist (SLP) to monitor (Duffy 2013; Yorkston, Beukelman, Stand, & Hakel, 2010). Oral, nonverbal apraxia can be described as problems in making volitional oral movements in the absence of significant paralysis or paresis. For example, the patient may have great difficulty when asked by the clinician to pucker his or her lips but may have no difficulty kissing his or her spouse as they part for the day. Apraxia of speech and this oral, nonverbal form of apraxia may coexist or may occur independently of each other.

Case History Oral Exam and Prognostic Factors

As with any evaluation, we collect case history information on the patient suspected of having apraxia of speech. Rarely do we know ahead of time that we are going to evaluate a patient with apraxia. More often than not, we are asked to evaluate a patient who sustained brain damage, and a language assessment is of foremost importance. During the testing for aphasia, we may become aware of some motor speech impairment and test further to diagnose the specific nature and extent of the impairment. Appendix A is a resource for examining the oral peripheral mechanism; Appendix B includes standard reading passages for clinical use. The Motor Speech Evaluation template from the American Speech-Language-Hearing Association (ASHA) can be found online (www.asha.org/).

Case history information, marital status, place of residence, social networks, and the like, may influence treatment. Prognostic significance has been attributed to some biographical data, such as age, education, premorbid handedness, occupational status at onset and highest occupational level achieved, and premorbid education level and intelligence.

Medical information helpful in making a differential diagnosis includes evidence of localized damage to the third frontal convolution and the presence of right hemiplegia. Medical data suggestive of a favorable prognosis are damage from a single episode (no previous history of brain damage), a small lesion confined to Broca's area, recent onset, and absence of coexisting medical or health problems.

The Evaluation of Apraxia

As mentioned, seldom do we know ahead of time that a patient is apraxic. The speech-language referral merely mentions a brain-damaged adult (e.g., degenerative disease, cerebrovascular accident [CVA]/stroke, tumor, trauma), so a multitude of coexisting problems *could* be present: aphasia, intellectual impairment, dysarthria, apraxia, and other possibilities. The job of the SLP is to evaluate the patient thoroughly to identify problem areas as well as strengths. In this way, a diagnosis will be based on the patient's characteristics. The clinician should plan a battery of measures but maintain flexibility so that as the patient's performance unfolds, planned tests can be altered, and additional items can be added to the battery. A typical starting point is elicitation of a spontaneous speech sample and the administration of an aphasia test (see Chapter 8 for possibilities). As hints of motor problems emerge in the patient's speech attempts, the clinician alters testing plans to investigate in detail the possibility of a motor disorder. Both formal and informal measures can be used. Table 9–1 lists areas to include in a thorough evaluation. Diagnostic questions should unfold in the mind of the clinician: Is there a clinically significant motor speech problem? If so, is it an apraxia or a dysarthria? Which type of apraxia does the patient have? Does the patient have mixed types of apraxia? Which kind of dysarthria is present? Are coexisting motor disorders present?

TABLE 9–1
Typical Assessment Battery for the Evaluation of Adult Apraxia of Speech

Aphasia test	Cognition, intelligence, memory tests, as needed
Apraxia battery	Oral peripheral examination
Articulation test	Spontaneous and reading speech samples
Specialized tasks (count, repeat, increase word length)	

Several of the aphasia tests evaluate the articulatory agility, melodic line, phonemic difficulties, and oral-nonverbal skills of patients. The inclusion of a word fluency test is good. The Boston Diagnostic Aphasia Examination (Goodglass, Kaplan, & Barresi, 2000) and the Western Aphasia Battery (Kertesz, 2006) are examples. A spontaneous speech sample should be analyzed, and an articulation test may be given as well. Of extreme importance is the oral-motor examination. The general oral peripheral examination is supplemented with motor and articulatory tasks to reveal volitional programming deficits. Such tasks or tests should address oral-nonverbal apraxia and apraxia of speech.

Let us now walk through this evaluation process as it relates to apraxia. Although several so-called tests of apraxia exist, few have adequate psychometric properties and normative data. Therefore, these tools should be considered informal yet insightful rather than as formal, standardized tests. Some tests available for evaluating apraxia of speech are listed in Table 9–2. Let us highlight the components of a few.

Early, modern attempts to evaluate oral and limb apraxia assessed rudimentary skills with instructions such as these: "Stick out your tongue," "Whistle," "Show how you would kiss someone," and the like. Groundbreaking work at the Mayo Clinic in the 1970s advanced the understanding of all motor speech disorders, yet assessment was refined very little. Duffy (2013) continues this Mayo Clinic tradition of expanding our clinical understanding of intervention with motor speech discords. Several forms attributed to the Mayo Clinic can be found on social media by searching for the Neurologic Speech and Language Examination (motor speech exam), Assessment of Apraxia of Speech, Assessment of Non-Verbal Oral Apraxia, and the Rating Scale Form for Deviant Speech Characteristics.

Over the years, many research clinicians published informal test protocols for apraxia of speech with rudimentary scoring procedures without norms. Patients were instructed to say lengthening words and phrases to stress the articulatory system. Now-famous assessment stimuli of increasing word length included "gingerbread," "statistical analysis," and "zip–zipper–zippering." Some also included tasks of vowel prolongation and imitation of syllable sequences, as well as the production of words and phrases. Responses were scored and analyzed for phonemic and prosodic errors. Informal testing for apraxia of speech using these classic stimuli is still done by many speech-language pathologists. Commercially available instruments include similar stimuli and are making strides at standardization.

Dabul (2000) designed the popular Apraxia Battery for Adults (ABA-2) to measure AOS and to rate its severity. Apraxia of speech is an acquired condition following brain damage in a specific area, so it is worth noting that the ABA-2 is reported to be useful with adolescents and adults. The battery includes six subtests: diadochokinetic rate, increasing word length, limb apraxia and oral apraxia, latency time and utterance time for polysyllabic words, repeated trials, and an inventory of articulation characteristics of apraxia. Various of methods are used to score these subtests; scores are then used to complete a checklist of apraxia features and to rate the severity on a Level of Impairment Profile. The Quick Assessment for Apraxia of Speech (Tanner & Culbertson, 1999)

TABLE 9–2
Differential Diagnosis of Dysarthria and Adult Apraxia of Speech

	Dysarthria	Apraxia
Definition	There are distinct patterns of speech resulting from weakness, slowness, and uncoordination of speech muscles. Oral movements are disrupted and reflect different types of neuropathology.	There are articulation errors in the absence of muscle slowness, weakness, and uncoordination resulting from disruption of cortical programming for the *voluntary* production of speech sounds.
Oral peripheral examination	There is obvious defectiveness: slow, weak, and uncoordinated. *Vegetative* functions (sucking, chewing), as well as speech movements, are disturbed.	There is no obvious dysfunction except when person is asked to execute *voluntary* movements. Vegetative functions are performed adequately.
Articulation	There is simplification: a. Distortions b. Substitutions Errors are consistent. More complex units (clusters of consonants) are more difficult. There are more errors in final position. Errors are consistent with neurological record. Severity is related to extent of neuromuscular involvement.	Complications are: a. Transpositions, reversals b. Perseverative and anticipatory errors c. Fewer distortions, more substitutions, intrusive additions Errors increase proportionate to word weight (grammatical class, difficulty of initial consonant, position in sentence, and word length). There are fewer errors in spontaneous performance. Inconsistency is key sign.
Repeated utterance	Same performance obtained.	Person makes repeated attempts and may achieve correct performance. Person appears to grope or struggle for correct production.
Rate	There is deterioration of performance with increased rate. There is slow rate of speech.	Performance improves at faster rate. There are disturbances of prosody: stuttering-like struggle reactions; slow, labored speech during voluntary attempts.
Response to stimulation	Person may alter performance slightly to match auditory-visual model. Best response is demonstration of specific articulatory gestures.	Best performance obtained if person sees and hears model. Person does better if she or he is provided with one stimulation and given several chances to match the model.

is a 10-minute tool for determining the presence or absence of apraxia in adults. Detailed analysis of speech difficulties is lacking, however. The Motor Speech Evaluation (Wertz, LaPointe, & Rosenbek, 1984) is useful in detecting the presence of apraxia of speech or dysarthria and in rating the severity of the condition. The evaluation includes the following tasks: conversation, vowel prolongation, rapid alternating movements, repetition of multisyllabic words, repeated production of the same word, repetition of words that increase in length, repetition of monosyllabic words that begin and end with the same phoneme, repetition of sentences, counting forward and backward, picture description, and oral reading. Several methods of scoring are suggested by the authors; however, severity is rated on a scale of 1 to 7, with 1 being equivalent to mild and 7 equivalent to severe.

The Apraxia Battery for Adults (Dabul, 2000) and the Motor Speech Evaluation (Wertz, LaPointe, & Rosenbek, 1984) are probably the most widely used instruments for assessing apraxia of speech. Most SLPs supplement the diagnostic workup with a favorite test of articulation (see Chapter 6) and with other areas mentioned in Table 9–1. The novel reading passage "The Caterpillar" (Patel et al., 2013; see Appendix B) was designed for the assessment of motor speech disorders, such as apraxia. Among other features, it includes words of increasing length and complexity as well as prosodic emotional demands. In using evaluation tools to diagnose a patient, we need to remember the important maxim: A test does not make the decision; a clinician does. The clinician has a responsibility to evaluate and interpret the patient's efforts competently.

Differentiating Apraxia from Other Disorders

As we stated earlier, apraxia of speech often coexists with other disorders of communication. Differential diagnosis of the many components of a patient's problem is of paramount importance. Apraxia is often differentiated from aphasia on the basis of the patient's relatively normal auditory comprehension compared to oral expression difficulties. In actuality, this differentiation is clear-cut for some forms of aphasia but is quite muddled for others.

On occasion, patients with apraxia of speech have sufficient phrase length and grammatical form to appear somewhat fluent despite their prosodic and articulatory difficulties. Errors may mimic literal paraphasias. Table 9–3 summarizes symptoms that differentiate apraxia from fluent, conduction aphasia, as discussed by McNeil, Robin, and Schmidt (2008).

Apraxia is differentiated from the language of confusion and generalized intellectual deterioration on the basis of more intact orientation, memory, and learning abilities. The reader should refer to Table 8–5 in Chapter 8 for examples of cognitive tests that might be used to make such a differential diagnosis.

Apraxia is classically differentiated from dysarthria by the preponderance of phonemic substitutions compared to distortion errors and intact neuromuscular functioning, with the exception of facial weakness and hemiplegia. Current thinking is that this substitution-versus-distortion dichotomy is less straightforward than once thought; however, Table 9–2 provides information useful in making a differential diagnosis of dysarthria and apraxia of speech.

Patients with apraxia of speech can generally anticipate their errors and can also recognize them once made. Perhaps this explains, in part, the many retrials and false starts heard in the speech of those with apraxia. The effortful articulatory groping and repetitive attempts may, at times, be reminiscent of stuttering secondary behaviors. This raises the question of a relationship between neurogenic stuttering (see Chapter 7) and

TABLE 9–3
Differential Diagnosis of Conduction Aphasia and Apraxia

Conduction Aphasia	Apraxia
Repeated trials, attempts at self-correction	Groping, inconsistent trials
High proportion of sequencing errors	Low proportion of sequencing errors
Frequent and unpredictable substitutions	Frequent and predictable substitutions
Difficulty linked to planning load	Difficulty associated with word length
Intact prosody	Abnormal prosody
Easy speech initiation	Difficult, often struggled speech initiation
Association with posterior brain lesion	Association with anterior brain lesion

apraxia of speech. Although we do not know the nature of this relationship, if any, it is worth considering in making a differential diagnosis.

> Mr. Nils Elander was referred to the hospital-based speech-language pathologist for testing. Evidence from the neuroradiology department showed a left hemisphere thromboembolic infarct. Speech and language improvement was rapid during the 2 weeks postinfarct. A predischarge reevaluation was performed by the clinician. Mr. Elander presented with mild Broca's aphasia and a moderate coexisting apraxia of speech. Numerous techniques were tried on a trial-and-error basis to see what stimulation and assistance aided Mr. Elander in initiating difficult words that occurred randomly, as well as at the beginning of utterances. The clinician was able to refer Mr. Elander for outpatient treatment at another facility. The report forwarded to that facility included specific recommendations about the future direction of treatment. These recommendations included multimodality prestimulation, first phoneme cueing, and use of baton gestures or finger-tapping to impose rhythmical fluency.

CHILDHOOD APRAXIA OF SPEECH

Childhood apraxia of speech (CAS) is the preferred term for a perplexing disorder that previously was called developmental apraxia. Children with CAS typically have little or no intelligible speech. The hallmarks of this disorder include not only a severe speech-sound disorder but also motoric (praxis) deficits. Childhood apraxia may seem to have core motor speech impairments in common with adults who have apraxia of speech, yet these are distinct disorders. The key difference seems to be that the motor programming deficits are not acquired; rather, they are present from infancy and affect linguistic processing as well as phonological development. Emerging information on CAS points to genetic and/or neurological underpinnings—even relationships to food allergies. This had led some researchers to think of childhood apraxia of speech as a syndrome of issues in much the same manner as is current thinking on attention deficit disorders and autism spectrum disorders (ADVANCE, 2010).

ASHA's ad hoc committee on childhood apraxia of speech (American Speech-Language-Hearing Association, 2007) offers the following working definition of CAS:

> Childhood apraxia of speech is a neurological childhood (pediatric) speech sound disorder in which the precision and consistency of movements underlying speech are impaired in the absence of neuromuscular deficits (e.g., abnormal reflexes, abnormal tone). CAS may occur as a result of known neurological impairment, in association with complex neurobehavioral disorders of known or unknown origin, or as an idiopathic neurogenic speech sound disorder. The core impairment in planning and/or programming spatiotemporal parameters of movement sequences results in errors in speech sound production and prosody. (p. 6)

The ad hoc committee further states that there is no valid list of diagnostic features that comprise childhood apraxia of speech. Though recent strides in our dynamic assessment abilities have been made, differentiation of CAS from some childhood dysarthrias and/or severe cases of articulation/phonological disorders (presumably in the absence of programming deficits) remain problematic.

Differential Diagnosis

There is a growing consensus about the presence of three cardinal features in childhood apraxia of speech. According to the American Speech-Language-Hearing Association (2007), these three cardinal features are:

1. Inconsistent errors on repeated productions of consonants and vowels in syllables and words
2. Lengthened and disrupted coarticulations between sounds and syllables
3. Inappropriate prosody

A host of other symptoms can characterize childhood apraxia of speech and signal pervasive problems in speech, expressive language, and phonological foundations of literacy. There may be early signs as to the possible need for augmentative and alternative communication as well.

Classic information provided by Yoss and Darley (1974) remains helpful in recognizing childhood apraxia of speech compared to other forms of defective articulation. These predictors are as follows:

1. Neurologic findings, such as difficulty in fine motor coordination, gait, and alternating motion rates of the tongue and extremities (often manifested as a generalized dyspraxia)
2. Two- and three-feature articulation errors (for example, /p/ for /ð/ involves an error in place, voicing, and continuancy), prolongations and repetitions of sounds and syllables, distortions, and additions in repeated speech tasks
3. Distortions, omissions, additions, and one-place errors in spontaneous speech
4. Slower-than-normal rate on measurements of oral diadochokinesis
5. Poor maintenance of syllable sequences and shapes; polysyllabic words altered by addition, omission, or revision of syllables

Crary (1988) elaborates on the symptomatology, stating that children with apraxia exhibit slow and irregular alternating motion rates (diadochokinesis). They possess a reduced sound inventory, including vowels, and have obvious prosodic deficits, including slow rate, excess stress, prolonged sounds and pauses, postural/articulatory groping, and unusual intonational contours.

Other authors have cited nasal resonance and nasal emission as characteristics of developmental apraxia of speech (Hall, Hardy, & LaVelle, 1990). Presumably, the velopharyngeal mechanism performs inadequately during complex, rapid, sequential speech. Nasality, then, is more pronounced with conversational speech compared to single-word utterances.

In the diagnostic session of a child with the potential of CAS, the speech-language pathologist should determine, to the extent possible, the child's etiological factors through a case history and should thoroughly assess the child's oral-motor development, speech, language, and prosody so that the presence or absence of CAS signs and markers can be determined.

Case History Indicators

Square and Weidner (1981) reviewed case history information from parents of clients diagnosed with childhood apraxia and found commonalities. Parents reported that auditory responses of the infants seemed normal but that early vocal patterns were suspect. The parents reported that little, if any, babbling occurred. If babbling was done by the infant, parents expressed that its phonetic pattern was undifferentiated. The infant was often described as a quiet baby. Feeding differences were also reported by the mothers. Babies were said to prefer liquids and soft foods. Some were described as lazy chewers. With regard to general motor development, reports suggest clumsiness, developmental immaturity, and possible soft neurological signs. When these children were toddlers, there remained little or no attempt to imitate sounds or words.

From this we can conclude that in a case history interview, the SLP must inquire about the child's health (and hopefully results from neurological testing), history of infant babbling, prosodic patterns of early vocalizations (see Appendix B for developmental milestones), a description of the infant's temperament (quiet versus fussy), and history of any feeding difficulties (covered in Chapter 10). These sorts of historical questions are repeated in the interview to collect the current status of the child. A full description of the child's speech, prosody, language, cognitive status, and general motor coordination (speech and nonspeech) are in order. This is the type of child that can benefit from an interdisciplinary team approach. Certainly, input from a neurologist, neuropsychologist, and speech-language pathologist is at the core of a diagnostic workup. Additional questions regarding motor coordination, health and neurological issues, and any chewing or eating concerns (and the textures and types of food the child prefers) need to be raised. Some commercially available CAS assessment instruments provide case history suggestions as well.

Assessing Childhood Apraxia

Recognizing the ill-defined nature of childhood apraxia of speech, it is not surprising that the assessment of CAS is a process of excluding other disorders and including, or identifying, apraxic signs and symptoms. The medical evaluation seeks to exclude other causes of the motor impairment, such as neoplastic disease, degenerative conditions, cerebral palsy, acquired central nervous system (CNS) damage, and the like. The neuropsychological evaluation excludes general intellectual deficits, autism (as does the SLP), and behavioral-emotional problems (however, it is recognized that behavioral problems are often a consequence of the child's apraxia). The primary sensorimotor evaluation excludes problems of muscular tone, strength, speed, and sensation. The SLP also should perform his or her own detailed oral motor examination (see Appendix A).

Instruments are commercially available for the SLP's communicative assessment, but the evidence on which most are based is still emerging. Examples include the Screening Test for Developmental Apraxia of Speech (Blakeley, 2001), which screens expressive language discrepancy, vowels and diphthongs, oral-motor movement, verbal sequencing, motorically complex words, articulation, transpositions, and prosody. A screening instrument, though, is not adequate for diagnostic assessment and for treatment planning. Crary (1988) and Square and Weidner (1981) suggest important areas for the SLP to tap in the assessment of childhood apraxia of speech. We have summarized these areas in Table 9–4; Table 9–5 lists some suggested nonspeech oral movements for the child to perform.

It is highly desired, however, that the SLP use diagnostic tests with standardized norms and indexes of reliability and validity. McCauley and Strand (2008) reviewed various diagnostic tests of childhood nonverbal oral and speech motor performance for psychometric properties and content characteristics. All examined tests were found to be in need of refinement; reliability measures were particularly lacking. However, we list a few of the well-known diagnostic tests for CAS in Table 9–6. But because of the

TABLE 9–4
Four Key Areas for Assessing Childhood Apraxia

Motor Assessment
Facial/limb praxis
Oral apraxia on simple and complex tasks
Lingua-mandibular and labial-mandibular synkinesis
Velar function
Oral reflexes
Facial mimicry tasks

Motor Speech Assessment
Diadochokinesis
Nasal resonance (and further tests, if noted)
Standard articulation tests
Phonological analysis (distinctive features and phonological error processes)

Prosody Assessment
Stress patterns
Intonation patterns
General fluency and articulatory flow

Language Assessment(s)
Auditory memory assessment

TABLE 9–5
Instructions for Nonspeech Tasks for Assessing Childhood Apraxia

Volitional Oral Movements
Stick out your tongue.
Try to touch your nose with your tongue.
Try to touch your chin with your tongue.
Bite your lower lip.
Pucker your lips.
Puff out your cheeks.
Show me your teeth.
Click your teeth together.
Wag your tongue from side to side.
Clear your throat.
Cough.
Whistle.
Show me that you're cold by making your teeth chatter.
Smile.
Show me how you would kiss a baby.
Lick your lips.

Sequenced Volitional Oral Movements: Two Items
Puff your cheeks, then smile.
Pucker your lips, then wag your tongue.

Sequenced Volitional Oral Movements: Three Items
Puff out your cheeks, show me your teeth, then pucker your lips.

complex and multifactorial nature of childhood apraxia of speech, we caution SLPs that no single test score should be used to diagnose childhood apraxia of speech. The decision rests with information from an entire team of professionals and with the skills of an experienced clinician. Only then can the overdiagnosis of CAS be curtailed (American Speech-Language-Hearing Association, 2007).

TABLE 9–6
Some Diagnostic Tests for Childhood Apraxia of Speech

Dynamic Evaluation of Motor Speech Skills (DEMSS) (Strand et al., 2013):
ages 36 to 79 months
Marshalla Oral Sensorimotor Test (MOST) (Marshalla, 2008):
ages 4:6 to 7:11 years
Nuffield Center Dyspraxia Programme, Third Edition (NDP3) (Nuffield Speech and Hearing
Center, 2004): ages 3 to 7 years
Preschool Motor Speech Evaluation and Intervention (Earnest, 2001):
ages 18 to 60 months
*Verbal Dyspraxia Profile (*Jelm, 2001):
ages birth to 2 years
Screening Test for Developmental Apraxia of Speech, Second Edition (STDAS-2) (Blakely,
2000): ages 4 to 12 years
Verbal Motor Production Assessment for Children (VMPAC) (Hayden & Square, 1999):
ages 3 to 12 years
The Apraxia Profile (Hickman, 1997):
ages 3 to 13 years
Kaufman Speech Praxia Test for Children (KSPT) (Kaufman, 1995):
ages 2 to 6 years

In this regard, a newer research/clinical tool shows great promise. The Dynamic Evaluation of Motor Speech Skills (DEMSS) is proving to be reliable and valid, and it does not overdiagnose CAS (Strand et al., 2013). The DEMSS is recommended for use with children who exhibit severe phonological impairment and severe motor deficits. In other words, it is the instrument of choice for cases of suspected childhood apraxia. The DEMSS uses dynamic assessment in which multiple attempts are elicited from the child for scoring, as the SLP provides cueing or other strategies (e.g., slower rate, simultaneous production) to facilitate the child's performance. The DEMSS uses a point values scoring system and rates four areas: overall articulation, vowel accuracy, prosody accuracy, and consistency. Before closing this topic, we also wish to cite a valid and reliable subjective measure of articulatory intelligibility useful in CAS, the Intelligibility in Context Scale (McLeod, Harrison, & McCormack, 2012).

THE ADULT DYSARTHRIAS

Dysarthria, or more accurately the dysarthrias, is a collection of motor speech disorders due to neurological abnormalities in strength, speed, range of motion, steadiness, tone, or accuracy of movement (Duffy, 2013). Dysarthria, particularly in adults and adolescents, may be due to trauma (e.g., automobile wreck, stroke, gunshot or blast explosion to the head, near poisoning) or disease state (e.g., muscular dystrophy, myasthenia gravis, tumor invasion, multiple sclerosis, encephalitis, inherited degenerative disorders, etc.). The same issues may occur in children; in addition, cerebral palsy from infancy is a typical cause of dysarthria. Regardless of the cause or age of onset, damage or disease can affect the neuromotor system and the processes of respiration, phonation, articulation, and resonation (not to mention feeding and swallowing, which will be covered in Chapter 10). More specifically for our purposes, the dysarthrias are neuromuscular speech disorders arising from motor pathway damage at single or multiple sites from the cortex to the muscle. The entire speech production mechanism, including respiratory, phonatory, articulatory, and resonatory processes, may be affected (as in Parkinson's disease). Likewise, disruption may be confined to specific musculature (as in Bell's palsy of the face).

Differential Diagnosis

The subfield of dysarthrias of speech was advanced greatly by researcher-clinicians at the Mayo Clinic in the 1970s. This tradition continues in the writings of Duffy (2013) and others (Freed, 2012; Yorkston et al., 2010). Novice clinicians often have difficulty differentiating the two motor speech disorders: apraxia of speech and dysarthria. The underlying neuromotor impairment is clearly different, and site of lesion knowledge will go far in sorting out the two possibilities. Relying only on clinical (behavioral) signs that the patient displays does not make the diagnosis nearly as clear-cut, as many textbooks imply. Review Table 9–3, which lists distinguishing characteristics of patients with apraxia of speech and dysarthria. Complicating the differential diagnosis is the fact that the two disorders can co-occur.

Differential diagnosing also involves categorizing the patient's symptoms by type of dysarthria. Again, this often proves to be a difficult task for many clinicians, not just the novice student. The type of dysarthria demonstrated depends on the site of the lesion within the motor pathways. The landmark investigation that delineated the types of dysarthria, prominent speech dimensions, and neurological disruption was conducted at the Mayo Clinic in the 1970s. This expertise continues through the writings of Duffy (2013). An understanding of the types of dysarthria is paramount to the assessment process and the differential diagnosis. We present a synopsis of the characteristics of each type of dysarthria, but we are assuming that the reader has an understanding of the nervous system and neuroanatomical terminology. In addition to Duffy's other texts on motor speech disorders, we recommend those by Freed (2012), Love (2000), and Yorkston et al. (2010).

Flaccid Dysarthria

Flaccid dysarthrias result from disorders (or lesions) of the lower motor neuron system. The muscle-movement problem may be progressive, as in myasthenia gravis, or it may affect the bulbar motor units, as in the bulbar palsies. In bulbar palsy, a common form of flaccid dysarthria, the muscles are weak, hypotonic (flaccid), and hyporeflexive and may be atrophied. Spontaneous twitches or dimpling of the skin over the muscle may be noted (fasciculations and fibrillations). Often the bulbar palsy is due to damage of one cranial nerve, and the muscular problems are confined to the body region or group of muscles served by that nerve. For example, in facial palsy (also known as Bell's palsy), the damage to one of the facial nerves (cranial nerve VII) results in a drooping facial expression, inability to raise the corner of the mouth during a smile, infrequent blinking, lowering of the eyebrow, and inability to wrinkle the forehead on the affected side. In hypoglossal palsy, there is damage to cranial nerve XII, and the tongue becomes flabby, atrophied, shrunken, and wrinkled. The client is unable to perform many of the tongue maneuvers asked during the oral peripheral examination. Damage may be due to multiple cranial nerve involvement as well. This type of flaccid dysarthria is known as generalized bulbar palsy. It would not be uncommon in this condition for the lips, tongue, jaw, velum, pharynx, and larynx to be affected to varying degrees.

Speech abnormalities that are often observed in the bulbar palsies include hypernasality, imprecise articulation of consonants, breathiness, monopitch, and nasal emission. Other characteristics are certainly seen in these patients. We have only attempted to highlight some of the most prominent.

Spastic Dysarthria

Spastic dysarthrias result from disorders of the upper motor neuron system—in particular, the pyramidal system. As a result, there can be whole extremity damage (as in cortical lesions) or generalized damage (as from lesions of the internal capsule). The damage may be unilateral, as is often seen following a stroke where the patient has aphasia and hemiparesis, or the damage may be bilateral. If it is bilateral, we often use the classification *pseudobulbar palsy* because the bulbar system is affected indirectly. Muscular symptoms include spasticity, weakness, limited range of motion, slowness of movement, and hyperreflexia.

Deviant speech dimensions include imprecise consonant articulation, monopitch, reduced stress, harsh voice quality, monoloudness, low-pitched voice, and slow speech rates. Again, we have attempted to list only some of the more prominent and severe symptoms.

Ataxic Dysarthria

Disease or damage to the cerebellum can result in ataxic dysarthria. In ataxia, there is inaccuracy of movement (affecting force, range, timing, and direction of movements), slowness of movement, and hypotonia (flabby muscles). Speech characteristics include imprecise consonant articulation, use of excess and equal stress patterns, and irregular articulatory breakdowns, among others.

Hypokinetic Dysarthria

Disorders of the extrapyramidal system, such as in the basal ganglia complex, often result in hypokinesia, a reduction of movement. A commonly encountered disease causing hypokinesia is Parkinson. There seem to be six characteristic signs of hypokinetic dysarthria: (1) slowness of movement; (2) limited range of motion; (3) paucity of movement, where the patient may have difficulty initiating a movement and may experience false starts, arrests of movement, or even immobility; (4) rigidity or hypertonicity (may be intermittent); (5) loss of automatic aspects of movement; and (6) presence of rest tremors. Deviant speech dimensions often seen in patients with Parkinson highlight the movement difficulties of the hypokinetic dysarthrias. The most deviant are monopitch, reduced stress patterns, monoloudness, imprecise consonant articulation, inappropriate silences, and short rushes of speech. Other, less deviant characteristics exist as well. We highlight Parkinson because this progressive disease occurs in 1% of the population over age 60. However, Parkinson is underserved by SLPs despite its impact on cognition, communication, speech, voice, swallowing, and more. The ASHA portal on Parkinson disease also is a good source of assessment issues (search www.asha.org).

Hyperkinetic Dysarthrias

Hyperkinetic dysarthrias result from disorders of the extrapyramidal system. The hallmark of these disorders is the presence of abnormal involuntary movements—some are quick movements and others are classified as slow. In the short space we have in this text, we cannot describe completely the numerous forms of both quick and slow hyperkinesias. The interested reader is urged to study further; however, we do summarize some of the most distinguishing and deviant speech characteristics, averaged over the various subtypes, including imprecise consonants, variable (or perhaps slow) rate, monopitch, harsh or strained voice quality, inappropriate silences, distorted vowels, and excess loudness variation.

Mixed Dysarthrias

Mixed dysarthrias, as the name implies, result from involvement of several motor systems. Mixed dysarthrias are often associated with syndromes or particular diseases, such as amyotrophic lateral sclerosis (ALS), multiple sclerosis, and Wilson disease. Because of the mixed nature of these dysarthrias, it is almost impossible to summarize characteristic speech disturbances. We highlight ALS, which is also known as Lou Gehrig's disease, given the public awareness of this progressive and devastating motor neuron disease. The brilliant physicist Stephen Hawking continues his research in spite of suffering from ALS, which has stripped him of motor muscle abilities and makes him dependent on computer-generated speech and a wheelchair for locomotion. A good review of dysarthria in ALS, with mention of some dedicated ALS assessment scales, is by Tomik and Guiloff (2010). The ASHA portal on ALS is also a good source of assessment issues (search www.asha.org).

The Appraisal of Dysarthria

As evident from the various speech characteristics associated with the types of dysarthria, the patient may have difficulty with any or all of the speech production processes. Consequently, the clinician must assess features of respiration, phonation, articulation, and resonation. Such an appraisal follows along the lines of the oral peripheral examination (discussed in Appendix A) and focuses also on themes discussed in Chapters 11 and 12, on voice disorders and resonance disorders, respectively. While articulation/phonology testing (see Chapter 6) augments specialized motor speech testing described here, we also remind the reader that Appendix B provides some adult (and child grade-level) reading passages that help unmask issues of resonance, articulatory imprecision and slurring, intelligibility, performance declines with repeated readings, and such. Let us elaborate on a few aspects of assessing adult dysarthria.

As with apraxia of speech, the hallmarks of the motor speech dysarthrias can best be elicited and observed through a motor speech examination. We recommend the Motor Speech Evaluation template, which is available online from ASHA (search www.asha.org). Another motor speech exam worthy of special mention is the Neurological Speech and Language Examination that is attributed to the Mayo Clinic and found on social media, as mentioned earlier. Also at this site are forms to help the clinician differentiate apraxia of speech from dysarthria, and a scale to help rate the deviancy of speech characteristics (in pitch, loudness, voice quality, resonance, intelligibility, bizarreness, respiration, prosody articulation, and other attributes such as alternating motion rates [AMRs]). Methodically evaluating such a variety of speech characteristics is essential not only for diagnosing the presence of dysarthria but also for discovering *which* dysarthria (together with case history information and various medical tests, of course).

Suffice it to say that we need to take note of any inhalatory noises, poor breath support, poor management of the air stream, abnormal vocal loudness and stress patterns, abnormal vocal pitch and inflectional patterns, and abnormal vocal-resonatory qualities. Of particular interest is analysis of the sustained phonation during the "ah." With proper instrumentation, detection of irregularities in shimmer and jitter may be quite suggestive. Tanner (2001) notes that progressive neurological diseases, such as ALS, multiple sclerosis, and Parkinson, can be detected early and monitored through minor changes in voice irregularities. Respiratory and/or phonatory dysfunction is often a hallmark of speech dysarthria, an area for perceptual and instrumental assessment, and a focus in behavioral management. A systematic review of evidence-based practice for respiration and/or phonation dysfunction is provided by Yorkston, Spencer, and Duffy (2003).

Regarding the articulatory impairment that is often present in the dysarthrias, the clinician should analyze a sample of spontaneous speech and/or have the patient read aloud. Standard articulation tests, either single-word or sentence versions, are also useful in documenting phoneme errors. Standard reading passages, such as "My Grandfather," are commonly used in clinical assessment of motor speech in adults and older children (see Appendix B). Distortion is the most common articulatory error in dysarthric speech. Unlike the difficulties seen in apraxia of speech, the imprecision of consonantal articulation is fairly consistent in dysarthria. In essence, intelligibility is a key speech measure in the diagnosis and continuing evaluation of a person with dysarthria. The Quick Assessment for Dysarthria (Tanner & Culbertson, 1999) includes diagnostic questions and checklists for swiftly assessing respiration, phonation, articulation, resonance, and prosody. An evidence-based practice review of oral motor exercises is provided by McCauley, Strand, Lof, and Schooling (2009).

The Frenchay Dysarthria Assessment (FDA-2) (Enderby & Palmer, 2008) is a well-established tool for both clinical and research purposes, with norms for adolescents and adults (ages 12 to 97). The Frenchay profiles oral-motor performance for the various diagnostic categories, such as spastic–upper motor neuron, flaccid–lower motor neuron, extrapyramidal, cerebellar, and mixed neurological lesions. Clinicians may find this helpful in differential diagnosis decision making. Patient performances are rated on eight functions: reflexes, respiration, lips, palate, larynx, tongue, intelligibility, and other influencing factors.

The Assessment of Intelligibility of Dysarthric Speech (AIDS) is available commercially (Yorkston, Buekelman, & Traynor, 1984) and is also one of many dysarthria assessment tools described in the textbook by Yorkston et al. (2010). The AIDS has the patient read words and sentences. Several measures can be derived, including intelligibility for single words, intelligibility for sentences, speech rate, rate of intelligible speech, rate of unintelligible speech, and a communication efficiency ratio. Classification by type of dysarthria is also possible with this test. Also available from these authors is the Computerized Assessment of Intelligibility of Dysarthric Speech. The software provides for efficient quantifying of single-word intelligibility, sentence intelligibility, and speaking rates without tedious stimuli selection or computation.

The Dysarthria Examination Battery (DEB) (Drummond, 1993) evaluates responses to 23 tasks spanning the areas of respiration, phonation, resonance, articulation, and prosody. Responses are rated on a scale of 1 to 5. Administration of the DEB requires the use of a stopwatch, audio recorder, dry spirometer, laryngeal mirror, bite block, and a few other more standard items.

One diagnostic task that many authorities consider important is that of diadochokinetic (DDK) or alternating motion rate (AMR) testing (refer again to Appendix A and to the assessment tools already cited for this task). The rhythm and speed with which alternating motion rates can be performed are helpful in sorting out the various types of dysarthrias. Differential diagnosis may be difficult from only a conversational sample of speech. DDKs, on the other hand, seem to "stress" the motor system and thus reveal the difficulties of movement more clearly. The instructions to the patient should stress this notion of "fast and even." Information that is important to the clinician includes the rate, regularity, and duration of the alternate movements of the articulators. A slow, regular diadochokinetic rate is highlighted in spasticity. For ataxia, alternate motion rates underscore the irregular breakdowns in articulatory precision. It is characteristic to hear fluctuating changes in the intervals between syllables as well as variations in their duration and loudness. Rate of syllable production varies from normal to slow. In hypokinetic Parkinson, alternate motion rates may begin at a slow rate and then accelerate to a rapid yet usually regular rhythm. Imprecise articulation due to limited excursions of movement (i.e., hypokinesia) may produce the sound of a continuous blur. Hyperkinetic dysarthrias take on many different forms; AMRs are usually irregular, slow, and perhaps interrupted by arrests of speech.

We offer one final note about appraisal. The patient with dysarthria is not expected to have language, cognitive, intellectual, memory, or learning deficits unless such deficits are associated with the disease process that produced the dysarthria. The clinician should be alert to deficits in these areas, however, and should include appropriate language-cognitive tests in the assessment battery, if necessary.

CEREBRAL PALSIES AND DYSARTHRIA IN CHILDREN

Brain damage sustained before, during, or shortly after birth can produce movement disorders known as *cerebral palsies* (CPs). Movement can be mildly affected or severely limited. When the muscles underlying speech are affected, we may say that the person has dysarthria (a motor speech disorder) subsequent to the cerebral palsy. Cerebral palsy is a static encephalopathy, meaning it does not worsen by spreading or degenerating. The causes of CP may include anoxia (lack of oxygen to the brain at any time), trauma during delivery, faulty genetics, maternal infection, infectious disease during early childhood, and a traumatic injury during childhood.

Although various classification systems for cerebral palsy have been proposed through the years, most typical is to classify CP according to both distribution and type. Terms describing distribution include the following:

- *Hemiplegia* is the most common form of distribution; an arm and leg (and perhaps speech muscles) on the same side of the body are affected but not necessarily to the same degree.
- *Paraplegia* is where both legs are affected (the speech muscles are not affected unless in the torso/respiratory area).
- *Quadriplegia* results from widespread brain damage where both arms and legs (and probably many speech muscles as well) are affected.

Often the types of cerebral palsy are classified into six principal symptoms:

1. Spasticity is characterized by hyperactivity of the stretch reflex. It is secondary to a lesion in the cerebral cortex and causes a loss of control and differentiation of fine voluntary movements with increased muscle tone.

2. Athetosis is involuntary writhing or squirming movements that are irregular, coarse, relatively continuous, and somewhat rhythmic. It is secondary to damage in the extrapyramidal system, often the basal ganglia complex.

3. Cerebellar ataxia is lack of coordination and poor balance owing to cerebellar dysfunction.

4. Rigidity is a "lead pipe" characteristic of affected muscles and often resembles a severe form of spasticity.

5. Tremors, either athetoid or rigid, involve generalized trembling of the extremities.

6. Flaccidity, as a form of cerebral palsy, is due to damage to the sensorimotor cortex. Affected muscles are unable to contract except reflexively.

Perhaps 90% of the cases of cerebral palsy are of the first three types, with spasticity overwhelmingly the most common.

The Assessment of a Child with Cerebral Palsy

All authorities on cerebral palsy strongly advocate the multidisciplinary approach to assessment, diagnosis, and intervention. From birth, it may be apparent that the infant with CP has a weak cry, respiratory issues, and sucking/feeding difficulties, or the neuromuscular impairments may unfold over the first year or so. Either way, the SLP will not assess motor function and abnormal reflexology without the aid of a neurologist, physical therapist, or other healthcare professional. Collaborative information is needed to shape the feeding and prespeech stimulation programs that the infant may need as well as the handling and positioning techniques that may facilitate optimal feeding, prespeech rehabilitation, and later speech-language intervention. The team working with a high-risk infant or pediatric patient with CP usually includes a pediatrician, neurologist, physical therapist, orthopedist, occupational therapist, speech-language pathologist, and possibly others, for example, nutritionists, orthopedic surgeon, otolaryngologists, and more. The child with cerebral palsy typically presents with a host of impairments—orthopedic, sensory-perceptual, cognitive, feeding, and swallowing (see Chapter 10), socioemotional, speech-voice-language, and so forth. Some early classification schema no doubt will be applied to the child, although this may evolve over time with growth and maturation (regardless of CP being a nonprogressive disorder). The Gross Motor Function Classification System (GMFCS) is a simplistic but commonly used five-level classification schema based on walking and gross-motor movements (Palisano et al., 1997). Of interest for the SLP is the assessment of communication skills and deficits. A review of the literature clearly documents that children with cerebral palsy (particularly the athesosis type) have higher auditory detection thresholds, poorer speech reception thresholds, and poorer speech discrimination than do typically functioning children. Thus, a complete audiological evaluation should be part of every evaluation session.

It is estimated that more than 50% of the CP population show some degree of cognitive impairment, while the rest possess typical intellectual capabilities. Impaired language development, learning difficulties, and academic problems often occur in children with cerebral palsy. Etiological reasons may be numerous. Certainly, the SLP must assess cognitive development and linguistic attainment in a CP client. Language assessment procedures discussed in Chapters 4 and 5 should be utilized.

Speech is a dynamic process requiring highly skilled coordination of the articulatory movements for the production and sequencing of sounds into utterances. It is of no surprise, then, that speech impairments are common among children with cerebral palsy. About 70% of CP children exhibit speech disorders; athetoid and ataxic forms seem to be particularly detrimental to speech. However, there appears to be insufficient evidence for the notion that these speech impairments are so distinctive as to justify the concept of *cerebral palsied speech*. This myth was laid to rest in Chapter 6 when we discussed articulatory and phonological speech disorders. The assessment tools discussed in that chapter are certainly applicable to the child with cerebral palsy. Respiration, phonation, and rhythm are likely to be affected as well and must be assessed by the clinician. The ultimate measure of speech effectiveness is its intelligibility; a severity rating scale may be part of the assessment battery. Last (although likely done first by the SLP in a diagnostic session), we remind the clinician that an oral peripheral (oral-motor) examination is of critical importance (see Appendix A as well as resources in Appendix B). The SLP may find the ASHA practice portal on assessment issues in CP a helpful resource (www.ncepmaps.org/Cerebral-Palsy-Assessment-Diagnosis.php). The SLP may also need to consider the need for augmentative or alternative communication.

ASSESSING AUGMENTATIVE AND ALTERNATIVE COMMUNICATION NEEDS

If a motor speech disorder precludes the production of serviceable speech—whether in an adult or a child—the SLP may need to consider the appropriateness of either augmenting the patient's meager communication method or training an alternative method of communication. The vast area of alternative and augmentative communication (AAC) strategies may be divided into unaided and aided types. In unaided strategies no external materials or equipment is used to assist the patient with communication. Examples of unaided AAC include gestures, body language, and formal or informal sign language. In contrast, aided communication systems require the use of tools or equipment to convey the message. Aided communication methods range from low-tech (such as paper-and-pencil writing or picture board to point at message ideas) to computerized high-tech speech-generating devices (SGDs). Electronic communication aids, in a variety of types, may allow a patient to use picture symbols, letters, and/or words and phrases to create messages. Some devices cost thousands of dollars; affordable tablet applications are increasingly available and no-cost picture, word, and letter communication boards and notebooks can still be made for free. The complex body of literature on AAC system options, assessment of patients for their use (and reevaluation of patient's changing needs over time), plus the training of patients and significant others in AAC use and troubleshooting is the subjects of many good books (Beukelman & Mirenda, 2013; McCurtin & Murray, 2000).

Likely candidates for using an AAC device include children with cerebral palsy but also children and adults with acquired disabilities. Permanent and stable etiologies might include spinal cord injuries, traumatic brain injuries, and cerebrovascular accidents; permanent but degenerative etiologies might include dementias, acquired immune deficiency syndrome (AIDS), and some of the diseases and associated dysarthrias covered in this chapter (e.g., amyotrophic lateral sclerosis, multiple sclerosis, Parkinson, Huntington Chorea, Fredrich ataxia). Clearly the motor speech dysfunction, bodily motor dysfunction, developmental age, and cognitive abilities of each patient are paramount in an SLP's assessment and system considerations. Some of our thoughts on this process include the following:

1. Assess current communication needs and uses. What is the patient's current method of communication and is it adequate? Grunting and gesturing one's needs may be serviceable in some environments, but a student in a classroom will need more communicative skill. An adult's level might span only basic needs to social interactions, to theoretical physics research (as with Dr. Stephen Hawking, who was mentioned earlier).

2. Assess cognitive and language abilities. Include language comprehension and production (vocabulary, grammar, etc.) but also spelling and writing mechanics.

3. Assess voice, speech, and intelligibility.

4. Understand the underlying etiology. If the condition is degenerative, should the communicative support begin at a minimum but increase over time (e.g., treatment strategies to improve intelligibility evolving to a dependence on a speech-generating device)? Even in stable, nonprogressive etiologies, the cognitive/educational needs of the patient may improve in sophistication (or decline), which means that the AAC methodology must be reevaluated periodically.

5. Assess full body motor abilities and limitations because this determines the device type and switch access. For example, can the patient type on a computer keyboard with coordination, or must the device be preprogrammed by the SLP or significant

other for patient activation with eye gaze scanning movements, a respiratory puff of air into an activation tube, or the like?

6. Keep current with the types of AAC devices, from low-tech to high-tech and everything in between. Stay abreast of funding and reimbursement issues (Kander & Satterfield, 2014). Gain expertise through conferences and colleagues who work in the subfield of AAC. This is a large and burgeoning technical field that cannot be learned in a day!

CONCLUSION AND SELF-ASSESSMENT

This chapter covered motor speech disorders, including the adult apraxias, childhood apraxia of speech, the adult dysarthrias, and the childhood dysarthrias affiliated with cerebral palsy. This chapter was also a logical place to mention the diagnostic assessment and periodic reevaluations of a patient with an augmentative or alternative system of communication; we have but scratched the surface of information available to the SLP. Yorkston et al. (2010) remind us that all clinicians can be guided in their decision-making processes by following a model of disablement for understanding the broad range of motor speech disorders. The World Health Organization's International Classification of Functioning, Disability and Health (ICF) model is a disablement model (World Health Organization, 2002). Figure 9–1 presents this model for the motor speech disorders discussed in this chapter.

FIGURE 9–1
Assessment of Motor Speech Disorders Using the World Health Organization's International Classification of Functioning, Disability and Health (ICF)

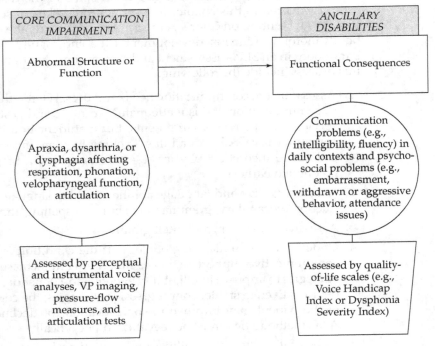

The American Speech-Language-Hearing Association (2004) preferred practice patterns for assessing motor speech are consistent with the framework provided by the World Health Organization, and are a concise conclusion to our chapter. They state that motor speech assessment is conducted to identify and describe:

- Underlying strengths and deficits related to structural and physiologic factors that affect motor speech and swallowing performance
- Effects of the motor speech (and swallowing disorder) on the client's activities, both capacities and performance, in everyday contexts
- Contextual factors that serve as barriers to or facilitators of successful communication (and swallowing) in individuals with motor speech disorders

After reading this chapter you should be able to answer the following questions:

1. In adults, differentiate apraxia of speech from the dysarthrias.
2. Name at least four types of speech dysarthria in adults, and include the neuroanatomical site underlying each.
3. Cite characteristics that differentiate childhood apraxia of speech from a typical articulation/phonology disorder.
4. What is cerebral palsy? Why might a child with CP need the services of an SLP?
5. What is AAC? Provide some examples.

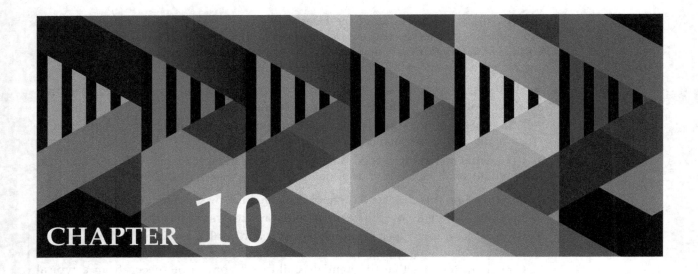

CHAPTER 10

Adult Dysphagia and Pediatric Feeding and Swallowing Disorders

LEARNING OUTCOMES

After reading this chapter you will be able to:

1. Explain aspiration and why it matters in adult and pediatric patients.

2. Describe events along the vocal tract that typically occur in each "phase" of the adult swallow.

3. Name two types of imaging studies used with swallowing and the advantages and limitations of each type.

4. Describe how to perform a "sip test" in an adult patient.

5. Name at least four medical disorders in infancy and childhood that are high probability for disorders of feeding and swallowing.

6. List at least eight questions to explore with a parent of a toddler wondering if his or her child has a feeding/swallowing disorder.

The role and scope of practice in speech-language pathology includes the burgeoning area of evaluation and treatment of swallowing disorders, or *dysphagia*. Clinicians tend to specialize their practice into adult or pediatric dysphagia based on employment setting. Disorders of dysphagia emerge as a consequence of many types of conditions, often medically related and potentially life-threatening. Newborn infants to older adults can have dysphagia, as will be seen in this chapter. Issues related to feeding, chewing, and swallowing also have social and psychological consequences no matter what the patient's age. The 15-minute dysphagia documentary with personal perspectives, available on YouTube, is recommended viewing for students and clinicians alike (www.youtube.com/watch?v=MrbEUDO6S5U).

Dysphagia includes many medical conditions and terms with which the speech-anguage pathologist (SLP) should become familiar. The American Speech-Language-Hearing Association (ASHA) offers a useful glossary online (go to www .asha.org and search for the dysphagia Glossary of Terms and Conditions for Infants). This chapter addresses diagnostic and evaluation issues for both adult and child. As a foundation for clinical insight, we begin with typical physiological events in nondisordered adults. A brief tutorial of a typical swallow that shows images from a modified barium swallow study can be viewed on YouTube at www.youtube.com/watch?v=xu_YYOAlZEw.

DEGLUTITION IN TYPICAL ADULTS

The purpose of *deglutition* (swallowing) is to transport food and other materials from the oral cavity to the stomach without allowing entry of substances into the airway. Safe swallowing entails precise coordination of neuromuscular events, including the brain, brainstem, cranial nerves, and the muscles of the oral cavity, pharynx, larynx, and esophagus.

Swallowing is considered a three-phase process by most authorities: the oral phase, the pharyngeal phase, and the esophageal phase. However, the first phase may be subdivided for clinical utility into the oral preparatory stage and the oral transit (or transport) stage. It is not uncommon, therefore, to describe four phases in the swallow.

The Oral Phase, Including Preparation and Transit

Feeding begins with the oral phase, specifically the oral preparation, which is under volitional control and so may be manipulated in a therapeutic regime. Oral preparation reduces food to a consistency appropriate for swallowing. Lips are closed to contain the food and saliva, the tongue manipulates the food in the mouth as muscles of mastication move the jaw in rotary and lateral maneuvers, the teeth tear and crush the morsels, and saliva is mixed with the mass of food, forming a cohesive *bolus*. Duration of oral preparation is highly variable, depending on the consistency of the food and the time spent tasting it. Oral preparation provides much of the pleasure from eating, and so it is an important psychological consideration when working with a patient with dysphagia. (Liquid diets, for the most part, bypass this pleasurable aspect.) The time devoted to this is highly variable and depends on food types and textures, muscle speech and strength, and desired amount of taste and pleasure.

Tension in the cheek muscles increases to prevent food particles from falling into the sulcus between the mandible and the cheeks. The velum is pulled anteriorly and rests against the back of the tongue to help keep food particles in the oral cavity. When readied, the bolus is manipulated by tongue muscles away from the front and center portions of the oral cavity and is compressed against the hard palate, pushing it in an up and back motion toward the posterior part of the oral cavity, near the faucial pillars (tonsil area). This oral transit stage comprises the second part of the oral phase, and it too is considered under volitional control primarily by way of the hypoglossal cranial nerve XII. The *swallowing reflex* is believed to be triggered by tongue action as the bolus passes the anterior faucial pillars, although little is understood of this elicitation. Triggering of the swallow is crucial to a safe swallow, but the importance of healthy tongue manipulation cannot be underestimated. Effective tongue manipulation sets the entire stage and keeps to a bare minimum any food dripping down into the pharynx prematurely, where it either comes to rest in the valleculae or pyriform sinus for another swallow attempt or, worse, aspiration into the lungs.

The Pharyngeal Phase

As the swallow is triggered, multiple, rapid, and sometimes concurrent pharyngeal responses last about 1 second. This fast duration is regardless of the person's age and gender, or the consistency of the food being swallowed. Events in the pharyngeal phase are automatic but can be influenced to some extent by behaviors of the swallower. Much is mediated by the glossopharyngeal (IXth) cranial nerve and the brainstem. In the pharyngeal phase, there is velopharyngeal closure to separate breathing from swallowing. This is aided by retraction of the tongue in an up and back direction and elevation of the velum itself. The larynx elevates and is pulled forward to tuck safely out of the line of the food trajectory, aided by the hyoid bone with its own elevation and anterior movement. Inversion of the epiglottis, bending back and down, also hovers over and reduces the laryngeal opening. Three sphincter actions also constrict the internal larynx and further provide protection to the airway entrance: the aryepiglottic folds constrict, the ventricular (false) folds approximate, and the true vocal folds adduct. Meanwhile, coordinated pharyngeal contraction—first the superior muscle fibers, then the middle constrictor, followed by lower constrictor muscles—create a "stripping wave" to propel the food bolus downward with the help of gravity.

Initiation of the Esophageal Phase

Relaxation of the muscles encircling the lower segment of the inferior pharyngeal constrictor muscle (e.g., cricopharyngeus fibers) and the top of the esophagus permits the bolus to enter the esophagus, on its way to the stomach and digestive tract. This area may be referred to as the pharyngeal-esophageal segment (PES) or the upper esophageal sphincter (UES). There is no volitional control of the esophageal phase, although its duration, from esophageal entry to the lower esophageal valve, may extend 8 to 20 seconds and often lengthens with age.

From this description of the many coordinated events that occur in a typical adult swallow, the astute reader will discern areas of behavioral assessment and variables to manipulate systematically in the evaluation and treatment of a person with dysphagia.

ADULT DYSPHAGIA: CAUSES AND ASSESSMENT GOALS

Dysphagia in adults can occur in the oral, pharyngeal, esophageal, or a combination of phases in the swallowing process. Often some medical event occurred or some condition developed in a previously typically functioning adult. Swallowing difficulties can emerge as a consequence of many neurologic conditions. In order of frequency, these conditions include stroke, traumatic brain injury, spinal cord injury, and tumors of the brain (Cherney, Pannelli, & Cantiere, 1994). Dysphagia can also result from progressive neurologic diseases (e.g., Parkinson, dementia, motor neuron disease), head and neck cancers or their treatment, vocal fold paralysis, various conditions of the upper aerodigestive tract, and more. Knowing the cause of dysphagia can shape the direction of assessment and intervention. For example, the SLP may approach a case of stroke-related dysphagia differently from a case of cancer-related dysphagia; research on evidence-based practice points to different outcomes. For additional information on adult dysphagia and its management, the interested reader is referred to books on the subject (Groher & Crary, 2010; Swigert, 2007).

When an SLP, as part of a medical team, approaches the assessment of an adult with suspected or known dysphagia, he or she should have certain goals in mind. Determine if the current oral manner of feeding is safe. Is there evidence of aspiration (food or liquid entering the airway and lungs; the sensation of a trickle usually triggers a cough to expel it) or of silent aspiration (food or liquid entering the airway without detection or protective action)? What are the risks? Can behavioral strategies and/or changes in food types and consistencies reduce the risks? In some cases, the assessment goal is to ascertain whether the patient can safely change from one feeding method (e.g., tube) to another (e.g., oral), and to what degree. The overarching, desired goal of a specialized assessment is to get the patient eating "something" quickly and safely. To attain these goals, the SLP begins with the collection of important, insightful information.

BEDSIDE, GENERAL, AND NONINSTRUMENTAL ASSESSMENT OF THE ADULT

The patient suspected of suffering from dysphagia warrants assessment and management by a team of medical professionals. Team members may include the physician (perhaps a laryngologist, gastroenterologist, and/or neurologist), radiologist, nurse, dietician, occupational therapist, pulmonologist/respiratory therapist, SLP, and others as warranted. The clinician's bedside evaluation of an adult in a hospital, or the initial assessment in a related setting, begins with the SLP's thorough review of the patient's medical chart. What were the presenting complaints and medical diagnoses? What has the physician noted? What insights about feeding and swallowing are in the notes from the nurse, dietician, and social worker? What is the current method of nutrition?

Screening or Testing of Communicative Abilities

Because of likely concurrent medical conditions, some causative and others not, the SLP will want to screen the adult with dysphagia for other communication issues. A **hearing screening** should be performed. In addition, the patient's **cognitive and receptive and expressive language skills** need either to be screened or tested in detail (recall Chapter 8). Because stroke is the leading cause of dysphagia in adults, a complete aphasia diagnostic evaluation may be necessary. The medical background (e.g., stroke, dementia, Parkinsonism, head injury, and so forth) may be a guide for determining cognitive and communicative testing details.

Oral Peripheral Testing

An oral peripheral examination that emphasizes oral-sensory and oral-motor abilities is certainly relevant to the oral preparatory stage of the swallow. Refer to Appendix A for conducting this exam. The integrity of cranial nerves V, VII, IX, X, and XII is particularly relevant to chewing and swallowing. A video sample of a speech-language pathologist demonstrating an oral mechanism examination bedside (part I adult dysphagia) can be viewed on YouTube (see www.youtube.com/watch?v=-xJvYPVhCxs).

Case History and Sensory Symptom Information

Whether in an interview room or bedside, the SLP methodically ascertains as much history as possible directly from the patient. Spouses or caregivers can help complete the history intake. Some SLPs provide a preliminary check sheet or written questionnaire of possible symptoms in advance of the interview. Two symptom surveys we find useful are the following. First, the Eat-10 Swallowing Screening Tool (Belafsky et al., 2008) has the patient rate, from 0 (no problem) to 4 (severe problem) 10 behavioral impact statements. Scores of 3 or higher may suggest problems swallowing efficiently and safely. The Nestlé Nutrition Institute provides the one-page Eat-10 online (see www.nestlenutrition-institute.org/Documents/test1.pdf).

A second survey we find useful is the Sydney Swallowing Questionnaire (SSQ) from the Department of Gastroenterology of the St. George Hospital and University of New South Wales. It can be found online for clinical and research use (go to stgcs.med .unsw.edu.au/ and search for the SSQ). In addition to stroke and generic patients, this questionnaire has been used with oral and oropharyngeal cancer patients treated with primary surgery (Dwivedi et al., 2012). This three-page questionnaire of 17 items has the patient rate functional statements from "no difficulty at all" to "unable to swallow at all." No scoring scale is provided, but insights are gained.

In face-to-face interviews, the SLP should explore questions about issues such as the patient's eating habits, amount of time spent eating a meal, frequency of meals in a day, items in the diet, any weight changes, and the like. According to Schindler and Kelly (2002), patients with feeding problems secondary to cognitive difficulties may eat sporadically and for short periods and thus lose weight. Patients with primary dysphagia often require longer feeding periods (and may use compensations like multiple swallows, smaller bites, and prolonged chewing) and may feel self-conscious about their slow feeding or be fearful of coughing or choking. There is even the likelihood of weight gain because such patients gravitate to more processed and high-caloric foods (e.g., milkshakes and dietary supplements). Question further about any differences noted among solid, semisolid, and liquid swallowing. Patients with fixed obstruction (such as webs, strictures, or neoplasms) often complain of solid rather than liquid dysphagia. Patients who complain of difficulties with liquids are more likely to have neurological conditions that weaken the pharyngeal musculature or result in discoordination of the swallowing reflex. Associated symptoms of nasopharyngeal regurgitation and dysarthria may point to the level of the lesion. Breathy hoarseness may suggest glottic incompetence (and a risk for aspiration), so check for a poor cough. Although wet vocal quality is commonly thought to be a symptom of swallowing incompetence, controversy exists over its importance. (Wet quality alone often reveals adequate swallow in imaging studies, but wet quality with onset after stroke is a likely warning sign.)

All in all, the case history interview leads the SLP methodically into a perceptual voice assessment (see Chapter 11) and, to supplement the oral examination, attention should be directed to the integrity of the oral mucosa and to the quality and quantity of saliva (which helps form the bolus and trigger the swallow).

Ask about current medications because these may point to other conditions affecting appetite, feeding behavior, salivation, and/or swallowing. Detailed information on medications that can affect swallowing is available (Carl & Johnson, 2006; Gallagher, 2010; Puntil-Sheltman, 2002); some are highlighted in Table 10–1.

In evaluating the patient, the most important determination is the risk of aspiration. This risk determines the patient's feeding method (bolus unrestricted, bolus restricted, some alternative to oral intake). Of course, the evaluation also strives to determine the need—or not—for swallowing treatment and what compensatory strategies might be used to improve the safety of the patient's swallow.

Books by Groher and Crary (2010) and Swigert (2007) provide sample questionnaires and recording forms. Various published assessment programs include case history questionnaires as well. The following succinct topics of inquiry have served us well:

- What are your swallowing concerns?
- How long ago did these concerns begin? How have these difficulties changed over time?
- Describe your current health issues and what medications you take.
- What types of food and liquid do you currently eat and drink? Which of these seem to cause the most problems? Which seem to cause the fewest problems?

TABLE 10–1
Partial List of Medications That May Affect Swallowing

Decreased Saliva (Dry Mouth)
Diuretics (e.g., Edecrin)
Oxybutynin (Ditropan)
Diphenhydramine (Benadryl)
ACE inhibitors (e.g., Capoten, Prinivil)

Gastroesophageal Reflux and Esophageal Dysmotility
Nifedipine (Procardia)
Albuteral

Impaired Chewing and Swallowing Movements
Haldol
Thorazine
Risperidone

Impaired Cognition and Attention
Diazepam (Valium)
Lorazepam (Ativan)

Distorted Taste
Chemotherapeutic drugs
Tetracycline

Improved Ability to Focus on Tasks Such as Eating
Ritalin
Provigil

- Describe any sensations you feel when eating and swallowing (pain [odynophagia], lump, blockage, chocking, coughing, dryness of mouth, drooling, regurgitation, etc.).
- How stable has your weight been this year?
- What has your doctor told you about your swallowing?
- What do you hope we can do about your swallowing? Do you have a particular wish or eating goal?

Noninstrumental and Brief Bedside Swallow Assessments

It is critically important to assess the patient's danger of aspiration from food particles, liquids, or his or her own saliva. An inward flow or suction of food or liquids into the airway and lungs can cause *aspiration pneumonia* in patients with dysphagia, and the condition can be life-threatening. It is precarious to test a patient's ability to swallow safely without *seeing* this process that occurs in the neck because of the choking hazard to the patient and the potential legal issues for the clinician. Imaging studies, which are discussed shortly, are necessary. Still, a brief and carefully executed noninstrumental preliminary assessment is sometimes appropriate to establish whether dysphagia is present (the problem versus no problem determination), the extent of the dysphagia, and the plans for appropriate detailed testing.

Stanford Medicine offers various online tutorials. Its Bedside Swallow Screen depicts the SLP performing a quick, efficient adult screening. Available on YouTube, this tutorial consists of a cognitive (one-stage command), oral-motor, and 3-ounce water sip/swallow screening (see www.youtube.com/watch?v=x_sssJErd6U). SLPs may also have the patient swallow small bits of foods of varying consistencies while monitoring—albeit imperfectly—the patient's swallow: feeling for laryngeal elevation, feeling for the trigger of the swallow reflex (or multiple swallows), watching for any patient response (e.g., squinting or enlarged gaze), listening for any patient response (e.g., coughing or gurgling sounds), and so forth. We repeat that such methods are unreliable indicators of swallowing or aspiration and should be used with caution. A YouTube example of a bedside food trial that involves a teaspoon of water, a sip of water, pudding, diced fruit, and bite of a sandwich can be seen at www.youtube .com/watch?v=Sh6fiO8N_PA. During each food trial presentation, the SLP palpates the patient's neck for cues of laryngeal elevation and swallow trigger, checks the oral cavity for any food residue left behind, and listens for any patient coughing or gurgling sounds. Also, ASHA offers a thorough Clinical Swallowing Evaluation Template that can be found online at www.asha.org.

CLINICAL AND INSTRUMENTAL ADULT ASSESSMENTS

Many protocols exist for detailed clinical assessments and for imaging studies with the adult dysphagia patient. Table 10–2 is a representative list of resources in wide use. Some of these will be highlighted.

The Mann Assessment of Swallowing Ability (MASA) (Mann, 2002) was designed for use as a bedside evaluation of patients with dysphagia. It purports to be brief (to take 15 to 20 minutes to administer), but it contains 24 clinical items that are scaled according to severity. Normative data have been established, and MASA scores have been segmented into severity groups that consider both severity and aspiration features. While the MASA has been a popular assessment tool, a shorter version now exists. The Modified Mann Assessment of Swallowing Ability (Antonios et al., 2010) is known as the Modified MASA. In this assessment, no food trial is given, and the assessor (e.g., SLP, nurse) has specific task instructions. The number of tasks is reduced to 12, and the

TABLE 10–2
Some Adult Dysphagia Case History Forms, Sensory Scales, Assessment Programs, and Imaging Protocols Available Commercially or from Professional Sources

Bedside Evaluation of Dysphagia (BED) (Hardy, 1995)
Bedside Swallow Assessment (EATS) (Courtney & Flier, 2009)
Burke Dysphagia Screening Test (BDST) (DePippo, Holas, & Reding, 1992)
Clinical Evaluation of Dysphagia (CED) (Cherney, Pannelli, & Cantiere, 1994)
Dysphagia Evaluation Protocol (Avery-Smith, Rosen, & Dellarosa, 1997)
Eat-10: A Swallowing Screening Tool (Belafsky et al., 2008; also Nestlé Nutrition Institute at www.nestlenutrition-institute.org/Documents/test1.pdf)
Gussing Swallow Screen (GUSS) (Trapl et al., 2007)
Mann Assessment of Swallowing Ability (MASA) (Mann, 2002)
Mann Assessment of Swallowing Ability–Cancer (MASA-C) (Carnaby & Crary, 2014)
Massey Bedside Screening (Massey & Jedicka, 2002)
M.D. Anderson Dysphagia Inventory (MDADI) (search M.D. Anderson Cancer Center at www.mdanderson.org)
Modified Mann Assessment of Swallowing Ability (Antonios et al., 2010)
Northwestern Dysphagia Patient Check Sheet (Logemann, Veis, & Colangelo, 1999)
Standardized Swallowing Assessment (SSA) (Perry, 2001)
Swallowing Ability and Function Evaluation (SAFE) (Ross-Swain & Kipping, 2003)
Swallowing Quality of Life Survey (SWAL-QOL) (McHorney et al., 2000)
Sydney Swallowing Questionnaire (SSQ) (St. George Hospital and University of New South Wales; search for SSQ at http://stgcs.med.unsw.edu.au/)
Toronto Bedside Swallowing Screening Test (TOR-BSST) (Martino et al., 2009)

scoring system is displayed on a one-page form that is more straightforward. The total score ranges from 0 to 100, where a value equal to or greater than 95 suggests the patient may have an oral diet, as tolerated. Scores 94 and lower warrant the no food or liquid intake by mouth directive that is known simply as "nothing per oral" and abbreviated NPO. The medical status of NPO should trigger physician orders for a full SLP consult. A related instrument has been designed for use with cancer patients. The Mann Assessment of Swallowing Ability–Cancer (Carnaby & Crary, 2014) is known as the MASA-C. This version has a similar approach and scoring system, with some items adapted for this patient population.

The Gussing Swallow Screen (GUSS) (Trapl et al., 2007) includes a semisolid, liquid, and solid food trial in its screening protocol, and instructions are clear. A severity scoring system is provided and covers deglutition, coughing, drooling, and voice changes.

SAFE: The Swallowing Ability and Function Evaluation (Ross-Swain & Kipping, 2003) guides the SLP through the three stages of evaluation identified as (1) the evaluation of general information relative to swallowing, including cognitive and behavioral factors; (2) examination of the oropharyngeal mechanism; and (3) a functional analysis of swallowing with attention to the oral preparatory, the oral, and the pharyngeal phases of the patient's swallow. The SAFE seeks to provide "a definitive diagnosis or label of dysphagia" in adolescents to adults and provides suggestions for treatment planning.

The Clinical Evaluation of Dysphagia (CED) from the Rehabilitation Institute of Chicago (Cherney, Pannelli, & Cantiere, 1994) outlines the areas to assess for the SLP. Typically, a prefeeding evaluation is done first, when a patient is at high risk for aspiration (e.g., patients who are not yet eating orally or those with tracheostomies). The evaluation of prefeeding skills on the CED includes collecting a history of the problem and observing oral, pharyngeal, and laryngeal structures and functions. From this, the SLP decides the patient's potential for oral intake and the need for further evaluation and referral. The CED's prefeeding evaluation form guides the clinician in the collection and documentation of important information. While daunting for the novice clinician, we feel the CED's outline of key observations becomes second nature to the experienced SLP. These key observations include (1) medical/nutritional status; (2) respiratory status (e.g., breaths per minute, coughing, shortness of breath); (3) history of aspiration; (4) type and size of tracheostoma, if any; (5) level of alertness and ability to follow directions; (6) behavioral characteristics; (7) current feeding methods (e.g., oral, nasogastric tube, gastrostomy tube, percutaneous endoscopic gastrostomy), when tube was placed, frequency and amount of food intake; (8) positioning (e.g., of body, head, and neck), any motor control problems, best feeding position without giving food (maximal airway protection is upright at 90 degrees with head tilted forward), and what is needed to achieve that position comfortably (use of wedges, pillows, other supports); (9) observation of oral motor, pharyngeal, and laryngeal functioning (perform a thorough oral motor examination and include observations on quality and strength of the voice); (10) presence or absence of both involuntary and elicited coughs; (11) gag reflex and its strength bilaterally; (12) ability to perform a dry swallow on command (feel and watch for laryngeal elevation); (13) presence of drooling, mouth odors, any abnormal reflexes that may affect feeding; and (14) response to stimulation (e.g., adequacy of lip closure, lip protrusion, response to touching by a spoon, and the like).

Although it may be determined after this assessment that a patient should remain NPO (nothing per oral), nutrition must be accomplished through other means. Treatment may be recommended to improve prefeeding skills with the anticipation of improvement and future reassessment. The CED clinical or bedside evaluation of dysphagia can continue on patients who can tolerate at least one food consistency. The nature of this

TABLE 10–3
Foods and Food Consistencies Used in Evaluating Dysphagia

Thin liquids: such as water, apple juice
Thick liquids: such as tomato juice, cream soups, yogurt
Puréed foods: such as applesauce, puréed canned fruit, pudding
Ground foods: such as rice, scrambled eggs, canned tuna, ground chicken, hamburger
Chopped solids: such as tender bites of meats, vegetables
Regular solids: usual table foods

evaluation differs substantially for patients of differing levels; Cherney, Pannelli, and Cantiere (1994) provide guidelines for patients with severe dysphagia, those with a tracheostomy, and those receiving an oral diet. Like many assessment programs, the CED guides the SLP in observing (or inferring) and rating behaviors during swallowing. Six different food consistencies can be evaluated; Table 10–3 lists sample foods.

In a national survey of dysphagia clinicians, the top preferences of clinical/bedside methods in current use were discerned (McCullough, Wertz, Rosenbek, & Dinneen, 1999). Table 10–4 lists the top seven methods per area. On a cautionary note, Martino, Pron, and Diamant (2000) state that only two bedside findings have been proven to help in predicting aspiration, as seen by videofluoroscopy: (1) reduced unilateral pharyngeal sensation and (2) coughing with the 50-mL water swallow procedure. Consequently, an imaging study should follow the bedside examination of any patient. The patient's performance on various diagnostic tasks serves as a dynamic assessment. What tasks were difficult or unwise for the patient? What tasks facilitated improved swallowing? What, if any, consistencies, positions, and techniques were revealed in the assessment that might be the basis for treatment? Some of these same clinical questions need further exploration using objective instruments to judge improved and safe swallowing best. It bears mentioning that some cases do not warrant oral feeding and swallowing, a topic that is beyond the scope of this text.

TABLE 10–4
Dysphagia Clinicians' Top Seven Preferred Methods in Bedside Evaluations

History	**Trial Swallows**
Patient reports	3-oz swallow
Family reports	150-mL test
History of pneumonia	Other thin liquid
Neurological insult	Thick liquid
Nutritional status	Pudding
Gastrointestinal history	Purée
Structural (nonsurgical) history	Ice chips
Oral Motor	**Voice**
Rapid alternating speech	Variations in pitch and loudness
Tongue strength and range	Breathiness
Lip seal and pucker	Harshness
Jaw strength/lateral	Wet/gurgly
Soft palate movement	Strained/strangled
Palatal gag	Dysphonia/aphonia
Pharyngeal gag	Resonance

Imaging Adults to Assess Swallowing

A range of technologies is useful in studying various aspects of the swallow. Ultrasonography involves the use of transducers to observe structural movements (e.g., of the tongue and hyoid in adults, or to study infants' suck and oral transit). Surface electromyography records electrical activity in an area where various muscles are involved in swallowing. There also is scintigraphy, which may be referred to as radionuclide milk scanning in the pediatric population Some of the more popular methods, such as videofluoroscopic and endoscopic assessments of swallowing, allow dynamic visualizations.

Videofluoroscopic Swallowing Study or Modified Barium Swallow

The traditional barium swallow concurrent with radiography is useful in visualizing upper airway anatomy and perhaps observing lesions and neoplasms. To see a swallowing sequence of motions, however, the barium consistency is modified and a videofluoroscope is used. A modified barium swallow (MBS), also known as a videoflouroscopic swallowing study (VFSS), provides a dynamic view of swallowing, from the oral cavity through to the lower esophageal sphincter. As a procedure, then, it does involve some radiation, is performed at a hospital (nontransportable), and can be costly. Still, the MBS/VFSS provides a good anterior-posterior view of the entire process, from food intake through a portion of the esophagus. The SLP and radiologists need to work cooperatively. The patient swallows purée, liquid, and/or solid food consistencies that have been mixed with barium for fluoroscopic imaging. For the oral/pharyngeal portion of the exam, liquid barium may be given and the patient can be asked to hold it in the mouth for 10 seconds before swallowing. Any incidence of leakage before the swallow is observed for insight into oral-pharyngeal muscle coordination. Observations also include volume of the swallow, leakage into the nasal cavity, and entry into the laryngeal vestibule. The modified barium swallow is useful in assessing the patient's ability to protect the airway versus penetration and threat of aspiration. Note that the barium is distasteful and must be mixed with food and/or liquids for the examination. Even in healthy adults, the presence of barium (versus no barium) affects the person's taste sensitivity and swallowing behavior (Nagy, Steele, & Pelletier, 2014), so the MBS study is but a glimpse into a patient's abilities.

Images during an MBS study while a patient swallows pudding, with the SLP talking to the patient and instructing about head position changes, can be viewed on YouTube (see www.youtube.com/watch?v=sM6uxd1uS6M). An excellent step-by-step assessment outline for conducting a VFFS/MBS swallowing study is provided on ASHA's website (see www.asha.org and search for Videoflouroscope Swallowing Examination Template).

There are many events for the SLP to attend to during each phase of a patient's swallow on the VFFSS/MBS image, but we find focusing on the bolus critical. Stop or replay the recorded image, as needed, and note the following in particular. Before the swallow is initiated, observe the oral anatomy/physiology for any abnormalities and movement issues. Watch the anterior-posterior (A-P) propulsion of the bolus closely. As the swallow is initiated (recall typical landmark anatomical events), does the bolus move consistently or with hesitation? If there is a delay, how long does it last? Does the bolus (or any part of it) appear to enter the airway before, during, or after the swallow is triggered? During and after the swallow, observe bolus movement through the pharynx and into the esophagus (PES/UES area). After the swallow, look for any residual bolus matter in the oral cavity, valleculae, pyriform sinuses, and/or along the posterior pharyngeal walls.

Often the clinican needs to modify the imaging procedures and try various strategies to elicit the best and safest swallow from a patient. With knowledge of the patient's issues, it is best to preplan these before the barium thickener is introduced. Consider what head position and body posture should be used. What food types and textures will be tried? Be ready with prompts instructing the patient to cough, swallow again, or swallow hard to help clear remaining bolus particles that threaten the airway and cause aspiration. Was the cue successful in clearing the bolus as seen in the image?

Fiberoptic Endoscopic Evaluation of Swallowing (FEES)

The flexible endoscopic evaluation of swallowing (FEES) also provides the SLP with a dynamic view of swallowing and, some would argue, a more thorough view of the entire swallowing process. However, the FEES lacks the anterior-posterior (A-P) perspective that the MBS/VFSS affords and has a split second of white-out when the image disappears in the pharyngeal swallow. Clearly, some facilities prefer one method over the other and have equipment for one method; however, some large medical facilities have both imaging options and indeed find both kinds of information insightful on a single patient. In FEES, the equipment can be rolled to the patient's bedside. The flexible nasopharyngoscope is passed thought the nose and into the nasopharynx. This allows visualization of the anatomy and function of the palate, pharynx, larynx, saliva pooling, and sensation. It is good to observe the patient during phonation such as saying "ka-ka-ka" and singing a vowel up and down the scale. Then swallowing is assessed with varying consistencies of food (such as a bit of cracker or applesauce) and with a small amount of liquid (grape juice or water with green food coloring rather than tinted blue dye aids visualization). It is very important to observe any pooling of secretions or bolus residue in the pyriform sinuses, valleculae, and laryngeal vestibule because this can indicate an aspiration danger. This is similar to the detailed observations with the previous method of VFSS/MBS.

A FEES demonstration by an SLP and physician that includes a brief patient explanation can be viewed on YouTube (see www.youtube.com/watch?v=M-TbMp_63Yc). This clip mentions some advantages of FEES and uses colored liquids and food consistencies. We also suggest the excellent and detailed tutorial on FEES on YouTube (see www.youtube.com/watch?v=OxzrQsBpjx4). Both novice and seasoned clinicians will appreciate this level of training. In addition, ASHA has a detailed Endoscopy Swallowing Examination Template on its website (search www.asha.org).

Imaging Probes and Trial Swallowing Strategies

We want to remind the reader that the evaluation, especially the imaging evaluation, is a time to probe elicitation techniques of the patient's best and safest swallowing method(s). Indeed, preplanned methods are ideal for visualizing patients "at their best swallow" to make an informed judgment about immediate feeding recommendations and potential for improvement through intervention.

Based on medical documents, patient's case history, symptom checklist, and general clinical or bedside assessment in advance of an imaging study, the SLP should have an informed idea of what strategies should be tried with the patient during the imaging examination. What head position and body posture should be used? Is any external pressure needed (such as cues to hold the lips closed or chin a certain way)? What foods and foods consistencies should be tried or not tried? Can the patient remember cues or follow them when verbally reminded? Does or can the patient swallow twice consecutively or swallow harder to clear residue? Can the patient spontaneously cough or be cued to cough? The SLP's insights into these types of questions guide clinical recommendation about current and hoped-for feeding options and whether treatment is warranted (and, if so, directions to take in rehabilitation).

Bolus Flow and Aspiration

The SLP must always remember that the ultimate concern in swallowing is for the patient's safety. Aspiration that can lead to aspiration pneumonia (also called penetration pneumonia) can be life-threatening. In imaging studies, the gaze of the SLP should concentrate on "following the bolus." Various measures of bolus flow exist and often involve timing the patient's oral transit duration, pharyngeal phase duration, and total swallowing duration (e.g., from start of the posterior bolus movement through entry into the UES). Rosenbek and colleagues (1996) proposed an 8-point rating scale still in popular use. The Penetration/Aspiration Scale (PENASP) describes numerically whether and to what extent a patient's airway is compromised during bolus swallowing. The eight category ratings about what occurs with any bolus particles in a given patient are as follows:

> Scale 1: No bolus particles enter the airway.
>
> Scale 2: Some bolus enters the airway, remains above the vocal folds, and is ejected.
>
> Scale 3: Some bolus enters the airway, remains above the vocal folds, and is not ejected.
>
> Stage 4: Some bolus enters the airway, contacts the vocal folds, and is ejected.
>
> Scale 5: Some bolus enters the airway, contacts the vocal folds, and is not ejected.
>
> Scale 6: Some bolus enters the airway, passes below the vocal folds, and is ejected into larynx or out of the airway.
>
> Scale 7: Some bolus enters the airway, passes below the vocal folds, and is not ejected from the trachea despite effort.
>
> Scale 8: Some bolus enters the airway, passes below the vocal folds, and no effort is made to eject.

Scale scores of 2 to 5 indicate some degree of penetration, whereas scale scores of 6 to 8 indicate aspiration. Also, patients scaled 7 or 8 are in danger of silent aspiration because the bolus residue is penetrating/aspirating without effortful and successful ejection and airway protection (via strategies such as repeat swallows, coughs, and so forth). These insights may be clues to rehabilitation potentials and/or food restrictions.

Penetration aspiration is a major concern with dysphagia patients, and additional detection techniques continue to be developed and refined. The Fiberoptic Endoscopic Evaluation of Swallowing with Sensory Testing (FEESST) (Aviv et al., 1998) combines the FEES assessment of swallowing with a technique for determining a patient's laryngeal-pharyngeal sensory discrimination threshold. In the FEESST, pulses of air of varying strengths are delivered by endoscope to the upper laryngeal area (served by the sensory superior laryngeal nerve of vagus CN X). Visualized laryngeal responses, or lack thereof, to certain air puff strengths are proving to be good predictors of aspiration in patients.

FUNCTIONAL OUTYCOMES AND QUALITY OF LIFE IN ADULT PATIENTS

The Functional Oral Intake Scale (FOIS) was developed for use with dysphagia patients following stroke (Crary, Mann, & Groher, 2005). It describes the diet level at which a patient functions safely and with acceptable nutrition and hydration. The seven levels serve as outcome measures to describe the patient's attainment following rehabilitation or at the time of discharge. It also is a useful reassessment tool for tracking a patient's progress or lack thereof. A similar and simple use of the FOIS is to document the patient's level pre- and post-feeding intervention. The seven levels are as follows:

Level 1: No food or liquids taken by mouth (NPO).

Level 2: Dependent on tube feedings with minimal food or liquid permitted.

Level 3: Dependent on tube feedings with considerable food or liquid permitted.

Level 4: Oral diet of a single consistency.

Level 5: Oral diet of multiple consistencies requiring special preparation or compensations.

Level 6: Oral diet of multiple consistencies without special preparation but with specific food limitations.

Level 7: Oral diet without restrictions.

Quality-of-life measures are consistent with the concerns of the World Health Organization and are frequently obtained following some degree of intervention in patients with dysphagia. The Swallowing Quality of Life *Survey* (SWAL-QOL) (McHorney et al., 2000) contains 11 subscales, each having the patient rate items on a scale of 1 to 5. It was designed specifically for use with dysphagia patients and appears to be the scale of choice in dysphagia research and for clinical utility. The M.D. Anderson Dysphagia Inventory (MDADI), which can be found at the M.D. Anderson Cancer Center website (search www.mdanderson.org/) is a quality-of-life tool that was designed for use with patients following stroke to test their swallowing. It has also proven to be a valid instrument for use with head and neck cancer dysphagia patients (Chen et al., 2001).

PEDIATRIC FEEDING AND SWALLOWING DISORDERS

Pediatric dysphagia encompasses disorders of sucking, feeding, and swallowing in infants and children. Some segment *feeding disorders* as issues of eating food or liquid with or without concomitant swallowing problems and may encompass disruptive meal-time behaviors, refusal, rigid food preferences (including types and textures), difficulty with age-appropriate utensil or self-feeding, and poor growth related to limited intake. In this segmented view, *swallowing disorders* are problems in one or more of the swallowing phases, and, admittedly, the distinctions of feeding and the entrance of food/liquid into the mouth for oral preparation can be fuzzy. For clarity, it is best to consider *pediatric dysphagia* as the umbrella term for both feeding and swallowing disorders; indeed medical coding and billing for both feeding and swallowing are under dysphagia. Pediatric dysphagia, naturally, is assessed relative to developmental, age-appropriate behaviors. The anatomy and physiology of suckling, sucking, chewing, and swallowing differ between pediatric and adult populations; for detailed pediatric aspects, the SLP is referred to books by Arvedson and Brodsky (2002) and Swigert (1998).

The phases to assess in pediatric cases are oral preparation, oral transit, pharyngeal, and esophageal. Pediatric dysphagia can occur in any phase of the swallow. In addition, in infants and toddlers, feeding and swallowing can focus on preliminary aspects of the oral preparation phase with regard to optimal handling and positioning, nipples, and manipulation of utensils. The acts of feeding and swallowing are both motor, but they are also sensory. Behavioral elements can affect the process as well.

Perhaps more than 25% of typically developing children have had a feeding/swallowing problem. Infants and children with various medical conditions, such as cerebral palsy, cleft lip and/or palate, and autism spectrum disorders, are at high risk of

TABLE 10–5

Causes and Conditions Associated with Pediatric Dysphagia

Neurological disorders: cerebral palsy, meningitis, traumatic brain injury, face/neck muscle weakness, cerebrovascular accident, progressive encephalopathy (e.g., multiple sclerosis, HIV).
Neuromuscular coordination factors or disease: prematurity, low birth weight, motor neuron disease (e.g., polio, progressive bulbar paralysis of childhood), myasthenia gravis, muscular dystrophy.
Neurosensory-behavioral or psychosocial issues: autism spectrum disorders; institutional deprivation; behavioral refusals; parent–child interaction difficulties, especially at mealtime.
Other medical diseases: gastroesophageal reflux disease (GERD), heart disease, pulmonary disease.
Structural malformations: cleft lip and/or palate, laryngomalcia, tracheoesophageal fistula, orofacial anomalies (e.g., Pierre Robin syndrome).
Medication side effects: dryness of mouth, decreased appetite, drowsiness.

dysphagia. Conditions of childhood associated with feeding/swallowing disorders are cited in Table 10–5.

With such a complex population, it is likely that assessment and intervention will involve a team approach. Various physician specialists, dieticians, nurses, SLPs, occupational therapists, and physical therapists are but some expected team members. Nutrition is essential for life, and pediatric dysphagia can have long-term consequences if it is not diagnosed and addressed. Long-term effects of dysphagia may include malnutrition and failure to thrive, poor weight gain, aspiration pneumonia, regurgitation, dehydration, and other negative consequences.

PEDIATRIC ASSESSMENT GOALS

Pediatric assessments vary widely depending on causative factors but also on the child's age, development (including reflexes, muscle tone, posture), cognitive ability, and such. The ultimate goal of a feeding and swallowing assessment is to develop a management plan that enables safe and efficient feeding and is enjoyable for both the child and the caregivers. Adequate nutrition and hydration goals must be achieved without compromise of airway safety (Groher & Crary, 2010). The medical team and indeed the SLP should remember this at all times. While a key focus in the SLP's assessment of the child will be his or her ability to protect the airway and the practicality of the child using oral feeding (versus the need for alternative, safer methods of nutrition), a secondary purpose of a feeding/swallowing assessment is to establish baseline clinical data. The Oral-Motor Feeding Rating Scale (Jelm, 1990) may be useful in tracking the progress and skills from 1 year of age; other tools are useful for nursing infants or older (eating) youth.

To accomplish these goals, pediatric feeding and swallowing evaluations should include these primary components:

- Review of medical documents and careful case history intake from the parent and from the child, if appropriate
- Screening of hearing, speech, and language/cognition, as appropriate for age
- Examination of the oral motor mechanism
- Observation of a trial feeding and/or observation of parent feeding session
- Collection and review of specialized imaging studies, as clinically indicated

PEDIATRIC DYSPHAGIA CASE HISTORY

Medical records help identify medical, neurological, developmental, and etiological factors that predispose the child to dysphagia. Likewise, knowledge of medications, syndromes, and systemic problems (e.g., cardiopulmonary and respiratory distress) that increase demands on pharyngeal function and boost nutritional requirements is necessary.

The mother or primary caregiver/feeder can provide details of the feeding history. The SLP needs to know the child's current oral feeding patterns: types of food and liquids tolerated, manner of presentation, feeding position, duration of meals (10 to 30 minutes is best), frequency of meals, total intake, and the like. If the client is tube fed, the SLP needs details on the type of feeding tube, when it was initiated, formula amount per feeding, feeding schedule, position during feeding, and use of and response to oral stimulation. In addition to these face-to-face interview questions, the SLP might collect in advance a parent/caregiver checklist of behavioral indicators. An example of such a checklist is shown in Table 10–6.

ORAL MOTOR EXAMINATION

The SLP should observe the child at rest, noting body tone and posture. If the child is in an acute care setting, baseline respiratory rates, heart rates, and pulse oxygen levels can easily be obtained (changes in these physiologic patterns during feeding may indicate general intolerance or airway compromise). Look for clinical signs of oral or pharyngeal dysfunction, such as drooling, coughing, and upper aerodigestive tract noises. As discussed earlier in this chapter, a thorough oral motor examination is performed. The lips, tongue, and velum are evaluated for precision, strength, range, and symmetry of movement. Cranial nerves screened for oral phase function include V, VII, X, and XII. The pharyngeal phase of deglutition depends on muscles innervated by cranial nerves IX, X, and XI. Oral sensations and laryngeal functions are also assessed. Appendix A provides information on conducting an oral motor exam. Appendix B cites resources on developmental milestones that are clinically useful.

TABLE 10–6
Checklist of Behavioral Indicators and Symptoms of Pediatric Dysphasia

Check all behaviors typical of the infant or child:
____ Reflux of liquid or food out of the nose or mouth
____ Spitting up or vomiting when fed
____ Coughing or choking during or after feeding
____ Taking small sips or overly small bites
____ Lack of weight gain
____ Weight loss
____ Packing food in mouth with swallowing
____ Prolonged feeding session; too slow
____ Gagging or coughing during or after feeding
____ Drools excessively (not due to teething, after teething stage)
____ Refusal behaviors when trying to feed (e.g., squirming, clenching mouth, crying, hitting)
____ Difficulty chewing certain foods or textures (provide a list if yes)
____ Difficulty swallowing certain foods or textures (provide a list if yes)
____ Noisy or wet vocal quality during or after feeding

DEVELOPMENTAL AGE ASPECTS OF ASSESSMENT

There is great heterogeneity of pediatric dysphagia cases, from birth through adolescent, and from newborn suckling to "picky" solid food chewers in school. We wish to subdivide this vast range by developmental feeding/swallowing stages based on where the child *is* performing, relative to where the child *should* show skills. The assessment performed by the SLP certainly will be shaped by such factors. Here we provide some appraisal issues to include in the total assessment.

Infant Assessment Considerations

Newborn infants, especially those with obvious orofacial or neuromuscular deficits, present an immediate concern to the medical team, including the hospital-based SLP. In such cases (including premature births), nutritional needs may be met by tubes and other options. The SLP, however, has assessment responsibilities for prefeeding and feeding readiness, as well as with family support and training. It is important for the SLP to assess early the infant's oral peripheral mechanism for both structural integrity and motor skill. Check for the rooting reflex, where the infant's mouth should open and his or her head should turn toward a stroked check. Can the infant get emotional pleasure and oral exercise from *nonnutritive sucking*, as with a pacifier or finger? Do the infant's jaw and tongue create pressure and suction against the pacifier? Assess the infant's *nutritive sucking* during a breast- and/or bottle-feeding session with a parent or nurse. For an elaborate instrumental quantitative evaluation of nonnutritive and nutritive sucking, see Lau and Kusnierczyk (2001). Observe the sucking pattern, efficiency (volume per minute), endurance on task, and any other infant responses.

Toddler Assessment Considerations

The evaluation of toddlers, ages 1 to 3, builds on what is done in infant assessments. Added emphasis is placed on the home environment, behavioral dynamics, and especially interactions between child and parent (or significant others) involved in feeding. Keen observation is given to the toddler's use of implements (sippy cup, glass, spoon or fork) or lack thereof, and the foods consumed (types, textures). In short, identify the toddler's strengths as well as any feeding/swallowing difficulties, according to the child, the parent, and your own SLP observations. For this age, feeding/swallowing assessments must also consider—and assess—the toddler's communicative-cognitive abilities, social skills, and motor development.

Preschool and School-Age Assessment Considerations

The evaluation of preschool and school-age youth covers a wide population, from 3 to 21 years of age, with great diversity of expected feeding/swallowing skills. The SLP likely has past documentation and medical records to review on a case. Gather current home environment information and parental perspectives. Collect teachers' observations about feeding/swallowing and their concerns noted during snacks or mealtimes. Collate parent and teacher impressions of the youth's strengths and limitations in the realms of behavior, motor skills, communication, academics (cognitive), social, and mealtime. With this age group, input from the client is important and insightful, as is his or her cooperation to assess and intervene. As with other age groups, the SLP should observe the client eating. We now return to our generic, controlled assessment outline.

ASSESSMENT SCALES, OBSERVATION OF A TRIAL FEEDING, AND INSTRUMENTAL ANALYSIS

The diagnosis and management of pediatric feeding and swallowing conditions has exploded in the past few decades. Clinicians are fortunate to have many research-based and clinically useful assessment guides at their disposal. In particular we wish to mention the pediatric dysphagia practice portal of ASHA and its section on assessment evidence maps (go to www.asha.org and search for Pediatric Dysphagia Assessment). Journals and commercially available assessment programs, scales, and forms exist to aid the clinician. Some are shown in Table 10–7, and we highlight the utility of a few.

Representative of Swigert's (1998) numerous pediatric dysphagia assessment instruments, the Feeding and Swallowing Evaluation (birth to 4 months) guides the SLP along observations to make and responses to elicit from the infant (or children in other age groups). This step-by-step guide allows the SLP to collect information (medical, feeding history) and videofluoroscopic testing of trial feedings and explains what detailed observations to make during each phase of the swallow.

TABLE 10–7
Some Available Pediatric Feeding/Swallowing Assessment Questionnaires, Forms, Scales, and Templates

Assessing Nutritional Patterns and Methods of Feeding (Lefton-Greif, 1994)
Bottle-Breast Feeding: Neonatal Oral Motor Assessment Scale (NOMAS) (Palmer, Crawley, & Blanco, 1993)
Brief Autism Mealtime Behavior Inventory (BAMBI) (Lukens & Linscheid, 2008)
Endoscopy Swallowing Examination (ASHA, search www.asha.org)
Feeding and Swallowing Evaluation (birth to 4 months) (Swigert, 1998)
Feeding and Swallowing Evaluation (4 months to 5 years) (Swigert, 1998)
Feeding and Swallowing Evaluation (5 to 18 years) (Swigert, 1998)
Infant Feeding History and Clinical Assessment Form: Infant 6 Months and Younger (ASHA, search www.asha.org)
Montreal Children's Hospital Feeding Scale (Ramsay, Martel, Porporino, & Zygmuntowicz, 2011)
Multidisciplinary Feeding Profile (MFP) (Kenny et al., 1989)
Neonatal Oral-Motor Assessment Scale (NOMAS) (revised by Case-Smith, 1988)
Oral-Motor and Feeding Evaluation (Arvedson & Brodsky, 2002)
Oral-Motor Feeding Rating Scale (Jelm, 1990)
Pediatric Eating Assessment Tool (Pedi-EAT) (Thoyre et al, 2014)
Pediatric Feeding History and Clinical Assessment Form: Infants 6 Months and Older (ASHA, search www.asha.org/)
Pre-Feeding Skills, Second Edition (Morris & Klein, 2000)
Preterm Infant Breastfeeding Behaviour Scale (PIBBS) (Nyqvist, Rubertsson, Ewald, & Sjödén, 1996)
Rehabilitation Institution of Chicago Parent/Caregiver Questionnaire and Pre-Assessment Form (Perlin & Boner, 1994)
Screening Tool of Feeding Problems Applied to Children (STEP-CHILD) (Seiverling, Hendy, & Williams, 2011)
Videoflouroscopic Swallowing Study of Infants (consuming liquids only) (ASHA, search www.asha.org)
Videoflouroscopic Swallowing Study of Infants and Children (consuming liquids, purées, etc.) (ASHA, search www.asha.org)

By contrast, the purpose of the Montreal Children's Hospital Feeding Scale (Ramsay et al., 2011) is a brief 14-item screening to identify feeding problems in children through parent report. This bilingual tool covers topics including oral motor, oral sensory, appetite, maternal concerns, mealtime behaviors, maternal strategies, and family reactions.

Observation of a Trial Feeding

While it is optimal for the SLP to observe a regularly scheduled mealtime, it is more practical to arrange or contrive this event. The SLP should observe the parent feed the child using foods, utensils, special adaptations (to the nipple, to the thickness, etc.), and positioning equipment used at home. The SLP should monitor the child for clinical signs associated with aspiration. This includes any tendency to cough, choke, or gag, plus any change in vocal quality, upper digestive tract noises, or other signs of distress. Observation of a trial feeding allows the clinician to define patterns of oral intake, positioning, and optimal stimuli for feeding (i.e., bolus characteristics of size, texture, and temperature). Specific forms have been developed to guide the clinician through the case history intake and other prefeeding observations (recall Table 10–7).

Lefton-Greif's form for Assessing Nutritional Patterns and Methods of Feeding (Lefton-Greif, 1994) and Arvedson's Oral-Motor and Feeding Evaluation (Arvedson, 1993) warrant mention, and others were cited in Table 10–7. The SLP observes the infant/child during feeding again during any imaging study medically ordered. Other tools for special mention that cover a wide variety of purposes include the Neonatal Oral-Motor Assessment Scale and the Multidisciplinary Feeding Profile. The Neonatal Oral-Motor Assessment Scale (NOMAS) (Case-Smith, 1988) yields semiquantitative information for the identification of oral-motor dysfunction by 40 weeks' gestational age. The scale rates tongue and jaw responses during nonnutritive and nutritive sucking. The Multidisciplinary Feeding Profile (MFP) is a comprehensive feeding disorder assessment package for patients who are dependent feeders (Kenny et al., 1989). Scaled numerical ratings are made on physical/neurological factors (posture, tone, reflexes); oral-facial structure, sensation, and motor function; ventilation/phonation; and a functional feeding assessment.

Indications for Specialized Studies

When to proceed with special tests and imaging procedures is a decision reached by the multidisciplinary team. The child must be medically stable (and able to risk an episode of aspiration); usually there is some prognosis for change in the current feeding regime. As discussed in the adult section, the videofluoroscopic swallowing study (VFSS), also known as a modified barium swallow (MBS), and the fiberoptic endoscopic evaluation of swallowing (FEES) are common imaging procedures, even with children. The SLP typically conducts the swallow study in conjunction with the radiologist and/or other physician. Monitoring of physiological stress to the infant or child can be done concurrently by tracking cardiac, respiratory, and oxygen saturation levels, as well as other indirect clues such as skin color change, nasal flaring, change in fidgeting/fussiness, and coughing/choking (though not necessarily trustworthy). Imaging studies show the movement of the liquid or solid bolus dynamically from the beginning phase of oral intake, preparation, and propulsion backward into the pharynx, areas near the all-important larynx, and the upper esophageal segment (UES) leading toward the stomach. Whether with the VFSS/MBS or the FEES (though differences in the details seen do exist, and possibly the age of the child will affect toleration), the SLP visually assesses events that do or do not happen along the vocal tract.

Many factors affect oral and pharyngeal performance, including the rate and manner of food presentation (which can be mixed with barium for image enhancement). The evaluation itself often manipulates bolus characteristics (texture, amount, temperature), manner of presentation (bottle, spoon, cup), and special adaptations (positioning, specific modifications of feeding devices). Test protocols and assessment forms are available in the literature and in Table 10–7. SLP tips for analyzing the dynamic image may include the following laundry list of observations:

1. What lip, tongue, and mandible movements does the sucking infant display? Is there left-right symmetry in any movement? Is liquid lost out the mouth?

2. How does the toddler or child use articulatory muscles to remove food from a utensil?

3. Observe mastication/chewing of food. Assess quality, duration and symmetry of movement.

4. Observe bolus formation. Does the tongue push it out of the mouth? Does the bolus spread loosely over a wide area or form into cohesive mass? When is the bolus nestled (centrally on tongue, lateralized)?

5. Assess oral transit maneuvers (process less than 3 seconds) and the quality and symmetry of tongue movement to propel the bolus back. Does some of the bolus remain behind, and if so, where in oral cavity?

6. For triggering of the safe swallow, assess velopharyngeal contact/closure. Is there any (or excessive) posterior tongue elevation (tongue humping) toward the velum? Does the soft palate elevate symmetrically? If so, when does it do so relative to the timing of other events? Is there any nasal leakage/regurgitation? Observe if and when the larynx moves "up and forward" under the chin and tongue. Look for indications of ventricular (false vocal) fold closure, downward and back folding of the epiglottis, and closure of the (true) vocal folds. Is there any premature leakage of some liquid or food (before swallow trigger of the main bolus) into the laryngeal area (valleculae, pyriform sinuses)?

7. Assess pharyngeal phase danger signs. Did some of the bolus penetrate into the airway after the swallow and leave any residue? Did aspiration occur before or after the swallow? Was any residue cleared with the next swallow or not?

8. Observe initiation of the esophageal phase. Is the bolus transit into the upper esophageal segment (UES) slow or rapid? Is any residue left around UES area? Is there any reflux from the UES back into the pharynx?

During the imaging study, the SLP should, based on observed concerns, attempt to assess trial therapy strategies or see whether the safety of the child's swallow can be improved by posture, head position (tilt or turning), strength of swallow techniques akin to those mentioned with adults, bolus consistency and texture effects, and so forth. This is but another reminder that a key goal in dysphagia assessment is determining whether the child can swallow certain types and textures of foods safely and without undue risk of aspiration.

Observations such as the eight listed above warrant multiple looks at the recorded swallowing study after the fact. Detailed insights provide clues about the actual disorder, locus of concern, and also strengths the child has in the act of feeding/swallowing. Positive behaviors of what is working well should be conveyed in the SLP assessment report as well as to the family and the medical team.

We leave the reader with one sobering note of caution when working with clients with multiple handicaps. Rogers et al. (1994) conducted a study of 90 infants with cerebral palsy and multiple disabilities. Videofluoroscopic swallow examinations showed that almost all patients had abnormalities of both the oral and pharyngeal phases of deglutition. In particular, tongue control abnormalities and oral phase delays were present, along with delayed, multiple swallows and pharyngeal pooling. In addition to these observations, some 38% of the children aspirated in the absence of coughing or choking (silent aspiration). The clinician's work with dysphagia patients of any age is both dangerous and rewarding. The SLP should seek in-depth training in this area of specialization.

CONCLUSION AND SELF-ASSESSMENT

This chapter covered adult dysphagia and pediatric feeding and swallowing disorders. We have provided assessment direction for the SLP working in these areas, but we admit that we have barely scratched the surface with regard to instrumental assessment and imaging analysis. The SLP is advised to study further both MBS and FEES (or as appropriate to one's employment setting). Conferences are particularly useful for training the analysis process because one can view many patient videos with a wide variety of feeding and swallowing issues. As for dysphagia in general, Yorkston, Beukelman, Stand, and Hakel (2010) remind us that clinicians can be guided in their decision-making processes by following a model of disablement that provides a framework for understanding the broad range of sensorimotor speech and swallowing disorders. The World Health Organization's International Classification of Functioning, Disability and Health (ICF) disability model (refer to Figure 9–1) applies to adult and pediatric dysphagia as well.

This chapter covered a broad expanse of clinical and professional issues in both adults and the diverse pediatric population. Dysphagia indeed encompasses disorders of feeding, chewing, and/or swallowing *safely.*

After reading this chapter you should be able to answer the following questions:

1. Explain aspiration and why it matters.
2. Describe events along the vocal tract that typically occur in each phase of the adult swallow.
3. Describe the image seen in a VFFS/MBS swallow study. What are some advantages and limitations of this method?
4. Describe the image seen in an FEES study. What are some advantages and limitations of this method?
5. Name some common causes of adult dysphagia.
6. Names some medical disorders in infancy and childhood that are likely to include disorders of feeding/swallowing.
7. List at least eight questions to explore with a parent of a toddler in an initial evaluation session.

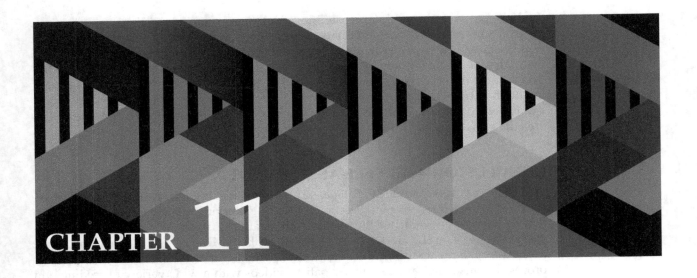

CHAPTER 11

Laryngeal Voice Disorders

LEARNING OUTCOMES

After reading this chapter you will be able to:

1. Discuss how some disorders and diseases affect voice production.
2. Explain three or more parameters of the voice.
3. List some perceptual-acoustic measures used to assess each voice parameter.
4. Explain how the speech-language pathologist assesses maximum phonation time and why.

There were major changes in the assessment and treatment of voice disorders in the last hundred years. The speech-language pathologist (SLP) became involved in the processes of diagnosis and remediation, which were previously the province of physicians and singing teachers. Recently, there has been increased research in the area of normal and disordered vocal physiology, and assessment and treatment are being changed further by advances in technology. Instruments are available for diagnosis and treatment that help to measure behaviors that were previously unobservable and fleeting. It is an exciting time for clinicians who deal with voice disorders.

The proliferation of new instrumentation and research, should not, however, obscure the fact that we have developed some very effective clinical procedures over the years that do not require equipment. Many authorities continue to believe that the listening skill and judgment of the well-trained clinician are the most important tools in a voice evaluation. Measured vocal components help SLPs track areas of aberrance and therapeutic changes with precision—something welcomed by third-party payors and those of us concerned with evidence-based practice. Voice diagnosis combines the subjective and the objective, as does all clinical work, and the clinician must be able to shift from the mental set of the scientist to that of the artist, and back again. In this chapter, we will touch on both subjective and objective aspects of vocal assessment.

Many adults and some children are referred to the SLP by their physician (often an otolaryngologist/ear, nose and throat doctor [ENT]) for voice disorders resulting from medical difficulties or surgical intervention. The clinician also frequently comes in contact with children as the result of screening large numbers of youngsters in school settings or by teacher or parent referral. Prevalence figures for voice disorders among school-age children vary considerably in the literature, but these figures probably hover around 6% (Duffy, Proctor, & Yairi, 2004). From our experience, it would appear that substantially less than 1% of school-age children are presently receiving voice therapy, and this is usually for chronic hoarseness. The prevalence of voice disorders among adults tends to be higher than in children, especially among certain vocally demanding professions like teaching (Remacle, Morsome, & Finck, 2014; Yiu, 2002).

THE NATURE OF VOCAL DISTURBANCES

The imprecision of labels, which is the bane of voice study, begins with the term *voice* itself. Some definitions restrict the term to the generation of sound at the level of the larynx; others include the influence of the vocal tract on the generated tone; and still others broaden the definition to include aspects of tonal generation, resonation, articulation, and prosody. In this chapter, we will limit our discussion of voice to disorders affecting the laryngeal mechanism. While this topic includes cancer of the larynx, Chapter 13 will focus on alaryngeal rehabilitation and reevaluation. Disorders of resonance along the vocal tract will be discussed in Chapter 12.

A framework for conceptualizing voice and voice disturbance is shown in Figure 11–1. The auditory characteristics of pitch, loudness, and quality constitute one dimension of our paradigm. These are the primary perceptual attributes of the voice and relate generally to the fundamental frequency, amplitude, and complexity of the signal.

FIGURE 11–1
Organizational Schema of Voice Disorders

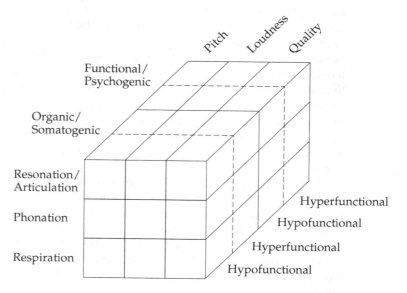

Pitch that is too high, too low, too invariant, or inappropriately variant for the speaker or the circumstances constitutes a voice disorder. The loudness of the speaking voice is usually judged according to the speaking circumstance, with the aberrant ranging from the total lack of voice (aphonia) to the inappropriately loud. For our purposes, the term *quality* refers to the perceived pleasantness, or appeal, of the voice. Although this perception is linked to both the phonatory and resonatory characteristics of the speaker, we will consider only the disturbance of phonation in this chapter. Many terms have been used to describe vocal quality, yet roughness or hoarseness, and the term *breathiness* seem to be the two most widely accepted quality descriptors.

The physical systems that most directly influence vocal production are the respiratory, phonatory, and resonatory-articulatory systems, but they are not the only systems that influence the voice. The endocrine and neural systems may also have an impact on voice production.

The respiratory system provides the motive force for voice production, and ultimately the resultant air stream becomes the vibrator that embodies all of the characteristics that the ear eventually senses. The importance of the air stream to vocal production is not really the issue at this point, but there is some question about the influence of the respiratory mechanism on the various vocal characteristics. The serious reader is referred to companion articles on physically examining the abdominal wall and the diaphragm by Hixon and Hoit (1998, 1999). The respiratory mechanism must be capable of the following:

1. Providing an adequate amount of air so that the speaker can sustain speech with ease to allow for natural phrasing and prosodic factors.
2. Providing adequate control of the flow of air so that the mechanism can, when necessary, either initiate or arrest the speech signal.
3. Providing an air stream that is not so indebted to active muscle contraction that it encourages unnecessary muscle tension in the respiratory and phonatory mechanisms.

Knowledge of the elements of laryngeal function is crucial in guiding the diagnostic process. To be an efficient sound source, the larynx must perform a valving action on the flow of air that establishes alternate, regular pressure changes within the body of air. To do this, the vocal folds must be capable of (1) performing a wide range of valving actions, from completely open and unrestricted to closed and totally restricted; (2) valving completely along the length of the vocal folds; (3) closing and opening during phonation with just the right amount of energy to avoid extreme tension during the closing phase; (4) moving in a natural way that is free from superimposed and undue tension; and (5) making small, subtle, instantaneous adjustments, which are done continuously to alter the various vocal characteristics (these adjustments must allow for a variety of cyclic variations in the potential time of glottal opening and closing, from the long closing time of the glottal fry to the short closing time of the falsetto voice). The vocal folds must also be (1) of approximately equal size and shape so that they can move in synchrony with one another and (2) of appropriate size (length and mass) for the age and sex of the person.

The glottal tone is complex and rich in higher harmonics, but only through the resonant and damping effects of the vocal tract do the speech sounds achieve their identity. For the resonating chambers of the vocal tract to be efficient, they must be flexible in size, shape, texture, and relationship to one another.

The term *functional* should imply more than the simple absence of measurable organic deviation; it should imply that the diagnostician has found some active agent of etiology and that the agent is nonorganic. *Functional* has unfortunately come to mean diagnosis by default.

Figure 11–1 identifies functional/psychogenic and organic/somatogenic as clinically meaningful categories. In this figure, *functional* refers to those disorders where the learned, psychic, or maladaptive behavior has resulted in faulty vocal production but not in physical alteration. If physical change has resulted from the functional cause, however, the proper designation is *psychogenic*. Similarly, if the original factor was physical or organic, then the term *organic* is justified; but if the physical difference results in behavioral change—that is, emotional response or faulty compensatory adjustments—the term *somatogenic* is appropriate. The terms *hyperfunctioning* and *hypofunctioning* refer, respectively, to an excess or insufficiency of laryngeal tension and, as such, could apply to a wide variety of organic or functional disorders. *Voice disorders*, then, refers to abnormal pitch, loudness, or vocal quality according to the sex, age, status, temporary physiological state, purpose of the speaker, and elements of the speaking circumstances. Vocal disorders may be primarily organic or functional, and may be affected by any of the primary systems.

THE DIAGNOSTIC PROCESS

Before beginning our discussion of diagnosis and evaluation of voice production issues, let us restate that this chapter will not cover the many and varied types of voice disorders; such information is available in other sources (see, for example, Boone, McFarlane, Von Berg, & Zraich, 2014; Rubin, Sataloff, & Korovin, 2006; Sapienza & Ruddy, 2013; Stemple, Roy, & Klaben, 2010).

Screening for voice disorders is perceptual. A critical ear is required of the SLP as he or she listens to the speaker's pitch, loudness, quality, and other parameters to make a judgment of normalcy and age appropriateness. The speech sample judged may be conversation, picture description, a reading sample (see Appendix B), or utterances elicited in conjunction with articulation and language screening tasks. Often a voice screening is conducted on individuals who are part of a group for mass screening. Young children are screened in the public schools for various vision, hearing, and speech-language concerns. Lee, Stemple, Glaze, & Kelchner (2004) provide a *Quick Screen for Voice* suitable for kindergarten through grade 5. From a 2- to 3-minute elicited sample of speech, the examiner responds to a checklist of observations of respiration, phonation, and resonance. There are also a few habitual pitch and loudness tasks for which norms are provided for ages 3 to 18+. Failure on one or more productions constitutes a failed screening and the need for medical referral (and presumably a later detailed voice evaluation by the SLP). We also wish to mention that the article provides a parental guide, "Your Child's Voice," that the SLP may find useful when a child has failed the voice screening.

Another example of a voice screening tool, but for adults, is provided by Ghirardi, Ferreira, Giannini, and Latorre (2013). These researchers developed a scorable "Screening Index for Voice Disorders (SIVD)." Administered to adults in high-risk vocal professions, such as classroom teachers, this is a 13-item written questionnaire about vocal symptom.

Our major focus will be on the actual planning, preparation, and execution of vocal appraisals. Diagnosis is intended to assess the parameters of the voice; determine the etiology and/or perpetuating factors; and outline a logical course of intervention, if warranted. Key components of the evaluative process include:

- Case history (including referral input, client interview, client's own impact ratings)
- Preliminary screenings (hearing, oral-motor, speech-language)
- Perceptual vocal assessment
- Acoustic analyses (low- and/or high-tech)

FIGURE 11–2
Assessment of Voice Using the World Health Organization's International Classification of Functioning, Disability and Health (ICF)

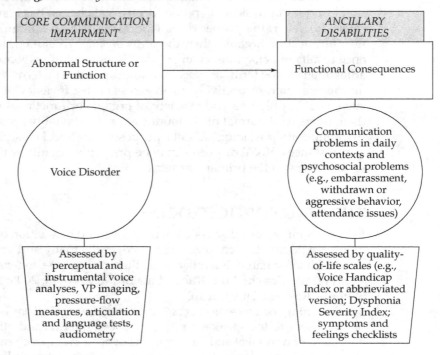

- Aerodynamic analysis (when available)
- Visual assessment
- Trial therapy probes

This process, then, addresses both vocal function and consequential impacts of the disability as advocated by the World Health Organization (2002). This is shown in Figure 11–2.

The Total Case History

The diagnostic process begins with a careful scrutiny of the original statement of the problem as provided by the referral source. Four perspectives guide our evaluation of this information: Who? What? When? and Why? This is followed by case history questionnaires and interviews, and also the gathering of patient impact ratings.

Sizing up Referral Information

It is important to know *who* presents the original complaint about the client's voice. We have found that the "best" source, from a motivational standpoint, is the client, but any individual who might have a significant impact on the client may be a satisfactory referral source. If the client does not consider her or his voice to be a problem, treatment may not be in order or, if it is, this denial may necessitate counseling and education as precursors to the actual voice treatment.

In the schools, it is often the classroom teacher who notices a vocal difference in a student and makes a referral to the SLP. Awareness training may be necessary in the early sessions with the client here, too. It should be pointed out, however, that without prior training, such as listening experiences during inservice programs, classroom teachers are not particularly good at recognizing and referring students with voice disorders.

Next, consider *what* is described as the problem. When a description of the problem comes from the person with whom we will be working, we listen not only to the actual words spoken but also to the way in which they are presented. One of the best sources of information about the impact of the problem on the individual is the way in which it is described. Case history questionnaires invariably ask for a description of the voice problem: when it started and what might have caused it.

In considering *when* the referral was made, three factors are of concern. First, it is important to know when in the sequence of the development of the problem the referral was made. Is this a long-standing problem that has only recently become serious, or is it a relatively new phenomenon that has been detected early? Second, what is this person's age and maturational level? Certain vocal changes are to be expected before puberty and would be considered normal, but a similar vocal quality at a later maturity level may be abnormal. Third, does this problem appear in cycles? For example, the client may suffer from this vocal change only during "hay fever" season. The time of year of the referral may provide some important diagnostic information.

Why was the referral made? The reason may vary from something as simple as an impending trip ("I just have to sound better than this by the first of August") to fears of serious medical problems. In evaluating the reasons for referral, it is important to keep in mind that contacting a speech clinician is often seen as psychologically safer than going to medical doctors or psychologists. This underscores the importance of secondary referrals.

Sometimes the SLP refers the individual to other specialists for their input into the total assessment process; referrals work in both directions. Laryngologists often refer clients to SLPs for behavioral vocal intervention. Equally often, persons with voice problems seek the help of SLPs without first seeing a doctor. In most cases of phonatory voice disorders, some type of referral for medical or psychological evaluation will be necessary. We must remember that SLPs diagnose the voice and its characteristics, whereas medical doctors—particularly laryngologists—diagnose the vocal mechanism per se. It is not within the province of the SLP to diagnose nodules, inflammation, cancer, or the like. The SLP does assess the parameters of the voice that may or may not reflect such structural changes. Voice disorders may be caused by life-threatening situations such as carcinoma of the larynx or something as simple as vocal misuse. The importance of medical referral, then, is obvious. Structural changes such as ulcers, polyps, tumors, or nodules may be detected by the laryngologist through laryngeal examination and confirmed by tissue biopsy. Auditory symptoms such as hoarseness or harshness of the voice and/or sensory complaints (e.g., laryngeal pain, lumps, and the like) should prompt the SLP to make the referral. Hoarseness lasting beyond 14 days, particularly in persons over the age of 40, should be referred on a suspicion of being a serious, life-threatening condition until proven otherwise. The need for a medical diagnosis cannot be underestimated because of the life and health implications for the client, the legal implications for the practicing clinician, and the requirement of third-party reimbursement agencies that services provided be "medically necessary."

It is widely accepted that the SLP and the laryngologist should ideally cultivate a close working relationship when dealing with voice cases. Each professional can provide significant information to the other, and *voice treatment* that attempts to alter one or more parameters of the voice, such as pitch, should not begin without a laryngological examination. A *vocal hygiene* program, which does not alter the voice but teaches care of it, can begin with many clients prior to laryngoscopic examination. Thus, waiting for medical examination in cases of vocal abuse should not be used as a reason to postpone enrollment in an intervention program.

During an examination by a medical specialist (often the otolaryngologist in conjunction with the SLP), indirect laryngoscopy will be accomplished via a mirror, or direct laryngoscopy may be accomplished by use of a rigid or flexible endoscope. In cases of infants or preschool children, for whom such procedures are difficult, the laryngologist may use direct laryngoscopy under anesthesia. Videostroboscopy is also available in many laryngolists' offices and sophisticated voice centers. Videostroboscopy allows real-time observation of the condition and function of the vocal folds. This method will be discussed later in the chapter. The SLP will be interested in the findings of the laryngeal examinations for several reasons and may wish to view the folds personally to better understand the reported findings and diagnosis. Many SLPs perform videostroboscopy.

First, the examination can document any physical alteration to the vocal mechanism (e.g., nodules, polyps) that may account for vocal differences. Second, the speech pathologist will want to have the extent of any vocal fold pathology documented as baseline information if voice therapy is indicated so that alterations in the client's voice over time, as the result of treatment, might be correlated with concomitant organic changes that show in future laryngological examinations. Forms containing drawings of the vocal apparatus have been recommended so that the physician can make notes indicating the size and location of abnormalities, or the image may be stored in a computer file. Either way, this could become part of the client's record and be used for comparisons over time as evidence of intervention effectiveness.

A third reason the speech pathologist will be interested in the laryngeal examination is that surgical intervention may be recommended as the treatment of choice for a particular patient. A dialogue between the clinician and the doctor may be necessary to discuss this decision and to discuss recommendations regarding the appropriateness of follow-up voice therapy.

Finally, the absence of organic deviations on the laryngoscopic examination may suggest more functional bases for the client's disorder. Such knowledge would have direct implications for the direction of voice treatment and may also indicate that other referrals by the speech pathologist (e.g., to a psychologist) are in order.

A general medical evaluation or specific neurological or endocrinological examination may be indicated in certain cases. When dysfunction of the peripheral or central nervous system appears to be a possible contributing factor to the voice disorder, as in dysarthria (see Chapter 9), referral is indicated.

During a routine screening of all college students entering the teacher education and certification program, Susan came to our attention. Susan's voice was weak, and she had difficulty projecting it louder or trying to shout when requested to do so. On questioning, it was revealed that her voice tires easily throughout the day, and a slight hoarseness is typical. This prompted us to inquire further—trying to unravel the mystery of Susan's voice problem and wondering about a possible endocrinological basis. Suspicions of a hyperactive thyroid gland became stronger when Susan complained of nervousness and irritability, generalized muscle weakness, and fatigue—making it difficult for her to complete her aerobics routine at the local gym (one day her legs trembled and were so weak she could not rise from a squat), excessive sweating, weight loss—which she was happy about even though she still ate lots of food, and insomnia, and had irregular menstrual periods. Her once-radiant skin had turned sallow in recent months. Referral to a physician was made and hyperthyroidism (Grave's disease) was diagnosed.

Case History Questionnaire and Interview

The SLP should interview the client directly and, in the case of a child, the parents, teachers, and others of significance should be consulted as well. Much information about daily use of the voice, possible phonotraumas (abuses), and functional impacts can be gathered from informants. There are many excellent sources for guidance in taking an adequate case history with an emphasis on voice disorders, and many of these sources provide forms for the clinician's use (see, for example, Boone et al., 2014; Rubin et al., 2006; Sapienza & Ruddy, 2013; Stemple et al., 2010). The American Speech-Language-Hearing Association (ASHA) provides a useful general-purpose adult template for collecting demographic and case history information as well as a version appropriate for children (search for these templates at www.asha.org/). The interested reader is encouraged to consult social media because many university clinics and publishers make their case history forms available online at no charge.

Sample case history questions that we routinely ask during a client interview are shown in Table 11–1. In addition, Table 11–2 may be used as a checklist on which the client indicates any coexisting sensory symptoms. In the following section, we will elaborate on the case history topics most relevant to vocal diagnosis and subsequent intervention, but it is helpful to realize that the information in both these of tables opens the exploration into how the voice is affecting the client's quality of life.

Family Data

For a young client, information regarding parental occupation, number of siblings, history of family adjustment, other voice problems within the family, and general health pattern of the family tells us a great deal about the young client's social and physical milieu. Generally, the following characteristics may be considered potentially remarkable and should be explored further: (1) too much or too little structure and organization in the home, (2) premium placed on verbal competition, (3) interparental friction, (4) unusual sibling competition, (5) history of voice disorders, (6) poor parental adjustment, (7) history of extended recurrent health problems, and (8) general level of concern for physical and health problems. For the adult client, we are interested in many of the same issues, particularly occupation,

---

TABLE 11–1
Sample Questions to Ask in the Case History Intake

1. What are your voice concerns?
2. When did these voice issues begin?
3. Did this begin suddenly or develop slowly?
4. What do you think may be the cause? What conditions surrounded the onset of your voice issues (cold, illness, surgery, personal problems, etc.)?
5. When is your voice better (e.g., morning, night)? When is it worse (e.g., morning, night)?
6. Describe the daily use of your voice (typical weekday behaviors and job demands on the voice; typical weekend activities).
7. Are there specific situations when voice trauma occurs? (Inquire about the frequency of common misuses and abuses such as excessive crying, throat clearing, coughing, smoking, screaming, etc.).
8. Describe your general health (sinus problems; allergies; illnesses; injuries to the head, neck, or scrotum; endocrine disorders; heart disease; surgery; fatigability; smoking and/or drinking habits; etc.).
9. What medications do you take?
10. What has your doctor told you about your voice? Why has the doctor referred you?

TABLE 11–2
Checklist of Sensory Symptoms

Mark (with an X) all symptoms associated with *your* voice.

_____ 1. Frequent throat clearing
_____ 2. Frequent coughing
_____ 3. Vocal fatigue that progresses with use of the voice
_____ 4. Irritation or pain in the voice or throat
_____ 5. Strain, bulging, or tender neck muscles
_____ 6. Swelling of veins/arteries in the neck
_____ 7. Feeling of something or a lump in the throat
_____ 8. Ear ache, irritation, or tickling
_____ 9. Frequent sore throats
_____ 10. A burning sensation in the throat or base of tongue (worse during which foods and/or drinks?)
_____ 11. Scratchy or dry throat
_____ 12. A feeling that talking is an effort
_____ 13. Pain or difficulty swallowing

number of persons living in the home, and health problems or communication disorders among those living in the home.

> Barbara was a 32-year-old mother of twins. Both 4-year-old boys were described as rambunctious, and Barbara was the archetypical housewife. She also cared for her mother-in-law, who was hard of hearing, a bit senile, and lived in the same home. Barbara just could not understand why she had developed bilateral vocal nodules and why the doctor insisted on her enrolling in voice therapy.

Clearly, family information of this type suggests etiological factors of vocal abuse and provides behavioral change as a direction for treatment.

Onset of the Problem   In many instances, the beginning of the voice problem will have great diagnostic significance. It is important to investigate not only the nature of the onset but also the circumstances surrounding it. Physical or psychological trauma may have equally instant effects on voice production. In some cases, extended questioning may be necessary because it is common for clients to repress uncomfortable incidents of the past. A sudden onset within hours suggests the high probability of a conversion vocal disorder or a neurological origin (such as stroke), whereas many other types of vocal disturbances develop gradually (mass and approximation lesions, degenerative disease, etc.).

Although the abrupt onset of a vocal disorder is traumatic and startling, most voice disorders are of insidious origin. Many people cannot pinpoint the exact date of the onset and tend to indicate when people first noticed or remarked about their voices. A gradual onset is not necessarily specific to organic or functional etiologies, so the examiner must look to other data for final answers. Probably more important than the rate of development is information on coincident factors such as the client's general health and emotional state.

Course of Development   A careful description of the developmental stages of the voice disturbance may provide helpful diagnostic information. The course of the development of the voice disorder may be found to parallel a chronic medical problem, cumulating vocational stress, certain periods of physical maturation, changes in family relationships, or developing financial crises. We want to know how the problem has changed since its onset, and we want to know about any circumstances surrounding variability of the voice disturbance. For instance, were there changes in the voice disorder during its development that might be correlated with changes in personal habits (e.g., smoking, use of alcohol), work conditions (e.g., excessive noise, stress), or medical conditions (e.g., sinus, allergy)? The clinician will want to keep in mind that, once a voice disorder has been firmly established, only a minimal amount of tension, misuse, or abuse will be necessary to perpetuate the problem.

Description of Daily Vocal Performance and Problem Variability While the course-of-development questions seek a historical perspective, we need information on factors that influence the voice at the time of the evaluation. For instance, we might ask the client to describe his or her daily routine and relate it to talking. Does the problem become worse through the day? Does it become better as the day progresses? It is especially important in cases of childhood vocal pathology to obtain an accurate picture of the youngster's typical use of voice and instances of misuse or abuse.

Social Adjustment Assessment of the personality characteristics of the individual may assist the diagnostician in interpreting other information. Formal personality testing is not within the jurisdiction of the speech pathologist, but each clinician is expected to be perceptive and sensitive to clues about the client's basic adjustment to life. Classification of voice characteristics with specific personality types has not provided overwhelming evidence of definite relationships, but the personality and the voice do interact in a complex fashion, and this results in many symptomatic characteristics.

Vocation We are interested in the vocation of our voice client for two reasons. First, we must determine if the occupation demands a great deal of talking and if that talking is under adverse conditions. Not all teachers develop "teacher's nodules," however, and the vocation must be judged in relation to the person. Several writers have postulated that there is a personality type that develops vocal nodules. We have found many people who develop nodules to be tense, energetic, high-strung, and verbally aggressive. Place this type of person in an occupational setting that demands a great deal of speaking under tension, and combine this factor with a bit of poor judgment in choosing adaptive procedures, and the chances of finding an individual with vocal nodules could be greatly enhanced.

A second factor in our evaluation of the vocation of an individual is to assess the possibility of changing aspects of the client's job routine or behavior at work if the vocation has a deleterious effect on the voice disorder.

> We worked with a college professor who taught several large lecture classes to groups of over 150 students. His vocal abuse and misuse during his class presentations had resulted in small nodules for which voice therapy was recommended. In an effort to be audible, dynamic, and authoritative, he had been speaking loudly, with a lower pitch, and excessive tension. We explored the possibility of his using a lavalier microphone in the large lecture rooms, and this effectively eliminated an abusive situation that was vocationally related.

Health

Realizing that the voice is influenced by many physiological systems, a complete medical history and examination are necessary in many instances. A history of the general health and physical development of the client should be obtained, along with information about specific illnesses, surgeries, and medications. The clinician should also obtain data concerning the client's general energy level and health-related habits, such as smoking, drinking, and drug use.

Patient Impact Ratings The last part of the case history phase of assessment seeks to ascertain, from the client's perspective, the degree of impact that the voice is having on the client's daily functioning. Currently, these assessments are referred to as quality-of-life scales. Such topics evolved in the interview questioning (recall Table 11–2 and Figure 11–2 with regard to daily performance, social adjustment, and vocation) but now need to be objectified with scoreable tools that are normed, reliable, and valid. Instruments of this type can be used pre- and post-treatment to assess effectiveness and change in quality of life (Awan & Roy, 2009; Hakkesteegt et al., 2010). In this sense, quality-of-life scales and assessments are evaluative probes and reevaluations that monitor change and the impact of intervention. A list of quality-of-life and patient symptom assessment scales is presented in Table 11–3. A few are also discussed here.

The Voice Handicap Index (VHI) and abbreviated versions of the VHI are now in common clinical use. The 30-question VHI (Jacobson et al., 1997) explores three patient domains using a rating scale of 0 to 4. In the physical domain, the client rates statements such as "I feel as though I have to strain to produce voice." The functional domain statements tap into daily impacts, such as "My voice makes it difficult for people to hear me." An example of a statement in the emotional domain is, "My voice problem upsets me." Seven- and 10-question abbreviated versions of the VHI exist in experimental form. However, the literature suggests that the 30-item VHI is statistically sound, and clinicians often administer the VHI in the initial diagnostic session and periodically thereafter to monitor treatment progress, both physically and behaviorally. A shorter 10-item version is the Voice Handicap Index, the VHI-10 (Rosen, Lee, Osborne, Zullo, & Murry, 2004); however, we believe the original 30-item VHI is in dominant use among clinicians. A pediatric version of the Voice Handicap Index (pVHI) exists as well (Zur et al., 2007) and will be mentioned in Chapter 12.

Although specific to unilateral vocal fold paralysis cases, a validated 36-item Voice Outcomes Survey is available (Gliklich, Glovsky, & Montgomery, 1999).

The Dysphonia Severity Index (DSI) is another handicap scale in popular use (Wuyts et al., 2000). The DSI features more of a focus on severity as a function of perceived vocal quality. It weighs a combination of actual acoustic measures: the highest vocal frequency (fundamental frequency expressed in Hertz), the lowest intensity (in dB), the maximum phonation time (MPT, in seconds), and jitter (percentage derived from requisite equipment). The index is scored between +5 for a normal voice to −5 for a severely dysphonic voice. The more negative the client's index, the worse the vocal quality. The DSI is normed and valid according to the authors and is highly correlated with the Voice Handicap Index.

To assess the impact of a voice disorder, quality-of-life measures may be taken of an adult both pre- and postintervention. Here we highlight the Voice-Related Quality of Life (V-RQOL) scale (Hogikyan & Sethurama, 1999), which ideally is rated by the patient 2 weeks before the diagnostic appointment. This is a brief 10-item questionnaire (rated on a scale of 1 = no problem through 5 = problem as bad as it can be) for various social-emotional and physical-functional aspects of the voice problem. Example aspects include the patient's trouble speaking loudly, running out of air, depression, using the telephone, and so forth.

TABLE 11–3
Some Quality-of-Life and Symptom Impact Scales for Children and Adults

Iowa Patient's Voice Index (IPVI) (Karnell et al., 2007)
  A simple three-item patient perception questionnaire developed by Verdolini and colleagues at the University of Iowa and studied for reliability by Karnell.
Dysphonia Severity Index (DSI) (Wuyts et al., 2000)
  See text for description.
Patient Questionnaire of Voice Performance (PQVP) (Carding & Horsley, 1992)
  Patient self-rates aspects of his or her own vocal performance to yield an impact score (e.g., 12 = normal functioning, 60 = severe dysphonia); often used with nonorganic dysponic cases.
Pediatric Voice Handicap Index (pVHI) (Zur et al., 2007)
  Assesses physical, functional, and emotional attributes.
Pediatric Voice Outcomes Survey (pVOS) (Hartnick, Volk, & Cunningham, 2003)
  Assesses physical, social, and school attributes in children ages 2 to 18.
Pediatric Voice-Related Quality of Life (PVRQOL) (Boseley, Cunningham, Vollk & Hartnick, 2006)
  Assesses physical and social-emotional attributes.
Singing Voice Handicap Index (SVHI) (Cohen et al., 2007)
  Subjective assessment useful with patients who sing,
Voice Activity and Participation Profile (VAPP) (Ma & Yiu, 2001)
  Assesses perception of voice problem, activity limitation, and social participation restrictions at work and play in a 28-item questionnaire.
Vocal Disability Coping Questionnaire (VDCQ) (Epstein, Hiran, Stygall, & Newman, 2009)
  Assesses information-seeking, avoidance, and social support attributes.
Vocal Impact Profile (VIP) (Martin & Lockhart, 2005)
  Assesses potential impact of factors like health, vocal history, voice care and status, anxiety/stress, social/environmental factors, and vocal demands.
Voice Handicap Index (VHI) (Jacobson et al., 1997)
  Assesses physical, functional, and educational attributes in 30 questions.
Voice Outcome Survey (VOS) (Gliklich, Glovsky, & Montgomery, 1999)
  Assesses functional, social, and work attributes; was designed for used in cases of unilateral vocal fold paralysis.
Vocal Performance Questionnaire (Paul Cardin, Freeman Hospital, United Kingdom; search online at https://entuk.org/)
  Twelve multiple-choice, scoreable questions; available online by searching above site.
Voice-Related Quality of Life (V-RQOL) (Hogikyan & Sethurama, 1999)
  Assesses physical and social-emotional attributes in a 10-item questionnaire designed to be completed 2 weeks prior to the voice evaluation.
Voice Symptom Scale (VoiSS) (Deary, Wilson, Carding, & Mackenzie, 2003)
  Assesses the voice and patient reports of communication problems, throat infections, psychological distress, voice sound and variability problems, and phlegm.

Preliminary Screenings

Before progressing deeper into the initial diagnostic session, it is important for the SLP to rule in or out other factors that may have an impact on the client's communication status. Whether this can be done in a cursory manner or whether it necessitates a detailed approach is determined by the clinician's impression of the patient based on a review of the referral documents, early access to the patient's completed case history form (best if obtained prior to the appointment), the patient's age (child/adult), and skilled clinical impressions when greeting and chatting with the new client. At a minimum, the SLP determines whether each communication attribute is "judged to be within normal limits for age and gender" or additional screening or testing measures are warranted. Aspects of communication needing assessment include an oral-motor exam (see Appendix A), a hearing screening (see Appendix B), speech articulation/phonology and intelligibility (see Chapter 6), as well as language reception/expression (see Chapters 4 and 5 for children and Chapter 8 for adults).

PERCEPTUAL, ACOUSTIC, AND AERODYNAMIC ASSESSMENT

The first step in voice analysis is simply listening to the client in an analytical manner. Obviously, this listening process is largely judgmental. Much of what we do in a routine voice assessment is perceptual and subjective. Rating scales, profiles, checklists, and assessment outlines are thus the order of the day. A generic 7-point rating scale, such as the one shown in Table 11–4, may guide the clinician in a cursory appraisal of the various characteristics of the voice. What is important to assess is not the overall voice but a decomposition of the voice into its various attributes of pitch/frequency, loudness/intensity, quality, and myriad other features that vary with the rating scale used. Many voice assessment tools (rating scales, profiles, checklists, open-ended observation forms, and the like) are available. Table 11–5 lists some commonly used resources. It must be stated, however, that the reliability, validity, and standardization norms of such tools are disappointing, if not lacking. Unfortunately, this is true of the two widely used scales, the GRBAS and the CAPE-V, which were developed to avoid such shortcomings (Biddle, Watson, Hooper, Lohr, & Sutton, 2002). We provide a brief word about each.

The GRBAS Scale was developed by the Japanese Society of Logopedics and Phoniatrics for rating hoarseness and was first described in English by Hirano (1981); see also Omori (2011). GRBAS is an acronym for the parameters of grade (where hoarseness is scored on a scale of 0 to 3); roughness, breathiness, asthenia, and strained are also scored but on a scale as follows: 0 = normal, 1 = slight degree, 2 = medium degree and 3 = high degree. Rough hoarseness is described as a raspy or rattling sound in the voice. Breathy hoarseness has a whisper component to the voice. Asthenic hoarshness is a small or weak voice. Strained hoarseness exhibits throat constriction. While GRBAS is an auditory-perceptual evaluation, the measure of MPT is a key barometer in the last three (breathiness, asthenia, strain) aspects of this hoarseness scale.

MPT is a frequently collected data point in *any* type of voice evaluation. MPT represents the maximum length of time a client can sustain vocalization of a vowel (such as "ah") following a maximum inhalation of air. The attempt is timed, and the best of three tries can be used. A rule of thumb is that 10 seconds or less is abnormal, and 5 seconds or less very probably interferes with activities of daily living. While age and general health affect MPT, the vocal impact with these rule-of-thumb times tends to hold true clinically.

Another widely used rating scale, said to be "more objective" than most, was developed by the Voice Special Interest Division 3 of ASHA. It is called Consensus Auditory Perceptual Evaluation–Voice, or CAPE-V. In CAPE-V, the voice is assessed in sustained vowel production, sentence production, and conversational speech. The clinician describes how consistently the voice is produced and assigns a severity rating of consistent, mild, moderate, or severely deviated. This rating is done for each vocal attribute: roughness, breathiness, strain, pitch, loudness, and overall quality. Access to CAPE-V is limited to members of ASHA through its website (www.asha.org), and member login is necessary.

TABLE 11–4
Generic Rating Scale of Vocal Characteristics

Pitch

1 2 3 4 5 6 7*

Description		Severity				
Too high	1	2	3	4	5	6	7
Too low	1	2	3	4	5	6	7
Invariant	1	2	3	4	5	6	7
Pitch breaks	1	2	3	4	5	6	7
Diplophonia	1	2	3	4	5	6	7
Repetitive pattern	1	2	3	4	5	6	7

Loudness

1 2 3 4 5 6 7*

Description		Severity				
Excessive	1	2	3	4	5	6	7
Inadequate	1	2	3	4	5	6	7
Uncontrolled variation	1	2	3	4	5	6	7
Repetitive pattern	1	2	3	4	5	6	7
Invariant	1	2	3	4	5	6	7
Tremulous	1	2	3	4	5	6	7

Quality

1 2 3 4 5 6 7*

Description		Severity				
Hoarseness	1	2	3	4	5	6	7
Harshness	1	2	3	4	5	6	7
Breathiness	1	2	3	4	5	6	7
Hypernasal	1	2	3	4	5	6	7
Hyponasal	1	2	3	4	5	6	7
Other (describe)	1	2	3	4	5	6	7

Judgment of Vocal Tension

1 2 3 4 5 6 7*

Aphonia/whisper

Breathy phonation

Normal

Hypertension

Hypertension/intermittent phonation

Overall Judgment of Voice

1 2 3 4 5 6 7*

*Note: 1 = normal; 7 = severely disordered.

TABLE 11–5
Annotated List of Some Available Rating Scales and Evaluation Materials

Boone Voice Program for Adults, Third Edition (Boone, 2000)
   Both diagnosis and remediation procedures for vocal disorders are contained in this kit.
Boone Voice Program for Children, Second Edition (Boone, 1993)
   Screening, evaluation, and referral instructions are included in a manual with this
   remediation kit. Also provided are the necessary forms and stimulus materials.
Systematic Assessment of Voice (SAV) (Shipley, 1990)
   This is a comprehensive inventory of tasks, strategies, and guidelines for assessing
   functional and organic voice problems in children and adults. It contains reproducible lists
   of words, phrases, sentences, passages for oral reading, case history forms, letters to
   parents, and so forth.
Voice Assessment Protocol for Children and Adults (Pindzrh, 1987)
   This protocol directs and quantifies clinical observations of voice. The following vocal
   parameters are assessed: pitch, loudness, quality, breath features, and rate.
Voice Diagnostic Protocol (Awan, 2000)
   This manual compiles methods of low-cost vocal analyses, including history taking
   and perceptual analysis of vocal frequency, intensity, quality, examination of structures,
   evaluation of respiratory and phonatory control, and effects of excessive muscular tension.
   Each diagnostic procedure is explained, and normative data and interpretations of results
   are provided. Includes a CD.
CAPE-V
   See text for description.
GRBAS Scale for Hoarseness
   See text for description.

The research literature is robust in assessing reliability and validity of perceptual voice scales and quality-of-life scales. A case in point is the work by Karnell and colleagues (2007). The clinician-rated vocal attributes of GRBAS and CAPE-V perceptual scales were compared, and both were found to be reliable, though CAPE-V was said to be more sensitive to small vocal differences. However, these two scales showed less agreement with the patient-administered vocal attributes and quality-of-life impact scales of V-RQOL and IPVI (see Table 11–3).

Let us now turn our attention to a discussion of the vocal parameters and how they are routinely assessed. As in evaluating other communication disorders, the clinician must realize that the type of sample obtained affects how "ecologically valid" it is. For instance, in the case of a child with vocal nodules who is suspected of being a voice abuser, it would be ideal to observe the youngster in a play situation with others, during school activities, and in the home environment. Most often, a variety of sampling activities is used in the evaluation, and these activities range from conversation to counting, coughing, singing the scale, and prolonging isolated speech sounds. The point here is that the clinician should be aware that a broad sampling of vocal performance is needed in order to make correct judgments on any parameter of the voice.

Five voice areas of pitch, loudness, quality, breath features, and rate/rhythm are routinely assessed in clients through a marriage of perceptual and simplistic acoustic analysis, as with a stopwatch and pitch pipe or piano keyboard. More sophisticated technological appraisals are also becoming routine in a variety of clinical settings. Let's review the five areas of vocal assessment from perceptual, acoustic, and aerodynamic vantage points.

FEATURE ASSESSMENT
Pitch

Clinicians routinely evaluate various pitch characteristics of the client's voice. Pitch is a perceptual phenomenon that correlates with the valving rate of the vocal folds. Rightly or wrongly, clinicians interchange the terms *pitch* and *frequency* when talking about a client's voice. *Pitch determination* of the speaking fundamental frequency, also known as habitual pitch, can be accomplished with musical-matching methods using low-tech (pitch pipe or keyboard) or high-tech instrumental analysis, as shown in Table 11–6. The client's speaking fundamental frequency can then be compared to normative data, based on age and sex. Table 11–7 shows average fundamental frequencies, synthesized from the literature, for a representative sample of ages.

Pitch determination methods can also be used to locate a client's optimal pitch. *Optimal pitch* is a controversial concept that supposes each person has an optimal or natural pitch range at which he or she *should* be speaking. If we accept the premise of optimal performance, habitual pitch may need to be raised or lowered in treatment when optimal pitch does not match habitual pitch. The determination of optimal pitch is by no means precise. In addition, it should be emphasized that optimal pitch is not a single note but a range of notes where the vocal mechanism appears to function best

TABLE 11–6
Some Available Software for Vocal Assessments

Computerized Speech Lab (CSL) **(http://www.kaypentax.com/)**
This website contains purchasing information for models of expensive, freestanding equipment. Considered the gold standard for research and clinical analysis of voice, the CSL includes popular components such as the VisiPitch and the Multi-Dimensional Voice Program.

Multi-Speech **(http://www.kaypentax.com/)**
This website contains purchasing information for this low-cost, Windows-based speech analysis software system akin to the CSL; performs a variety of voice analyses.

Praat: Doing Phonetics by Computer **(http://www.fon.hum.uva.nl/praat)**
Allows for various free spectral, pitch, and format analyses as well as for jitter and shimmer; popular with students and clinicians alike.

Sona-Speech II **(http://www.kaypentax.com/)**
This website contains purchasing information for affordable models that are alternative to the VisiPitch for measuring speech and vocal behaviors.

Speech Analyzer **(http://www.sil.org/computing/speechtools/speechanalyzer.htm)**
Free downloads of Speech Analyzer allow viewing sound files such as waveform, pitch plot, spectrum, or various F1 versus F2 displays. Updated software is also available at low cost.

Speech Filing System **(http://www.phon.ucl.ac.uk/resource/sfs/)**
The Speech Filing System (SFS) is free software that is powerful for assorted speech analyses; suitable for research and clinical purposes.

The Voice Diagnostic Protocol (Awan, 2000)
Part of a commercially available assessment package, this protocol contains a CD for the clinician's computer when a microphone is added. Information on available software and using equipment also is provided.

Voiceprint **(http://www.visualizationsoftware.com)**
Voiceprint is useful for spectrographs. A trial version can be accessed for free, but the full program is inexpensive.

Waveform Annotation Spectrograms and Pitch (WASP) **(http://www.phon.ucl.ac.uk/resource/sfs/wasp.htm)**
WASP is a free download; the program allows for recording and analyzing speech signals. It displays features like spectrograms and fundamental frequency easily for students and clinicians alike.

TABLE 11–7
Average Fundamental Frequencies and Nearest Musical Note for Selected Ages

Age (in Years)	Sex	Mean Fundamental	Musical Note
1–2	Either	445 Hz	A4
3	Either	390 Hz	G4
6	Either	320 Hz	E4
10	Male	235 Hz	A3#
15	Male	165 Hz	E3
20–29	Male	120 Hz	B2
50–59	Male	118 Hz	A2#
60–69	Male	112 Hz	A2
80–89	Male	146 Hz	D3
10	Female	265 Hz	C4
15	Female	220 Hz	A3
20–29	Female	227 Hz	A3#
50–59	Female	214 Hz	G3#
60–69	Female	209 Hz	G3#
80–89	Female	197 Hz	G3

with the least muscular tension. Various vegetative (natural, involuntary, and non-speech sounds) and range-singing techniques have been proposed for eliciting optimal pitches from clients; once elicited and recorded, the value of the optimal pitch can be determined musically or instrumentally. Table 11–8 summarizes some of the more commonly used methods for eliciting a client's optimal pitch. Later in the chapter, we will discuss how these techniques are useful as probes or facilitators of voicing abilities.

The normal voice is characterized by *pitch variability*, also known as *intonation* or *inflection*. The voice is abnormal when there is a lack of pitch variability or when pitch fluctuations are excessive. Dysarthrias may be characterized by monopitch, where a limited range of notes are used monotonously. Monopitch and restricted pitch ranges are also associated with superior laryngeal nerve paralysis, additive lesions, and other disorders. Excessive pitch variability or prosodic excess may be heard in the dysarthrias, particularly spastic, ataxic, and hyperkinetic forms (Duffy, 2013). Dysarthria voice samples often exhibit frequency variations, especially on sustained vowel productions. Hearing-impaired and deaf speakers often utilize excessive pitch fluctuation.

Diplophonia refers to the presence of two or more simultaneous pitches or tones in the voice and may be caused by separate or unequal vibratory sources. Possible causes include a paralyzed vocal fold vibrating at a rate different from the healthy one, a vibration of a growth or lesion, simultaneous adduction of the ventricular folds and true folds, and even an innocuous saliva globule.

Pitch breaks most often occur in a person using an inappropriately low-pitched voice. Intermittently, the pitch will suddenly break upward toward a more optimal level. Any condition that adds to the mass or size of the vocal folds may alter their vibratory characteristics. Pitch breaks may be one symptom of additive lesions such as, but not limited to, nodules, polyps, and tumors.

To summarize our discussion of pitch, the clinician must observe the client, measure pitch features, and seek answers to the following questions: What is the client's habitual pitch (speaking fundamental frequency), and is this pitch appropriate for the person's age, sex, and body stature? What is an optimal level for the client to use? Is a normal amount of pitch variability present in the speaking voice, or is the voice

TABLE 11–8
Some Techniques for Determining Optimal Pitch

Resonance-Swell Method
Have the client hum at the same intensity up the scale, and note whether the voice becomes louder or swells in a given range of pitches. The client and/or the clinician should listen for this swell in loudness.

Loud-Audible Sigh
The client should take a deep breath and produce /a/ as a loud sigh. Listen most carefully for the pitch at the onset of the sigh because one tends to lower the pitch during the sound. Optimal is said to be the onset tone.

Yawn-Sigh
The client should yawn and sigh audibly in a relaxed manner. Yawning opens the throat and minimizes the constriction around the larynx.

Vegetative Techniques
Listen to the natural, spontaneous laugh, cough, throat clearing, or grunt of the client. These vegetative forms of phonation may be representative of optimal pitch.

Inflection Methods
Have the client say "um hum" using a rising inflection with lips closed, as though he or she were spontaneously and sincerely agreeing with what was just said. In addition, the clinician could have the client say "hello" in a natural, spontaneous, and sincere way. An automatic affirmative utterance often approximates optimal pitch. A related method is to have the client say "hello" with rising inflection, as though asking a question. The slight inflection may reveal a more optimal voice.

Pushing or Pulling Techniques
The client should attempt to phonate /a/ of optimal quality while pushing down or pulling up on his or her chair. This method may be particularly useful for clients with disordered closure of the vocal folds.

Pitch Range Methods
The type of phonation may be do-re-mi or ah-ah-ah or one-two-three, and so on. The client phonates the entire vocal range from the lowest sound that can be produced to the highest, excluding falsetto. One-third of this range should represent optimal pitch. An alternate and popular method is to have the client phonate his or her entire vocal range from the lowest note to the highest, including falsetto. The total range is then divided by one-fourth to locate the optimal. For example, calculate the number of full-step notes in the client's range and then locate the note that is one-fourth of the way from the bottom.

monotone or widely varying and sing-song in pattern? Are pitch breaks present? Is diplophonia present?

Loudness

Perceptual judgments of vocal loudness are common, but instrumentation is available for measuring intensity (e.g., sound level meter, CSL). Of interest during the assessment is whether the *loudness level* is appropriate for the speaking situation. In normal conversational speech, when a person is 3 feet from the speaker, the average sound intensity is 65 dB (range of 55 to 75 dB). Typical loudness levels may be abnormal in various pathologies. Adults with dysarthria may speak too softly (as in Parkinsonism) or with a booming voice (as in some spasticities and dystonias). Lack of vocal loudness is characteristic of paralyzed cords and psychogenic disorders. Clients suffering from vocal abuse often speak with excessive effort and loudness, at least in some situations; the end result, however, may be hypofunctional loudness.

The clinician should also note if the typical loudness level can be maintained comfortably, without trailing off, or whether there is a *degree of effort*. Listen for loudness that trails off at the end of a sentence, which may be typical in vocal fold paralysis, dysarthrias, or obstructive lesions. *Phonation breaks* or momentary skips of loudness are abnormal and may indicate difficulty maintaining vocal fold adduction and vibration.

A certain amount of *loudness variability* is normal and is reflected in the stress patterns of the language. In addition to listening critically to conversational speech, we often ask the client to read "with feeling" sentences such as the following:

> Get out of here! Get out of here!
> I don't know! I said I don't know!
> I need more money, Dad, I'm broke!
> Where did she go? I can't find her.
> Will you cut that out!

We have observed that lack of loudness variability may take two differing forms of monoloudness: Excess and equal stress patterns are typical of many dysarthrias, whereas the monoloud but weak and "bland" voice is typically seen in affective disorders and some forms of dysarthria.

The clinician may wish to have the client demonstrate his or her *loudness range,* from soft to maximal levels. Whispering and shouting can be requested. One method is to ask the client to count, beginning softly and increasing in loudness with higher and higher numbers. Restricted loudness range is often seen in clients with respiratory involvement, particularly the dysarthrias.

Loudness abuse is one example of phonotrauma that may be situation-oriented. For instance, conversational levels may be appropriate, but frequent loud talking or screaming (as in lectures, sermons, cheerleading, playground activities, etc.) may be perpetuating a vocal disorder. Questions asked in the interview should probe the client's daily uses of the voice with the purpose of discovering situational abuses.

After appraising the client's voice, the clinician should then have answers to the following questions about loudness: Is the loudness level that is used appropriate for the speaking situation? Can the level be maintained comfortably without undue strain? Can the level be maintained throughout the entire utterance or does it begin to trail off? Are loudness breaks present? Is the loudness variable in order to reflect stress and emphasis patterns of English or is the client monoloud? Can loudness vary from minimal (whispered) to maximal (shouted) levels? What, if any, situations are frequently encountered in which loudness abuse occurs?

Quality

The descriptive terminology used with disorders of vocal quality reflects the perceptual nature of the judgments. It can be argued that the clinician's ear is the best tool for describing the quality of a voice—and many clinicians use just that. However, rather sophisticated equipment is also available to study, categorize, and "objectify" acoustical parameters of the voice. Technology is available to measure periodicity of vocal fold vibrations, changes in amplitude (shimmer, which is proving to be an important, objective measure to ascertain), changes in frequency (jitter), and opening–closing characteristics. The Computerized Speech Lab from Kaypentax has many software options (recall Table 11–6) for voice measures. Still, deciding whether a voice is breathy, harsh, or hoarse is done most efficiently by critical listening.

Vocal quality is affected by the manner of vocal fold vibration. Many terms of vocal quality appear in the literature, including *breathy, harsh,* or *hoarse*; hoarseness is the most prevalent. Designations such as *strident* and *husky* are used less frequently. With the popularity of CAPE-V, standardized terms are often limited to *roughness, breathiness,* and *strain.*

The breathy voice is characterized by an audible escape of air through partially closed folds. The lack of firm adduction may be due to obstruction by a mass or lesion, a paralyzed cord, or muscular incompetence.

The voice displaying effort and force is the harsh voice. Harshness is usually perceived in a phonatory milieu of hard glottal attacks, low pitch, intensity problems, and overadduction of the vocal folds. Equivalent terms are *roughness* and *unpleasantness,* although *strident, coarse, grating, rasping, rough, metallic,* and *guttural* have been used as synonyms for *harshness.*

The hoarse voice incorporates the features of both breathiness and harshness. As such, turbulent air flow, rough/aperiodic vibrations, low pitch, and neck muscle strain may be evident. Hoarseness is a common symptom of many vocal pathologies and should be recognizable by all SLPs. In particular, the public school clinician should be familiar with the auditory symptoms of hoarseness as a warning sign of vocal abuse and related lesions in children. The clinician must make medical referrals as appropriate. In addition, the clinician must educate teachers through inservice programs to recognize voice disturbances in students so that teacher referrals to the SLP will be accomplished.

The perception of vocal quality is also affected by *glottal approximation.* The hard glottal attack refers to an abrupt impact or strong initiation of speech. Extra effort is used to start the vibrations of tightly adducted folds. Presumably, then, prior to phonation there is too much tension in laryngeal muscles. Conversely, soft attack is an abnormally weak glottal approximation. Breathiness usually precedes this phonation. The astute clinician is listening for symptoms of an inappropriate glottal approximation.

The measures of jitter (frequency perturbation) and shimmer (amplitude perturbation), typically on a sustained vowel, are becoming more common because of jitter's and shimmer's utility in early detection of pathology, even when the laryngologist sees no obvious lesion or tissue change. Speech pathologists working with laryngologists are called on to obtain measures of jitter and shimmer for their patients. The sound spectrogram has long been a favorite piece of equipment for the voice scientist and clinician. Isshiki, Yanigahara, and Morimoto (1966) proposed that narrowband analyses can provide measures of hoarseness. They described four types:

- Type 1 shows the slightest degree of hoarseness, where the distinct harmonic component is mixed with the noise component, which is limited within the formant region of the vowels; vowels to use are /u, o, a, e, i/.

- Type 2 shows a slight noise component in the high-frequency region (3,000 to 5,000 Hz). The noise components predominate over the harmonics, most noticeable for the vowels /e/ and /i/.

- Type 3 shows only noise in the second formant of /i/ and /e/; there is an additional intensification of noise above 3,000 Hz.

- Type 4 is characterized by noise in the second formant of /e/, /i/, and /a/ and in the first formant of /a/, /o/, and /u/. In these formant regions, the harmonic components are hardly noticeable.

The clinician can use the typing system of Isshiki, Yanigahara, and Morimoto for baseline, objective documentation of a patient's hoarseness. Spectrographic reassessments and retyping could be used as a barometer of improvement through treatment. Quality can also be affected by resonance imbalances. These disorders will be discussed in Chapter 12.

Breath

Breathing variables affect laryngeal function in general, and vocal loudness and rate of speech in particular. Several features of the respiratory system and breath management are typically assessed in a voice evaluation. In this section, an overview of the following assessment techniques is presented:

- Observation of breathing
- Vital capacity measures
- Attention to noises
- Words (or syllables) per breath
- Maximum phonation time (MPT)
- Maximum exhalation time (MET)
- S/Z ratio
- Mean flow rate (MFR)
- Phonation quotient (PQ)
- Phonation threshold pressure (PTP)
- Subglottal pressure measure

Any or all of these measures aid in the clinical decision process.

The clinician may first want to observe the *predominant region* used for breath support. The diaphragm is the principal muscle of inhalation, and various thoracic muscles assist when needed in expanding the lung-thoracic unit. Diaphragmatic breathing involves descent of the diaphragm and expansion of the abdomen during inhalation. Although quite normal—and a preferred way of breathing for both song and speech—it is difficult if not impossible to observe in a clothed, seated client. Expansion of the chest, not the shoulders, in a slight heaving motion is more observable; this type of thoracic breathing is used by many people. Clavicular breathing, in contrast, is characterized by shoulder elevation, upper thoracic tension (in the area of the clavicle or collarbone), and neck muscle strain. Clavicular breathing is an inefficient method of lung expansion for inhalation because it involves too much effort for too little breath. The clinician should try to observe the region predominately used for breathing by clients; many hyperfunctional voice cases employ this inefficient form of breathing.

The maximum amount of air that can be exhaled following maximal inhalation is called *vital capacity*. The relationship of vital capacity to speech production is somewhat a matter of conjecture at this point. Vital capacity is apparently related to several factors, such as body size, physical condition, and sex. There is little or no research to vindicate those who have worked to increase the vital capacity of their voice clients. On the other hand, it is logical to assume that an individual with an extremely small amount of available air would find it difficult to sustain phonation and might resort to increased laryngeal tension and forcing to maintain normal or near-normal phrasing. It is probably not so much the volume of air as it is the individual's ability to control the air flow.

Equipment, such as the spirometer, is necessary to measure vital capacity. Clinically, however, we have found that a vital capacity insufficient for normal speech purposes was so obvious from normal observation that further formal testing was not necessary. Vital capacity measurements may be of particular concern in cases of emphysema, later stages of Parkinson disease, and cerebral palsy in children. Related to lung volume are indications of the client's tidal volume, inspiratory reserve volume, expiratory reserve volume, and air flow rates, which some authorities recommend measuring clinically (Boone et al., 2014).

Inhalation for speech should be quick and quiet. The clinician should listen for *associated noises* such as gasps and vocalizations during inhalation as the client speaks. Rating scales may also prompt the clinician to judge the conspicuousness or severity of gasps and vocalizations. *Inhalatory stridor* refers to noticeable phonatory sounds during inhalation and may be common in cases of vocal fold paralysis and dysarthrias.

When respiratory support is inadequate for normal speech, clients may breathe more frequently. In addition, fewer words (or syllables) may be spoken per breath group. These two factors contribute to the perception of "choppy" speech. The clinician should assess *words per breath;* a patient who can utter only six or so words per air charge is displaying poor breath support. Occasionally, a patient may say an excessive number of words per breath group. Research about what constitutes excessive, however, is lacking. Perhaps upward of 12 or 13 words per breath group is typical of normal speakers. Increased speaking rates and loss of intelligibility may be the negative by-products of too many words per breath.

Of interest in a voice evaluation is the maximum duration that a client can sustain sound plus air. MPT is typically measured with a stopwatch as the client prolongs certain voiced phonemes, such as /a/ or /z/. This surprisingly simple assessment is quite sensitive to vocal dysfunction along the glottal edge, and so it is a must in any voice evaluation. Speyer et al. (2010) have shown its reliability across various methods of assessment. A similar measure is MET, where a voiceless phoneme such as /s/ is used. The clinician should provide several trials, instruct the client to use a deep breath, and record the longest sustained attempt. A general rule of thumb that is easy to remember and clinically useful is that elementary-school-age children (6 to 10 years old) should be able to prolong /a/ for at least 9 seconds, regardless of sex; adult males average 25 to 35 seconds MPT; adult females average 15 to 25 seconds MPT; and persons over age 65 average 12 seconds MPT. Related to the measures of MPT and MET is the clinical procedure of computing the *S/Z ratio.* The S/Z ratio is a quick-screening device used to determine how much of a voice problem may be related to respiration control and how much may be the result of laryngeal problems. Clients who have laryngeal pathology have less control of the air stream during the production of a prolonged /z/. Two trials are given for the prolongation of both the voiceless /s/ and the voiced /z/ phonemes, which are measured using a stopwatch. The best or longest /s/ and the longest /z/ are used in calculating the S/Z ratio. If the S/Z ratio is greater than 1.2 for a child or 1.4 for an adult, a laryngeal pathology, especially of the glottal edge, may exist (Boone et al., 2014). Gelfer and Pazera (2006) discuss various methods of elicitation and ratio calculation for optimal reliability. We wish to reiterate that the physical examination of the abdominal wall and diaphragm (Hixon & Hoit, 1998, 1999) is worth considering by the SLP, and straightforward assessment forms are provided by Hixon and Hoit.

Aerodynamic tests can assess properties of phonation, including subglottal pressure, supraglottal pressure, glottal impedance, and the volume velocity of the air flow at the glottis. Hirano (1981) states that the values of these four parameters vary during the opening and closing maneuvers of the glottis and may be difficult to measure. For example, the determination of subglottal pressure necessitates an invasive approach (such as a tracheal puncture), and glottal resistance must be calculated mathematically because it cannot be measured directly. The measure of MFR, however, is often done as an office procedure.

The MFR of a sustained vowel, such as /a/, spoken at a natural pitch and loudness level, has been used clinically to evaluate phonatory function. The patient sustains the vowel for a maximum period of time while wearing a mask fitted tightly to the face or using a mouthpiece with the nose clamped. The mask or mouthpiece is coupled to a spirometer, pneumotachograph, or hot-wire anemometer. The MFR is obtained by dividing the total volume of air used during phonation by the duration of phonation. Normal values of MFR range from 40 to 200 ml/sec in adult males and females. The MFR is greater than normal in cases of recurrent laryngeal nerve paralysis. Values for MFR in cases of nodules, polyps, polypoid swelling (Reinke's edema), and neoplastic tumors also exceed the normal range but are not as marked as with recurrent laryngeal nerve paralysis. In contrast, MFR values are typically within normal limits for the conditions of laryngitis, contact granuloma, and spastic dysphonia. Therefore, MFR is diagnostically important and may be used to probe or reevaluate progress in treatment.

Another aerodynamic measure that may be calculated is that of *phonation quotient (PQ)*. Hirano (1981) calculates the phonation quotient (PQ) by dividing the vital capacity (VC) by the maximum phonation time (MPT):

$$PQ = \frac{VC}{MPT}$$

He also reports that the phonation quotient has a high positive relationship to MFR and therefore is a reasonable, clinical substitute for MFR when no equipment for air flow measurement is available. Normal values of PQ in adults and children are typically between 120 and 190 ml/sec. High phonation quotients are associated with recurrent laryngeal nerve paralysis and additive lesions of the folds, such as nodules, polyps, polypoid swelling, and neoplasms.

Subglottal and phonation threshold pressure measures are also aerodynamic and may be ascertained with a special face mask to be less intrusive. Normal values of subglottal pressure during habitual phonation are typically 5 to 10 cm H_2O, but these values change with variations in vocal intensity and fundamental frequency. Pressure values are abnormally high in laryngeal carcinoma, recurrent nerve paralysis, laryngocele, and perhaps even in functional dysphonias. Phonation threshold pressure (PTP) is the amount of air pressure necessary to set the vocal folds in motion at the lowest intensity level. Often this is 2 to 3 H_2O pressure, though humidity and a host of other variables can affect PTP values. As reviewed by Plexico, Sandage, and Faver (2011), there is a need to standardize methods of measuring PTP because it is a sensitive measure of glottal edge dysfunction. Excess vocal fold mass, bowing during approximation, and paralysis of movement require higher amounts of PTP than do healthy larynges.

Rate and Rhythm

Although traditionally not part of vocal evaluations, the *rate* at which a client talks should be assessed because rate can affect or be affected by other variables of speech and the voice. Excessive rates are often related to poor breathing features and improper phrase groupings. The client may try to say too many words on one breath, giving the perception of an excessive rate of speech, as in Parkinsonism. The converse may also occur. Frequent air intakes may give the perception of choppiness—the client may be able to say only a few words, then breathe, then say a few more words, then breathe, and so forth. The result is not only a choppy *rhythm* but an overall slowness of speech from the increased pause time. Rate changes may also interfere with intelligibility, as is so typical of the dysarthrias.

Rate is typically expressed as words per minute (wpm) or syllables per minute (spm). It can be quite cumbersome to measure an entire speech sample for the determination of rate. Therefore, we offer the following efficient and clinically useful estimation method (recording for later playback is recommended): Count the number of words in a 60-second sample of "connected" speech. If no connected 60-second samples are available on the recording, then count the number of words in whatever connected sample is available and mathematically calculate words per minute. For example, if a 20-second speech sample contains 50 words, then, on the average, the person is talking at 150 words per minute (60 seconds ÷ 20 seconds = 3, and 3 × 50 words = 150 wpm). An alternative method, useful for determining rate of speech during reading, is to give the client a reading passage with prenumbered words. Allow the client to read aloud for 1 minute, as timed with a stopwatch, and note how many of the words were read.

Conversational speech rates for children and for adults were discussed in Chapter 7. At the present time, we do not know what constitutes a speech rate that is "too fast" or "too slow," and so the clinician's judgment of normalcy is important. Rate determinations may be most necessary with neurological voice disorders.

VISUAL ASSESSMENT

Technological advances have permitted us to view laryngeal function, and much of this technology is in clinical application: fiber-optic, videostroboscopy, and laryngographic techniques are proving useful in the assessment of neurologic dysfunction, vocal fold lesions, morphologic changes of the folds, and abnormal phonator function. While much has been done to standardize the clinical examination of the larynx (e.g., stroboscopy analysis by Poburka, 1999), we need to remember that it is the purview of the physician and/or otolaryngologist to *diagnose any laryngeal pathology*. As mentioned earlier in the chapter, the physician or the otolaryngologist in many settings performs the visual examination, often before any referral to the SLP. But in many voice centers, the SLP performs a videostroboscopic examination of vocal fold to augment his or her other perceptual and acoustic analyses. Visual findings of vocal fold membrane status and function, presented in the videostroboscopy evaluation report, help shape the appropriateness of any behavioral treatment.

Vidstroboscopy examples are readily available on social media. An SLP explaining basic vocal fold mobility and the process of videostroboscopy can be viewed at www.youtube.com/watch?v=mJedwz_r2Pc. An example showing a patient with a paralyzed vocal fold can be seen at www.youtube.com/watch?v=8Y0SHkwDC3w. Equipment-based visual approaches require costly and specialized instrumentation, expertise, and patient cooperation. The SLP lacking these may find referral to a voice center in a nearby university clinic or medical center prudent. Many SLPs assess the visible larynx, often with a videostroboscope, so we offer the following assessment information.

In viewing the videostroboscopic image of a patient's larynx, the primary focus is logically on glottal closure patterns and the status of the leading edges of the vocal folds, but other observations also shape clinical impressions and possible directions for any behavioral vocal treatment. By recording the videostroboscopic session, the SLP can review the visual information repeatedly for confidence in his or her assessment findings. While books on voice disorders, especially that by LeBorgne (2011), are instructive on this subject, we offer the following observational scheme, which proceeds through the anatomical-physiological region. The clinician may also use the following as a helpful reporting guide:

Supraglottic Observations:

1. Comment on (or rate) the degree of tension in the entire region above the folds.

2. Comment on any compression observed in the ventricular (false) folds.

3. Comment on left-right symmetry of the laryngeal ventricles.

Glottal Observations:

1. Describe the color of laryngeal tissues.
2. Observe the symmetry of movement and opening during breathing versus sustained vowel phonation.
3. Observe the pattern of glottal closure and describe or rate it. Descriptors might include whether glottal closure is completely achieved along the entire length, there is closure except for a triangular anterior gap, the folds are bowed open or spindle-shaped in the middle area during closure attempts, closure occurs along the anterior segment of the folds but a triangular gap is apparent posteriorly, or the folds are unable to approximate at all. In the latter case, comment further on which fold or both fail to meet in the midline.
4. Observe left-right fold symmetry of lengthening and shortening during vowel pitch glides.
5. Judge motility of each fold; rate each as to normalcy or to degree of difficulty with addiction and abduction (e.g. normal motility, limited motility, fixed motility).
6. Assess status of vocal fold edges, both left and right; attend to how smooth and straight to how rough and irregular each edge is.
7. Observe size and location of any mass on the left or right fold.

Vibratory Observations:

1. Assess movement: the extent or amplitude of the left and right fold during phonation.
2. Assess mucosal wave smoothness or stiffness.
3. Assess the movement pattern of each fold during pitch glides up and down the musical scale.
4. Describe the open/closed quotient.
5. Observe the presence of a nonvibrating portion of each fold.

Other Observations:

1. Comments.
2. Overall impressions (e.g., normal, hypofunctional disorder, hyperfunctional disorder, etc.).

INFORMAL ASSESSMENT PROBES

We have now explained both the perceptual-informal and the technological-formal methods of voice appraisal for a variety of situations (see Figure 11–3). Many SLPs operate in work settings with limited instrumentation available. Over the years, clinicians have developed effective behavioral techniques for assessing, probing, treating, and reassessing laryngeal voice disorders. Indeed, the process of voice therapy is behavioral; that is, we as clinicians use strategies, techniques, devices, and even psychological "tricks" to change or alter a client's voice. Of course, this presupposes that the changes are somehow better for the client—the voice sounds better, less effort is expended in its production, further damage is not being inflicted on the vocal mechanism, and so forth. But just completing a voice evaluation where deviant vocal parameters have been analyzed, in and of itself, does not suggest how to proceed clinically. As clinicians, we want to know what we can do to make the client's voice "better." Here we enter the world of trial therapy—a necessary component of assessment—and the use of facilitating

FIGURE 11–3

Critical Assessment Process in Vocal Disorders

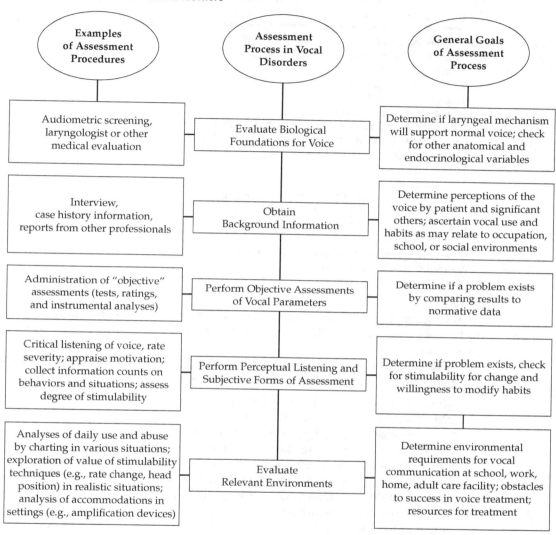

techniques to probe the client's potential to alter his or her voice for the better. Let us now highlight some of these probe techniques in the hope that clinicians will identify the client's ability to modify and improve parameters of the voice during the initial diagnostic evaluation. By doing so, the clinician will be able to accomplish two important goals: a meaningful prognosis and a direction for intervention.

Patients with hypofunctional voice problems often show improved phonatory abilities by increasing glottal tension. The clinician should probe which maneuvers, if any, are successful in improving the voice. Do any of the so-called optimal pitch techniques help, such as grunting, pushing, pulling, throat clearing, or coughing (see Table 11–8)? An intentional hard glottal attack, even if accompanied by increased tension in the arms and trunk while pushing forcefully, may facilitate approximation of the vocal folds. Used this way, these maneuvers may be thought of as hypertonic techniques rather

TABLE 11–9
Some Circumlaryngeal Reposturing and Resonant Facilitating Techniques for the Improvement of Voice as Trial Therapy

To improve adduction and phonatory abilities:
    Gutzmann lateral compression of thyroid lamina
    Head turning or tilting
    Pushing or pulling concomitant with voicing
    Hard glottal attacks
To alter pitch and/or quality:
    Gutzmann frontal compression of thyroid prominence
    Any/all of the optimal pitch techniques (Table 11–8)
    Change in loudness
    Change in speech rate
    Soft glottal attacks
    Relaxation of musculature/reduction of tension
    Lip bubbles and tongue trilling
    Easy, resonant counting
    Singing, humming
    Slow, exaggerated nasal words (*noon, moon*)
    Alteration of respiratory patterns

than as techniques to achieve optimal pitch. Table 11–9 presents a useful sampling of techniques used by many clinicians over the years that may facilitate, or improve, voice production.

Two case examples may illustrate how the use of hypertonic probe techniques in the evaluation affected treatment recommendations:

> Mrs. Hernandez was involved in a rather messy divorce settlement after 22 years of marriage. Over the past few months, she has experienced periodic losses of voice—sometimes during heated conversations but occasionally for an afternoon or an entire day. Mrs. Hernandez indicated that the voice was reduced to a whisper during these episodes and was not hoarse as with laryngitis. The current episode of voice loss, and the reason she was seeing a speech-language pathologist, had lasted over a week. The clinician was not able to get Mrs. Hernandez to speak above a whisper in the evaluation; she showed no potential to talk, sing, or shout. The clinician was able to elicit, rather quickly, a cough and a throat-clearing maneuver that contained true phonated sound. A diagnosis of hysterical aphonia was made and, because of the rehabilitation potential displayed for phonation, treatment was recommended immediately. After three sessions of behavioral shaping, beginning with vegetative eliciting techniques, the client was speaking normally. Referral was then made for psychological support services.

> Mrs. Osborne, age 42, presented with unilateral vocal fold paralysis subsequent to thyroid surgery. The laryngologist referred the patient for voice improvement therapy. Teflon injection was contraindicated because it would further compromise the reduced glottal airway. The patient presented with stridor during physical exertion; the speaking voice was hoarse and of limited loudness. Hoarseness diminished and loudness improved when the speech-language pathologist exerted medial pressure against the thyroid lamina on the side of the paralyzed fold (a rendition of the Gutzmann medial compression technique). Other hypertonic facilitating techniques were also helpful in

improving Mrs. Osborne's voicing abilities. With medical management contra-indicated, the clinician felt compensatory strategies involving increased muscular effort and glottal attack were appropriate and realistic. Treatment was recommended along these lines.

Vocal quality improvements can also be brought about by changes in the manner of speaking. Adjustments in the respiratory, phonatory, and articulatory processes have an impact on the overall perception of the voice. We provide one case example here:

> Greg was a college student referred to us by the university infirmary. Greg had gone to see the doctor, with general complaints of not feeling well, simply in an effort to get a medical excuse for missing a class exam for which he had not studied. The doctor could find nothing wrong with Greg but was concerned by his "gravel-sounding, hoarse voice." Indirect laryngoscopy revealed normal structures and referral was made to our speech clinic. Greg's voice was pitched abnormally low and the quality was indeed abnormal. The aberrant quality was the more conspicuous problem. He indicated that his voice always sounded like this and gave him no trouble other than fatigue after any day of heavy talking. Part of our evaluation session was spent with trial-and-error attempts to change Greg's voice. Some things we tried had no effect, others made him sound more harsh, and a few techniques seemed to bring out a "better" voice. In particular, raising Greg's pitch slightly decreased the harshness. The higher pitch, he assured us, felt comfortable. We hypothesized that Greg was using an inappropriately low and harsh voice, perhaps to project a more masculine image, and that the functional disorder would remediate quite well. Treatment was recommended to improve the harsh quality by raising pitch.

Prognosis

Prognosis has several aspects. First, there is the question of spontaneous remission of the presenting symptoms. Will this individual display an improvement in voice without intervening therapy? Second, how much improvement can be expected following the prescribed clinical program? That is, to what degree will the voice therapy, as projected, be effective? Third, how permanent will the gains shown in therapy be? Is the vocal improvement such that continuous therapy will be necessary to maintain optimal voice performance? (Medicare and most third-party reimbursement agencies will not fund so-called maintenance therapy.) Finally, would some other clinical procedure be of greater benefit to the client?

A variety of factors have potential prognostic value in voice cases. Some of the variables are directly observable and subject to quantification; others are much more subjective. The factors appear to fall into three broad categories: characteristics of the disorder, the person, and the environment. Factors with potential prognostic value include:

1. *Duration of the problems.* Generally disorders of long duration have greater resistance to clinical treatment.

2. *Etiological factors.* Two factors are relevant here. First, is the cause of the problem identifiable? Second, is the cause of the problem alterable? And if so, is the type of necessary habilitating service available?

3. *Degree of secondary psychological components.* Generally, the greater the degree of psychological disturbance, the poorer the prognosis.

4. *Variability and general flexibility of the voice.* Generally, the more the client is able to alter his or her vocal behavior, the better the prognosis. This underscores the

importance of probing for vocal change with facilitating techniques during the initial session.

5. *Auditory and imitative skills.* The better the client is at hearing differences in quality, pitch, and loudness, coupled with the ability to imitate these differences, the more favorable the prognosis.

6. *Impact or degree of disability.* The greater the impact of the voice difference on the individual, the better the chances for cooperation and motivation. Generally, if the family of the client is supportive, the outlook is more favorable. This relates to the World Health Organization's emphasis on impact (see Figure 11–2).

7. *Structural integrity of the vocal mechanism.* Clearly, the more the speech mechanism is disrupted anatomically or neurologically, the more limited the prognosis will be.

CONCLUSION AND SELF-ASSESSMENT

This chapter has covered a great deal of information. But what are a reasonable number of measures important to track pre-, peri-, and post-treatment as evidence of progress and outcome? The measures we try to collect on each client include the following:

- Patient, family, and SLP ratings of the voice (e.g., features of pitch, loudness, quality, and so forth)
- Perceived sensory symptoms, including phonatory effort
- Average fundamental frequency during reading and monologue
- Frequency range utilized during reading and monologue
- MPT of a vowel
- Jitter (expressed as a percentage)
- Laryngeal appearance

Certainly more can be added to this list, but we feel comfortable that these are reasonable measures that can be reevaluated often to document change—or lack of it. Evidence of this type also satisfies our accountability to the client and to third-party payors.

The evaluation of voice disorders is a challenge to the speech-language pathologist. It requires the ability to deal with older adults as well as young children. The clinician must often work closely with medical personnel and other allied health workers, which necessitates knowing procedures and terminologies that are peripheral to speech-language pathology. The clinician must also remain abreast of current technological developments in electronics, surgery, and medical technology. Finally, the clinician must keep interpersonal clinical skills finely honed so that psychological aspects of vocal disorders can be detected and dealt with through treatment or referral.

After reading this chapter you should be able to answer the following questions:

1. Name and explain perceptual aspects of the spoken voice.
2. List five or more case history questions important to ask a child, parent, or teacher of a new voice referral for a child in fifth grade.
3. List five or more sensory symptom questions important to ask a new adult voice referral.
4. Describe the collection of a client's MPT.
5. Select and research an available published voice assessment tool. Discuss aspects that it covers or does not cover and how to use it.

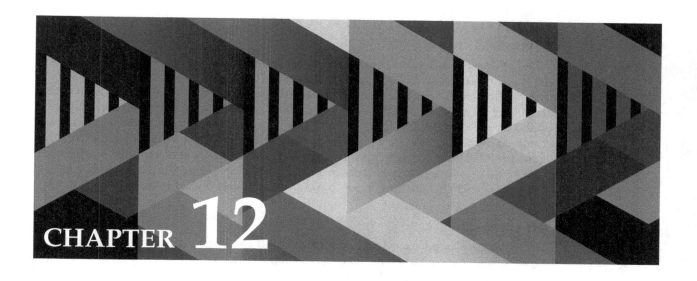

CHAPTER 12

Assessment of Resonance Imbalance

LEARNING OUTCOMES

After reading this chapter you will be able to:

1. Describe these types of abnormal resonance: hyponasality, hypernasality, nasal emission, cul-de-sac, and thin/effeminate resonance.

2. Name some speech stimuli to differentiate perceptually hyponasality from hypernasality.

3. Explain expected findings in a nose-occluded versus a nose-unoccluded assessment task.

4. Explain nasal emission and how to "see" it.

5. Differentiate velopharyngeal insufficiency from velopharyngeal incompetence.

6. Explain at least three instrumental assessment tools (acoustic or physiologic).

Disorders of vocal quality may be due to faulty transmission of sound through the vocal tract (the pharyngeal, oral, and nasal cavities). Sound generation at the level of the larynx occurs normally and so these are not laryngeal voice disorders, which were discussed in Chapter 11. Rather, there is a perceived oral-nasal imbalance of resonance. Problems of resonance may be classified as hyponasality, hypernasality, cul-de-sac resonance, or mixed types. The behavioral and instrumental assessment of resonance disorders will be the focus of this chapter, along with special comments about those with clefts of the palate.

TYPES OF ABNORMAL RESONANCE
Hyponasality

The hyponasal voice lacks the normal nasal resonance expected on /m/, /n/, and /ŋ/ in English. These articulatory distortions often resemble /b/, /d/, and /g/, respectively. The vocalic elements may also take on the characteristics of talking with a head cold; indeed, the term *denasal* is an acceptable synonym of hyponasal speech. Hyponasality usually results from some blockage or obstruction in the nasopharynx or nasal cavity. This obstruction may stem from congestion, nasal polyps, or various structural deformities. The speech of children with cochlear implants also may display inconsistent hyponasality on vocalic speech elements and the normally nasal consonants of /m/, /n/, and /ŋ/, making them sound denasal (Teoh & Chin, 2009).

Hypernasality

Hypernasality is an excessive amount of nasal resonance during the production of vowels and vocalic elements. The nasal cavity is not adequately separated from the oral cavity during speech. When an underlying cause for the abnormal velopharyngeal function is not yet known or is behaviorally modifiable, one of two generic terms may be used to describe the situation: *velopharyngeal dysfunction (VPD)* or *velopharyngeal inadequacy (VPI)*. When poor movement of the velopharyngeal structure can be attributed to a neuromotor or physiological disorder, the term of choice is *velopharyngeal incompetence (VPI)* (Kummer, 2013a). Congenital clefts of the hard or soft palate are obvious examples of structural/functional defects frequently leading to velopharyngeal (VP) incompetence. Not only can hypernasality result from clefts of the hard or soft palate, it can also result from submucous clefts, short velums, or pharyngeal dimensions that are too large. A neuromuscular deficit, such as a paralyzed or paretic velum, or dysfunction of the pharyngeal constrictor muscles may be attributed to trauma-induced dysarthria or disease-related dysarthria. Diseases such as myasthenia gravis, muscular dystrophy, and poliomyelitis often affect velopharyngeal functioning.

Hypernasality may be pronounced or only slightly apparent; in addition, it can be continuous or intermittent. In mild intermittent cases, the excess nasality on vowels may be most noticeable in the context of nasal consonants. This represents assimilation nasality and indicates a velum that can function but moves too slowly during connected speech.

Nasal Emission

During hypernasal speech of some but not all persons, the phenomenon of nasal emission may occur. Nasal emission is an audible escape of air out the nose (through the nares) during the production of pressure consonants, such as plosives, fricatives, and affricates. Implicated in this condition is an incompetent closure of the velopharyngeal mechanism. Nasal emission is different from the resonance imbalance of hypernasality, although the two problems may co-occur. Nasal emission is often phoneme-specific and may be attributed to faulty articulation patterns (Kummer & Lee, 1996).

Nasal Rustle

Also known as turbulence, a nasal rustle is a loud and distracting form of nasal emission. The nasal rustle has been attributed to a large amount of air being forced through a small velopharyngeal opening, with the result of a friction or rustling sound of air (Kummer & Lee, 1996).

Cul-de-Sac Resonance

This type of *resonance* or reverberation occurs in the oropharynx, perhaps because of posterior tongue retraction, a large tongue, or enlarged tonsils/adenoids. This resonance imbalance is heard as a muffled and hollow-sounding voice with a pharyngeal focus. It also has been described as "potato-in-the-mouth" (Kummer & Lee, 1996). Peterson-Falzone (1982) states that cul-de-sac resonance can also result from an anterior nasal obstruction and a posterior aperture (opening). Cul-de-sac resonance associated with tongue retraction often occurs on a functional basis, as well as in patients with deafness, flaccid and spastic dysarthria, athetoid cerebral palsy, or oral verbal apraxia (Boone et al., 2014). The degree of this nasality may be reduced in hearing-impaired individuals with increases in speaking rates (Dwyer, Robb, & O'Beirne, 2009).

Mixed Resonance

Both hypernasality and hyponasality resonance can, in fact, co-occur in a speaker. Mixed hyper-hyponasility might be present when the client exhibits both velopharyngeal insufficiency (causing hypernasality) and a nasal blockage, as by a polyp growth, that impedes the flow of air in the nose (causing hyponasality).

Thin Vocal Resonance

Thin vocal resonance, once known as an *effeminate voice quality* because it more often occurs in males than females, seems related to an anterior tongue posture. The habitually high and excessively anterior tongue position is almost always due to functional, not organic, reasons; the voice sounds very weak and lacking in resonance, particularly for the back vowels. Speakers, intentionally or unintentionally, articulate with a minimal oral opening and with little range of movement of the jaw. Often, the speaker's vocal pitch is elevated slightly, which adds to the perception of vocal effeminacy. Following assessment, treatment may be geared to altering these patterns for a stronger and gender-appropriate vocal quality. Conversely, speech-language pathologists (SLPs) working with male-to-female transgender clients may seek to alter oral resonance patterns, thus creating the thinner voice (Carew, Dacakis, & Oates, 2007).

CASE HISTORY AND GENERAL VOICE ASSESSMENT

The evaluation of a resonance disorder is often an outgrowth of a general voice evaluation; the clinician may not know beforehand the specific nature of a patient's problem. Consequently, the evaluation session proceeds along the lines described in Chapter 11. First, a case history interview is done. Routine information is gathered, but particular questions need to be asked concerning the patient's description of the voice problem and known or suspected causes of the disorder. Oronasopharyngeal injuries, structural defects, and any surgeries need to be thoroughly discussed. In the case of clefts of the palate in infants and children, it is important to ask not only about surgeries that have occurred but also any known timeline of planned future surgeries. Second, the oral peripheral examination is crucial to the evaluation of resonance; third, all parameters of the voice must be assessed. Infants and children with clefts of the hard or soft palate require a more extensive velopharyngeal assessment, so we will devote a section on this topic later in the chapter.

Samples of questionnaires for use in voice/resonance case history intakes abound online, in textbooks, and in commercial materials. Whether the client is an adult or we are interviewing the parent of a pediatric case, questions follow those discussed in Chapter 11. In particular, the SLP notes the following: the client's current communication concern, when was this first noted, and when and how the voice/resonance varies; developmental history; medical history (vocal and general); and so forth. Reflecting on types of resonance imbalance and typical causes of each is a good guide to case history questions beyond the general.

Any of the assessment tools mentioned in Chapter 11 are appropriate to use. A Voice Assessment Protocol for Children and Adults (Pindzola, 1987) is useful in assessing a multitude of vocal parameters. It evaluates the resonance of the patient's voice on a severity continuum. The patient may be scored as exhibiting normal resonance balance, cul-de-sac resonance, hyponasality (slight or intermittent versus moderate to severe), hypernasality on vocalic elements (slight, intermittent, or assimilative versus moderate versus severe), and any presence of nasal emission on pressure consonants (slight or intermittent versus moderate to severe).

The American Speech-Language-Hearing Association (ASHA) provides an in-depth (adult) Voice Evaluation template, which the reader can find at www.asha.org/. To this particular template is added the PDF form of the Consensus Auditory-Perceptual Evaluation of Voice (CAPE-V), although CAPE-V may be accessed only by ASHA members. CAPE-V is a measuring tool sponsored by ASHA's Special Interest Division 3, Voice and Voice Disorders. The article by Kempster et al. (2009) also is a good source for the instrument and for documentation forms. CAPE-V rates six voice quality features: overall severity, roughness, breathiness, strain, pitch, and loudness. The astute reader will note that resonance is not among these attributes. The CAPE-V form includes two unlabeled scales allowing the SLP to document other salient perceptual features; here, the clinician can rate the type and degree of nasality (or any other vocal features desired). CAPE-V also advocates using a standard reading passage in the evaluation of voice. See Appendix B for reading passages that can be used in any evaluation and with readers of various ages.

Various commercially available treatment programs include an assessment instrument. An example pertinent to resonance is found in *Hypernasality Modification Program: A Systematic Approach* by Ray and Baker (2002). This product includes a Resonance Evaluation to profile resonance in 16 structured phonetic contexts and purports being useful for children ages 6 and up and for adults. After a thorough, overall voice assessment, emphasis is given to the appraisal of the resonance imbalance. Resonance quality deviations are, first and foremost, perceptual judgments (which may or may not have clear acoustic and physiologic underpinnings). Perceptual judgments necessitate a "good clinical ear" and so require no or low-tech materials for assessment. Figure 12–1 displays the assessment process we recommend.

Assessment Techniques and Probes for Resonance Imbalance

In this section, we discuss techniques requiring little or no instrumentation that the SLP can and should use to assess the various resonance imbalances. Before concluding the evaluation, we feel very strongly that the clinician should experiment, or probe, to see what improvements, or changes in general, can be effected in the patient's voice. Some writers have called this *stimulability*. The ability of a client to produce a clear resonant voice on stimulation means that behavioral treatment has a good chance of being successful.

Hyponasality

Denasality is often due to obstruction in the nasal cavity; thus, an examination of the nasal region is in order during the oral peripheral part of the assessment. During the case history intake, the patient may indicate knowledge of having a deviated septum,

FIGURE 12–1

Critical Assessment Process for Determining Resonance Imbalance

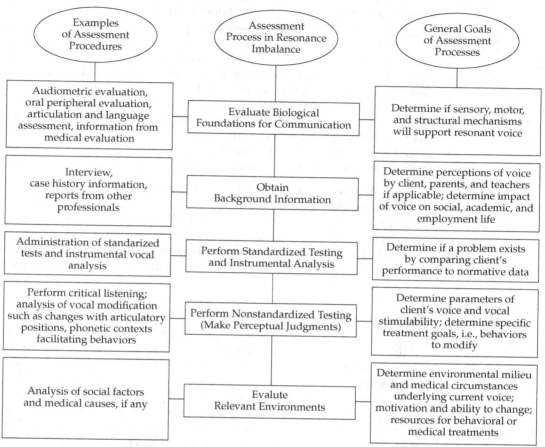

nasal polyp, enlarged adenoids, and the like. On the other hand, the basis of a patient's hyponasality may be neuromuscular and may reflect improper timing of velar movements. Case history questions should probe for trauma- or disease-related etiologies.

To evaluate a patient for hyponasal voice quality, SLPs rely on critical listening. While the patient is conversing or reading a standard paragraph, the clinician listens carefully for denasality shadowing the vowel portions of speech and, in particular, listens for the articulatory distortions or substitutions of b/m, d/n, and g/k. By using specially constructed phrases, sentences, or paragraphs that have a preponderance of nasal phonemes, the clinician has a heightened opportunity to perceive denasal resonance. Suggested stimuli include the following examples, some of which we have devised or borrowed from the literature:

> Mama made some lemon jam.
> I know a man on the moon.
> Many a man knew my meaning.
> Mike needs more milk.
> My mom makes money.
> When may we know your name?
> I'm naming one man among many.

Having the patient count aloud from 90 to 100 is also contextually appropriate. The following word pairs are useful in detecting hyponasality: bake/make, rib/rim, dine/nine, mad/man, wig/wing, bag/bang. In hyponasality, nasal resonance would be lacking and so, for example, the bake/make pair would sound like bake/bake.

Another clinical task that is helpful in revealing hyponasal speech is to have the patient read a list of words initiated with the /m/ phoneme. Bzoch (2004) suggests these 10 words: *meat, moat, mit, moot, mate, mut, met, Mert, mat,* and *might*. While the patient is reading, or repeating, each word from the list twice, the clinician alternately compresses and releases the patient's nostrils. In normal velopharyngeal function, the resonance becomes hypernasal when the nares are occluded, but no resonance change is heard in true hyponasality. Bzoch counts the number of words with no change in resonance and uses this figure as an index of hyponasality. Operating on this same principle is the humming technique. The inability of a patient to hum or to hum clearly is suggestive of hyponasality.

> Carmen Perez has fluctuating hyponasality. The severity of her hyponasality changes on a daily basis, but there is a more noticeable fluctuation with the seasons. Carmen's ear, nose, and throat doctor observed nasal cavity characteristics typical of allergic inflammation: tissue coloration changes and hypertrophy of the nasal turbinates secondary to edema. The planned course of treatment involved use of prescribed antihistamines and the option of undergoing a lengthy allergen tolerance program.

Hypernasality

Judgments about resonance are truly judgments of a perceptual nature; a well-tuned clinical ear is essential—and adequate—for the SLP. The SLP, of course, appraises nasality relative to the local norm; the amount of acceptable speech nasality is highly variable among geographical regions and diverse cultures. Critical listening by the clinician while the patient converses and/or reads a passage can be supplemented by rating the severity of the hypernasality on a rating scale. Let us highlight a few other methods.

Classical methods rate the severity of hypernasality from mild to very severe. A typical perceptual system categorizes speech into five levels of nasal severity, as follows:

- *Normal nasality.* Speech has enough nasality to sound normal but not so much as to call attention to it unless the SLP is specifically listening for it.
- *Mild nasality.* Nasality is apparent as the person speaks. It is somewhat greater than that of most speakers but would probably cause little or no distraction if the SLP is not listening for it.
- *Moderately nasal.* Nasality is obviously present and is moderately distracting to the listener.
- *Severely nasal.* Nasality is prominent, is a highly distracting feature in the speech, and makes listening to the message difficult.
- *Very severely nasal.* Nasality is so distracting that it dominates all aspects of speech and makes hearing the message extremely difficult.

The Buffalo III Resonance Profile (Wilson, 1987), though dated, is circulated on the Internet and in use by various school systems. It is a 12-item supplement to Wilson's more general Buffalo III Voice Profile and is used when a patient has been rated 2 or higher on the nasal or oral resonance items of that voice profile. The profile for resonance uses a 5-point rating scale, with 1 equal to normal and 5 equal to very severe. Twelve parameters are then so rated: hypernasal resonance, hyponasal resonance, oral resonance, cul-de-sac resonance, nasal emission, facial grimaces, language level, articulation, speech intelligibility, speech acceptability, velopharyngeal competency, and overall resonance rating.

The SLP can use a "listening tube" to heighten the perception of a patient's hypernasality, thus facilitating its recognition. We have used a makeshift listening tube fashioned from the plastic headsets provided by the airlines for in-flight movies, or one constructed from 2 to 3 feet of hardware tubing. The ultimate low-tech device described by Kummer (2013b) is a bendable drinking straw. When using any such device, insert one end in or near the patient's nostril and the free end of the tube into the clinician's ear. With this in place, even the slightest degrees of hypernasality (and also nasal emission) can be detected in the patient's speech. Comercial devices with a plactic nasal olive, tubing, and stand include the Oral and Nasal Listener from Super Duper Publishing, available online at www.superduperinc.com, and the See-Scape from Pro-Ed, available online at www.proedinc.com.

The SLP may try a simple procedure sometimes known as the nasal flutter test. Have the patient repeat in an alternate fashion the vowels /a/ and /i/ while the clinician alternately compresses and releases the patient's nostrils. It is presumed that if velopharyngeal closure is adequate, there will be no noticeable difference in vowel quality as the nostrils are pinched. Conversely, if the clinician hears an increase in the nasal resonance during the nose-occluded condition, velopharyngeal incompetence may be suspected. The resonance quality change has also been described as a flutterlike sound—hence the name of the test procedure.

Bzoch (2004) recommends a similar nose-occluded–nose-unoccluded test procedure using plosive-vowel-plosive syllables. Ten vowels are tested in a /b—t/ context: *beet, bit, bait, bet, bat, bought, boat, boot, but,* and *Bert*. In a person with normal velopharyngeal closure, the nose-occluded and nose-unoccluded conditions sound the same.

Articulation tests involve both consonants and vowels and so can be fair measures of velopharyngeal closure, nasal emission, and hypernasality. Consonant environments influence the amount of nasality perceived on vowels. From least influential to most influential, these are /z, v, d, g, f, s, t, k/. It would seem, therefore, that nasality on vowels should be studied in these consonantal environments.

The perception of hypernasality can be heightened by using context-controlled stimuli. Having the patient count aloud from 60 to 100 is an insightful, yet simple assessment procedure. We offer the following summary of the counting task, which is a useful indicator of velopharyngeal incompetence and the symptoms of hypernasality, nasal emission, and hyponasality:

1. The 60 series of numbers may reveal velopharyngeal incompetence and nasal emission due to the frequent occurrence of the /s/ pressure phoneme.

2. The 70 series may reveal assimilative hypernasality because of the embedded /n/ phoneme.

3. The 80 series should reveal normal or near-normal articulation and resonance.

4. The 90 series should sound normal when produced by a patient with hypernasality because of the frequent production of nasal consonants. The patient with hyponasality may display the articulatory substitution of d/n.

The SLP can test for sound confusions in cases of suspected velopharyngeal incompetence. Have the patient read or repeat word pairs, such as bake/make, rib/rim, dine/nine, mad/man, wig/wing, bag/bang. In a patient with VPI, both sounds are hypernasal, making the bake/make pair, for example, sound like make/make.

Instrumentation is also available that purports to detect or measure hypernasality. We maintain that hypernasality is a perceptual phenomenon and must be assessed perceptually. Attempts to measure hypernasality "objectively" are really attempts to measure velopharyngeal function, oral and nasal air flows, and the like. Although these data certainly relate to judgments of hypernasality, they are not measures of hypernasality per se. We will discuss instrumentation used to measure aspects of velopharyngeal function later in this chapter when we discuss the cleft palate population.

Once the SLP has determined that the patient exhibits some degree of hypernasality, the evaluative session should turn to discovering what, if any, techniques and manipulations lessen the perception of nasality. Together, the patient and clinician should experiment to find what works and, in doing so, they can arrive at a prognosis for change and map the direction of future treatment, if warranted.

The variability of the hypernasality as it relates to phonetic context should be explored. Does the perception of hypernasality diminish or worsen in sentences loaded with high vowels? With low vowels? With numerous nasal consonants? With many pressure consonants?

Does the degree of hypernasality improve when the patient speaks with open-mouth articulation, where there is exaggerated mouth opening, and where speech sounds are enunciated with exaggerated movement? Air takes the path of least resistance, so by opening the anterior oral cavity wider, air tends to flow outward rather than through the narrower but opened velopharyngeal port.

The SLP should also probe for possible improvements in hypernasality with changes in speaking rate, pitch, and loudness. These may be prime areas of manipulation in compensatory treatment programs. It is likely that perceived hypernasality is lessened at higher pitch and intensity levels. The role of muscular fatigue can also be explored by having the patient determine whether nasality is better or worse at various times during the day.

At the beginning of the second grade, Belinda Johnston was noticed by the SLP during schoolwide screenings. The child's voice was hypernasal, and nasal emission occurred inconsistently on words starting with /s/, /f/, and /p/. Belinda failed this brief screening, and the SLP followed up on the case. In a telephone conversation with Belinda's mother, the clinician learned that Belinda had a tonsillectomy and adenoidectomy during the previous Easter break because of frequent ear infections and sore throats. The mother stated that Belinda's voice has sounded "unusual" only since the surgery, but she was told by the doctor that it would improve with time. The first-grade teacher confirmed that Belinda's voice sounded normal the previous year. Six months had elapsed since the surgery, so the SLP and Belinda's mother agreed to initiate appropriate school system procedures for a formal speech evaluation and subsequent intervention. In the evaluation, hypernasality was confirmed and its severity rated, as was the consistency and severity of nasal emission. The oral peripheral examination revealed several indicators of submucous clefting. There was a midline notching of the uvula (slight bifidity), an anteriorly placed velar dimple, midline translucency of the palate, and a highly vaulted hard palate. Velar movement occurred symmetrically, but contact with the posterior pharyngeal wall could not be observed with certainty. Air came out the nose when the SLP used the modified tongue–anchor technique, and Belinda was unable to blow up a balloon.

The SLP wondered whether traditional adenoidectomy should have been done on this child: The oral exam revealed several factors that would contraindicate a routine removal (Finkelstein, Wexler, Nachmani, & Ophir, 2002). (The adenoid's bulk compensated for the child's VPI.) The school SLP desired objective confirmation of the suspicions of VPI, available with sophisticated instrumentation, and expert opinions of the proper behavioral course of action, if any. Belinda was referred to the craniofacial team at a metropolitan hospital a hundred miles away.

The SLP at a rehabilitation hospital received Delondo Hayes as a transfer patient from an acute-care facility. Mr. Hayes is a 22-year-old automobile crash victim who had sustained brainstem and spinal cord injuries. The clinician noted in the initial speech consult that Mr. Hayes was partially paralyzed and used a wheelchair. His conversational speech was slow, slurred, and excessively hypernasal. In the oral examination, the speech pathologist also noted absence of gag reflex and weak lingual muscles. The patient was diagnosed with the motor speech disorder of flaccid dysarthria. Early treatment efforts would be directed at oral muscle mobility and precision of articulation. Slow speech rates would be accepted—indeed, encouraged—as a means of achieving target articulatory placements, including velar gestures. The hypernasality would be monitored for 4 to 6 weeks of rehabilitation before considering further alternatives.

Nasal Emission

Nasal emission and hypernasality can both be due to poor or absent velopharyngeal closure, so it makes sense that they often co-occur; yet we must keep in mind that the two problems are separate entities. Nasal emission is not a resonance issue per se.

The assessment of nasal emission involves looking and listening. The expulsion of air through the nostrils may be so obvious as to flare the nares of the speaker. In contrast, in an attempt to decrease the outward flow of air, the person may constrict the nares. The clinician, then, looks for facial (nasal) grimaces.

Critical listening is crucial for the SLP to diagnose the presence of nasal emission accurately. Sometimes the emitted air is obviously noisy; in fact, *nasal snort* is a descriptive term encountered in this body of literature. At other times, the nasal emission is barely audible or is detectable only with special techniques, as we shall see.

A frequent way to assess the presence of nasal emission is by administering a single-word articulation test. Attention should be directed toward production of pressure plosives, fricatives, and affricates. The results of the articulation test should answer the following questions for the clinician:

1. Does the speaker misarticulate fricatives, plosives, and affricates that have been demonstrated to require high intraoral breath pressure?
2. Do the misarticulations involve audible nasal emission?
3. Is there evidence of facial grimacing during the production of these consonants?
4. Does occluding the nostrils (preventing an air leakage) result in normal production of the consonants?
5. Regarding nasal emission, are voiced consonants less defective than their voiceless cognates? Typically, the required amount of oral air pressure is greater for voiceless phonemes.
6. Are single consonants less affected than blends?
7. Are consonants in the initial or final position in words articulated correctly more often than are medial consonants?
8. Does the patient use compensatory articulation patterns, such as glottal stop, pharyngeal stop, mid-dorsum palatal stop, pharyngeal fricative, posterior nasal fricative, and so forth?

In addition to, or in place of, a formal articulation test, the clinician may listen for nasal emission in specially designed words and sentences. Have the patient read or repeat stimuli loaded with pressure consonants, such as the following clinical favorites:

Pick the peas.
Pappa piped up.
Polish the shoes.
Bessie stayed all summer.
We'd better buy a bigger dog.
Follow Sally, Charley.
People, baby, paper, Bobby, puppy, bubble, pepper, B. B., piper, bye bye.

Likewise, the clinician can listen carefully as the patient counts aloud. The numbers between 60 and 79 are especially evocative of nasal emission.

The SLP can use simple items to enhance the detection and monitoring of nasal air emission. A small mirror held under the patient's nostril will fog as air escapes. We have used a dental mirror with its convenient handle or a small lipstick mirror. Fog on the mirror during the patient's attempts at prolonging fricatives, repeating vowel-consonant-vowel (VCV) syllables containing pressure consonants (such as /ipi ipi ipi/, /upu upu upu/), or saying the pressure-loaded sentences previously listed is strongly suggestive of velopharyngeal incompetence. These same procedures may be done with wisps of cotton on a wooden tongue depressor held beneath the nose when a mirror is not available. We find the cotton's sensitivity less reliable, though.

The listening tube, described previously (whether made or commercially bought), is also useful for assessing nasal emission. Note that devices used to detect and visualize the nasal emission of air are useful for client feedback in treatment as well as in assessment.

After determining that a patient has nasal emission, the clinician should probe for techniques that diminish air escape. If none are found, behavioral treatment may be contraindicated, and physical management may be necessary. Here are some techniques the SLP can try:

1. Have the patient use light articulatory contacts on pressure consonants—the plosives, fricatives, and affricates.

2. A complementary technique that may diminish nasal emission is that of open-mouth articulation, which was also suggested for hypernasality.

3. Perhaps having the patient extend the vowel portions of speech will lessen the emphasis placed on pressure consonant articulation and so improve nasal emission.

4. The fluency-enhancing techniques that involve vowel/syllable prolongations, found in many stuttering approaches, may prove useful with some patients.

5. Reduced rates of speech may also be useful, especially in patients who show velar movement potential but suffer from sluggish timing maneuvers.

Cul-de-Sac Resonance

The hollow voice quality of this disorder is typically due to hyperfunction of the tongue. Speech is produced with the tongue posteriorly positioned in the oral cavity and oropharynx regions. The SLP should try to observe this posterior retraction when possible; having the patient phonate an open vowel, such as /a/, may facilitate viewing of the posterior tongue placement.

De facto diagnosis may come from probing for improvements in cul-de-sac resonance. Experiment by having the patient read sentences or word lists loaded with phonemes that promote anterior tongue placement and inhibit lingual retraction. The following phonemes are suggested for developing clinical stimuli:

Tongue-tip: /t/, /d/, /s/, and /z/

Front vowels: /i/, /I/, and /e/

Front consonants: /w/, /hw/, /p/, /b/, /f/, /v/, /θ/, and /l/

It has been noted in the literature that hearing-impaired and deaf speakers often use too slow a rate of speech. The slow rate of speech seems to alter syllable durations, which in turn adversely affects speech intelligibility and voice quality. Increasing the speaking rates of hearing-impaired persons may improve their perceived hypernasality or their cul-de-sac resonance and should be attempted by the SLP.

Thin Vocal Resonance

The thin, effeminate voice quality is usually related to anterior tongue carriage, and thus the oral resonance of vowels and consonants is affected. By moving the place of the primary articulatory constriction more forward in the oral cavity, energy loci are shifted to higher frequencies, and vocalic formats are likewise elevated. The perception of effeminancy may be increased by the patient's use of an elevated fundamental frequency and/or exaggerated use of the upper range for pitch inflections. Pitch as well as quality should be evaluated in these patients. To assess thin resonance, have the patient read sentences or word lists containing many back vowels and back consonants (such as /k/ and /g/). Note whether there is an improvement in resonance with this probe technique.

ASSESSMENT ASSOCIATED WITH CLEFT PALATE AND VPI

In addition to the information already presented on assessing hypernasality and nasal emission, we would like to elaborate on the diagnostic process used with patients who have clefts of the hard or soft palate or who have had repairs—either surgical or prosthedontic—to their structures. The dramatic improvement of surgical and other rehabilitative procedures for the individual with a cleft has been encouraging. The SLP needs to assess the adequacy and sufficiency of the velopharyngeal mechanism for speech. We recommend the tutorial article on the nature, assessment, and treatment of velopharyngeal dysfunction by Dworkin, Marurick, and Krouse (2004). Textbooks also provide thorough coverage of these topics (Berkowitz 2013; Howard & Lohmander 2011; Kummer, 2013a). Clinicians also may find the Web resources listed in Table 12–1 of interest.

In the diagnosis of communication problems associated with cleft palate, the SLP is typically a member of a team. The craniofacial team is a well-accepted clinical entity and, in many communities, represents the ultimate in interdisciplinary cooperation among SLPs, audiologists, psychologists, surgeons, otolaryngologists, radiologists, prosthedontists, orthodontists, pedodontists, and educational personnel. The SLP is expected to inform the team members about the patient's communication abilities and disabilities, predict the effects of contemplated rehabilitative procedures, serve as the primary agent for change in the patient's speech-language skills, and stay up-to-date with how any communication differences or disorders may be affecting the person's daily life. As discussed by Boone et al. (2014), if there is tissue deficiency or velar weakness with reduced range of motion, behavioral therapy alone will not normalize the velopharyngeal anatomy and function. Realistic intervention, they say, must begin with a thorough

TABLE 12-1
Web Resources of Interest Concerning Cleft Lip, Cleft Palate, and Pharyngoplasty

http://www.widesmiles2.org
This detailed website has much usable information for the parent of a child with a cleft, including newborn feeding, emotional support with chat rooms, before-and-after surgical photos, and other helpful information. The SLP will benefit as well from viewing the general information and the explanations of primary and secondary surgeries. Pertinent also is material comparing and contrasting the three surgical options for velopharyngeal incompetence: pharyngeal flap, the double-reversing Z-plasty (Furlow), and the sphincter pharyngoplasty.

http://www.plasticsurgery.org//Reconstructive-Procedures/Cleft-_Lip-_and-_Palate
The website of the American Society of Plastic Surgeons provides simple illustrated explanations of surgeries for clefts of the lip and palate.

http://www.google.com
Do a video search on Google for cleft palate speech to see and hear samples before and after surgery, including change following pharyngeal flap surgery.

http://www.ich.ucl.ac.uk
Search the Institute for Children's Health, located in the United Kingdom, for a variety of cleft-related information. Of particular interest is the information on speech appliances, shown with pictures, including speech bulbs and palatal lifts.

http://www.cleftline.org/
The Cleft Palate Foundation presents parents with information, factsheets, feeding tips, and publication resources.

evaluation, not only a perceptual speech and voice analysis but aerodynamic studies, acoustical analysis, and videoendoscopic studies to judge the velopharyngeal mechanism accurately. The SLP should endeavor to evaluate, or have evaluated at an appropriate facility, many aspects of velopharyngeal functioning and communication such as those outlined in Table 12–2. We acknowledge this is a bit of a laundry list; still these are aspects (and options) that may need assessment attention. Similar areas of study have been suggested by Kummer (2013b) and via the ASHA Practice Portal on Cleft Lip and Palate (search www.asha.org). We also urge the SLP to keep in mind the framework of Figure 12–2, which is provided by the World Health Organization (2004), so that any impacts on daily life, education, and socialization are not overlooked.

TABLE 12-2
Areas Appraised, as Appropriate, by the SLP and the Medical Team in Suspected Cases of Velopharyngeal Dysfunction

Case history
Articulation and intelligibility—formal tests, informal stimuli, rating scales
Voice/resonance—perceptual judgments, rating scales, low-tech devices (listening tube)
Oral peripheral examination—subjective observation
Acoustic studies—nasometry, spectrography
Aerodynamic studies—pressure-flow analysis
Structural imaging—cephalometry (still, lateral X-rays), computerized tomography (CT), magnetic resonance imaging (MRI)
Movement imaging—endoscopy (nasopharyngoscopy), videofluoroscopy
Stimulability testing (probes)—for example, for resonance quality, articulation
Feeding/swallowing abilities
Other pertinent areas—language, cognition, hearing, dental
Impact/quality-of-life scale

FIGURE 12–2

Assessment of Speech Associated with Cleft Palate and Velopharyngeal Incompetence Using the World Health Organization's International Classification of Functioning, Disability and Health (ICF)

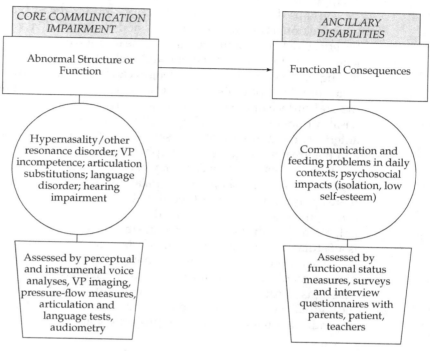

Case History

The routine case history data may need to be augmented for the cleft palate patient. Knowledge of the type and extent of cleft, as well as a description of the surgical, prosthodontic, orthodontic, and other rehabilitative procedures performed, is helpful. Some statement of the patient's current medical status and plans for future intervention procedures also helps direct the evaluative process. Most likely, the patient is pediatric and the informant is a parent. Case history questions about feeding issues, nasal regurgitation, and nutrition (e.g., weight gain) are in order (see Chapter 10). The attainment of developmental milestones (see Appendix B), and impressions of the child's language/cognitive development, sound and speech development, and psychosocial adjustments are pertinent lines of inquiry with this type of case. If the clinician is not a formal member of a craniofacial team, copies of reports from other professionals who have dealt with the patient should be obtained.

Oral Peripheral Examination

Although velopharyngeal closure cannot be visualized in an oral examination, it is important to examine the orofacial region of patients who manifest resonation disorders. The examination is an initial step in determining the general relationships among all structures in the vocal tract. For instance, the clinician can get a gross picture of palatal shape, total and effective velar lengths, movement ability and symmetry of movement of the velum, and dimensions of the pharynx, and can determine if any defects, such as fistulas of the palate, are present. If the SLP has any concerns regarding structure or function, the physician should be consulted.

Procedures for appraising the structure and function of the oral and peripheral regions are described in the literature (Dworkin & Culatta, 1996; St. Louis & Ruscello, 2000). General information on conducting an oral peripheral examination is provided in Appendix A. We offer a few special comments here.

Perhaps the most important observation for the SLP to make with the naked eye when velopharyngeal incompetency and/or insufficiency is suspected is to determine the effective length of the velum and the location of the velar dimple. The effective velar length is that portion of the elevated velar tissue used in closure of the nasopharynx during phonation. The effected length can be estimated from intraoral inspection of the velar dimple during phonation relative to nasopharyngeal depth. The velar dimple on the oral surface of the velum is an indication of the point of maximum elevation on the nasal surface of the velum. It typically occurs at 80% of the total velar length. The more anteriorly the dimple is placed (say, at the 50% mark), the less the effective velar length and the greater the degree of velopharyngeal incompetence.

Examination of the palate may reveal oronasal fistulas that are not always readily visible. What is the shape of the palatal vault? Is the coloration a healthy pink, or do there appear to be white or blue-tinted regions? Is there a palatal translucency observed during the oral exam when, in a dark room, a flashlight is shined into a nostril? Upon palpation, does the bony substructure feel firm and have normal posterior edges? If there is a fistula, the degree to which it affects articulation or resonance should be explored.

When overt clefting is present, the type and extent can be appraised. Many hospital-based craniofacial teams have devised specialized oral examination forms that contain diagrams of the lips and palate on which to mark the patient's features. The use of an individualized diagram not only documents the extent of the cleft but also facilitates communication among the team professionals.

Perceptual Assessment of Nasal Resonance and Voice

Resonance issues and other voice concerns are frequently heard in individuals with intraoral clefts or history of surgical repairs. The informal and formal perceptual assessment processes described earlier in this chapter certainly apply to the diagnostic workup of a child or adult patient. Any quality aberration is possible in persons with clefts of the palate (including hoarseness or harshness as a result of laryngeal compensation maneuvers) but disorders with the highest probability are hypernasality and nasal emission because both are related to velopharyngeal closure issues. The SLP should seek to determine how closely the resonance imbalance is related to functional factors such as tension, fatigue, and leakage (velopharyngeal incompetence); to organic factors such as neurological dysfunction; or to a structural defect that cannot be overcome through behavioral intervention (velopharyngeal insufficiency). Thus, instrumental acoustic and physiologic studies are important. We wish to restate, however, that critically listening to the patient's vocal and resonance parameters remains a fundamental aspect of diagnosis and evaluation. There are many rating scales to quantify a clinician's perception of hypernasality (and VPI). A straightforward 3-point rating scale for VPI resonance evaluation is 0 = competent, 1 = marginally competent, 2 = incompetent (Lohmander et al., 2009). For clients of reading age, use of nasal-loaded reading passages may help the SLP's perception (see Appendix B).

Articulation/Phonology and Intelligibility Testing

The initial interaction between clinician and young patient should occur as soon as possible when a cleft is detected. Prebabbling age is not too soon so that parents can be advised of speech and language stimulation approaches. The goal is to foster a phonetic inventory that minimizes nasal substitutions and glottal stops and encourages use of oral consonants (Hardin-Jones, Chapman, & Scherer, 2006). Not only does this develop good articulation and prevent development of stubborn and inappropriate articulation, it also helps prepare the toddler for eventual imaging evaluation of the velopharyngeal mechanism. With a conversational patient, the SLP must apply critical listening skills to assess the individual's total communicative effectiveness. This involves systematically shifting perceptual sets from one aspect of the patient's speech to another. The SLP should listen for the presence of a resonance imbalance (such as hypernasality, hyponasality, nasal emission, or a combination) and rate its severity. The clinician should also listen to and rate the speech intelligibility. Regarding evidence-based practice and the lack of speech intelligibility consensus procedures, the serious reader is referred to Whitehill's (2002) critical review of intelligibility assessment in speakers with cleft lip and palate.

Next, the SLP should assess the general articulatory pattern. Is there an obvious preponderance of a particular type of error (such as glottal stops or pharyngeal fricatives)? Does the articulation appear to alter with differing communication situations, speech, or stress patterns? (Note that in young children we may have a hybrid of articulation issues overlapping with rule-governed phonology issues as errors become ingrained in a child's linguistic system; this topic was discussed in Chapter 6.) Also, listen to the language of the patient, particularly if he or she is a young child, and check for appropriate word choice, sentence complexity, and structure. The rate and rhythm of the patient's speech should be noted. Are there any other vocal quality differences (such as hoarseness)? Is there a facial grimace, constriction of the nares, or any other behavior that detracts from the individual's total communicative effectiveness?

After formulating a general impression of the patient's speech patterns, detailed phonology and articulation testing should be done. Standard articulation or phonology tests may be satisfactory for an individual with cleft palate, but several considerations may best be examined by specialized articulation tests and context-controlled stimuli. Production of oral pressure consonants, either by informal elicitation words and sentences (which were suggested earlier in this chapter) or via formal testing (see Chapter 6), merits particular clinical attention. Oral pressure consonants include /p, b, t, d, k, g, f, v, s, z / and others.

Certainly, all of the functional, perceptual, and sensory factors that affect the typically developing person could be active, but in individuals with cleft palate and VPI there are added possibilities. Most important are the degree of velopharyngeal closure and the resultant air flow and intraoral pressure. The deviant geography of the oral cavity may contribute to this problem, which is complicated by the fact that the oral structure may well have undergone several architectural changes within the first few years of life. The SLP must keep in mind that this individual has been trying to produce standard sounds with a nonstandard structure, and under these conditions unique compensatory adjustments may have been made. The patient may have increased the air flow in order to build up adequate oral pressure, or the patient may have minimized it to lessen nasal escape (in the latter case, we say that the patient is producing weak pressure consonants).

Many patients with velopharyngeal incompetency/insufficiency adopt compensatory articulations, including glottal stop substitutions, pharyngeal fricatives, velar fricatives, and aspirant productions of vowels and consonants. Other, more unusual compensations may also be used, such as double articulations that may involve glottal or pharyngeal constriction simultaneous with valving at the lips or in the linguapalatal region; other labial-lingual double articulations may exist (Gibbon & Crampin, 2002). A wide variety of unusual speech-sound errors may exist in the population of clients.

Common articulatory/phonatory errors have been classified by some based on the individual's cleft-type characteristics (CTC; John, Sell, Sweeney, Harding-Bell, & Williams, 2006; Prathanee, 2010). Error patterns according to CTC include the following:

1. Anterior oral CTCs: dentalization/interdentalization, lateralization/lateral-palatalization/palatal

2. Posterial oral CTCs: double articulation, back to velar/uvular

3. Nonoral CTCs: pharyngeal articulation, glottal articulation, active nasal fricatives, double articulation

4. Passive CTCs: weak and/or nasalized consonants, nasal realization of plosives and/or suspected passive nasal fricatives, gliding of fricatives/affricates

5. Noncleft speech immaturity/errors

Keep in mind that it is entirely possible for the compensatory habits that developed before the final surgical adjustments to persist after competence of the velopharyngeal mechanism is established and the patient can make the correct articulatory movements. Stimulability probes therefore are important in determining the patient's prognosis for change. Articulation errors may also be related to an existing or prior hearing loss.

In summary, the clinician analyzes speech samples, elicited productions, and phonetic inventories for overall intelligibility and analysis of patterns, keeping in mind the main goal: to distinguish speech errors that may be due to faulty velopharyngeal or other structural deviations from speech errors that are compensatory or developmental. Trost-Cardamone and Bernthal (1993) provide a chart of guidelines for deciding on a direction for intervention based on these analyses.

Instrumental VP Assessment: Low-Tech

As previously indicated, the oral peripheral examination does not allow for definitive judgments to be made about velopharyngeal adequacy. In addition, an articulation test, whether published or informal, is but an indirect measure of the client's velopharyngeal function. Other techniques, many involving instrumentation, are available to assess, directly or indirectly, the velopharyngeal mechanism. We maintain that no single measure is adequate for appraisal of velopharyngeal function; we also believe that articulation testing and resonance assessment *must* be part of any diagnostic process. Despite advances in so-called objective acoustic measures of hypernasality (e.g., one-third octave spectra analysis), perceptual judgment remains the primary means for assessing levels of nasality (Vogel, Ibrahim, Reilly, & Kilpatrick, 2009). Let us describe some of the other assessment procedures that are available for routine and/or sophisticated diagnostic sessions.

The SLP, even with limited access to sophisticated instruments, can start with simple techniques, such as the listening tube described earlier (self-constructed or commercially available, but a bendable drinking straw will do) to emphasize the presence of hypernasality or nasal emission. Another is the tongue-anchor technique (Fox & Johns, 1970), which is still used to estimate static closure ability. For this the patient is required to maintain intraoral pressure by puffing the cheeks. If this procedure is accomplished, the patient is asked to protrude the tongue and then puff the cheeks (to prevent lingual valving). The clinician holds the patient's nostrils while this exercise is done to aid in impounding pressure. If no air escapes when the nostrils are released, it is assumed that velopharyngeal closure is adequate.

A long-standing clinical method for subjectively visualizing a VP leak, hypernasality, and also nasal emission has been to observe whether a small mirror held beneath the patient's nostrils fogs during special speech attempts. This low-tech fog test has been elevated to aerodynamic status called the Glatzel test (Van Lierde, Muyts, Bonte, & Van Cauwenberge, 2007). The degree of fogging or circumference of condensation is rated during the production of vowels and reading passages on a scale of 0 to 4, with 4 = severe condensation. (See Appendix B for grade-level passages and also a nasal-loaded passage.)

Another low-tech indicator of velopharyngeal leakage (and likely hypernasality and nasal emission) is to observe movement of small wisps of cotton or facial tissue held beneath the patient's nostrils during speech. Words and phrases loaded to elicit cotton or tissue movement should be used (plosives, and others presented earlier in this chapter) as well as observations during nose-occluded/nose-unoccluded speech conditions, though the area under the nostrils gets very crowded when doing so.

Instrumental VP Assessments: Acoustic

Attempts to translate perceptual judgments of hypernasality into objective, acoustic measures are ongoing and fraught with inconsistencies. We will highlight two types of acoustic measures here.

Spectrography

The coupling of the nasal cavity to the oral during both normal (when intended) and disordered articulation affects the sound spectrum. Nasality enhances the amplitude of low frequencies and absorbs the energy at higher frequencies. Typical characteristics seen on a sound spectrogram, say, of a vowel segment, include dark (intense) fundamental and first formant frequencies with excess energy absorption (lighter striations) in middle and higher formant regions. Quantification and perceptual correlation difficulties affect the popularity of regular spectrographic analysis in clinical practice. Clinicians that perform spectrographic speech analysis often rely on the Computerized Speech Lab (CSL) equipment and software from KayPENTAX (www.kayelemetrics.com).

Nasometry

The study of oral and nasal sound pressures during speech constitutes nasometry. It is a popular assessment tool for SLPs working in medical centers, voice clinics, and university clinics. Decades of research have shown the measure known as nasalence to be highly correlated with perceptual judgments of nasality. KayPENTAX (www.kayelemetrics.com) markets a Nasometer for coupling to its CSL computer-based system. Clinical assessment with the Nasometer is noninvasive and entails a microphone and a headset positioned to collect sound pressure levels at the nostrils and mouth as the patient speaks controlled phonetic syllables or words or reads a standard passage (see Appendix B). The oral and nasal measures form the oral-nasal acoustic ratio, which may be analyzed to provide a nasalance score, expressed as a percentage. To calculate this percentage score, the measured nasal acoustic energy is divided by the nasal acoustic energy plus the measured oral acoustic energy and multiplied by 100. Software with the Nasometer performs calculations, provides statistical measures, and displays the percentage of nasalence changes over utterance duration. A rule of thumb is that normal nasalance does not exceed 10% to 20% above baseline. Use of a Nasometer is quite feasible with young children, who are not bothered by the special headset and microphone.

Although the nasalance score has been shown to be a reliable correlate of nasality, Prathanee (2010) maintains that differences in resonance acceptability among multicultural and internal populations suggest the need for local norms. Available diversity information includes English (Seaver, Dalston, Leeper, & Adams, 1991), Flemish (Van Lierde et al., 2007), and Thai (Prathanee, Thanaviratananich, Pongjunyakul, & Rengpatanakij, 2003).

We believe the SLP will find it important to have objective analyses via nasometry done before and after any medical, prosthodontic, and behavioral speech-language treatments of a patient. This conforms with our philosophy of periodic reevaluations of patients. Note also that the Nasometer is a useful tool in treatment, providing the patient with visual feedback from the monitor during speech attempts. Again, the SLP can repeat the measure over treatment sessions because the nasalence score can be an objective indicator of improvement or lack thereof to satisfy third-party payors.

Instrumental VP Assessments: Aerodynamic

Air pressure and air flow analyses during speech tasks have ranged from the straightforward to the complex over the last 60 years. Aerodynamic instrumentation for pressure and flow studies also varies according to the clinical work setting, with sophisticated velopharyngeal analyses likely found in medical centers, specialized voice clinics, and some university clinics. Physicians and plastic surgeons are often keenly interested in aerodynamic estimates of the size of any velopharyngeal orifice, nasal air flow measures, and the ability of the patient to generate oral air pressure. The SLP too sees the utility of this information for determining a patient's competence or insufficiency for improved speech/resonance through behavioral methods. Here we provide some historical highlights and a cursory mention of high-tech options.

Manometry

The oral manometer is an affordable piece of equipment and is helpful in discriminating between persons with good and poor velopharyngeal closure. The patient either blows into or sucks from, as forcefully as possible, a mouthpiece. The exhalation task yields a positive pressure reading from the manometer gauge, while the inhalation task gives a negative reading. A ratio is obtained by comparing pressures achieved in the nostrils-open and nostrils-occluded conditions. A normal ratio of 1.00 is suggestive of velopharyngeal closure adequacy, particularly if an open bleed valve was used to inhibit compensatory maneuvers, such as tongue-palate valving. Ratios less than 1.00 may be indicative of VPI, hypernasal speech, and reduced intelligibility in cleft palate patients; ratios less than 0.89 are particularly poor indicators.

Air pressure and air flow techniques are based on the fact that VPI results in a decrement of intraoral air pressure and an increase in air flow through the nose. Consequently, pressure and flow measurements can be part of the total diagnostic workup; they are often used for research purposes. Pressure transducers, such as strain gauge transducers, are used to measure air pressures, while air flow meters are used to measure volume rates of air flow. Types of flow meters include warm-wire anemometers, pneumotachographs, and thermistors. The pneumotachograph is perhaps the most commonly used and requires the use of a face mask to collect the air flow and direct it through a sensing screen. Air pressure and flow instrumentation is expensive and complex. However, Realica, Smith, Glover, and Yu (2000) adopted a common U-tube manometer using a Y-connector to measure oral and nasal air flow as well as pressure quantitatively. This is a simple means of assessing velopharyngeal incompetence.

Nasality Severity Index

The Nasality Severity Index (NSI) is listed here, although it is a combination of three parameters developed using multivariate analyses by Van Lierde et al. (2007). Often using single sounds, oral text readings, or oral-nasal weighted text passages (see Appendix B), the patient's index score is derived from an equation that weights (1) the patient's nasalance score as an acoustic measure, (2) the perceptual rating of the patient's nasality on a 5-point scale (mild to very severe hypernasality), and (3) the patient's aerodynamic capacity. The aerodynamic part of the assessment consists of determining the patient's maximum duration time (MDT) for sustaining the voiceless sound /s/ at habitual loudness while seated. The Glatzel test is also used to visualize any nasal air flow on a small mirror placed below the patient's nares (as mentioned, this uses a rating scale of 0 to 4). To calculate a patient's Nasality Severity Index, the following weighted formula is used: NSI = −60.69 − (3.24 × percentage oral text) − 13.39 × Glatzel value "/a/" + [0.244 × maximum duration time (seconds)] − (0.558 × percentage "/a/" + (3.38 × percentage oronasal text). The more negative the patient's index, the worse his or her nasal quality (e.g., −24.0 is slight hypernasality, whereas normal nasality averages +4.9).

Instrumental VP Assessments: Imaging

Instrumentation exists to provide the medical team with sophisticated visualization of velopharyngeal structures and functional movements. Imaging studies help determine the direction of intervention: Can the patient's hypernasality improve through behavioral intervention (voice/speech therapy), or is the VP mechanism incapable of doing so (i.e., it is insufficient) without surgical/prosthodontic intervention? The medical team (especially the surgeon) is keenly interested in imaging information, but the ethical SLP also needs to know the appropriateness of providing services. We will highlight a few of the structure and movement imaging options from Figure 12–2. The SLP may or may not conduct the imaging study but certainly will be interested in interpreting communication impact and potential. Also, it important to have objective imaging analyses done before and after any medical, prosthodontic, and behavioral speech-language treatments; such data have become *de rigeur* as outcomes evidence.

Lateral Cephalometry

With radiographic methods that involve low doses of radiation, still images of the head and neck bones (hard tissues) and the velopharyngeal structure (soft tissues) can be visualized. The still X-ray of the lateral vocal tract allows for standardized measurements (depth and distance calculations, structural orientations, structure oddities). Lateral cephalometry, like other types of structural images (e.g., CT, MRI), provides only a static image, not functional movement of the velopharyngeal mechanism.

Nasopharyngoscopy

Direct visualization is easily accomplished through an invasive but tolerated technique that uses a viewing device called an endoscope (in particular, the nasopharyngoscope). Rigid forms of endoscopy useful in observing velopharyngeal closure are the oral pan-endoscope and the nasal endoscope. Flexible endoscopes use a thin tube of fiber-optic bundles to transmit the image. We again remind the reader that closure, or lack of it, is best viewed from above, and so the flexible fiberscope inserted through a nostril is used to view oro-nasal and pharyngeal structures plus movement of the velopharyngeal mechanism. In particular, the VP port and associated constriction of the lateral and medial pharyngeal walls and the up-back movement of the velum can be viewed during activity. This nasal cavity perspective affords a view of the completeness or incompleteness of VP closure in all dimensions. Speech tasks are the activity of choice for judging the sufficiency of VP closure (e.g., sounds, syllables, words, sentences). VP patterns of closures during nonspeech tasks (sucking, blowing) are different than during speech tasks.

Many hospitals; ear, nose, and throat (ENT) physicians; and voice clinics have the necessary endoscopy equipment, including those equipped with state-of-the art stroboscopic lighting and video capabilities (e.g., videolaryngoscopy). The SLP may perform the scoping procedure in many work settings. Cooperative patients can be examined while seated and performing speech and nonspeech tasks. Even young children tolerate well a flexible optic tube placed nasally (Hay, Oates, Giannini, Berkowiz, & Rotenberg, 2009). Various rating scales exist to standardize reporting of information from nasendoscopy and related images. Examples include Tieu et al. (2012) and the international Golding-Kushner scale (Golding-Krushner et al., 1990) which quantifies movement of the velum; lateral and posterior pharyngeal wall; and the size, shape, symmetry, and location of any VP gap noted on the image.

Magnetic Resonance Imaging

MRI technology is used widely in hospitals and medical centers and can provide a static, three-dimensional measurement of the head, neck, and velopharyngeal mechanism. Movement can be inferred, particularly when MRI is combined with other imaging techniques; still many physicians advocate MRI to view static structures. The use of dynamic MRI to access levator veli palatini muscle activity at rest and during speech is growing (Ettema, Kuehn, Perlman, & Alperin, 2002). Though MRI protocols have been standardized for studying the velopharyngeal mechanism in adults at rest and during speech, there is a lack of standardization for children, though research efforts are under way (Tian et al., 2010). MRI is noninvasive and can often be performed without general anesthesia in some children. The popularity of this imaging technique is sure to grow.

Other Assessments Important with Cleft Palate and VPI Cases

Typically, in major hospitals and medical centers, once an infant is born with an orofacial anomaly, the work of a multidisciplinary team is set into motion. The SLP, as part of the team, will wish to see the infant as soon as possible while working closely with the parents—through counseling and training—to prevent future communication problems. Areas in need of early and ongoing, periodic assessments by the SLP include the following.

Feeding Issues

The infant with a cleft of the palatal may have mild to severe issues with nursing, feeding, and weight gain. This subject was touched on in Chapter 10, so it will not be repeated here. This may be an area of assessment for the SLP and the medical term.

Auditory Issues

The high incidence of hearing problems and chronic ear infections (related to the altered anatomy) among children with cleft palate has been well documented. For this reason, it is essential that every patient have a hearing examination and continued follow-up over time. These examinations should include both air and bone conduction testing and should be a part of every speech diagnosis. Periodic monitoring and reevaluations help to prevent other speech and language problems.

Language Assessment

During early, initial contact, the parents of an infant can be informed about the need for normal speech-language stimulation, what to expect from their child regarding speech and language production, and the need for frequent language testing over time. Some speech clinicians use established language stimulation programs as a preventive measure with these children, especially because vocabulary expansion tends to develop slowly in these toddlers (Hardin-Jones, Chapman, & Scherer, 2006). Subsequent child language assessment measures may parallel issues discussed in Chapters 4 and 5.

Self-Esteem and Daily Impact

Children with clefts, nasal emission, and nasality issues often find in playgroups and in school that they are the brunt of teasing, ridicule, and social exclusion because they may look and sound different. Parents, teachers, SLPs, and other healthcare team members need to anticipate these reactions and take steps to minimize their psychosocial impacts on the child. Indeed, a goal of medical and speech-voice intervention is "to fix" the structures and functions to the extent possible so that other negative consequences do not occur. The framework of the World Health Organization that was depicted in Figure 12–2 is helpful to remember. Although assessing the quality of life following intervention is an emerging body of literature, we wish to mention some tools that show promise for SLPs as well as surgeons.

Boseley and Hartnick (2004) administered a Pediatric Voice Outcomes Survey (PVOS) to the parents of children (mean age 5 years) pre- and postsurgery for velopharyngeal incompetency. They specifically compared outcomes between sphincteroplasty and superiorly based pharyngeal flap and found the PVOS to be a valid tool for functional impact. The SLP might well use the PVOS to track daily-living changes and perceived functional adjustments as a function of speech treatment.

Two systematic reviews of the literature on quality of life among children treated for cleft lip and/or palate found no single instrument of choice, though numerous and diverse clinical instruments exist. Also no consensus of perceptions and impacts emerged among the children (Klassen & Tsangaris, 2012; Raposo-do-Amaral et al., 2011).

PROGNOSIS ASSOCIATED WITH RESONANCE IMBALANCE

Let us now return to our general discussion of resonance imbalance and list some of the prognostic indicators for the treatment of resonance. We freely admit that much is speculation or opinion or is simply based on assumptions of etiology. Research documenting clinical effectiveness is sorely needed.

1. It has been stated that voice treatment for cul-de-sac resonance is not usually successful in patients with neurologic involvement of the articulators, which includes conditions such as oral apraxia, athetoid cerebral palsy, flaccid dysarthria, and spastic dysarthria. Patients with functional cul-de-sac resonance and, to a lesser extent, deaf speakers can benefit from intervention directed toward anterior positioning of the tongue.

2. Thin resonance, with its assumed functional etiology, is remediated easily only in patients motivated to change. Treatment efforts should be directed toward correcting tongue carriage. The clinician may benefit from knowledge of male–female communication differences when assisting a patient to reduce the effeminate aspects of speech. The emerging literature on communication treatment for transsexuals may be used as a resource.

3. Hyponasality, when due to some nasal obstruction, necessitates physical management. Speech treatment alone is not likely to be beneficial.

4. The patient's motivation to change is paramount in predicting the outcome of voice treatment.

5. A favorable prognosis for treatment is indicated if the clinician was able to elicit a better voice resonance from the patient during the assessment. This phase of activity may be termed the probe, stimulability, or trial therapy phase where various techniques are tried with the patient to assess potential for change. Indeed, it is on this basis that treatment should be prescribed.

There are several indications and contraindications to resonance and speech treatment for individuals with cleft palate and VP insufficiency. Kummer (2013b) provides some practical auditory and visual probes and techniques. We cite some treatment indicators below (though many apply to cases of hypernasality and nasal emission in the absence of a cleft):

1. Speech treatment is contraindicated for patients with clearly inadequate velopharyngeal closure; physical management is warranted. As discussed in this chapter, evidence of velopharyngeal inadequacy should come from a variety of sources, including articulation testing showing consistent hypernasality and nasal emission, observation of nasal grimacing, imaging evidence, oral examination findings of an anteriorly displaced velar dimple and/or excessive nasopharyngeal dimensions, and pressure-flow measures.

2. Because home programs are essential in most therapeutic approaches, motivated and cooperative patients and their parents are a requirement for enrollment in a speech intervention program.

3. Speech/resonance treatment is not warranted, or is a low priority, when the patient needs language and communication improvement.

4. Patients with borderline velopharyngeal closure may not be good candidates for speech treatment, and the risk of developing inappropriate articulatory and laryngeal compensation is real. Likewise, nasality treatment is contraindicated if the patient presents with hoarseness, although hygiene treatment directed at reduction of hoarseness may be in order.

5. Patients who demonstrated improvement during the assessment probes are good candidates for speech treatment. Especially favorable are reduced hypernasality when employing exaggerated, open-mouth articulation and a marked difference in velar activity when gagging and phonating.

6. Some patients with inadequate velopharyngeal closure cannot benefit from further physical management. The SLP may opt to provide compensatory treatment. The goal, then, is not normal-sounding speech but the best speech of which the patient is capable. Tasks used in the assessment probes may be appropriate treatment techniques in that the perception of hypernasality is reduced by their use. These tasks include increased mouth opening, low and forward placement of the tongue, auditory training, exaggerated articulation movements, light and quick articulatory contacts, overall slowed rate of speech, and altered pitch and/or loudness levels.

CONCLUSION AND SELF-ASSESSMENT

Information has been presented in this chapter in agreement with the profession's preferred practice patterns for resonance and nasal air flow assessment (American Speech-Language-Hearing Association, 2004b). The evaluation of resonance disorders is a challenge to the SLP. The clinician must often work closely with medical personnel and other allied health professionals, which necessitates knowing procedures and terminologies that are peripheral to speech-language pathology. The clinician must also remain abreast of current technological developments in surgery and medical technology. Finally, the clinician must keep interpersonal clinical skills finely honed so that psychosocial aspects of vocal/resonance disorders can be detected and dealt with through treatment or referral.

After reading this chapter you should be able to answer the following questions:

1. Evaluate oral/nasal resonance and velopharyngeal function for speech without purchased tests or instrumentation.

2. Identify and describe various communication areas to assess regarding an individual's strengths and weaknesses.

3. Explore any effects on the individual's participation in everyday activities related to the resonance disorder.

4. Identify any contextual factors that serve as barriers to or facilitators of successful communication in affected patients.

5. Explain some clinical findings from a thorough assessment suggesting that services needed by the patient are medical, rather than behavioral, in nature.

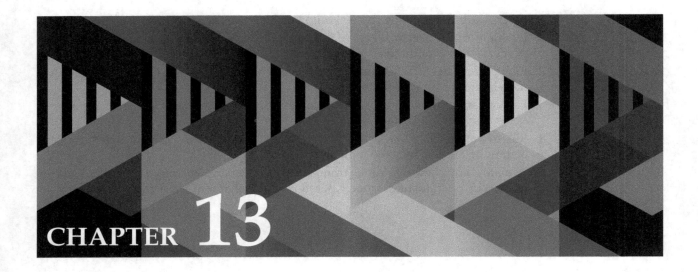

CHAPTER **13**

Cancer and Alaryngeal Voice Disorders

LEARNING OUTCOMES

After reading this chapter you will be able to:

1. Describe the altered anatomy when a total laryngectomy is performed.

2. Explain important *functional* changes a person experiences as a result of a total laryngectomy.

3. Compare and contrast the source of vibrations for speech production in speech with an electrolarynx, traditional esophageal speech, and in speech with a tracheoesophageal puncture.

4. Troubleshoot or assess some reasons for speech failure in a tracheoesophageal puncture (TEP) patient just fitted with a valve prosthesis.

The impacts of head and neck cancers represent an expanding area of practice for speech-language pathologists (SLPs). When cancer occurs anywhere along the vocal tract, speech and swallowing may be affected—even after life-saving measures by physicians (surgeons, oncologists, radioncologists, etc.). The medical treatments, whether surgical excision, radiation, chemotherapy, or a combination of these approaches, may further affect the patient's speech, swallowing, and psychosocial functioning. As part of the team of healthcare professionals working with cancer patients and cancer survivors, many SLPs have developed expertise in optimizing communication outcomes. Going beyond the physician's diagnosis of cancer and planned medical intervention, the SLP assists the patient in honing one or more methods of postintervention communication. This chapter provides an overview of laryngeal cancer, speech rehabilitation options, and the continuing assessments (reevaluations) of the patient's communication progress.

LARYNGEAL CANCER PRIMER

When a malignancy starts in the larynx, it is called a laryngeal cancer. Laryngeal cancer can be classified further by region affected. Three regions of laryngeal cancer are recognized. Cancer arising on one or both vocal folds is glottic cancer. Cancer in the glottal area is a common form and can range from a small spot to all-encompassing. Glottic cancer can be detected early as symptoms of vocal hoarseness, chronic cough, noisy breathing, sensation of a throat lump or pain, and/or difficulty swallowing. Supraglottic cancer is located above the vocal folds and may affect laryngeal structures such as the arytenoids, aryepiglottic folds, false vocal folds, and epiglottis. The least common of the three regions for laryngeal cancer to occur is below the level of the vocal folds; these subglottic cancers often have delayed symptom awareness that allows significant growth or spread before the person seeks medical attention. Early detection of any cancer is best, when less intrusive medical interventions are often an option. All laryngeal cancers may spread, or metastasize, to adjacent laryngeal areas, areas of the neck, or distant sites throughout the body (such as the lungs or liver). Metastasis occurs when malignant cells are carried from the primary site via the lymphatic system (the neck has a concentration of lymph nodes) or via the bloodstream to other locations; metastasis is always a serious concern.

Physician Assessment of Cancer and Prognosis

When presented with a new patient, the physician augments his or her office interview (initial complaint and case history), general physical examination, and laryngeal examination (such as by indirect laryngoscopy, endoscopy, or perhaps videostroboscopy to view the structures) with subsequent diagnostic procedures performed at a medical center. These may include imaging (magnetic resonance imaging [MRI] or computerized tomography [CT]), laboratory tests, tissue biopsy, and others. Squamous cell carcinoma accounts for the vast majority of laryngeal cancers. Descriptions of imaging techniques were presented in previous chapters and also may be found in voice disorders texts (e.g., Sapienza & Ruddy, 2013).

The cumulative medical findings, when positive, are used to describe the cancer. One of three staging/grading systems may be used with laryngeal cancer. The TNM staging system summarizes the key features of the **t**umor (how much of the larynx is affected), the **n**ode (whether the lymph notes are affected), and **m**etastases (whether it has spread to another part of the body)—hence the acronym of TNM. For example, the definition of a supraglottic primary tumor labeled T3 is a "tumor limited to larynx with vocal cord fixation and/or invades any of the following: postcricoid area, pre-epiglottic space, paraglottic space, and/or inner cortex of thyroid cartilage." The regional lymph node description for an N1 example is "metastasis in a single ipsilateral lymph node, less than or equal to 3 cm in greatest dimension." Distant metastasis rated as M0, for example, indicates that the cancer has not spread beyond the larynx. The interested reader can find more TNM information as applied to laryngeal cancer at the website of the National Cancer Institute (www.cancer.gov/cancertopics/pdq/treatment/laryngeal/HealthProfessional/page3).

In the number staging system, laryngeal cancer is categorized as either Stage 0, I, II, III, or IV. For example, Stage 0 describes a cancer where cancer cells are in the lining of the larynx (in situ). Stage IV describes a cancer where the cancer has spread beyond the larynx (into large lymph nodes, surrounding tissue, and/or other parts of the body).

The grade of the cancer gives an idea of how quickly it might develop based on its cellular composition. In Grade 1 (low grade), the cancer cells tend to grow slowly, appear similar to normal cells, and may be less likely to spread. In Grade 2 (moderate grade), the cells look more abnormal and tend to grow a bit quicker. In Grade 3 (high grade), the cells look very abnormal, tend to grow faster, and are more likely to spread.

According to Brook (2013), the potential for recovery from laryngeal cancer depends on aspects such as: (1) the extent to which the cancer has spread (the stage); (2) the appearance of the cancer cells (the grade); (3) the location and size of the cancer; and (4) patient attributes such as age, general health, and gender. No doubt, the SLP should be familiar with such information as well. The stage and grade of the cancer are key components in shaping the recommended course of intervention by the medical team. For example, a small, noninvasive caner might be surgically excised, leaving the area mainly intact, or it might be treated with radiation. Larger cancers and those that have spread may necessitate extensive surgery, radiation, chemotherapy, or a combined approach.

Surgery to remove the larynx is termed a laryngectomy. Depending on the stage, size, and location of the cancer, a partial, subtotal laryngectomy may be used to excise a small area, such as one vocal fold or half of the larynx, with plastic surgery reconstruction for a modified but functional larynx. In a total laryngectomy, the entire larynx is sacrificed. With metastasis into the neck, the surgeon may opt for a total laryngectomy with radical neck dissection on one side of the neck. In this chapter, the focus will be on a total laryngectomy. The patient who has undergone a laryngectomy procedure may be referred to as a laryngectomee; notice the change of spelling. Medical treatment for cancer of the larynx may involve surgical excision, radiation to kill cancer cells, chemotherapy to kill or inhibit the growth of cancer cells, or a combination of these approaches. A sobering statistic shows a two-decade increase in the use of nonsurgical treatments (i.e., radiation, chemotherapy) yet the return of the cancer and an increase in morbidity rate (Hoffman et al., 2006).

Regardless of the medical approaches used, Brook (2013) states that the effectiveness of treatment is decreased if the patient smokes or drinks alcohol during the medical treatment phase. The potential for recurrence is also heightened in those who continue smoking and drinking after treatment.

Prevalence of Laryngeal Cancer and Multicultural Issues

The Surveillance, Epidemiology, and End Results Program (SEER) of the National Cancer Institute (www.SEER.cancer.gov) estimated over 12,000 new cases of laryngeal cancer in the United States in 2013. Laryngeal cancers as a whole are not common, accounting for less than 1% of all cancers. SEER reports a two-decade decline in the prevalence of laryngeal cancers and attributes this to national declines in smoking. Although tobacco is a known cause of cancer, other contributors are said to be alcohol consumption, urban environmental (air) pollution, poor nutrition, and other unknown factors. There is speculation that these factors are more apparent in persons of low socioeconomic status and among minority groups. SEER data indicate higher rates of laryngeal cancer among African Americans and Native Americans, although cancer shows no boundaries.

THE TOTAL LARYNGECTOMY AND THE LARYNGECTOMEE

We now turn to a discussion of the loss of voice due to total laryngectomy (the suffix -ectomy refers to "removal of the structure"; the suffix -mee refers to "the person so affected"). The SLP must understand the altered anatomy, appreciate functional changes as a result of the surgery, assist the physician and others on the healthcare team with avenues of rehabilitation (speech, swallowing, other), and play a key role in the actual rehabilitation and ongoing assessments of the patient and the patient's family.

In a total laryngectomy, the surgeon first creates an alternate path for breathing by creating a hole in the neck below the surgical area of the larynx. Creating an opening into the trachea is a procedure called a tracheostomy, and the hole is called a tracheostoma (which can be shortened to stoma). The stoma will become the patient's permanent route for breathing, with inhaled and exhaled air bypassing the typical nose and mouth route and with concomitant loss of nasal heating, cooling, and filtering of the air breathed. These functional changes have rehabilitation implications. *It is critical to remember always that lung air is henceforward breathed in and out through the patient's stoma.* With so many functional changes, rehabilitation questions and options, and psychosocial quandaries the patient is feeling, it is often the SLP who provides early counseling and early communication assessments.

THE COUNSELING PROCESS

The evaluation seeks to determine a patient's rehabilitation potential and to provide information necessary to shape the direction of treatment. But the evaluation process also has the goal of providing information, support, and emotional release for the patient and the patient's family. The clinician must wear many hats. In this section, let us explore the clinician's role in the preoperative visit, family and spouse counseling, arranging or assisting with the visit by another laryngectomee, and postoperative counseling of the patient.

The Preoperative Visit

Ideally, the surgeon requests that a preoperative visit be made by the SLP. When the physician informs the patient of the cancer, a thousand thoughts must surge through the patient's mind: Will I die? Will I be disfigured? Will my family be able to look at me? Will I talk again? Will I lose my job? Private thoughts such as these may happen so forcefully and quickly that the patient does not absorb much of what else the physician says. We often see patients with only a small understanding of the surgery and its many consequences for daily living. Explanations offered by the physician, then, can be supplemented at a later meeting by the SLP. A preoperative visit is an ideal time to meet the patient, who can still talk, ask questions, express feelings and fears, and so forth. The clinician must be emotionally and professionally capable of dealing with the issues of this meeting. It can be a time when grown men cry, when women react with such anger as to order you out of the room, when denial is apparent, and/or when the patient needs desperately to hear some words of hope and optimism.

One goal of the first meeting, then, is to provide emotional release and support. The clinician must remember in the preoperative visit that the patient is facing a trauma unparalleled in his or her lifetime. The first confrontation is no social chat and may well demand all of the professional proficiency the clinician can muster. Occasionally, the clinician might find that the patient is not capable of dealing rationally with the topic immediately before surgery and, in these cases, it may be preferable to postpone detailed discussion until after recovery.

Another major goal of the first meeting is to provide some information about the operation and the implications for speech. After consultation with the physician, every attempt should be made to present a clear discussion of the anatomical changes. Charts and diagrams are helpful. Either in this session or later as rehabilitation begins, we like to inform the patient of some helpful booklets and online informational sources. Many practical guides are available at little or no cost. Table 13–1 lists some resources for the laryngectomized person.

TABLE 13–1
Some Useful Resources Every Laryngectomized Person Should Know

Organizations
American Cancer Society
Search for assorted information on cancer of the larynx and its treatment at
http://www.cancer.org.
International Association of Laryngectomees (IAL)
The IAL aims to assist with the total rehabilitation of persons who have been laryngectomized.
The IAL provides various resources and support, including print media and videos, as well as
the operation of local clubs throughout the country. Often these are called "Lost Chord" or
"New Voice" clubs. Information is available at http://www.theial.org/.
Web Whisperers
This group offers online support and guidance to laryngectomees and their families. It is an
especially useful site for newly laryngectomized persons to chat and seek advice on a variety
of topics. The link is http://www.webwhispers.org/.

Informational Booklets and Self-Help Guides
"First Steps: A Guide for New Laryngectomees," by the International Association of Laryngec-
tomees, is downloadable from its website at http://www.theial.org/.
"The Laryngectomee Guide" and "My Voice: A Physician's Personal Experience with Throat
Cancer" are both written by Izhak Brook (2013). The first is a thorough, all-topics covered,
170-page guide. Both booklets are endorsed by the American Academy of Otolaryngology
Head and Neck Surgery and are available as free downloads from the organization's websites:
http://www.entnet.org/HealthInformation/Laryngectomee.cfm and http://www.entnet.org/
content/ebooks. Both also are available as free downloads from the author's website at http://
dribrook.blogspot.com/, along with other helpful information such as videos and articles. Both
are also available in paperback or Kindle book form from Amazon.com.
"Self-Help for the Laryngectomee" is written by Edmund Lauder (1978), a laryngectomized
person. This long-popular guide covers assorted topics as well as how to get started with
esophageal speech. It is available as a paperback and spiral-bound book through Amazon
.com. A free downloadable PDF version has been donated by Lauder Enterprises to the Web
Whisperers; search for this book at http://.www.webwhispers.org/.

We explain that many communication avenues exist. At this time, we decide on an appropriate short-term method (e.g., writing, gesturing, pointing to pictures), depending on
literacy, vision, and manual dexterity abilities versus limitations. We arrange for the hospital, family, speech services, social services, or other department or agency to make the
necessary supplies available immediately after surgery (e.g., paper and pencil, wipe-off
writing boards, picture communication boards, synthetic speech devices, and so forth). We
may also introduce other methods that the patient may learn to use, such as esophageal
speech and speech with an artificial larynx unless tracheoesophageal fistula is planned.
The introduction must offer the optimism that the patient may actually speak again, but
care must be taken not to overwhelm the patient with too many details at this point.

Family and Spouse Counseling

Providing adequate information to the family can have far-reaching clinical implications. The spouse and immediate family must also understand the anatomy of the operation. Often, clinicians stress what the laryngectomee will be unable to do, and although
this information is important, it is also important to stress to the family what the patient
will be able to do. We generally attempt to have a frank discussion with the spouse about
the typical reactions of the family. If a problem can be identified before it develops, it
may be easier to control. The tendency to dominate the silent mate (or parent) must be

controlled, as must the inclinations to infantilize, overindulge, and pity. Often we have to warn the family not to shout at the patient—they may think that someone who cannot talk also does not hear well. Some families readily admit to a feeling of repulsion because of the physical changes; this can be easily conveyed to the patient. The silent mate is sometimes excluded from conversation and decision making in the family. The clinician must be sensitive to the fact that the spouse will have significant concerns. The fear of death, reduced income, new responsibilities, social changes, and alterations in the marital (and sexual) relationship may be topics for discussion. One of the primary purposes of the clinician's visit with the family members is to let them know that their feelings are understood. It is expected that the clinician will be warm, sincere, and insightful, but we resist the temptation to dictate any specific attitude beyond this because each patient will require a somewhat different approach. Some need to be dealt with gently, others straightforwardly and frankly. Find the level and type of interaction your patient and his or her family respond to best and use it.

Materials available from the IAL (see Table 13–1) are useful in spouse and family counseling. Many different pamphlets can provide the family with information and inspiration. We also like to arrange a viewing of one or more videos; the patient should attend with the family. The IAL film list should be consulted for something appropriate. Family counseling, then, seeks to ensure that the family is emotionally and physically ready to assist in the rehabilitation program and care of their loved one.

Laryngectomee Visitation

It is ideal when the surgeon and/or the SLP can arrange for the patient to be visited by a laryngectomee either before or after the surgery. The laryngectomee visitor, by his or her sheer presence, offers the patient hope: Here is a person who survived cancer, survived the operation, learned to talk, perhaps returned to work, and generally has gotten back into life. The laryngectomee can offer to the patient sincere understanding of the emotional turmoil—he or she has been down that road—and may be the best paraprofessional to offer advice and empathy. The laryngectomee visitor is also a model of alaryngeal speech. The patient hears firsthand what practiced alaryngeal speech (of some type) sounds like. Visitors are also great at explaining the importance of personal drive and daily practice. The International Association of Laryngectomees offers a "Laryngectomee Visitor Program Manual" that is available on its website (see Table 13–1).

Postoperative Counseling

If preoperative referrals were not made, the postoperative meetings will offer the opportunity for emotional release, support, and information sharing. All that we have described in the previous sessions needs to be accomplished now. If preoperative visits were done, then postoperatively the SLP is ready to move forward with the rehabilitation program, which involves a balance between treating and reassessing the patient's emotional, physical, and speech status.

The first few postoperative days may be the emotional low point for the patient. Frequent and brief visits may provide the support needed. The SLP should also ensure that the patient has a means of communicating. Earlier we mentioned planning for written messages, picture communication boards, and the like. The clinician, with physician knowledge, may introduce artificial larynx devices for immediate speech if a primary tracheoesophageal fistula was not created for speech. The interested reader is urged to consult any of the many excellent sources describing the available devices, their types, and how to begin training a patient in their use. Also of interest in postoperative counseling is that Rogers, El-Sheikha, and Lowe (2009) developed a Patient

Concerns Inventory to help reveal areas in which head and neck cancer patients wanted more consultation. The 45-item online questionnaire indicated that main issues of concern included chewing and eating, saliva, swallowing, and speech and voice.

INITIAL ASSESSMENT THEMES

The assessment of a person who has undergone a total laryngectomy is inherently different from the initial assessment of persons with other communication disorders. We do not approach the initial session to solve the problem/no problem issue. When we get a referral to see a laryngectomee (we may or may not have seen the person for a preoperative visit), we immediately know that the ability to speak has been lost—there is a problem and the speech disorder diagnosis is obvious. We also know that some form of intervention will be necessary to reestablish a means of communication for the patient. What needs to be assessed is the current status of the patient (physically, psychologically, and the like), the potential for rehabilitation, and the direction(s) that the intervention program should take. We maintain that the evaluation of the newly laryngectomized patient began with the first meeting and continues through all subsequent treatment contacts: Their needs and their progress are in continual flux.

Background and Current Status Information

In preparation for the initial meeting and case history interview, the SLP should review available medical documentation. Background information that holds particular interest for us includes the initial patient symptoms and complaint, the medical report (including stage or grade of cancer), the surgical report (especially in relation to structures removed or altered, type and extent of surgery, and plans for any secondary surgery), the daily notes by the nursing staff (if available, for hints about patient compliance, difficulties and progress encountered postsurgically), and the report from social services (with regard to family status and support).

In determining the potential for speech, a thorough case history is helpful with laryngectomized patients. Three facets are particularly crucial. It is important to know the extent of the surgery, the degree of involvement of related structures such as the tongue or pharynx, general health of the patient, and medical prognosis. The second critical area is the individual's vocation and interests. We find it most helpful to plan our clinical work around the patient's preferred activities. It is also important to know if the person will be able to continue in those vocations and hobbies that involve communication. A third variable related to the patient's potential for learning traditional esophageal speech is attitude and motivation. Some patients are depressed, discouraged, and unmotivated, while others evidence a high level of interest in recovering their communication abilities. This is a subjective judgment on the clinician's part, but it is one of those intangible variables that certainly relates to the potential of the patient to speak again.

Some voice disorders texts or specialized alaryngeal books discuss the types as well as medical and background information helpful in planning a rehabilitative program (e.g., Sapienza & Ruddy, 2013; Salmon, 1999). Table 13–2 lists themes and questions that guide us in the collection of information on a patient. In addition to shaping the treatment program, such information provides prognostic insights.

A necessary part of the evaluation concerns the current status of the patient's oral-motor abilities. Consult Appendix A for general information on conducting an oral examination. We thoroughly evaluate the tongue, lip, and jaw mobility because these muscle areas may be affected by the extent of the surgery. Articulation may be affected if surgery involved the hyoid bone, which is an anatomical connection for many muscles

TABLE 13–2
Laryngectomee Case History Outline

1. *Surgical Factors*
   Date of surgery
   Extent of surgery
   Postoperative complications
   Irradiation and other treatment procedures
2. *Physical and Mental Factors*
   General physical condition
   Upper respiratory health
   Status of oral structures
   Hearing acuity
   Other physical factors or conditions
   Cognitive-mental clarity
   Educational background
3. *Emotional Factors*
   Level of negative emotion or depression
   Level of motivation
   Degree of dependency on spouse and family
   Other personality traits or problems
4. *Social Factors*
   Home and family situation
   Occupational aspects
   Hobbies and pastimes
   Smoking and drinking habits
   Social network and sociability
   Family attitudes and acceptance

of the tongue, mandible, and pharynx. In addition, it is not uncommon that surgical alterations were necessary to contain concomitant oral, lingual, or lymph node cancers. Screen or test the patient's articulatory skills (see Chapter 6). Word, sentence, and/or reading passages (see Appendix B) may prove useful in assessing articulation, speech intelligibility, and speech dysarthris (see also Chapter 9). Some information about the previous articulation, speech, and language patterns of the patient is helpful for comparisons. For example, we have had poor success with alaryngeal speech intelligibility in cases where, premorbidly, the patient was edentulous and seldom wore dentures. Do not overlook a language/cognitive screening (see Chapter 8).

The SLP should also screen the patient's hearing (see the guidelines in Appendix B). A high percentage of laryngectomized persons are over the age of 55, so it is common to find a presbycusic hearing loss. Further hearing acuity assessments might be needed. A moderate to severe hearing loss may hinder the alaryngeal speech learning process and, of necessity, shape the direction of the rehabilitation program. The same can be said about the influence of the spouse's hearing ability; some methods of alaryngeal speech are louder or softer than others even in home environments.

This is also the opportunity to screen for dysphagia, as discussed in Chapter 10. The anatomy disrupted in a laryngectomy affects both oral and pharyngeal muscles and tissues and so can lead to issues with chewing, swallowing, and health risks. Physiological changes in the swallow in this patient population were systematically reviewed by Wall, Ward, Cartmill, and Hill (2013). The SLP clearly needs to screen for dysphagia and potential aspiration. Do an oral motor examination and trial feedings, and ask the patient about any known eating and swallowing concerns. Be familiar with the medical documentation, which may also point to issues of dysphagia. With this population of patients, detailed swallowing assessments will often be necessary (see Chapter 10).

Mr. Wayne Johnson, a 61-year-old white male, was admitted with a 6-month history of hoarseness. Examination by otolaryngologist revealed a hard mass in the neck at the angle of the jaw (at the area of the middle one-third of the left anterior lymphatic chain), and dysplasia involving the left aryepiglottic fold, false fold, and true fold. Biopsy confirmed locations with the finding of squamous cell carcinoma. A left radical neck dissection and total laryngectomy were performed.

Background information, contained in the report from social services, included mention that Mr. Johnson was a salesman and lived in an affluent resort community on a lake and golf course. He and his wife golfed several times a week and enjoyed all water sports, including skiing.

The speech pathologist, after reading the medical chart, began to wonder about the quality of life for Mr. Johnson following laryngectomy. Communication and meeting the public are necessary parts of his job as a salesman. Will he return to work? Will he experience a loss of earnings from lost commissions? (The public might not buy from an unusual-sounding person.) Will the company "urge" him to take early retirement? Could the company shift his duties from sales force to office work? To be sure, questions such as these were not only going through the mind of the speech pathologist but also that of the patient and his wife. The clinician felt that an impending return to work would be a strong motivator for Mr. Johnson to speak. The clinician also had thoughts concerning his avocations and knew future counseling would have to deal with these issues. Mr. Johnson almost certainly would play golf again, but with a reduction in general strength, head-neck rotation abilities, and a less effective golf swing because of the radical neck dissection. The lake lifestyle posed particular dangers. Stoma breathers generally are advised to stay clear of water. Skiing is out for Mr. Johnson, as is swimming; riding in a motor boat carries a certain risk (accidents do happen). Will Mr. Johnson adjust to these restrictions? He could wade in the water and even try to snorkel with a special breathing device for laryngectomees, but clearly his lifestyle is in for a drastic change. Of prime importance, however, is the containment of cancer, his survival, and a return of the ability to communicate.

Determining the Direction for Speech

Today, patients who undergo total laryngectomy often—but not always—have a primary **tracheoesophageal fistula** created for speech. This also is known as a **tracheoesophageal puncture (TEP).** The surgeon may not deem fistulazation appropriate for the patient; this is not the only option for speaking. A detailed discussion of all alaryngeal speech options and their continuing dynamic assessments is beyond the scope of this text. Rather, some general evaluative thoughts on **artificial larynx speech** training and traditional **esophageal speech** acquisition will be presented. Clinical issues in the more common **tracheoesophageal speech (TES)** method via fistulazation/puncture will be discussed. Table 13–3 provides a summary of these approaches. Also, a 3-minute video clip that demonstrates electrolarynx speech, traditional esophageal speech, and tracheoesophageal speech can be viewed on social media; it includes a brief description of the methods as part of a training video for emergency medical services personnel (go to www.youtube.com/watch?v=Qdbg_DZqe3g).

TABLE 13–3
Overview of Three Forms of Alaryngeal Speech Rehabilitation

Esophageal Speech
- Vibratory sound source is tissue in the upper esophageal segment (UES) and/or where the trachea joins the esophagus (this is known as the pharyngo-esophageal or PE segment).
- Exhaled lung air cannot be delivered to this area; a different source of air must insufflate the segment.
- Techniques for generating this air include injection and inhalation.
- Injection uses articulators to increase air pressure and force a ball of air through the muscle sphincter at the top of the PE segment.
- Inhalation involves decreasing air pressure in a rapidly expanding thorax (below that of room air pressure) so that air insufflates the esophagus.
- Control of the egress of air is crucial for articulation intelligibility.
- Length of utterance (number of syllables) per air charge is limited
- Speech frequency is low and quality is rough in traditional esophageal speech.
- Main advantage: does not require purchase or maintenance of special equipment.
- Main disadvantage: difficult and slow to learn.

Artificial Larynx Speech
- Vibratory sound source is an external mechanism: either electronic (battery powered) or pneumatic (oral air to a rubber membrane).
- Placement of electrolarynx often on neck, chin, or cheek but intraoral tubing available to deliver sound into mouth, as is done in pneumatic type.
- Relies on resonance in the vocal tract and articulation of sound.
- Device usually held by nondominant hands.
- Speech quality often mechanical with strong volume.
- Electrolarynx speech phrasing can be continuous; training on pausing promotes intelligibility.
- Main advantage: easy to learn and provides immediate speech.
- Main disadvantages: requires use of one hand, is visually conspicuous, cost to purchase and to maintain (recharge battery).

Tracheoesophageal (TE) Speech (also abbreviated TES)
- Surgeon creates a puncture (fistula) in the wall separating the trachea and the esophagus. A one-way valve (prosthesis) is placed into the puncture site to allow exhaled lung air to pass into the esophagus. This air vibrates the PE segment for sound production.
- The one-way valve allows lung air to pass into the esophageal segment without food and liquids leaking into the trachea.
- Occlusion of one-way valve prosthesis with thumb or finger makes speech possible; often a prosthetic speaking valve is coupled to allow hands-free speech.
- Use of lung air affords speech that is near-normal in breath support and phrasing.
- Vibration of PE segment results in lower vocal frequency and rougher quality than in laryngeal speech.
- Main advantages: lung air is used for speech and, apart from healing time, speech is instantaneous or easy to acquire.
- Main disadvantages: additional surgical step is necessary for the puncture, some patients are not good candidates for TE speech, routine maintenance of all purchased devices is necessary, and the danger of aspiration exists if liquids leak through a malfunctioning valve.

Our evaluation process and our speech rehabilitation process are truly intertwined when working with an alaryngeal patient. What we find in the patient's background, current status, and screenings leads us to attempts with trial therapy, whether with an artificial larynx, speech via a surgically created tracheoesophageal fistula, or rudimentary attempts at esophageal speech (to be honed with practice). Does the patient follow directions and seem motivated to learn? How is the patient doing with this method? What modifications may be needed? Is it the right method for now (or to pursue later)? The clinician's insights, judgments, and competencies with trial therapy techniques are crucial because this evaluation session is also truly the initial treatment session.

Once the patient is talking (which can be a jump ahead in time), we maintain that it is important, subjectively and objectively, to appraise the quality of the patient's speech and aim for refinements. This is consistent with our philosophy of continuing assessments. Our patients deserve the best speech of which they are capable; SLPs need yardsticks with which to measure their progress and coach them further.

ASSESSING ARTIFICIAL LARYNX SPEECH

While a discussion of alaryngeal speech treatment options is beyond the scope of this text, an ongoing assessment process is or should be part of any alaryngeal speech rehabilitative method. The use of an artificial larynx, whether a pneumatic device (lung air collected at the stoma to vibrate the device's reed or membrane for sound) or a battery-powered model (electronic excitation of tissue, bone, and cavity air to generate sound), was more popular in the past. Still, the artificial larynx has its place in the clinician's toolkit. We posit that the SLP assesses and trains a patient for using an artificial larynx on three main occasions:

1. After the surgery, when the area is swollen and sore and/or the patient is not yet physically ready for the demands of other speech methods.
2. Ongoing use as the speaking method preferred by the patient.
3. As a backup to another primary speech method, such as during evenings and weekends when a person wishes to rest from another method (e.g., patient with a tracheoesophageal valve does not install the necessary adhesives and prostheses). An artificial device produces speech that is louder than other methods and so may be opted for in some situations.

Regardless of the circumstances, the user of an artificial larynx needs to be trained for optimal speech intelligibility and performance. The method generally is easy to learn and has the advantage (for some environments) of speech that is loud. Some users become "good" with this type of speech; others are not so proficient. A variety of speaking samples is available on social media, and the novice clinician is encouraged to watch a variety of speakers. One 5-minute example of an intelligible, conversational speaker can be viewed at www.youtube.com/watch?v=mnAq-M6Ldtw. In working with patients, the SLP must do ongoing assessments to know when tweaking of speech retraining is needed.

Early Artificial Larynx Attempts

We limit our discussion here to the electrolarynx. Brand models differ in price, size, pitch and adjustability, sound quality, and type of battery. The SLP provides an initial introduction to speaking with an artificial larynx and focuses on optimal placement of the device for the client's circumstances and best sound. Placement affects intelligibility, as does the patient's quality of articulatory movements to shape the sound. Advanced training refinements entail continuously reassessing patient maneuvers with the device switch; timing and pausing is crucial.

Given this overview, we initially proceed as follows, always monitoring (assessing) patient performance. Help the patient seek out the best placement for the device. How quickly will the patient learn to return the device's vibrating head precisely to that spot: in five trials or 50? Are other feedback cues necessary to learn this skill? If so, hints such as tactile stroking of the spot by the clinician before each attempt at placement may prove beneficial. Also, marking an X on the skin with a washable marker and having the patient practice placement drills in front of a mirror may be just what is needed. Explain and demonstrate the noisy effects of poor contact of the vibrating head with the skin. How efficiently will the patient absorb this knowledge and learn to place the device consistently in the correct spot with *firm* contact? Advise the patient to exaggerate articulation movements, especially in opening the mouth and moving the tongue. Will the patient quickly adjust to such pantomiming actions or persist in trying to "breathe for speech," only to have a noisy exhalation out the stoma? Explain and demonstrate the on-off mechanism and the precise timing needed to coordinate phrasing. How agile or clumsy will the patient be in manipulating the switch concurrent with phrases? Slow learners make one or more of the following mistakes: having the device on continuously and not stopping at grammatical junctures, turning the device on and off excessively and creating choppy speech, or turning the device on or off in a poorly timed fashion at the beginning and end of utterances. The result is that sounds or syllables are chopped off or buzzing noises occur when speech is not being mouthed. The point here is that during the early training in the use of an artificial electrolarynx device, the clinician should constantly evaluate the learning skills of the patient and adjust his or her treatment monitoring. Some patients can speed quickly through an SLP's early teachings, while others progress with painful slowness.

Further Assessing Artificial Larynx Speech

By setting goals and continuously monitoring progress, the SLP can help the electrolarynx user progress toward good-quality artificial laryngeal speech. Characteristic features of proficient electrolarynx speech, drawn from research spanning the 20th century (when this was a popular topic) include the following six themes: frequency range, speech rate, intensity variations, extraneous noise, inappropriate pauses, and consonantal differentiation. We will discuss each one in the following subsections.

Frequency Range

Proficient users of neck-type devices acquire a variety of techniques to alter the frequency output, such as "riding" the device on the neck using different pressures. They exhibit a frequency range, or pitch variability, between 13 and 20 Hz, with an average fluctuation of 16 Hz. In contrast, poorer speakers range from 6 to 15 Hz, with a mean of 11 Hz.

Speech Rate

Speech rate is perhaps the main feature that differentiates very good users of artificial larynges from poorer ones. Proficient users speak faster and appear more fluent. The mean rate of speech with an electrolarynx is around 125 words per minute.

Intensity Variations

Intensity variations contribute to perceptual stress or emphasis. Greater intensity variations characterize better electrolarynx speakers compared to more monoloud device users.

Extraneous Noise

Limiting extraneous noise from the device is a hallmark of a proficient user. Novice and poor device users frequently fail to achieve firm coupling of the vibrating device head and the target tissue area (often the neck), and leakage or buzzing occurs as a result. Proficient users have mastered firm and consistent coupling and do not leak extraneous noises.

Inappropriate Pauses

Instances when the electronic device is shut down during utterances occur more frequently with poorer users. Proficient speakers are better with their coordination of timing the on button with articulation and phrasing.

Consonantal Differentiation

Proficient device users employ buccal (cheek) air and precise timing of device activation to produce stops, fricatives, and affricates more effectively. Voiced–voiceless distinctions are also achieved perceptually by careful manipulation of buccal air and/or by varying the coupling pressure of the device with the tissue site (e.g., neck). Novice and poorer users have yet to master the nuances of consonant production with the electrolarynx.

ASSESSING ESOPHAGEAL SPEECH

Traditional esophageal speech, once a hallmark of an excellent, practiced alaryngeal communicator, has declined in popularity since the introduction of the easier-to-learn tracheoesophageal speech method in the late 1970s. Still, there are surgical circumstances (e.g., radiated PE segment likely to form undesired fistulas rather than the planned TEP) when acquiring traditional esophageal speech will be necessary, and some patients will want or need it. There are several methods for injecting a ball of air into the top of the esophagus (because, after laryngectomy, the person breathes through the stoma and there is no anatomical connection with the lungs to use pulmonary air for speech). This ball of air, on expulsion, vibrates the top area of the esophagus (recall the PES or UES) to produce sound. The PES (UES) functions in this manner as a pseudo-glottis. This esophageal-produced sound is then shaped into speech by the articulators. Learning traditional esophageal speech has challenged many persons over the years; it requires stamina, patience, and much practice to acquire. Some persons acquire excellent esophageal speech (though the reservoir of PES air is small and speech attributes are different), while others fail to acquire usable speech. Barometers of proficiency suggest treatment goals and continuing assessment for the SLP.

Audio and video clips of esophageal speakers, both good and not so good, are available on social media. A well-known champion of esophageal speech has been Edmund Lauder. His book *Self-Help for the Laryngectomee* (Lauder, 1978; see Table 13–1 for PDF download) has provided insight into learning esophageal speech and has self-help tips. A 32-minute audio on esophageal speech by Lauder demonstrating both proficient esophageal speech and how to start learning it is available on YouTube at www.youtube.com/watch?v=rtRetlucFeA.

Early Esophageal Speech Attempts

Regardless of the technique(s) being taught (injection, "inhalation," consonant injection, and so forth), the essence of learning esophageal speech involves getting air in and sound out, and this is no easy feat because pulmonary (lung) air is not available. As baseline data, the clinician can rate the patient's esophageal production abilities. Some fortunate patients will be successful in "eructating" simple sounds or words in the first session, others may occasionally get out a "burp," and still others may be unable to get any sound out and need much practice in performing air intake maneuvers. The dated but still useful 7-point acquisition rating scale shown here provides baseline and improvement tracking (Wepman, MacGhan, Rickard, & Shelton, 1953):

1. Automatic esophageal speech
2. Esophageal sound produced at will with continuity: word grouping
3. Esophageal sound produced at will: single-word speech
4. Voluntary sound production most of the time: vowel sounds
5. Voluntary sound production part of the time: no speech
6. Involuntary esophageal sound production: no speech
7. No esophageal sound production: no speech

No doubt, the baseline data for most patients will be a score of 7 or 6. This same scale can be used periodically to reassess and document the progress of the patient in producing reliable esophageal sound and speech.

Of interest in these early sessions is the learning skill and potential displayed by the patient following adequate instruction and demonstration. Early eructation abilities suggest a favorable prognosis for acquiring esophageal speech.

Further Assessing Esophageal Speech

Once a patient has begun using esophageal speech, some measure of current performance level is necessary. A clinician with critical listening skills is an efficient means of ongoing assessment, especially when attention is focused on specific parameters. The parameters of traditional esophageal speech on which we assess—and which we hone with our patients— are pulled from decades of research and are summarized in the following subsections.

Pitch Level

It has been said that an average male esophageal speaker has a fundamental frequency of about 58 to 65 Hz; this is about half that of a typical laryngeal-speaking male. Female esophageal speakers average about 87 Hz. The PE segment is comprised of thicker tissue than the vocal folds and accounts for the low rate of vibration. No esophageal speaker ever seems satisfied with her or his new, lower-pitch speech. While research has shown that esophageal speakers with higher-pitch speech tend to be judged as more acceptable than those with lower-pitch speech, a patient's undue effort in attempts to raise his or her pitch often backfires, causing more strain, tension, and voice failure.

Inflection

Pitch variation is difficult to achieve with the neoglottis (PES). Rate of frequency modulation varies over a range of about 8 tones per second in proficient esophageal speakers (compared to typical laryngeal speakers, whose values are I 7 or 18 tones per second). Still, esophageal speakers who acquire a degree of inflection (pitch variability) are perceived as speaking better by listeners, and pitch variability is a more achievable goal than undue attention to fundamental frequency, which was mentioned earlier. Perceived pitch fluctuations may be achieved through control of loudness, rate, length of time spent on a word, and the use of pauses. For example, an esophageal speaker may use greater volume to raise the pitch but less intensity to lower the pitch.

Quality

Esophageal speech quality is different from the premorbid laryngeal speech quality. A certain amount of hoarseness or roughness is characteristics of the thicker vibrating PE segment. Strain and tension adversely affect the quality of the speech produced, however. The clinician should take note of the ease with which the patient can insufflate or charge air into the esophagus for enhanced quality.

Excess Noise

Esophageal speakers exhibit some noise unique to their new method of speaking, but excess and/or distracting noises should not occur in proficient speech. Early distracting noises should be diagnosed early, when it is easily eradicated and before bad habits become entrenched. Excess noise can be associated with air intake or it can occur at the level of the stoma. When a patient injects air too rapidly into the esophagus, a klunking sound can occur. Some patients exhibit multiple klunks when they attempt more than one inflation before phonation. Another distracting behavior is stoma noise, or stoma blast, which is caused by the patient forcing exhalations through the stoma at the time he or she is phonating esophageal speech. The patient has not adequately learned that breathing for breathing and breathing for speech are two separate functions. Sometimes the stoma noise masks the esophageal speech to the point of affecting intelligibility.

Visual Mannerisms

Other, nonvocal aspects of communication can be distracting to the listener. Facial grimaces, including eye squinting, and head movements often occur when a patient is trying to learn an air intake method such as injection. The clinician should assess these types of behaviors in patients and seek to eliminate them early in the treatment program before they become habituated.

Rate of Speech

Perceptual studies suggest that rate of speech is the most important aspect that differentiates superior from poor esophageal speech. Proficient esophageal speakers often display speech that is around 113 words per minute, with a "good" range of about 85 to 129. The SLP should probe and continuously assess the patient's progress in rate of speech development.

Words per Charge

Compared to typical laryngeal speakers, esophageal speakers recharge their speaking air about three times more often when reading a passage (see, for example, the passages in Appendix B). Superior esophageal speakers utilize their air charge for 1 to 1½ seconds, during which they average 2.8 to 6.3 words. A satisfactory number of syllables read on a single insufflation is around 11 to 12 syllables. During connected speech, a lower rate of 4 to 9 syllables is more typical.

Latency of Air Charge

Superior esophageal speakers take air in at a rate of 0.4 to 0.8 second; some are even quicker. A good rule of thumb for setting goals is a latency of 0.5 second. It is easier for patients to take air in quickly than it is to take in large amounts of air. Also, we should point out that 0.5 second to recharge approximates a typical speaker's grammatical pause time.

Latency of Phrasal Pauses

In proficient esophageal speakers, phrase-limiting pauses are made longer than the pauses for air charging—approximately 1.4 times longer. Both typical laryngeal speakers and superior esophageal speakers pause for phrases, but the superior esophageal speaker pauses longer so that such pauses contrast with air charge pauses. In other words, practiced esophageal speakers have learned to use silent times differentially; this aids the listener in linguistic comprehension. For example, a patient who charges air in 0.5 second may use a phrase-limiting pause of 0.7 second.

Articulatory Intelligibility

Removal of the larynx and hyoid bone disrupts the muscular connections of the tongue, and so articulatory mobility may be affected. Most patients, however, compensate quite well. The surgery also shortens the effective length of the vocal tract, altering formant frequencies that perhaps affect vowel intelligibility. Lacking vocal folds (glottis) after surgery, the region that now can be set into vibration as a substitute glottic (neoglottis) is the pharyngoesophageal segment (PES). The PES, however, is not equipped for abductor-adductor coordination, and so the voiced–voiceless cognate phonemes, along with the impossible glottal fricative /h/, are often a perceptual problem for the listener. Clearly, then, articulation, differentiation, and speech intelligibility can be concerns, and they warrant special practice, drills, and compensations for the client to be perceived as an accomplished esophageal speaker.

EARLY SPEECH ATTEMPTS WITH A TRACHEOESOPHAGEAL PROSTHESIS

The evaluation may proceed differently with patients planning to have a tracheoesophageal fistula created surgically; this procedure is also called a tracheoesophageal puncture. In this procedure, the surgeon places a hole (puncture or fistula) in the membranous wall between the trachea and the esophagus, thus providing a connection between these two structures. This puncture hole, in turn, can serve as a route through which exhaled lung air (when the stoma is momentarily blocked) can travel into the esophagus (PES). Unfortunately, this route can also serve as a passage through which saliva, food, and drink can penetrate dangerously into the esophagus. A prosthesis placed in this opening allows for pulmonary air to flow into the top of the esophagus under certain conditions so that vibrated sound can be produced. Breathing is still done through the stoma (and through an open prosthesis). Aspiration of saliva, liquids, and foods is minimized by the one-way directionality of the prosthetic device. The conditions that allow for diverting exhaled air into the esophagus, rather than out the stoma, are digital occlusion of the prosthesis opening, located in the stoma, or the use of a valving device to reroute the air stream when desired.

With muscular effort, air diverted into the esophagus will be compressed and forced through the top of the closed esophagus, thereby setting the pharyngoesophageal segment (PES) into vibration. This segment is the sound source or neoglottis; articulation of the sound is accomplished in the usual manner in the upper vocal tract. In essence, tracheoesophageal puncture speech (TEP speech; also referred to as tracheoesophageal speech [TES]) is esophageal in nature yet supported by the pulmonary system. Tracheoesophageal speech obviates the need to learn traditional esophageal speech and is easily acquired. Furthermore, the use of lung air provides acoustic and perceptual advantages over traditional esophageal speech.

Bosone (1999) reports that many surgeons prefer to do a total laryngectomy, pharyngeal constrictor myotomy, and TE puncture at the same time, while the patient is hospitalized. Others prefer that the patient convalesce before puncture.

Screening for candidacy, fitting of the device, and instruction in the care and use of the device are often done solely by the speech pathologist, sometimes in concert with the nurse and doctor. Fluent conversational speech typically is acquired rapidly. The SLP, then, has a brief but vital role to play in the rehabilitation of tracheoesophageal puncture patients.

The success of any method depends in part on the proper selection of candidates for that method. Patient selection criteria and contraindications for tracheoesophageal puncture were established early by Singer and Blom (1980), Fagan and Isaacs (2002), and Elmiyeh et al. (2010):

1. Motivation to undergo the procedure and sustained motivation to care for the prosthesis on a daily basis.

2. Absence of physical limitations and cognitive/mental ability needed for daily care of the adhesives, fittings, and prostheses. In particular, the patient should have adequate vision and eye–hand coordination to place the prosthetic device while in front of a mirror. Manual dexterity (e.g., absence of arthritis) is necessary for the handling of the prosthesis and all associated materials (particularly if additional tracheostoma valves will be used).

3. Good general health. Weak, feeble persons do not do well with TE puncture devices; however, conditions such as chronic pulmonary disease, diabetes, and alcoholism do not necessarily rule out candidacy.

4. Concern for hygiene in cleansing of the device, in neck tissue care (adhesives used with the valve can be irritating to sensitive skin), and in touching/handling all materials.

5. Adequate stoma characteristics. In particular, the stoma must not be retracted behind the manubrium. The size of the opening should be a minimum of 1 cm across the axis, but for some procedures 2 cm are needed. An excessively large stoma can be corrected somewhat by tape.

6. Recovery from postsurgical radiation treatment, if any. Also, overly radiated tissue is more likely to break down, forming fistulas.

7. Absence of chronic tracheitis or ulceration.

8. Absence of a history of unplanned fistulas, pharyngoesophageal stricture (spasm), or flap reconstruction. The presence of any of these conditions, however, does not necessarily rule out TE puncture candidacy but suggests the need for a more detailed assessment. A barium esophagram may yield findings to suggest whether dilation may be necessary to maintain an adequate opening for air flow and voice.

We need to explain here that a common reason for failure with tracheoesophageal speech is spasms of the pharyngoesophageal segment. Spasms make the vibration and production of sound difficult, if not impossible. The spasms usually can be relaxed by surgically cutting some of the muscle fibers in the neoglottis. The need for this surgical procedure, called a myotomy, can be predicted with a simple screening test. The SLP, surgeon, or both perform an air insufflation procedure, where air is introduced into the esophagus and the patient is asked to phonate. Good phonation, of course, indicates that the patient's pharyngoesophageal segment is capable of vibration, and therefore a myotomy would not be needed. Such a patient is considered an excellent candidate for TE puncture and speech. As mentioned previously, some surgeons do a myotomy on all patients at the time of primary surgery, whether necessary or not. There is some evidence that this results in poorer speech in some patients (Bosone, 1999). An alternative to surgical relaxation of the pharyngeal constrictor muscles is the injection of Botox. It is always best to identify patients early who will benefit from middle and inferior constrictor myotomy. Henley and Souliere (2009) give a preoperative injection of Xylocaine to produce a partial blockage for speech to confirm that myotomy will benefit the patient. Getting a patient started in the use of tracheoesophageal speech is a complex issue. We will attempt to subdivide the tasks and provide an overview of each.

Prosthesis Fitting

The speech pathologist is often responsible for fitting the patient with a properly sized prosthesis. Brands differ in size, features, and design to optimize individual patient fit. We discuss the topic in generic terms in this text; however, the medical practice where the SLP works may be partial to using one brand over another. Here we will present only generic principles.

Following typical TE puncture surgery, a catheter is left in place for 24 to 72 hours to prevent closure of the puncture site. After that, a voice prosthesis of an appropriate size can be fitted by the SLP. Voice becomes possible; speech produced with a tracheoesophageal prosethesis often is referred to as TEP speech. The speech pathologist should recheck the patient in 4 to 5 weeks and refit the prosthesis, if necessary. Occasionally, after the edema subsides, a shorter prosthesis is more appropriate.

The process of fitting and inserting the prosthesis may vary with the brand used, but it is basically as follows. Instruct the patient not to swallow while removing the catheter that has been in place since the puncture surgery. Insert a depth gauge or the fistula measurement probe (either one comes with the brand's installation kit) through the stoma and into the puncture site; feel it pop into place. Pull out slightly until the retention collar is firmly against the puncture opening and read the distance on the imprinted probe. This indicates the length of prosthesis needed for the patient. Once the size of the prosthesis has been determined, insert it and apply double-faced tape on the flanges, if necessary (depending on the design). Once the prosthesis is in place, have the patient drink some water to make sure there is no leakage around or through the prosthesis. Demonstrate digital occlusion for the patient, and instruct him or her to try to talk on exhalation while the stoma/prosthesis opening is occluded with the clinician's thumb or finger. An animated insertion training video supplied by a particular brand can be viewed on social media. This straightforward, smooth insertion procedure (less than 2 minutes) is available at www.youtube.com/watch?v=5hH1YtB7ed0. Next, the reader is urged to view the following clip of an SLP inserting a new prosthesis into a patient: www.youtube.com/watch?v=TxS1TogpUIM.

If voice is not produced with an inserted prosthesis, assess the reason(s) why (see next section). If successful, continue talking and practice with the patient. Note also that in-dwelling prostheses, those placed by the physician or SLP and remain in place for about 6 months, are becoming popular. These eliminate some of the need for screening candidates with regard to manual dexterity, personal hygiene, and especially the need to insert the device and secure it in place daily.

Voice Failure Assessment

An example of a patient speaking with a prosthesis is available on social media at www.youtube.com/watch?v=K9sN10MU9RU. If the patient is unable to produce voice, however, the speech pathologist should try to assess whether the problem lies with the prosthetic device or with the patient. Common problems of voice failure stemming from patient factors include the following:

1. The patient may be using excessive digital occlusion (finger pressure) against the stoma.
2. The patient may be using inadequate expiratory air pressure. A weak, feeble patient is a poor candidate for TEP speech because of the energy necessary to overcome the air resistance of the plastic devices. Alternately, perhaps the patient simply needs to be instructed to use more effort and more air in speech attempts. Other devices (styles and brands) may be tried as well; each model differs in its air flow resistance. An ultralow-resistance model may work for the patient.
3. Salivary secretions may have accumulated and are thus blocking the pharynx. In this case, the speech will sound gurgly. Expectoration should solve the problem.
4. A most likely reason for the absence of voice is the presence of pharyngoesophageal spasm. Perhaps the air insufflation pretest was not done prior to TEP. At any rate, do the insufflation test to see if voice is possible with the prosthesis removed. A myotomy or Botox relaxing may be necessary to counteract the spasms.

Voice failure may be due to problems with the prosthetic device. These problems are often easily identified and rectified. In these cases, the patient would have voice without the prosthesis (with stoma digital occlusion or with the air insufflation test), but no voice with a faulty prosthesis in place. In particular, note the following:

1. The patient may be unable to produce voice because the prosthesis is inserted upside down. Remove and reinsert the prosthesis.
2. The valve slit may be stuck together on devices with a slit (duckbill) design.
3. Incorrect prosthesis length could be the reason for lack of voice. A device that is too long, particularly a device with a slit design that would be so impeded, may be touching the posterior wall of the esophagus. Refitting the patient with a shorter device and/or changing to a different design (nonslit, flap-door) is in order. A prosthesis that is too short would not have the tip residing in the lumen of the esophageal tube. A slit-design tip would be impeded from passing its air into the esophagus. Try rotating the placement a bit. A longer prosthesis may be necessary.
4. Occlusion of the port may block air flow and hence voice. Clearing of saliva (or other matter) is in order.

If the patient has used TEP speech for a period of time and begins to experience a change in the voice, or loss of it, troubleshooting to find and eliminate the cause is necessary. We recommend the works of Bosone (1999), Bunting (2004), and the review of Elmiyeh et al. (2010) for troubleshooting ideas. Telemedicine also is finding a place in the troubleshooting and assessment of speech, swallowing or leakage, and overall concerns in postlaryngectomy patients via cameras and remote technology (Ward et al., 2009).

Tracheostoma Valve

Talking with the voice prosthesis alone requires digital occlusion of the stoma (with finger or thumb). This is an unnecessary inconvenience; after some experience with the prosthesis (minutes or weeks, depending on the patient's progress), the patient may be a candidate for using a tracheostoma valve for hands-free operation (various styles and brands exist). The typical patient is trained with a valve at the same time the prosthesis is introduced. The valve is fitted into the stoma opening and held in place by some type of housing. Naturally, the patient still wears the voice prosthesis. Valve selection, fitting, and training are tasks within the purview of the SLP.

Some valves are termed heat and moisture exchangers (HMEs) because their design aids the laryngectomized person in regulating the air temperature and moisture content of the breathed (into the stoma) air. Typically people breathe through the nose (or mouth), where air is filtered and warmed or cooled to body temperature, and the mucous membranes add moisture so there is 100% humidity going into the lungs. Persons who breathe through the neck have no natural conditioners of the incoming air. The HME styles aid with this process; the hands-free HME model is a popular choice of tracheostoma valve. Zurr, Muller, de Jongh van Zandwijk, and Hilger (2006) provide a rationale and review for further study. An SLP adjusting an HME device may be viewed online; an 8-minute demonstration can be found at www.youtube .com/watch?v=PguhHUjBoW0.

Tracheostoma Valve Contraindications

The valve fits into a flexible circular housing that is attached to the skin area surrounding the stoma with nonirritating adhesive. When positioned over the stoma, the valve diaphragm remains in a fully open position during quiet breathing and routine physical activity. For speech, a slight increase in exhalation causes the valve diaphragm to close and divert air into the esophagus. The valve automatically reopens when exhalation decreases at the completion of an utterance. A tracheostoma valve must be maintained by the patient on a daily basis, and it is not worn during sleep. The valve is easily disassembled for cleaning, and the diaphragm can be replaced by the patient as needed.

Some contraindications to using a valve include the following: (1) Patients with high phonatory pressure may blow the seal often, (2) a very recessed or irregular stoma may not accommodate the valve, (3) patients with excessive tracheal discharge may occlude or dangerously hinder the operation of the valve, and (4) inadequate pharyngoesophageal segments preclude usable speech.

Valve Fitting

Select the diaphragm thickness that does not inadvertently close on the patient during routine physical exertion or heavier-than-usual exhalation. Conversely, do not select a diaphragm that is so thick that it requires excessive exhalation for the generation of voice. The patient can often detect quickly that a certain valve offers too much resistance and makes speaking too effortful. In this situation, try another, lighter-weight valve. Some SLPs assess the patient's valve with a stair-step test. Have the patient try a diaphragm's sensitivity while going up and down some stairs. The SLP and the patient should carefully watch for valve closure as breathing deepens during this exertion. If the valve closes, remove it and try the next-thicker size. Repeat the stair-step test until the proper diaphragm size has been determined. Some patients may wish to purchase two diaphragms: one for general use and a thicker one for use while dancing, exercising, and the like.

Patients should be instructed not to sleep with the tracheostoma valve in place. In addition, patients may find it helpful to remove the valve from its housing when they feel an urge to cough or forcefully exhale. This prevents blowing the seal and the necessity of cleaning and reapplying the adhesive. Some models contain a spring-action valve with a cough-relief valve.

ONGOING TEP SPEECH ASSESSMENTS AND REFINEMENTS

The acquisition of TEP speech is often instantaneous for patients, yet practice and attention to improvement are needed. Often with a couple of treatment sessions and with self-practice, speech can go from "present" to "good." Goals and ongoing assessments may focus on the proficiency attributes shown in Table 13–4. These skills and attributes are culled from the literature (Carpenter, 1999; Lewis, 1999; Siric, Sos, Rosso, & Stevanovic, 2012).

PROGNOSTIC INDICATORS FOR SUCCESS

After the initial evaluation sessions, the SLP should have obtained pertinent case history data, provided information to the patient and the family, and assessed function. After this work, he or she has a good idea about the patient's current communication needs and potential for acquiring speech through some means (artificial larynx, esophageal speech, TEP speech). In considering the person for TEP speech, we offer the following list of prognostic indicators for success:

1. The patient should have competent anatomical structures for the method or methods of speech chosen. For TEP speech consideration, the puncture site and the pharyngoesophageal segment must be adequate. Any tendency for esophageal spasms (as pretested) must be addressed. Close communication between the SLP and physician is important for success.

2. The severity, extent, and type of surgery seem not to be related to the acquisition of speech. Yet this assessment may be highly individualistic.

TABLE 13–4
Skills and Attributes of Proficient TEP Speech

Maximum Phonation Time: As an indicator of respiratory support, patients should be able to extend the duration of a vowel for 9 to 17 seconds.

Fundamental Frequency: Approximate the speaking frequency of laryngeal speakers of similar age and gender; special attention may be needed for the female laryngectomee. Can telephone listeners distinguish the speaker's gender?

Intonation/Pitch Variance: The patient should practice to achieve changes via air pressure differences below the neoglottic; she or he should practice at the word/sentence level and by humming/singing songs.

Overall Intensity/Speech Loudness: Adequate for communication; ability to increase when needed via changes in subneoglottic air pressure and flow rates. (*Caution:* Increased loudness may lead to extraneous noises and poor speech quality.)

Stress/Loudness Variability: Clarity of lexical stress (OBject versus obJECT) and of contrastive stress (BEV loves Bob versus Bev loves BOB).

Articulatory Precision: Proficiency with voiced–voiceless contrasts; intelligibility of problematic phonemes such as plosives, fricatives, and affricates especially when they are in the initial position (practice differentiating, e.g., "jip-chip-ship").

Speech Rate: Correlated with speech naturalness; measured either as syllable rate or as word rate; measured during both speaking (goal of 120 wpm) and reading (goal of 166 wpm); set rates to approximate laryngeal values as close as possible.

Fluency: Degree of momentary periods of aphonia, with a goal of zero; aphonic blocks often due to unwanted oral injection of air or by swallowing just prior to TEP speech attempt; disfluency can also be due to pharyngeal constrictor spasm.

Extraneous Behaviors: Prevention or minimalization of features such as stoma noise, air leakage, valve thumping, neck tension or unusual posturing, observable mucus, oral/stoma odors, and so forth.

3. Patients should be of good general health. Feeble patients generally do not do well in learning TEP speech, which requires energy to persist in the rehabilitation process.

4. While TE puncture can be done at any time, the date of the surgery relative to the enrollment in the speech rehabilitation program is important. The prognosis for proficient speech after waiting is affected by other habits that have developed and are difficult to break.

5. Patients with a positive attitude and motivation to practice often throughout the day tend to be successful.

6. Those planning to return to work seem to have an extra ounce of motivation to master speech and to do so more quickly than those staying home or in an institution.

7. Patients who have family support at home, willing communication partners, and people willing to participate in the rehabilitation program and to help with daily practice generally do quite well.

8. Patients who are literate and willing to read and study materials about laryngectomy rehabilitation seem to make good progress. They make good use of workbooks, stimuli lists, and the like, in daily practice.

The functional outcome and quality of life are issues central to healthcare. The numerous measures of quality of life for head and neck cancer patients often inadequately assess communication-related issues. The activities of voice and speech, eating, and swallowing figure prominently in a person's self-perception and willingness to engage in life. Some quality-of-life scales designed for use with other voice disorders have been applied to persons with total laryngectomy and who have acquired a method of speaking.

Eadie et al. (2013) explored the auditory perceptual speech outcomes of alaryngeal speakers with their quality-of-life measures. It is interesting and cautionary to note that persons rated with better and more acceptable speech were not necessarily those with higher quality-of-life ratings. In contrast is the opposite finding from Carpenter (1999), who observed that effectiveness measures and overall satisfaction of alaryngeal speakers were related. In this investigation the speakers rated whether they talk as "much" or as "well" as they "need" to and "want" to. The University of Washington Quality of Life (UM-QOL) scale has been used following total laryngectomy (Kazi et al., 2007). The European Organization for Research and Treatment of Cancer Quality of Life Questionnaire-C30 (EORTC QLQ-C30) has been used in following up head and neck cancer patients and with those who had been laryngectomized (Boscolo-Rizzo et al., 2008; Hanna et al., 2004; Relic et al., 2001).

Bornbaum, Day, and Doyle (2014) examined the construct validity of using the Voice-Related Quality of Life (V-RQOL; described in Chapter 11) with alaryngeal speakers. Results of this brief 10-question instrument were subjected to a factor analysis. Problems were revealed with two questions in which the intended domains ("physical") seemed the reverse of patient response reasons ("social-emotional" domain). The researchers proposed a scoring adjustment, thereby making the V-RQOL a quality-of-life tool for this clinical population.

CONCLUSION AND SELF-ASSESSMENT

In certain work settings, speech-language pathologists play an important and rewarding role in assessing and managing persons treated for head and neck cancer. While cancers in the laryngeal area may be treated medically through surgery, radiation, chemotherapy, or some combination, patients who have undergone total laryngectomy need the SLP's best efforts in speech and voice, swallowing, and counseling services.

In this chapter we have shown the multitude of complex issues involved in assessing, counseling, prognosing, rehabilitating, and reassessing laryngectomized persons. We have also discussed aspects of care and the ongoing assessments necessary to help a laryngectimized person achieve his or her best speech possible.

After reading this chapter you should be able to answer the following questions:

1. What anatomical changes typically occur in a total laryngectomy?
2. Where is the stoma and what is its function?
3. What is the vibrating source of sound in the following three speech methods: electrolarynx, traditional esophageal speech, and TEP speech?
4. Why can pulmonary (lung) air be used in TEP speech but not in traditional esophageal speech? What implications does this have for the speech produced in these two speech methods?
5. Name at least three acoustic-perceptual features of "proficient" speech for each of the following methods (each feature might also be a treatment goal): electrolarynx speech, traditional esophageal speech, and TEP speech.

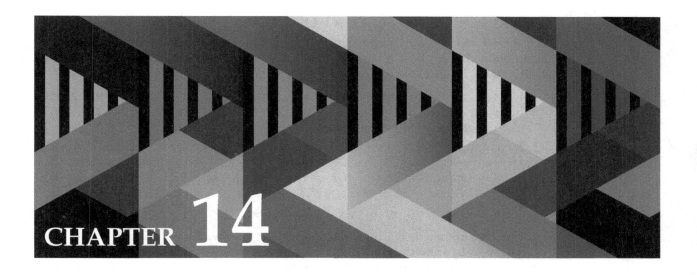

CHAPTER 14

The Diagnostic Report and Financial Essentials

LEARNING OUTCOMES

After reading this chapter you will be able to:

1. Describe some necessary components of a typical diagnostic report.
2. Defend the importance of clinical impressions in a diagnostic report.
3. Explain each component of a daily SOAP note when it is used to report a brief initial screening.
4. Explain what the FERPA and HIPAA public laws have to do with clinical reports.
5. Explain why the speech-language pathologist must know relevant medical codes.

Two very important phases of the diagnostic process remain. The speech-language pathologist (SLP) needs to prepare the professional diagnostic report, and, in this age of third-party full or partial payment, the document must contain the proper medical code. Shortly after the patient's assessment appointment, the SLP should put the clinical situation, the interview, testing methods, results, and impressions in writing as soon as possible. Never trust memory. Commit the details to paper or "electronic paper" in the protected software of the work facility while the facial characteristics and voice inflections can still be remembered. Make the report "alive" so that others can experience what occurred just by reading about it. The raw data are of limited value to the clinician or other readers (medical professionals, educators, agency employees, parents) until those data are assembled in a clear, precise, and orderly fashion. There is both an art and a technical skill to clinical report writing. Financial essentials, such as required data and the proper medical code, are necessary components to facilitate billing and reimbursement; the SLP needs to understand and include this information in the report.

THE REPORT AND FORMAT OPTIONS

A *diagnostic report* is a written record that summarizes the relevant information a clinician obtained—and how he or she obtained it—in his or her professional interaction with a client. It serves the following functions:

1. It acts as a guide for additional services to the client. It provides a clear statement of how the person was functioning at a given point in time so that the clinician can document change or lack of change.

2. It communicates the clinician's findings to other involved professionals. It provides answers to a number of clinical questions, including the following: Does the person have a communication (or cognitive or swallowing) disorder? Will treatment be helpful? Will referrals be necessary?

3. It serves as a document for research purposes.

The importance of the first function should be obvious: Intelligent clinical plans evolve naturally from carefully prepared reports. The second purpose of diagnostic reports is to answer questions about clients so that other professionals can plan and provide appropriate services. In addition to transmitting necessary information, a carefully prepared examination report also helps to establish the credibility of the SLP in the eyes of other professional readers. To state it another way, a written document is an extension of the diagnostician, and even minor errors in spelling or grammar may cast doubt on the accuracy and attention to detail with respect to substantive material. Although the clinician may be highly skilled in testing and interviewing, competence may be evaluated by the clinician's written communications. Clinical reports (whether electronic or on paper) are the principal way in which a clinician relates to other professionals.

There are several ways to organize a diagnostic report, and entire books are devoted to clinical documentation (Burrus & Willis, 2013; Goldfarb & Serpenos, 2013; Pannbacker, Middleton, Vekovius, & Sanders, 2001). Because reports may vary depending on the intended audience, no single schema is appropriate for all circumstances. In many instances, the format will be dictated by the agency the clinician serves. There appear to be three broad categories of report formats as a function of work setting:

- *University training programs and traditional clinics.* Student clinicians learn to write comprehensive reports that are robust in detail. These reports tend to be lengthy. They also typically contain numerous subheadings with a summary conclusion (and diagnosis) at the end of the report once all findings have been presented. This format also remains in wide use in most for-profit clinical settings because of its thoroughness of information, even when sections are written with brevity.

- *Medical setting.* Clinicians writing reports for health professionals use a concise, textual writing style, typically no more than one to three pages in length. Often the clinical summary (with communicative diagnosis, clinical impressions, and functional level) appears as the initial paragraph so that physicians and other healthcare professionals may read the gist of the patient's situation quickly. Another report style utilized in medical settings is a concise outline format, often patterned by the acronym SOAP (the example of SOAP will be presented later in this chapter). The outline allows the reader to locate easily routine types of information in a standard location. Alternately, there are standard report forms that may be required by the medical facility or government agency (as in the case of Medicare, Medicaid, etc.) that offer a fill-in-the-blank approach, with only abbreviated space for textual results. Such forms may combine an assessment summary with a plan of care (treatment) for physician approval. Reimbursement agencies have specific report elements. Forms from the Centers for Medicare and Medicaid Services (CMS) of the U.S. Department

FIGURE 14–1
Format for a Diagnostic Report

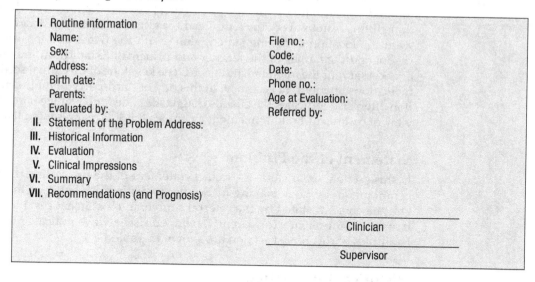

I. Routine information
   Name:
   Sex:
   Address:
   Birth date:
   Parents:
   Evaluated by:
    File no.:
    Code:
    Date:
    Phone no.:
    Age at Evaluation:
    Referred by:

II. Statement of the Problem Address:
III. Historical Information
IV. Evaluation
V. Clinical Impressions
VI. Summary
VII. Recommendations (and Prognosis)

_____
    Clinician

_____
    Supervisor

of Health and Human Services are of this type. The interested reader may search for various CMS forms online (www.cms.hhs.gov/).

- *School settings.* Clinicians prepare federally mandated reports that reflect required components. While the local educational agency may define an adopted format, the writing style tends to be concise, with the use of preprinted forms. A variety of school system samples can be found through social media.

Regardless of the format employed in work settings, a diagnostic report should be organized for easy retrieval of information and prepared in a manner that reflects high professional standards. Here are some criteria that the clinician should use to judge a diagnostic report: Is it accurate? Is it complete? Is it efficiently written (clear and with an economy of words)? Was it prepared promptly?

Figure 14–1 provides a generic format that we have found quite effective in university and traditional clinics and that we recommend to the beginning clinician. It contains several major sections, which can be written in longhand for later typing into a computer or stored as a template in a word processing program for ease of editing. Commercial software is available that provides a range of predesigned report templates (these can be found through an online search or from advertisements in SLP journals and professional magazines). Most medical facilities and clinics have documentation software that is required for use in the respective facility. Regardless of approach, the SLP must ensure that reports are confidential (and HIPAA-compliant; see the discussion later in this chapter) at all times. We join Swigert (2006) and urge that, when using time-saving technology, the clinician ensure the report is individualized as a picture of a particular client. A good report is always more than a citation of scores. Templates help ensure that all the necessary information (headings) are covered in a diagnostic report, but SLPs must guard against overdependence on prewritten text, which loses the individual and sounds generic for any John or Jane Doe!

Routine Information

In this section, we present basic identifying information—the client's name, sex, address, date of birth, telephone number, parent's name where relevant, and, of course, the date of the examination; an undated report is of very little use. In addition to these routine data, we generally identify the referral source (parent, teacher, physician), the evaluator, and (because it now matters on medical claims) the location where the testing was done if this is not part of the letterhead (or electronic banner). School systems also now want the location of testing stated, along with the name and location of the student's school and the names of the teacher and principal. Expand routine identification items as necessary for the intended audiences. The keystone of this initial section of the report is meticulous attention to accuracy. In this day of third-party reimbursement, this first section often also indicates the client's diagnostic code for coverage consideration. An overview of coding and reimbursement essentials for SLPs is presented later in this chapter.

Statement of the Problem

In this section, we include a succinct statement of the presenting problem. What is the complaint and who is making it? Be sure to distinguish between the client's complaint and the concern stated by the referral source. In most instances, the reason for referral is stated in the client's (or parent's) own words—always indicated by quotation marks. Examples of this report section are shown in Table 14–1.

Historical Information

Before seeing a client for evaluation, many clinicians request that the individual fill out a brief case history form. Alternately, this information can be gathered in a face-to-face interview. Rather than present a generic example of a case history form, we refer the reader to the case history information and forms cited in preceding chapters. Different information needs to be collected with specific disorders. Information obtained from referral letters, medical documents, the case history, and the intake interview are included in this section of the diagnostic report. Material regarding the client's development

TABLE 14–1
Examples of *Statement of the Problem* Sections from Diagnostic Reports

Example 1—from a child phonology case; this child is also a second-language learner:
As a result of classroom teacher (Ms. Wanda Kennedy) concerns and the child not passing the school's speech-language screening (Ellen Richman, SLP), Marcel Rojas, age 6 years 2 months, underwent a speech-language evaluation today (10-7-2014) at Central Elementary School. This evaluation was presumed an initial step toward determining Marcel's eligibility for special education services as speech-language impaired. A parent was not present, but previously the mother met with the clinician on 10-25-2014 and gave her consent. Ms. Rojas has limited English and so that interview was conducted in Spanish. She only indicated that Marcel's speech (in Spanish) was not as good as his two older sisters' had been. She had no opinion about his English speech skills.

Example 2—about a pediatric feeding/swallowing case:
Sierra Lucas, age 2 years 3 months, and her mother, Leona Lucas, were seen today (11-21-2014) at the clinic on the recommendation of her pediatrician. Dr. Kimbrel's referral letter indicates that Sierra's "weight is at the 60th percentile for her age and gender" and that the mother reported to him that "Sierra is a picky eater, unlike her other child." Ms. Lucas stated that Sierra often refuses to come to the table, either "running to hide or whining and squirms when made to sit." Sierra's preferred place to eat is on the couch in front of the TV where she "picks and nibbles for a long time." Sierra prefers to drink from her baby bottle and tends to "throw her sippy cup." Mrs. Lucas indicated she is "frustrated and worried" about her daughter.

TABLE 14–2

Examples of *Historical Information* Sections from Diagnostic Reports

Example 1—from an adult who will be diagnosed in this session with aphasia and apraxia of speech:

On July 5, 2014, Mrs. Martha Hickman fell at her home and was unable to get up and speak. She was transported by ambulance to Mercy Hospital, where she was attended by hospitalist Kyle Burke. Subsequent MRI [magnetic resonance imaging] scans indicated an infarct region in the left frontal cortex (Broca's area). Medical documents from both Mercy Hospital and later the Samaritan Rehabilitation Hospital indicated improved status over the past 3 months, during which she received both PT [physical therapy] and SLP services. Paralysis of the right leg and arm improved to pareses according to the reports, and at discharge she was ambulating with a walker but had limited use of her right hand and arm (difficulty dressing and unable to write). Over this time, her initial inability to speak and her limited comprehension improved. According to her son, Frank, she now lives at his house and is not getting additional speech therapy. He also says that his mother is "frustrated with her speech and usually talks in two- to three-word phrases." He also believes she "understands everything you say to her."

Example 2—from a young adult with head trauma:

Steve is a 20-year-old male who was assessed at the Shady Grove Rehabilitation Center due to concerns about speech and cognitive deficits resulting from a right-side parietal lobe brain injury. He was accompanied by his mother, Kathy, who supplemented Steve's case history. Steve experienced a closed head injury with a small subdural hematoma and a 2-mm right-to-left shift after being ejected from the passenger seat during a motor vehicle accident in September 2013. There was a loss of consciousness, and he was intubated at the scene of the accident. The accident resulted in a pulmonary contusion, bilateral frontal subdural hygroma, respiratory failure, and tracheostomy during his acute care stay. He also required PEG [percutaneous endoscopic gastrostomy] tube placement that has since been removed. Post-traumatic amnesia was estimated to be 9 weeks. Steve remained at Baptist Hospital, in Springfield, Illinois, from the time of the accident to October 14, 2013. He received inpatient physical therapy and speech therapy at Baptist Hospital from October 14 to November 11, 2013, for apraxia, dysarthria, and cognitive deficits, as well as left-side weakness and impaired coordination. Following his release, he received outpatient services from Baptist Rehabilitation Center from November 15 to April 11, 2014. Steve has regained most of his mobility but still experiences difficulty with fine motor skills such as fastening buttons, adjusting belts, and tying his shoes. Based on parent report, Steve's swallowing has improved, with difficulty only with large gulps of liquid (i.e., drinking from the milk carton) and select hard foods. He is frequently unintelligible to familiar listeners. Steve's speech difficulties cause difficulty among family members, and he gets frustrated easily when others do not understand him. He has a history of the following: alcohol abuse, marijuana use and tobacco use since high school, emotional lability, clinical depression, memory impairment, and learning disability. Steve currently takes Vyvanse for attention deficit disorder (ADD) and has recently discontinued prescribed Celexa for depression. He enjoys being outdoors hunting, fishing, and riding four wheelers. Steve's personal goal is to attend college, and he is currently auditing an English class at Frasier Community College.

(general and speech and language); medical, educational, and family history; and estimates of psychosocial and behavioral adjustments is summarized. Only the most pertinent items are included in the diagnostic report. Because most of the historical information is obtained by questioning the client, a parent, spouse, or other informants, we suggest that the clinician briefly describe the interview situation—type of rapport established, the frankness and completeness of the respondent's answers, and any other pertinent observations. Examples of this report section are shown in Table 14–2.

Evaluation

The results of the various tests and examinations are delineated in this section. Before describing the assessment procedures and results, however, we include an opening statement that describes how the client approached the clinical setting and the tasks used to evaluate the communication abilities: Was the client apprehensive, bored, fatigued, cooperative? The name of each test, an explanation of what it does and how it was administered, and the results obtained should be included.

Should the clinician include statements about communication skills that are judged to be within normal limits at the time of the evaluation? It is standard practice for a complete diagnostic report to mention, albeit briefly, all aspects of a client: hearing, speech (e.g., sounds, intelligibility, motor skills, voice, fluency), language (comprehension, expression), cognition, and swallowing abilities. Subsequent assessments can utilize the information as baseline observations. Collectively, nontested areas can be cited with the phrase "judged typical for the client's age," which is the more preferred language (compared to, for example, "judged to be within normal limits"). In this report section, many clinicians use subheadings to capture *all tested* areas. As an example for a stroke patient, subheads might include testing in the areas of hearing, oral peripheral exam, motor speech (apraxia and dysarthria), adult language (aphasia testing), cognition, and so forth. Expand the size of this section to present important testing information, but simply present the information; do not interpret it. Examples of this report section are shown in Tables 14–3 and 14–4.

Clinical Impressions

In this section, the SLP summarizes her or his impressions of the individual and the communication impairment. What type of speech-language-swallowing disorder, if any, does the client have? How severe is it? What might be the cause(s)? What factors seem to be perpetuating it? What impact has it had on the client and the client's family? How much does it interfere with everyday functioning? What are the prospects for treatment? Although we can offer interpretations here, we must still be able to support our impressions with information obtained during the interview, testing, and observations. Speculations based on previous clinical experience, such as similarity between the client and other cases the diagnostician has examined, should be clearly labeled as such. Examples of this report section are shown in Table 14–5.

TABLE 14–3

Example of the *Evaluation* Section from a Diagnostic Report in Which the SLP Performed a Separate Videostroboscopic Evaluation

---

Example—a 63-year-old male with poor vocal projection, short phonation duration, and rough vocal quality who just received a voice evaluation; here are the SLP evaluation findings from a videostroboscopic evaluation:

Laryngeal structure and function were assessed using a rigid 70-degree endoscope, which the patient tolerated without need for topical anesthetic. Laryngeal mucosa appeared white and well hydrated bilaterally. Bilateral vocal fold mobility was observed during a "heeheehee" task. During resting breathing, glottic margins were observed to be smooth and concave bilaterally. Sustained "ee" production, as examined under stroboscopic light at normal pitch and loudness, indicated intact edge pliability and typical mucosal wave bilaterally. Glottic closure pattern was persistently spindle-shaped. The glottic margins appeared to meet on-plane, and no supraglottic tension was observed.

TABLE 14–4

Example of the *Evaluation* Section from a Diagnostic Report on an Internationally Adopted Preschool Child with a History of Repaired Cleft Palate

Standardized tests used and their results were as follows.

Goldman Fristoe Test of Articulation–2 (GFTA-2)

George's speech and articulation were formally assessed using the *Goldman-Fristoe Test of Articulation,* Second Edition (GFTA-2). The *GFTA-2* is a standardized articulation assessment that uses picture stimuli to elicit consonant sounds and consonant blends. The Sound-in-Words subtest was administered by showing George a picture and asking him to say the word or words that correlate with the given picture. The scores listed below are from the Sounds-in-Words subtest:

Sounds-in-Words (Subtest of GFTA-2)	Raw Score	Standard Score	Percentile Rank	Test-Age Equivalent
	61	42	<1	<2.0

Speech Intelligibility Score

Known Listener with Familiar Context **(Single Words and Connected Speech)**	70% intelligible
Unknown Listener with Unfamiliar Context **(Single Words and Connected Speech)**	40% intelligible

The tables below show a list of the substitutions and omissions George exhibited for certain consonants on the *GFTA-2*:

Phoneme Production	Substitutions and Omissions (−) on the GFTA-2		
	Initial Position	**Medial Position**	**Final Position**
p	m		
n			−
g	n	−	i
k	n	−	−
f	m		p
d	n	−	−
ŋ			nd
j (**y**ellow)	n		
t	n	−	−
ʃ (**sh**ovel)	n	−	NE
t ʃ (**ch**air)	j	z	z
l	j	−	w
r	w	w	w
dʒ (**j**udge)	j	j	
θ (**th**umb)	d	j	f
v	b	b	−
s	n	−	−
z	n	n	−
ð (**th**is) voiced	d	d	

NE = nasal emission.

(Continued)

TABLE 14–4
Continued

Blend Production	Initial Position
bl	m
br	w
dr	w
fl	w
fr	w
gl	w
gr	w
kl	w
kr	w
kw	w
pl	w
sl	w
sp	p
st	n
sw	w
tr	w

George's errors produced during the assessment were substitutions, such as /m/ for /p/ and /n/ for /d, k, g/ in the initial position of words, as well as /j/ for /dʒ/ in both the initial and medial positions of words. On several occasions, he omitted phonemes in the medial and final positions of words, and other errors such as glottal stops, reductions, and substitutions of consonants in blends were produced.

The results of the *GFTA-2* reveal that George has established certain early sounds appropriate for his age level. These sounds include /m, w, h, and b/. According to the *GFTA-2* standardization sample, all of these sounds should be established no later than the age of 3. George has established correct production of these sounds, which shows strength in his ability to produce these consonants correctly in all positions of words for speech. Other correct productions of sounds that George exhibits, but has not established in all word positions, include /p, n, f, j, d, n, dʒ, and ŋ/. These sounds are in George's consonant inventory; however, these sounds were not exhibited in all positions of words targeted on the *GFTA-2*. Because George exhibits these sounds, there is strength in his ability to develop these sounds for complete establishment in all word positions. According to the *GFTA-2* standardization sample, George should exhibit complete establishment of the following consonants and consonant blends for his chronological age of 4 years, 11 months: /b, d, h, m, n, p, f, g, k, t, w/ and /kw/.

Based on George's scores from the *GFTA-2*, his articulation patterns are significantly below what is expected for his chronological age of 4 years, 11 months. The raw score is the sum of all errors made on the Sounds-in-Words subtest and can range from 0 to a total of 77. George's raw score of 61 is above the mean or average raw score for his chronological age, which indicates that he is producing more errors than expected for a child his age. George's standard score shows the distance between his performance and the average standard score from the normative population sample of the *GFTA-2*. The average standard score for the *GFTA-2* is 100, with a standard deviation (SD) of 15 from the average score. George's standard score of 42 indicates that his score falls almost four standard deviations below the average *GFTA-2* standard score of 100. The percentile rank on the *GFTA-2* specifies the percentage of individuals George's age who achieved his performance level or less than his performance level on the assessment. George scored less than the 1st percentile, which means that he performed the same or better than less than 1% of the normative population sample for his chronological age. The test-age equivalent is given to show the median or middle score of all the raw scores from the *GFTA-2* normative sample for George's chronological age. George's test-age equivalent of less than 2 years means that his raw score is below the median raw score for individuals who are 4 years and 11 months of age.

TABLE 14–4
Continued

Results from the *GFTA-2* indicate a significant articulation disorder characterized by omissions and substitutions of consonants in the initial, medial, and final positions of words. Some distortions of consonants, glottal stops, and hypernasality with nasal emission were also present in his speech when the assessment was given. George exhibited strengths in maintaining the number of syllable sounds in the adult form of target words, as well as the number of vowels found in each word. Although George's scores are below those expected for his chronological age, his scores reflect the presence of a repaired bilateral cleft lip and palate with a remaining fistula and VPI [velopharyngeal insufficiency].

Clinical Evaluation of Language Fundamentals–Preschool, Second Edition (CELF-P)

The *CELF-P2* was used to assess George's expressive and receptive language skills. The assessment was developed to identify, diagnose, or evaluate language deficits in children. The administrator can use the test to identify if a child has an overall language disability by administering three subtests to obtain a Core Language Score. A variety of other measures (Receptive Language Index, Expressive Language Index, Language Context Index, and the Language Structure Index) can be obtained and used to describe the nature of the language disorder if one is present. The clinician administered the following subtests: Sentence Structure, Word Structure, Expressive Vocabulary, Concepts and Following Directions, Recalling Sentences, Basic Concepts, Word Classes—Receptive, and Word Classes—Expressive. George's scores on the *CELF-P2* are as follows:

Subtest	Raw Score	Scaled Score	Percentile Rank	Age Equivalent
Sentence Structure	9	7	16	3.2
Word Structure	6	5	5	<3.0
Expressive Vocabulary	12	8	25	3.5
Concepts and Following Directions	6	7	16	<3.0
Recalling Sentences	5	6	9	3.0
Basic Concepts	12	7	16	3.5
Word Classes—Receptive	7	6	9	<4.0
Word Classes—Expressive	0	4	2	<4.0

Raw scores for each of the subtests are the sums of the scored items. The raw scores are then converted to a scaled score, which is used to provide the percentile rank. Both scaled scores and percentile ranks give insight into how George performed when compared to same-age peers. Scaled scores have a mean of 10 and a standard deviation of 3; therefore, a scaled score of 10 describes average performance. The Sentence Structure subtest measured George's ability to interpret spoken sentences. The target sentences gradually increase in complexity. The clinician instructed George to point to the picture that represented the sentence read aloud by the clinician. George achieved a raw score of 9, which is converted to a scaled score of 7. The corresponding percentile rank was 16. These scores indicate that George's performance is within normal limits.

The Word Structure subtest evaluated George's morphology and pronoun usage. The clinician instructed George to complete the end of a sentence that was read aloud by the clinician with the word that correctly described the picture. George's articulation difficulties were a factor during this subtest and were considered when interpreting the results. George had a raw score of 6, which is converted to a scaled score of 5 and percentile rank of 5. The scaled score falls more than one standard deviation below the mean, placing him in the low average range for a child his age.

(Continued)

TABLE 14–4
Continued

The Expressive Vocabulary subtest measured George's ability to label or name people, actions, and objects. The clinician audibly read a question aloud to George about a stimulus picture ("What is this?"), and he was instructed to identify the object, action, or person that was presented. George received a raw score of 12, which is converted to a scaled score of 8 and corresponding percentile rank of 25. His performance on this subtest also falls within normal limits.

The Concepts and Following Directions subtest evaluated George's ability to comprehend and interpret spoken directions of increasing length and complexity; identify an object from several choices; and remember characteristics, names, or order of mention. The clinician instructed George to point to the object that matched the description used by the clinician (e.g., "Point to the little cat"). George received a raw score of 6, which is converted to a scaled score of 7 and percentile rank of <3.0. These scores indicate that George's performance is within normal limits.

The Recalling Sentences subtest evaluated George's ability to listen to sentences that are read aloud and repeat the sentences back without changing the meaning or syntactic structure of the given sentence. George received a raw score of 5, which is converted to a scaled score of 6 and the corresponding percentile rank of 9. The scaled score of 6 falls more than one standard deviation below the mean, placing him in the low average range for a child his age.

The Basic Concepts subtest measured George's knowledge of concepts, including number, location, equality (sameness), and size. The clinician instructed George to point to the picture that represented what the clinician described (e.g., "Point to the boy who is sad"). George received a raw score of 12, which is converted to a scaled score of 7. The corresponding percentile rank of 16 indicates that George scored the same or better than 16% of his same-age peers. These scores indicate that George's performance is within normal limits.

The Word Classes subtest measured George's ability to identify semantic relationships between word classes (e.g., horn and drum) and provide the relationship (e.g., musical instruments). For the Receptive portion of this subtest, the clinician provided the client with an illustration of three objects, named the three objects, and asked the client to identify the two words that went together. George received a raw score of 7 for the receptive portion, which was converted to a scaled score of 6 and a percentile rank of 9. George's scaled score of 6 falls in the low average range. For the Expressive portion, the clinician asked George how the two words went together. George received a raw score of 0 for the expressive portion, which was converted to a scaled score of 4 and a percentile rank of 2. George's scaled score of 4 falls two standard deviations from the mean, placing him below normal limits for a child his age.

The above subtests are used to obtain Core Language and four index scores. Different combinations of scaled scores are added to create a Sum of Subtest Scaled Scores. These scores can be converted to a standard score, which indicates where George's scores lie when compared to the mean. The standard scores have a mean of 100 and a standard deviation of 15, so a standard score of 100 represents typical performance. George's Core Language Score and index scores are reported below:

	Core Language	Receptive Language	Expressive Language	Language Content	Language Structure
Standard Score	81	83	79	85	77
Percentile Rank	10	13	8	16	6

The Core Language Score is calculated by finding the sum of the scaled scores for the Sentence Structure, Word Structure, and Expressive Vocabulary subtests. The Core Language Score is used to determine if there is an overall language delay. George received a standard score of 81. George's standard score is converted to a percentile rank of 10. These scores indicate George performed better than 10% of his same-age peers, and his language abilities are considered low average, falling slightly over one standard deviation below the mean.

TABLE 14–4
Continued

The Receptive Language Index is a measure of auditory comprehension and listening. The score is determined by calculating the sum of the scaled scores of the Sentence Structure, Concepts and Following Directions, and Basic Concepts subtests. George received a standard score of 83, which is converted to a percentile rank of 13. These scores indicate that George performed better than 13% of his same-age peers, and his receptive language abilities are considered low average, falling slightly over one standard deviation below the mean.

The Expressive Language Index is a measure of the child's expressive language abilities. The index score is calculated by finding the sum of the standard scores of the Word Structure, Expressive Vocabulary, and Recalling Sentences subtests. George received a standard score of 79, which is converted to a percentile rank of 8. These scores indicate George performed better than 8% of his same-age peers, and his expressive language abilities are considered low average, falling slightly over one standard deviation below the mean.

The Language Content Index score measures semantic development. This includes vocabulary, comprehension of sentences both simple and complex, comprehension of the relationships among words, and concept development. It is calculated by summing the scaled scores of the Expressive Vocabulary, Concepts and Following Directions, and Basic Concepts subtests. George received a standard score of 85, which is converted to a percentile rank of 16. These scores indicate George's usage of semantics is considered average, within 1 standard deviation of the mean.

The Language Structure Index score measures the interpretation and production of different structures of words and sentences. The index score is calculated by finding the sum of the scaled scores of the Sentence Structure, Word Structure, and Recalling Sentences subtests. George received a standard score of 77, which is converted to a percentile rank of 6. These scores indicate George performed better than 8% of his same-age peers, and his basis for language structure is low average, falling slightly over one standard deviation below the mean.

The results of the *CELF-P2* indicate that George's language skills are slightly below those of his same-age peers. George's strengths include his expressive vocabulary skills, identification of several objects in pictures, and identifying related objects in pictures. Areas of weakness include expression of a word class relationship (i.e., telling how two items in a category are related), ability to repeat sentences verbatim, and use of a variety of word structures.

Velopharyngeal Assessment

The flexible endoscope was advanced into George's right nostril to the point where the velopharynx could be viewed. Copious, thick mucus was observed in the nasopharynx and obscured the view of the velopharynx until the endoscope was advanced beyond it. A clear image of the velopharynx was achieved, and George was asked to produce the following phrases: "Pet the puppy," "I see Suzy," and "Take it out." During these phrase productions, limited lateral wall and velar movement toward midline was observed. Little posterior pharyngeal wall movement was observed during these speech attempts. At no time during these speech attempts was George able to close his velopharynx adequately for balanced resonance production. The velopharyngeal port appeared largely adynamic with a persistent small gap. Given the nature of the velopharyngeal movement, additional phrases and co-articulatory contexts with nasals to assess velopharyngeal timing further, e.g., "hamper, hamper, hamper," were not completed.

Overall, George presented with moderately severe hypernasal resonance secondary to a largely adynamic velopharyngeal port 1-year status post–sphincter pharyngoplasty. Recommended that George consult with his plastic surgeon on the cleft palate team for further guidance on surgical options to restore balanced resonance.

(Continued)

TABLE 14–4
Continued

Nasometry

The Nasometer II was used to assess the percentage of George's nasalence, which is the acoustic correlate of perceived nasality. George was asked to produce sentences while wearing the Nasometer headset device. George's percentage nasalence across the three tasks is summarized below:

94% for a sustained nasal sound (expected = 95%, SD = 2)
48% for a nasal loaded sentence speech sample (expected = 61%, SD = 7)
36% for an oral (non-nasal) group of sentences (expected = 15.6%, SD = 4)

Scores for a nasal sentence are low, which is consistent with hyponasality perceived. Hyponasality is presumed to be the result of the mucus obstructing the sphincter orifice. Oral scores are in the marginal range and are lowered artificially because of glottal stops used in the repeated sentence sample.

Hearing

According to previous testing from 2010, George presents with bilateral conductive hearing loss. Otoscopy and tympanometry were performed in September 2012. This testing revealed excessive cerumen with no visualization of the tympanic membrane or tubes, along with Type B tympanograms for both right and left ears. In today's evaluation, pure tone air conduction thresholds were performed for both the right and left ears. Results indicated a mild hearing loss at 250 to 500 Hz, improving to within normal limits at 1,000 Hz, and increasing to a mild hearing loss at 2,000 to 8,000 Hz.

TABLE 14–5
Examples of *Clinical Impressions* Sections from Diagnostic Reports

Example 1—from a child language and literacy case:

Ben is a 12-year-old male who is in the sixth grade at Shipley Middle School, where he currently receives special education services. Based on initial parent report, concerns were raised about Ben's language, auditory processing, reading, and writing abilities. It was believed that they are having a negative impacting on his schoolwork and interactions with family and friends. During the evaluation, Ben was administered the following tests: The *Comprehensive Assessment of Spoken Language (CASL), the Test of Auditory Processing Skills III (TAPS-3), Token Test for Children (TTFC-2), and the Gray Diagnostic Reading Test-2 (GDRT-2)*. The results of the *CASL and TTFC-2* indicate that Ben has a severe impairment in receptive language. However, it was noted that when provided visual cues, Ben performed significantly better on all tasks presented to him. The *GDRT-2* was administered to assess Ben's current reading abilities. The results of this test indicates that he has a severe impairment in reading proficiency abilities. His ability to identify sounds associated with letters correctly suggests that he may have the potential to progress in his reading abilities. Overall, the test results highlighted Ben's difficulty with auditory memory, phonological segmentation and blending, grapheme–phoneme relationships, and general reading. Each of these should be targeted in therapy to help him increase his receptive language and reading abilities.

Example 2—from an adult following recent laryngectomy with secondary TEP [tracheoesophageal puncture]:

Subsequent to CA [carcinoma] of the larynx and total laryngectomy 3 weeks ago, today (11-20-2014) Dr. Guthrie performed a secondary TEP on Mr. Robert Weaver. This was followed in the office by this SLP fitting devices and assessing initial speech attempts. Mr. Weaver displayed good manual dexterity, comprehension of instructions, and tolerance of all procedures; he was also able to produce clear voice without strain. With two sessions of additional guidance in device care and placement, also with strategies for optimizing speech-language production, it is anticipated that Mr. Weaver will become a proficient speaker with TEP.

Summary

The summary section of a diagnostic report should be a concise (not more than a short paragraph) statement abstracting the salient features of the whole report. What is the communication disorder? What are the primary features of the disorder? What is the probable cause of the disorder? What is the prognosis for remediation (be it recovery or more limited achievements)? Examples of this report section are shown in Table 14–6.

Recommendations

The recommendations section is perhaps the most crucial portion of the report. We must now translate our findings into appropriate suggestions or directions that will help the client improve communication and related issues. Do we recommend additional speech and language evaluations? Is a medical referral necessary? Is treatment indicated? What direction should be taken in treatment or plan of care, and by whom, when, and how often? The task is to crystallize all the disparate interactions we have had with the individual, collate all the data, and then provide a flexible blueprint for further action (if any). We must attempt to answer the question: Where do we go from here? Try to make the recommendations specific and brief. Suggestions for treatment or a plan of care should be presented succinctly. (Any lengthy plan of care can be outlined in a subsequent document or agency form as a follow-up report.) Examples of this report section are shown in Table 14–7.

TABLE 14–6
Examples of *Summary* Sections from Diagnostic Reports

Example 1—a child on the autism spectrum with language and fluency disorders:
Based on formal and informal testing, Hannah's communication deficits are characterized by a mild articulation disorder (particularly an interdental lisp), a mild to moderate receptive language delay, a mild expressive delay, a severe fluency disorder, and pragmatic deficits commensurate with a formal diagnosis of autism spectrum disorder. She exhibits whole-word and part-word repetitions, with three to four iterations per stuttered event; prolongations; and blocks. The frequency of stuttering behavior is increased as she moves from scripted or echolalic speech to speech that is more novel or linguistically complex. Hannah's prognosis for improvement of language is good because of high parental involvement and foundational receptive and expressive language skills. Prognosis for improvement in fluency and pragmatics is fair to good with continued compliance with a regular therapy schedule and implementation of a home program. Collaboration with Hannah's ABA [applied behavioral analysis] therapist also will aid in Hannah's future success in therapy.

Example 2—from a kindergarten-age child who stutters:
Michael was very cooperative and eager to participate in the evaluation. Based on formal and informal assessments, Michael presents with a very severe fluency disorder. Throughout speaking tasks, he exhibited audible prolongations, silent prolongations (blocks), and syllable repetitions, which significantly affected the fluency of his speech. He also exhibited secondary associated behaviors accompanying his stuttering, such as bending over, stomping his foot, touching his mouth, and facial strain. Michael's responses during the evaluation, and specifically during the administration of the KiddyCAT [Communication Attitude Test for Preschool and Kindergarten Children Who Stutter], indicate that he is aware of his disfluencies and is embarrassed, bothered, and frustrated by them. His prognosis for improvement is fair because of the severity of his stuttering behaviors, maladaptive perceptions, and secondary behaviors that accompany his stuttering. Compliance with a regular therapy schedule and implementation of a home program will aid in Michael's future success in therapy.

TABLE 14–7
Examples of *Recommendations* Sections from Diagnostic Reports

---

Example 1—from an acute-care facility's adult stroke patient just reevaluated with FEES [fiberoptic endoscopic evaluation of swallowing]:
This patient presents with moderate impairment in receptive and expressive language skills and also with moderate oral dysphagia and mild to moderate pharyngeal dysphagia. Based on the FEES reassessment study (done 3-5-16) and the low but present aspiration risk, it is recommended to continue current swallowing precautions and methods of feeding with a modified mechanical diet until further notice.

Example 2—from a child language case:
It is recommended that Sarah enroll in speech-language services at a frequency of two times per week for 1-hour sessions. Treatment should focus on the following:

1. Using strategies to improve reading comprehension, such as skimming a text for important terms and/or information, and creating story maps and outlines of the text.
2. Utilizing the RAP strategy (**R**ead a paragraph; **A**sk yourself, "What are the main ideas and details of this paragraph?"; and **P**ut the main idea into your own words) to increase reading comprehension.
3. Utilizing the five steps in the SQ3R learning strategy (**s**urvey, **q**uestion, **r**ead, **r**ecite, and **r**eview) to increase reading comprehension abilities.
4. Increasing figurative and ambiguous language abilities.

Sarah should also receive classroom accommodations, such as sitting close to the front of the room, having notes printed before the class date, and possibly extra time to complete work.

One final warning: Do not recommend *specific* evaluations or remediation procedures to workers in other professions. It is improper, for example, to recommend a client for electroencephalography to a neurologist, or for dental braces to an orthodontist. After all, the SLP would be chagrined if a physician referred a client and recommended the administration of a specific test! Be sure that your referrals for additional assessment are based on sound evidence; it is expensive, time consuming, and stressful to the client for the SLP to make recommendations for comprehensive medical or psychiatric evaluation without serious and compelling reasons.

Early in the diagnostic session with 5-year-old Mark, we suspected the possibility of brain injury. Mindful of the family's limited finances, we wanted to document carefully all signs of apparent cerebral dysfunction before making a referral for a complete pediatric neurological evaluation. Observation revealed a number of serious symptoms: difficulty with motor coordination, labile emotions, rapid and slurred speech, perseveration, and blanking out spells. The necessity for referral was then obvious.

Recommendations and prognosis statements should not be misleading or unrealistic. A clinician's awareness of evidence-based practice can guide him or her in such matters. Consider, for example, the case of a 65-year-old female whose stroke occurred 10 years earlier. A clinician might report that Mrs. Tucker's enthusiasm for now receiving aphasia services suggests that prognosis in therapy might be good.

Why is this prognostic statement inappropriate? First, a client's degree of enthusiasm is not a reliable indicator of success. Second (and this factor is important), the amount of time that has elapsed since the stroke would warrant a more guarded prognosis because the aphasia literature is clear that recovery of function is time-sensitive. Third, the improvement of "what" is not specific.

THE WRITING PROCESS

Many students have difficulty writing reports. Most of them have found the task oner-ous, and a few are threatened and overwhelmed by the prospect of summarizing all that has been done. It has been our experience, however, that rather than have a writing deficiency, most of these students have a writing bias—they do not think they can do it. Of course, there are no quick and simple solutions, but we offer the suggestions in this section that have proven helpful to more than one beginning report writer.

Write on a daily basis. Each night—before retiring, for example—sit down and write a descriptive paragraph concerning something that happened to you that day. At the end of the week, review the writing you have done, edit, revise, and ask yourself what you meant by each word or phrase. The best way to learn to write, in our opinion, is to write.

Get the message out and revise it later. It is especially important in writing reports to begin as soon as possible while the material is still fresh in your mind. A common error that some beginning writers make is to attempt to produce perfect writing in the initial draft. It does not matter how it looks at this point; you can always edit or have someone help you edit. When you meet barriers or mental blocks, do not linger; jump over them and go on with the rest of the report. When you come back later, you will find that your mind has filled in the blank spots.

It is helpful to have someone read and comment on the initial draft of your report. Although it is difficult to submit one's prose for dissection, ask the reader to be frank and honest in his or her editing. So many times, a phrase that seems clear to the writer who conceived it is vague or obscure to an objective reader.

Style

In the interest of brevity, we shall simply enumerate several principles of style that we have found useful.

1. Make your presentation straightforward and objective, using a topical outline. Use simple, brief, but complete sentences. It is often helpful to write for a specific reader; picture the reader in your mind—the classroom teacher, physician, speech clinician—and then simply tell the story of what you observed and recommend regarding a par-ticular client. When in doubt about a reader's level of understanding, it is better to err on the side of simplicity.

2. Use an impersonal style. Some clinicians use the first person when writing diag-nostic reports, but in our view it is preferable to keep the "I" out of it; a reference to "the clinician" or "the examiner" is more in keeping with professional reports. We prefer to individualize the client described in the report, not the writer. We believe that an imper-sonal style not only helps to minimize the writer's verbal idiosyncrasies but also tends to encourage objectivity.

3. Edit the report carefully to make certain that spelling and use of tense, grammar, and punctuation are accurate. Errors, even trivial ones, undermine the confidence of the reader in the diagnostician. Remember, competence is judged to a great extent by the precision of your reporting.

4. Watch your semantics. Be wary of overused or nebulous words such as *nice, hope-fully, good,* and the like. Avoid pet expressions or stereotyped ways of phrasing informa-tion. One clinician used the phrase *in terms of* 13 times in a two-page diagnostic report. Another laced his reports with currently popular words like *input, interface,* and *scenario.* Some writers use the word *feel* inappropriately in statements like "The clinician felt the

client understood the diagnostic task." We believe (not feel!) that the word should be reserved for discussing emotions or tactile sensations. Use abbreviations sparingly. Avoid superlatives unless they are clearly indicated.

5. Avoid preparing an "Aunt Fanny" report—a bland written statement that could represent anyone or is so filled with qualifications (*perhaps, apparently, tends to*) that it reveals nothing—nothing, that is, except a timid diagnostician.

6. Make the report "tight." Do not leave gaps or ambiguity where it is possible to read between the lines. If findings in certain areas are unremarkable, always state this explicitly. Do not leave the reader to guess whether you have investigated all possible aspects.

7. A diagnostic report is no place to display your learning or to parade a large vocabulary. Pedantic reports are misunderstood or unread.

8. Stay close to the data until you wish to draw the observations together and make some interpretations. For example, tell the reader which sounds were in error instead of simply stating that the child sounds infantile.

9. The very essence of good style is the willingness to take the time and energy to write and rewrite the report until it communicates what the clinician did and what the clinician found in the diagnostic session.

Supervisory Writing Feedback

Clinical educators in university training programs as well as site supervisors of clinicians in externships or in their year as a clinical fellow all have a helpful role to play in mentoring clinical report writing skills. SLP supervisors in all work environments (university and general clinics, medical settings, school settings) but also SLP colleagues in the workplace are well positioned to acclimate students and new clinicians to the style of reporting and to the use of any formats, templates, or forms expected by the facility. This mentoring by all is important for the person's professional development.

The early and crucial report writing guidance occurs in university training programs where the clinical faculty member needs to be meticulous in shaping each future professional. Van Gilder and Street-Tobin (2011) developed a diagnostic report writing assessment rubric to help supervising clinical educators become more efficient in reviewing elements of a report. Their five-level standardized rubric for assessing diagnostic reports includes explanations and examples, and has both quantative and qualitative rating scales. The five dimensions and a sample of some subcomponents are as follows:

1. Content (40)—Completeness, Relevance, Accuracy, Interpretation
2. Style (20)—Organization, Conciseness, Precision
3. Professional Writing (15)—Formal language, Professional terminology, Differentiating between fact and opinion
4. Grammar and Proofreading (15)
5. Cohesion (10)—Coherence, Evidence for diagnostic conclusions and recommendations

We suggest that this supervisory rubric might also be used for self-appraisal before submitting a diagnostic report to a mentor or to a supervisor, or filed with the facility.

The Writing Audit

Another opportunity for honing one's report writing skills at any stage of career development is to have your reports audited. Voluntary diagnostic report audits performed by professional colleagues are a good check on one's writing clarity and attention to detail. Imposed, required audits can be stressful; clinicians who have participated in a mock audit are confident of their clinical quality and compliance and so have nothing to fear. Begin a voluntary, mock "diagnostic report audit" as a learning experience by suggesting that SLP colleagues (or perhaps others from allied disciplines) at the facility audit a sample number of diagnostic reports for format compliance. Of course, this first necessitates a review of the format expectations and expected details. Revisiting these periodically is always a good review for any diagnostic clinician.

Patient care audits are part of the national healthcare monitoring system for quality assurance. Patient care audits may focus on the quality of care provided patients through a variety of channels, including thoroughness of evaluation and diagnosis, treatment procedures, and audits of patient outcomes. The first item is pertinent to this chapter: Files can be analyzed retrospectively to see whether routine components are present in the diagnostic report. Before doing a patient care audit of the quality of reports, the clinician or agency must have specified minimal requirements beforehand—such factors as inclusion of the client's date of birth; mention of referral source, chart number, and date of evaluation; and performance of a hearing test, oral peripheral examination, and the like. Presetting some desired level of compliance is also necessary (e.g., "At least 90% of the audited reports will have . . ."). We recommend patient care audits, even if mock or self-administered, as a good spot-check of compliance with professional standards of information collection and reporting. When deficiencies are found, the clinician can target specific areas for needed improvement and/or adjust clinical procedures and expectations.

Confidentiality

In our view, confidentiality is basic to any helping profession. All reports and records (electronic and paper) should be kept secure so that no harm or embarrassment comes to the persons we serve. The privacy and security of documentation must be maintained in compliance with the regulations of the Health Insurance Portability and Accountability Act (HIPAA). When a diagnostic report is released, we prefer to mail it to a specific person rather than to the agency itself. Any transfer of electronic records must be done securely and conform with HIPAA regulations. HIPAA-compliant software (and protected server access) should now be in most or all clinical facilities. *A report with patient identifying information sent over the Internet as an email attachment is not secure; never do it!* Do not prepare patient reports on your home computer or laptop at a coffee shop that provides Wi-Fi because these public systems are not secure. Also, before releasing any information about a client, we secure the client's permission in writing; most speech and hearing centers and medical facilities have permission forms that are completed prior to or during the diagnostic session.

Because clients and parents have a legal right, according to Public Law 93-380, the Family Educational Rights and Privacy Act (FERPA) of 1974, to read any report containing information about themselves or their children, we often find it useful to send them a copy of the diagnostic report. Before mailing this report, we review our findings and recommendations with them. By going over the information that will be in the final report with clients or parents, we can be sure that they understand its contents.

Of interest is that Watson and Thompson (1983) researched parental perceptions of both diagnostic reports and conferences that followed the diagnostic session. Ninety percent of parents indicated understanding the clinical results as presented in a face-to-face conference. Likewise, 89% of the parents stated that they understood the conclusions of the written report. Although these figures are high, they suggest that there is room to improve clinicians' professional oral and written communication skills.

ADDITIONAL DETAILS FOR WRITING IN MEDICAL SETTINGS

Clinicians in medical settings may record their findings in a problem-oriented format (Kent & Chabon, 1980). Problem-oriented medical records (POMRs) feature a carefully defined and documented list of problems, which encompass all the significant difficulties a patient is experiencing. The list includes the presenting complaint as well as those problems identified by the members of the healthcare team. For example, a patient who suffered a cerebrovascular accident (CVA), or stroke, might have right hemiparesis and aphasia leading to problems with daily activities (e.g., feeding, dressing), locomotion, language, intelligibility, and the like. Ideally placed at the front of the patient's file, this list of problems generated by the multidisciplinary team points to areas needing further assessment and/or intervention. All available information about the person is then organized under the four headings shown in Figure 14–2. The four headings in the figure form the acronym SOAP. Popular for more than 40 years, the SOAP format can be used in daily chart documentations as well as diagnostic reports. Progress notes need to be concise. The SOAP format is employed by most medical disciplines and is an excellent tool for guiding professionals, including the SLP, toward brevity. The SOAP format ensures that key information on the day's (or week's) session is recorded. All that is necessary is a brief statement on the patient's level of cooperation, motivation, or frustration (Subjective); a citation of what tasks were attempted and at what levels of stimulation or cueing (Objectives); levels of accuracy to which tasks were performed (Assessments); and logical next steps in the rehabilitation program (Plan).

There has been a growing trend in healthcare toward the use of functional outcome measures, in which the patient's behaviors are assessed categorically relative to levels of function impact. Functional measures are required components of the patient's evaluation and subsequent report for many Medicare forms. SLPs in medical settings now routinely assess functioning in the initial diagnostic session; this provides a baseline for subsequent comparison by reevaluation after intervention or some period of time. In this manner, outcomes of services can be tracked, at least for some types of functions. Several functional outcomes instruments are in wide use.

The Functional Independence Measure (FIM) (State University of New York at Buffalo, 1993a) is an adult outcome measurement tool used by various healthcare professionals, including SLPs, especially those working in acute hospitals and rehabilitation settings. Comparison of pre- (initial diagnostic evaluation) and post- (later reassessment) scores provide the context for outcomes, while the content items focus on general functioning. The FIM is composed of 18 specific tasks that are often addressed in rehabilitation services. These tasks are grouped into six main categories: self-care, sphincter control, mobility, locomotion, communication, and social cognition. The FIM rates patient dependence-independence on each of the 18 items using a scale of 1 to 7, where 7 indicates complete independence in a particular activity and 1 indicates total assistance. The minimum total FIM score is 18; the maximum total score is 126. Ratings are made by a multidisciplinary team. Final scores can also be expressed as an adjective

FIGURE 14–2
SOAP Format for Medical Diagnostic Reports or Summaries

Subjective	Objective	Assessment	Plan
Interview and case history	Test results	Collation of subjective and objective information	Additional testing Treatment options

(e.g., total assistance needed, maximum assistance, moderate assistance, and so forth) or as a percentage of independence. Some facilities have used FIM levels to aid in patient selection and discharge decisions, and to track progress over time. The brevity of the FIM has led some agencies to more in-depth descriptors. For SLPs, having only one of the six FIM assessment areas for communication is too simplistic to reflect outcomes in functional communication; other detailed options exist.

Patterned along the same construct, but geared for young patients, is the Pediatric Functional Independence Measure (WeeFIM) (State University of New York at Buffalo, 1993b). The WeeFIM is intended for tracking outcomes (pre- versus post-rehabilitation services) in patients 7 years and younger. A provision of the WeeFIM states that children from birth to age 3 can be assessed by parental interview rather than actual task assessment. The 18 measures on the WeeFIM cluster into three domains: self-care (eating, grooming, bathing, etc.), mobility, and cognition (comprehension, expression, social interaction, problem solving, memory). A scoring system of 1 (total assistance) to 7 (complete independence) is used with the 18 WeeFIM measures. Again, we note the narrowness of this functional outcome tool for the communication disorders professional.

Three Functional Communication Measures (FCMs) are components of the American Speech-Language-Hearing Association's (ASHA's) National Outcomes Measurement System (NOMS) (American Speech-Language-Hearing Association, 1997–2014, retrieved from www.asha.org). The FCMs are a series of disorder-specific, 7-point rating scales that describe patient changes in communication and/or swallowing function over time (e.g., assessed pre- and postintervention). FCMs exist for three age groups: adults, children, and prekindergarten. Collectively, the specificity of these Functional Communication Measures should appeal to SLPs, whereas other tools mentioned in this chapter are too narrow to track functional outcomes adequately for the profession of communication disorders. The Center for Medicare and Medicaid Services has endorsed the use of FCMs in Medicare claims-based reporting. A Pathway format typically organizes patient information in columns representing phases or changes over time. Phase 1 entries critique the patient's status at the time of admission, often using FIM levels (rating scale of 1 to 7). A stroke Pathway might include items in medical/nursing, nutrition, swallowing, mobility, self-care, cognition, communication, and others completed by the team. Pathway's tracking also includes discharge planning and community reentry skills. Detailed Pathways can be appended by specific healthcare professionals for each area, as would be the case for a communication assessment by an SLP.

ADDITIONAL DETAILS FOR WRITING IN SCHOOL SETTINGS

Clinicians in school settings use specialized procedures and report formats with components mandated by law (i.e., PL 94-142, PL 99-457, and PL 105-17 IDEA-A). As part of the Individuals with Disabilities Education Act (IDEA) of 2004, a school's intervention assistance team (IAT), which includes a child's parents, may suspect that a child has a disability and so initiate testing. Testing is called a multifactored evaluation because it covers a wide range of skills (e.g., cognitive, language, academic, social-emotional, and visual-motor). The SLP is an important team member. Although there is no mandated format for the IAT evaluation report, four main sections are typical: (1) identifying information, (2) background information, (3) assessment results, and (4) intervention plans. When all components are compiled, the assessment team meets with the parent(s) to explain the results. Information about the student's learning strengths and weaknesses is discussed and, based on federal regulations, the student's eligibility for special education services is decided.

If the student (typically ages 3 to 21 but may include birth through 2 years) qualifies and the parents (or legal guardian) accept, the team determines how best to meet the student's educational needs. An individualized education plan (IEP) must be written to specify goals for the school year. The IEP process is where the SLP details the speech-language goals for the student and the best presentation method for addressing the goals (e.g., in the classroom, through consultation, individual or small-group pullout services, and so forth). The IEP is a student-focused plan devised by the team.

The updated standards to the Individuals with Disabilities Education Act (IDEA) require that IEPs include parent involvement, focus on the general curriculum (so an SLP *must* collaborate with classroom teachers), verify team members as qualified providers, mention needed accommodations, require assessments, and require progress reports. According to Blosser (2011) and the National Center for Learning Disabilities (2014), federal regulations specify the following IEP contents:

- Demographic information and a description of the student's communication impairment
- Present levels of performance (PLOPs) in the educational or curricular setting
- Measurement of annual goals
- Short-term objectives
- IEP team's choice of special education and related services (e.g., type, amount; include accommodations, assistive devices)
- Participation in general education (and extent of participation with students without disabilities)
- Projected dates for initiation of services and the anticipated frequency and duration of the services
- *Objective criteria and evaluation procedures* for progress reports; determining on at least an annual basis whether the short-term instructional objectives are being achieved

The IEP is a working document; the IEP team—including the parents—can make alterations or eliminate goals, as appropriate. Figure 14–3 displays a portion of an IEP prepared for a child with a phonological disorder.

The website of the American Speech-Language-Hearing Association provides assorted resources on the IEP and on SLP responsibilities when working in the schools (www.asha.org). IEP report examples can be found posted on social media. Also, the U.S. Department of Education has published IDEA information and model formats for the IEP; these forms describe the minimal content needed to comply with regulatory requirements. To download the IEP format models and related information, visit http://idea.ed.gov/. The SLP in the schools is also responsible for writing the individualized family service plan (IFSP). The assessment of infants and toddlers (birth to 3 years) presents special considerations in terms of record-keeping and evaluation procedures. Clearly, the family's as well as the child's health are targets of assessment and possible intervention. Public Law 99-457 requires a multidisciplinary team approach to assessment of this population because no single agency or discipline can meet the diverse needs of infants, toddlers, and their families. After assessment, the team is required by law to generate an IFSP that has the following components:

1. A statement of the child's present levels of development (cognitive, speech-language, hearing, motor, self-help, social)
2. A statement of the family's strengths and needs related to enhancing the child's development

FIGURE 14–3

Individualized Educational Plan for a Child with a Phonological Disorder

Student: David Grabowski
Parents: Gerard and Julie
Grade: First
IEP conference date: 9/12/14

Birthdate: 1/7/04 Address: 224 Orchard
District/School: Beaver Grove Schools
District of residency: Marquette County
Projected IEP review date: 9/10/15

Eligibility Statement: (What decision/description requires this service?)
David has difficulty with frictional manner of articulation production resulting in several substitutional errors: th/s, th/z, s/sh, ts/ch, dz/dj.

Current Educational Level: (Where is child currently functioning?)
David is enrolled in a developmental first-grade classroom.

Special Services

Goals	Objectives	Service description
1. David will produce s, z correctly at the word and sentence level. 2. David will produce sh correctly at the word and sentence level. 3. Progress reports will be sent to parents and teacher twice a year.	1. David will discriminate target sounds from other sounds with 90% accuracy. 2. David will produce target sounds at the beginning, middle, and end of single words with 90% accuracy. 3. David will correctly produce target sounds within sentences with 80% success.	Speech therapy

Dates of Services		Time in Programs	Responsible Individuals
Start	End	Daily	Speech-language clinician
9/19/14	5/1/15	Within small-group 20-minute sessions 2 times a week. In regular classroom rest of school week.	Supplementary aides: None

Evaluation Plan: (How is it planned to ascertain that goals have been reached?)
1. Goldman-Fristoe Test of Articulation
2. Pre- and post-therapy word list containing target sounds
3. Five-minute sample of spontaneous speech

IEP Committee Members:

Name	Position
Ellen Mattson	Teacher
Roy Brown, Jr.	Principal
Rebecca Clark	Speech-language clinician
Gerard and Julie Grabowski	Parents

3. A statement of major outcomes expected to be achieved for the child and family
4. The criteria, procedures, and timelines for determining progress
5. The specific early intervention services necessary to meet the unique needs of the child and family, including the method, frequency, and intensity of services
6. The projected dates for the initiation of service and the projected duration

7. The name of the case manager

8. The procedures for transition from early intervention into the preschool

One can readily see that the format of the IFSP has clear implications for assessment. First, it mandates family assessment, which forces the SLP to focus on the child's total environment. Second, it requires that judgments be made in a variety of areas that need multidisciplinary cooperation (e.g., cognitive, social, language, motor, hearing). Third, it requires the practitioner to recommend evaluation procedures to be used to determine progress. The clinician needs to be prepared to address the issues included in the IFSP when he or she participates in staff meetings with other professionals subsequent to his or her evaluations of these children.

IDEA and IDEA-A mandated that schools should plan for the transition of a student with disabilities from school to work or other postsecondary activities from age 14 onward. The assessment of students of this age must be comprehensive to determine and plan for educational, vocational, and social eventualities. The individual transition plan (ITP) is another report format, similar to the IEP, that school-based SLPs write. Blosser (2011) can be consulted for details.

FOLLOW-UP AND REASSESSMENT REPORTS

The clinician's responsibilities do not end when the diagnostic report is written and filed. A complete evaluation includes a final important task: careful follow-up. It is the examiner's professional obligation to determine that the diagnostic activities and recommendations are translated into action; it is useless, perhaps even harmful, to identify and describe problems unless the individual is seen for further testing or treatment (if warranted) as soon as possible. When the diagnostician is also the clinician, the follow-up transition of report information is straightforward. In an agency such as ours (a university speech and hearing clinic), however, we regularly refer clients to other SLPs and professionals for further assessment or treatment. We use the following questions as guidelines in implementing a follow-up program:

1. Did the intended readers receive the report? The best administrative support staff member occasionally misfiles a document, or the mail does not go through, so we generally call the referral source within a week after sending the diagnostic report to determine if it has arrived.

2. Does the reader understand the contents of the report? What questions did it raise, if any, about the client? We always log these phone calls in the client's folder or electronic file.

3. What is the disposition of the client? Is the client being seen for further testing? Is the client on a waiting list or being seen for treatment?

4. How is the client responding to treatment? We call the local professional servicing the client at least once to assess how the client is doing in treatment relative to our recommendations. Not only does this convey our interest and assistance, it also helps the diagnostic team evaluate the efficacy of its work.

Before leaving this discussion on follow-up, we wish to remind the reader that, after the initial diagnostic assessment, there are numerous opportunities to reevaluate the client. Indeed, this is the premise of this text, and it is reflected in its title. Subsequent formal evaluations, informal evaluations, probes, and progress documentation are necessary. The various formats we have presented are easily adapted to these purposes.

REPORTING FINANCIAL ESSENTIALS

Speech-language pathologists want to be reimbursed for their professional services. The days where clients paid independently and with cash for a diagnostic session (or for treatment) are now the exception rather than the rule. Whether the SLP works in a hospital, healthcare facility, community clinic, private practice, school, or other setting, he or she will rely on third-party payors for part or all of the fee due for delivered services. The reality is that SLPs must know the financial essentials of medical coding, and they must apply the accurate code to the "superbill" following services rendered and thereafter to the clinical report and/or form.

Various coding systems exist, and their use depends on the type of facility where the service was provided (acute inpatient, rehabilitation hospital, outpatient clinic, skilled care facility and such), what type of coverage applies to the client (Medicare Part B, Medicaid, etc.), and what services were provided (assessment, treatment, equipment, etc.). Codes may be further classified by the patient's disorder and refined by particular patient specifics (such as extent, onset, severity, and other details). The SLP in any work setting is expected to know details of coding appropriate to that facility and the services provided. This is crucial knowledge for clinicians employed in healthcare settings and those in private practice who bill third parties; SLPs in school systems also often provide services covered by Medicaid, Vocational Rehabilitation Services, and other agencies.

The billing and coding specialist at the facility is a great resource to the SLP; still, the clinician must be well versed in the codes he or she typically uses in the practice. Many books, social media resources, and workshops are available regarding the financial essentials of clinical practice. SLP colleagues in a particular work setting are invaluable mentors. Also, the American Speech-Language-Hearing Association offers information on many coding and reimbursement issues; visit its website at www.asha.org. The monthly ASHA magazine, *Advance,* is an excellent source of information to help members stay abreast of national changes. Here we provide a coding overview.

The ICD-10 System

On October 1, 2015, the United States transitioned to the International Classification of Diseases, 10th Revision. This ICD-10 replaced the outdated and limited ICD-9 system for coding *diagnoses* and also *inpatient procedures.* Widely used in Europe, the ICD-10 is owned by the World Health Organization, but the United States has expanded its features in two important ways.

Procedural Coding System

The procedural coding system, known as ICD-10-PCS, was developed by the U.S. Centers for Medicare and Medicaid Services (CMS). These codes are used in inpatient hospital settings. SLPs performing diagnostic (and treatment) services to inpatients use the ICD-10-PCS.

Clinical Modification

The clinical modification, known as ICD-10-CM, was developed by the Centers for Disease Control and Prevention for use in healthcare settings. It standardizes disease and procedure classifications throughout the nation and is the source for many U.S. health statistics. The ICD-10-CM suits the service delivery diagnostic needs of many speech-language pathologists. In fact, HIPAA requires the use of ICD-10-CM for billing and record keeping. The ICD-10-CM codes are based on an alphanumeric system. Codes are from three to seven characters long: the first character is alphabetic, the second is numeric, and the third and remaining characters are either alphabetic or numeric. These codes are important for use on the superbill and on the diagnostic report. Some example ICD-10-CM diagnostic codes used in speech-language pathology are shown below (additional digits are often added to further specify the patient's diagnostic status:

- F80.0—Specific developmental disorders of speech and language (e.g., phonological disorder)
- R47.01—Aphasia following cerebral cerebrovascular disease
- R49.21—Hypernasality

The Current Procedural Terminology System

Current Procedural Terminology (CPT) codes describe *procedures* that "are done" with the client as opposed to the diagnosis. CPT codes are necessary for reimbursement of services rendered. Most CPT codes in this field signify untimed service units, but a few procedures allow for timed billing. Some examples of both timed and untimed diagnostic procedural codes (there also are treatment procedural codes) are as follows:

- 92521—Evaluation of speech fluency (e.g., stuttering, cluttering)
- 92522—Evaluation of speech sound production (e.g., articulation, phonology, apraxia, dysarthria)
- 92523—Evaluation of speech sound production (e.g., articulation, phonology, apraxia, dysarthria with evaluation of language comprehension and production)
- 92524—Behavioral and qualitative analysis of voice and resonance
- 92520—Laryngeal function study (aerodynamic testing, acoustic testing)
- 92610—Evaluation of oral and pharyngeal swallowing function
- 92612—Evaluation of swallowing with fiberoptic endoscope (FEES)
- 92597—Evaluation for use and/or fitting of voice prosthetic device to supplement oral speech
- Assessment of aphasia—96105 per hour
- Standardized cognitive performance testing—96125 per hour
- Evaluation for speech-generating device—92607 first hour; 92608 each additional 30 minutes

These are just a few of the many CPT codes useful to describe diagnostic efforts. Many other CPT codes are used for treatment procedures; however, a discussion of these is beyond the scope of this text.

Other Codes of Note

CPT codes may be suplemeted by the Healthcare Common Procedural Coding System (HCPCS; Level I and/or Level II). Although some procedures are coded in this system, the HCPCS offen covers devices and supplies with E codes. E codes are alphanumeric. As mentioned earlier, SLPs may be required to report functional outcome measures regardless of work setting; for example, this is required for Medicare Part B beneficiaries. To indicate a postintervention outcome, SLPs must supply the baseline measure on the diagnostic report for future use. When using the ASHA NOMS system for a patient's Functional Communication Measure on a claim's form, the appropriate G code can be provided (G + four digits). A list of G codes can be found on the ASHA web site (www .asha.org). Clinicians providing treatment services need to report G code updates in the 10th session and again at discharge, so reevaluations are a necessity. We also wish to mention that the SLP working with some Medicare patients must supply the patient's severity modifier. Current modifiers are CH (0% impaired), CI, CJ, CK, CL, CM, CN (100% impaired). Details on these are available on social media and through the ASHA website.

Some other codes merit brief mention. Inclusion of a GN modifier specifies that the SLP performed a particular task (for example, the FEES study). Without this GN modifier, it is asumed that the physician, not the SLP, performed the procedure. Z codes may be used with ICD-10-CM to allow for additional findings beyond the current diagnosis of disease, injury, or cause. Z codes span Z00 to Z99. Last, DSM-5 codes are from the *Diagnostic and Statistical Manual of Mental Disorders* (Fifth Edition). Clinicians able to diagnose autism spectrum disorders (social/pragmatic communication disorders) need to know the DSM-5 codes.

CONCLUSION AND SELF-ASSESSMENT

As we close this chapter and this text, we wish to remind the reader that comprehensive assessment must be sensitive to cultural and linguistic diversity and also address the World Health Organization's concern for functional abilities–disabilities. This framework has guided much of the information presented in this text. This text has also shared ASHA's view on the clinical process of assessment: that it may be static (using procedures designed to describe current levels of functioning) and/or dynamic (using hypothesis-testing procedures to identify potentially successful intervention procedures). The comprehensive diagnostic—and report writing—processes presented in this chapter, and indeed in this text, echo the following aspects cited by ASHA as necessary and important:

- Collect and summarize the relevant case history, including medical status; education; vocation; and socioeconomic, cultural, and linguistic background.
- Review the client's auditory, visual, motor, and cognitive status.
- Interview the client and her or his family.
- Measure, with standardized and nonstandardized methods, the specific aspects of speech, spoken and nonspoken language, cognitive-communication, and swallowing function.
- Analyze associated medical, behavioral, environmental, educational, vocational, social, and emotional factors.
- Identify the potential for effective intervention strategies and compensations.
- Select assessment instruments with consideration for documented ecological validity.
- Follow up services to monitor communication and swallowing status and to ensure appropriate intervention and support for individuals with identified speech, language, cognitive-communication, and/or swallowing disorders.

Report writing in the profession takes many and varied forms, but succinct, accurate, clear, and grammatically correct documentation is a necessity and reflects well on the SLP. Preferred practice patterns of documentation (American Speech-Language-Hearing Association, 2004) were presented in this chapter and are summarized as follows:

- Documentation includes pertinent background information; results and interpretation; prognosis; and recommendations indicating the need for further assessment, follow-up, or referral. When intervention is recommended, information is provided concerning the frequency, estimated duration, and type of service (e.g., individual, group, home program) required.

- Documentation addresses the type and severity of the communication or related disorder or difference, associated conditions (e.g., medical or educational diagnoses), and impact on activity and participation (e.g., educational, vocational, social).

- Documentation includes summaries of previous services in accordance with all relevant legal and agency guidelines.

- Results of the assessment are reported, often within 1 to 3 days of the evaluation, to the SLP's work facility. A confidential copy may be provided, as appropriate, to any referral source and to the individual patient (or parent/caregiver if the patient is a minor).

- The privacy and security of documentation are maintained in compliance with HIPAA, FERPA, and other state and federal laws. The patient's consent in writing is recommended before any report dissemination beyond the referral source.

After reading this chapter you should be able to answer the following questions:

1. What are some necessary components (headings) of a comprehensive diagnostic report?
2. Why are clinical impressions important to formulate in a diagnostic report?
3. Explain each component of a SOAP note as used to report an initial screening.
4. Explain what the FERPA and HIPPA public laws have to do with clinical reports.
5. Defend the necessity of the SLP knowing relevant billing codes.

Appendix A

The Oral Peripheral Examination

To cover the diagnosis and evaluation of a multitude of clinical disorders adequately in this text, we have consolidated information on the oral exam here. Each disorder chapter references this appendix and also mentions salient information pertinent to that disorder. Regardless of the patient's age and the presenting complaint, the speech-language pathologist (SLP) should examine the oral peripheral structures and their functions. This can be a cursory look or a detailed appraisal, as warranted. Anatomical aberrations may underlie the communication disorder, as in a cleft of the lip and/or palate. Neuromuscular issues may result in speech-sound misarticulations or motor control difficulties (e.g., dysarthria, apraxia), but these issues also underlie nonspeech disorders of feeding and swallowing. Whether the SLP calls the exam the oral motor exam, the oral peripheral examination, or simply the oral exam, he or she clearly needs to be skilled at efficiently assessing the normalcy of each patient's intraoral, facial, and pharyngeal structures as well as his or her neuromotor integrity. With our territory now laid before us, let us begin our journey with the oral exam.

An examination of a client's oral cavity and surrounding area is a routine part of every speech-language evaluation. Regardless of the client's particular communication impairment, the findings of the oral peripheral examination may help shape a theory of etiology, diagnosis, and prognosis for change and provide a direction that the treatment should take. To avoid repetition in the chapters of this text, we thought it best to consolidate our discussion of the oral peripheral examination in one place. The oral peripheral examination not only looks at structures but also assesses the function of those structures from a motoric point of view, so we thought it most appropriate to include it in our discussion in this appendix. Indeed, the oral peripheral examination is often called the oral motor exam, a reflection of the importance of motoric integrity for normal speech production.

As we said, it is common practice to inspect a client's oral region to determine its structural and functional adequacy for speech. To provide an example of typical data gathered during an oral peripheral examination, we have included notes hastily scribbled during an evaluation of a 9-year-old boy with a hoarse voice and several articulation errors:

> Lips look okay. No asymmetry of face. Slight open bite; poor dental hygiene (lots of cavities and tartar buildup). Tongue has good mobility, no paralysis or sluggishness; can protrude, wiggle from side to side swiftly, and touch the alveolar ridge; can even curl and groove. Hard palate seems okay, no scars. Soft palate has good tissue supply; elevated fine, no asymmetry. Palatine tonsils are *really* enlarged, filling the whole isthmus between the fauces. Pharynx looks inflamed (possible postnasal drip?). Good gag reflex. Wonder why he has mandible thrust to left side on /ʃ/ and /tʃ/?

Note the systematic nature of the inspection. Although the period of observation was relatively brief—an oral examination is generally completed in less than 2 minutes—the clinician has a sound basis for making a referral to a laryngologist.

Now we shall present a rather detailed procedure for conducting an oral examination.

Tools You Will Need

You will need a light source; a small flashlight is good (we avoid the head mirror because it makes us look like physicians). Next, we obtain a supply of wooden tongue depressors; the individually wrapped ones are best for sanitary purposes. We also find the cherry-flavored tongue depressors are popular with children (you can find these supplies at www.superduperinc.com). Because we are living in the age of HIV/AIDS and other contagious diseases, the prudent clinician should wear sterile gloves, or at least use a finger cot, when palpating the roof of the client's mouth. Your examination kit should also include several pads of cotton gauze (for holding onto tongues), a small mirror that fits under the patient's nostrils, and perhaps a few candy suckers. For more elaborate or specialized examinations, additional materials may be needed, for example, cotton-tipped applicators, various flavor vials for taste sensation, oral stereognostic forms, bite blocks, a syringe and/or cup of water, some cookies or crackers, and the like.

Areas to Be Assessed

It is important to be *systematic* and *swift* when conducting an oral examination. This demands considerable practice. Use every opportunity to scrutinize normal-speaking persons of all ages, not only to perfect your technique and observational skills but also to establish a frame of reference on the range of normal structural and functional variation. The following list is presented as a basic guide for conducting a typical oral peripheral examination:

1. *Lips and Lip Movement.* Inspect the lips first for relative size, symmetry, and scars. Can the client smile, pucker the lips, and retract them? Can she or he close the lips tightly for the sounds /p/, /b/, /m/? Can the client utter the nonsense syllable *puh* at least once per second?

2. *Jaws.* Scrutinize the client's jaw in a state of rest; observe for symmetry. Can he or she open and close the mandible at least once per second? Does the mandible deviate to the right or the left on opening? Assess mandibular strength by having the client attempt to open or move his or her jaw laterally against resistance.

3. *Teeth.* Inspect the client's bite during a state of rest. A normal dental bite is characterized by the upper incisors overlapping the lower incisors by not more than one half of their vertical dimension. Is there an open, under-, or overbite? Does the client have cavities, jumbled teeth, gaps between teeth, or more than the normal complement of teeth? Does he or she wear a dental prosthesis?

4. *Tongue.* Note the size of the tongue relative to the oral cavity (macroglossia may suggest an endocrine disorder). Observe the tongue for symmetry of structure, and observe it during movement (in hypoglossal nerve palsy, the tongue deviates to the side of the palsy). Is there any scarring, atrophy, or fasciculations? (Fasciculations suggest motor neuron disease.) Can the client protrude and retract the tongue, wiggle it from side to side, and touch the alveolar ridge without random movement or extraordinary effort? Inspect the tip of the tongue and the frenulum for any evidence of tongue tie. See Kummer (2005) and Messner and Lalakea (2002) for discussion of ankyloglossia and speech. Some clients, especially those presenting with neuromuscular problems, may find it difficult to elevate the tip of the tongue to the alveolar ridge on command. Place a moistened piece of hard candy behind the upper incisors and encourage the client to go after it. (A spot of peanut butter or a tiny paper wedged high between the central incisors can also be used.) Can the client trill his or her tongue when the mandible is stabilized? Test for diadochokinesis by having him or her utter *tuh*; can he or she say this

TABLE A–1
Diadochokinetic Rate Assessment

Definition and Purpose

Diadochokinetic (DDK) rate assesses the client's ability to make rapid alternating speech movements. It is a maximum repetition rate task that is a form of alternating motion rates (AMRs), a term often used among neurology professionals. The speed of movement, along with the observed rhythm and coordination, are indicators of neuromuscular integrity. The premise is that DDK increases as a child ages and as the neuromotor system matures, and that there are expected declines in speed among the elderly. DDK rates outside the expected norm and patterns of any discoordination are helpful in the differential diagnosis of certain disorders.

Types of Stimuli Used

Single, double, and/or triple syllables may be used, for example, *puh-puh-puh, puh-tuh, puh-tuh,* and *puh-tuh-kuh, puh-tuh-kuh,* respectively. Triple syllables rapidly change place of articulation from anterior to posterior (bilabial, lingualveolar, linguavelar). Alternative stimuli for use with clients include words such as *pattycake* and *buttercup.*

Method of Measurement

Provide instructions, stressing the importance of doing the task as fast as possible. Allow practice. Use a stopwatch or similar instrument. For measuring DDK rate, it is typical to average three trials per type of stimulus (single, double, and triple syllables). Two methods of measurement are used clinically:

1. *Count-by-time method:* Count the number of syllables repeated by the client within a predetermined number of seconds. Example: The number of *puh* syllables uttered within 15 seconds.
2. *Fletcher time by count method:* Time the number of seconds necessary for the client to repeat a predetermined number of syllables. Example: The number of seconds needed for the client to produce 20 repetitions of *puh.*

Select one method, and take care to compare the client's results to normative data using the same method.

Norms

Use published norms appropriate for DDK method used. Selected sources include the following:

For children: Canning and Rose (1974), Fletcher (1972), St. Louis and Ruscello (2000), Yaruss and Logan (2002).
For adults: Dabul (2000), Prathanee (1998), Sonies at al. (1987).

Our Rule of Thumb

The client's level of effort, smoothness, and coordination matters as much or more than the count, although a syllable count below 5 is cause for concern for speech production at any age.

---

nonsense syllable at least once per second? Can the client say *pattycake* swiftly and repeatedly? Be sure to look for regularity as well as rate in any tongue movement task. This is important in patients suspected of motor speech disorders. Table A–1 provides more information on diadochokinetic rate testing. Is there any evidence of tongue thrust? (An open bite in a child might alert you to this possibility.) When the person swallows, does he or she have an exaggerated lip seal? Does his or her tongue protrude beyond the incisors? Is there no apparent bunching in the masseter muscle? (If the answers to these last three queries are positive, then the client may be a tongue thruster.)

5. *Hard Palate.* Note the shape (is it flat? high and arched?) and width of the hard palate. Are there any scars present? Is there any blue coloration to the palate (suggestive

of a submucous cleft)? Can you palpate solid bone under the tissues at the palatal mid-line? Can the client produce /r/ and /l/?

6. *Soft palate and velopharyngeal closure.* Inspect the velum for total size, scars, and symmetry of movement. Is it bifid? Look carefully for any variations in color, such as bluish borders or striations. Does the soft palate move back and up toward the posterior pharyngeal wall? What is the size of the velum relative to the depth of the pharynx? Can you visualize lateral movement of the velum? Can the client whistle or puff up his or her cheeks? (Chapter 12 presents details for assessing velopharyngeal competency as it relates to hypernasality and nasal emission.)

7. *Fauces.* Inspect the pillars for scars, the status of the palatine tonsils, and the width of the isthmus. Check the general condition of the oropharynx.

8. *Others.* Observe the client's breathing during speech and at rest. Is there an obstruction of the nasal passages? Is the client a mouth breather? Observe the facial muscles: Is a nasolabial fold flattened? Does an eyelid droop (ptosis)? Is one side of the face smooth and devoid of normal creases? Is there anything unusual about the appearance of the individual's head or spacing of the facial features?

The preceding list is typical of the methodical process that clinicians do, albeit swiftly, with all clients. Indeed, the oral peripheral examination can be done with the basics of a light, gloves, and tongue depressor and the clinical knowledge just listed. Obviously, with some types of clients, more attention to detail will be necessary. For instance, when working with a pediatric case exhibiting a cleft of the lip and/or palate, more time will be needed to document both structural aberrations and functional impact fully. With an adult exhibiting a neuromuscular disorder, additional tasks and details are help-ful in differentially diagnosing the type of disorder, which affects treatment planning. The consensus-based adult Motor Speech Evaluation Template, which is available from the American Speech-Language-Hearing Association (ASHA), is a detailed and useful resource. You can find the template at the ASHA website (www.asha.org).

Numerous oral examination checklists can be found online by searching social me-dia. We caution readers, however, because many of these checklists are cursory in na-ture, and many lack guidance about what constitutes normal and how observations are to be rated or scored. For the beginning clinician, we have found the Oral-Peripheral Exam tutorial (available online at http://firstyears.org) to be informative with regard to observations of the face, teeth and bite, tongue mobility, and the like, in children.

An excellent journal article regarding adult oral motor functioning is written by Sonies et al. (1987). These authors developed a scale to assess three areas: oral anatomy, physiology, and speech. Ten categories cover each area, and each is rated on a 4-point severity scale (1 = normal, 2 = mild, 3 = moderate, 4 = severe). Some weighting of measures is done to obtain a profile of performance. Anatomy ratings include assess-ment of the appearance of facial bones, tissues, and oral facial symmetry. Physiology ratings include assessment of range of motion; strength; precision; speed of lingual, labial, palatal, velar, and facial muscles; and oral sensation. Swallowing function, a sub-component of the scale, is assessed from a questionnaire, an ultrasound visualization of the swallowing act, mealtime observations, and a medical history. Speech ratings include articulation, voice, fluency, and diadochokinetic rate.

Commercially available tools also exist for conducting oral peripheral examina-tions. Some are general; others focus more on certain neuromotor or swallowing as-pects. Table A–2 lists some resources for the clinician. We will highlight a few.

A popular commercial product for use with clients between the ages of 5 to 77 years is the *Oral Speech Mechanism Screening Examination* (OSME-3) by St. Louis and

TABLE A–2
Commercially Available Oral Peripheral Assessment Tools and Their Use According to Age Range

Dworkin-Culatta Oral Mechanism Examination and Treatment (D-COME) (Dworkin & Culatta, 1996)—Can be tolerated at any age.
Oral-Motor Feeding Rating Scale (Jelm, 1990)—Age 1 year to adult.
Oral Speech Mechanism Screening Examination (OSME-3) (St. Louis & Ruscello, 2000)— Ages 5 to 78.
Screening Test for Developmental Apraxia of Speech (STDAS-2) (Blakely, 2001)—Ages 4 to 12.
Test of Oral Structures and Functions (TOSF-1) (Vitali, 1986)—Age 7 to adult.

Ruscello (2000). By using the scoring form and the demonstration audio CD training that is provided in the kit, the SLP may make more reliable judgments. Because it is a screening tool rather than a detailed diagnostic assessment, the OSME-3 provides little to no guidance for planning treatment.

The *Dworkin-Culatta Oral Mechanism Examination and Treatment* (D-COME) (Dworkin & Culatta, 1996) is a lengthy assessment for clients at any age because it takes 30 to 40 minutes to administer. It is particularly useful with organic cases (e.g., clefts, neuromuscular disorders). However, it does include a short Screening Test Checklist Form for quick use that can be copied and reproduced. The D-COME is available at www20 .csueastbay.edu/class/departments/commsci/files/docs/pdf/Dworkin-Culatta_ Oral_Mech_Exam.pdf.

Another commercial oral motor screening tool is the *Screening Test for Developmental Apraxia of Speech*, Second Edition (STDAS-2; Blakely, 2001). The STDAS-2 is appropriate for children between the ages of 4 to almost 8 years. Because it is a screening test, the reader is cautioned against using it to make a diagnostic decision, especially with regard to the complex disorder of apraxia.

It may be obvious to the reader now that some assessment instruments are more detailed than others and that some seem to weigh heavily certain aspects of the total oral peripheral examination. Specific oral examination protocols exist for individuals with cleft lip and/or palate, childhood apraxia, pediatric feeding and swallowing difficulties, stuttering, various adult neurogenic disorders, and so forth. Specific oral motor examinations may be covered in the disorders chapters. We suggest that the reader observe a variety of video examples of clinicians performing oral peripheral examinations; many are available online. Some social media samples are efficient screenings. Others demonstrate more detailed aspects, such as attention to hygienic principles, nasal emission fogging a mirror, oral motor strength and coordination, cranial nerve assessment, taste sensitivity, bedside swallowing screening, and more. We wish to cite the 9-minute *Extraoral and Intraoral Examination* from the West Los Angeles College of Dental Hygiene as an example of a thorough neuromotor and oral structural assessment (see www.youtube.com/watch?v=78r3d4qa9A0). Video clips of neurologists performing cranial nerve examinations are also beneficial for SLPs to watch, particularly because these examinations are similar to the way that SLPs elicit patient performance in swallowing and speech relative to the functioning of cranial nerves V to XII. One such example is at www.youtube.com/watch?v=G6FZR64Cq9U.

At some point in the not-too-distant future, the diagnostician may have instruments that measure tongue, lip, and other movements very precisely.

To conclude our discussion of the oral peripheral examination, we would like to remind the reader that one swallow does not make a summer, and one deviancy in the oral area does not necessarily cause disordered speech.

Appendix B

Assessment Resources

1. Developmental Milestones
2. Transcription Symbols Selected from the International Phonetic Alphabet
3. Screening the Client's Hearing
4. Hearing-Related Questions to Ask a Parent
5. Auditory Processing Disorder Considerations
6. Reading Passages Useful in Assessing Speech and Language

DEVELOPMENTAL MILESTONES

When assessing infants and children, the speech-language pathologist (SLP) collects information on attainment of developmental milestones. This may be done through a case history form completed by the parent or guardian and/or through a case history interview. The child's attainment of milestones in motor development, play, learning, speaking, social-behavior areas, and so forth, matters to the SLP doing a thorough diagnostic evaluation.

Resource information on developmental milestones, from birth to age 5, is available online from the Centers for Disease Control and Prevention at www.cdc.gov/ncbddd/actearly/milestones/index.html. Age-appropriate information can be selected from this site for the following developmental periods:

- 2 months
- 4 months
- 6 months
- 9 months
- 1 year

- 18 months
- 2 years
- 3 years
- 4 years
- 5 years

The SLP can also download a milestone checklist from this website. A video on milestones called "Baby Steps," which is suitable for parents, can also be accessed from the CDC's website.

TRANSCRIPTION SYMBOLS SELECTED FROM THE INTERNATIONAL PHONETIC ALPHABET

Commonly used English language phoneme symbols for consonants and vowels are shown in the following chart, along with sample allographs and place/manner of production.

Phoneme	Allograph	Description
/b/	*b*at, ra*bb*i, *b*ack*b*oard	Voice bilabial stop
/p/	*p*urse, *pupp*y, cu*p*	Voiceless bilabial stop
/d/	*d*og, *d*a*dd*y, shoul*d*	Voiced lingua-alveolar (apical) stop
/t/	*t*ry, *t*a*tt*oo, ca*t*	Voiceless lingua-alveolar (apical) stop
/g/	*g*oat, a*g*o, do*g*	Voiced lingua-velar (dorsal) stop
/k/	*c*up, oc*c*ur, la*k*e, fol*k*	Voiceless lingua-velar (dorsal) stop
/v/	*v*ase, ri*v*er, li*v*e	Voiced labiodental fricative
/f/	*f*ood, a*f*ter, sta*ff*	Voiceless labiodental fricative
/ð/	*th*is, *th*ey, fa*th*er	Voiced lingua-dental fricative
/θ/	*th*umb, ma*th*, wi*th*	Voiceless lingua-dental fricative
/z/	*z*oom, a*s*thma, pu*zz*le, bu*zz*	Voiced lingua-alveolar fricative
/s/	*s*afe, *c*ity, cu*s*p, pa*ss*	Voiceless lingua-alveolar fricative
/ʒ/	mea*s*ure, rou*g*e, apha*s*ia	Voiced lingua-palatal fricative

Continued

Phoneme	Allograph	Description
/ʃ/	*sheep*, *sugar*, *ocean*, *push*	Voiceless lingua-palatal fricative
/h/	*he*, *happy*, *who*	Voiceless glottal fricative
/m/	*moon*, *summer*, *poem*	Bilabial nasal
/n/	*new*, *knife*, *renew*, *sign*	Lingua-alveolar (apical) nasal
/ŋ/	*sing*, *finger*, *tongue*	Lingua-velar (dorsal) nasal
/l/	*loop*, *island*, *tall*	Lingua-alveolar lateral
/r/	*rude*, *carry*, *rhyme*, *right*	Alveolar rhotic or retroflex
/dʒ/	*judge*, *gem*, *bridge*	Voiced palatal affricate
/tʃ/	*chess*, *nature*, *watch*	Voiceless palatal affricate
/w/	*worn*, *one*, *wow*	Voiced labial and velar glide (semivowel)
/ʍ/	*which*, *while*	Voiceless labial and velar fricative/glide
/j/	*yellow*, *yes*, *onion*	Voiced palatal glide (semivowel)
/i/	*peep*, *she*, *beat*	High-front, tense, and unrounded vowel
/ɪ/	*hit*, *sitting*, *tip*	High-mid, front, lax, and unrounded vowel
/ɛ/	*set*, *bed*,	Low-mid, front, lax, and unrounded vowel
/e/	*cake*, *chaos*	Mid-front, tense, and unrounded vowel
/æ/	*had*, *cat*, *black*	Low-front, lax, and unrounded vowel
/ə/	*away*, *cinema*	Mid-central, lax, and unrounded vowel (unstressed)
/ʌ/	*cup*, *luck*, *bud*	Low-mid, back-central, lax, and unrounded vowel (stressed)
/ɚ/	*butter*, *teacher*	Mid-central, lax, and rounded vowel
/ɝ/	*bird*, *purr*, *her*	Mid-central, tense, rounded vowel
/u/	*blue*, *food*, *boot*	High-back tense, and rounded vowel
/ʊ/	*put*, *hood*, *could*	High-mid, back, lax, and rounded vowel
/o/	*hoe*, *stow*	Mid-back, tense, and rounded vowel
/ɔ/	*four*, *ball*, *frog*	Low-mid, back, tense, and rounded vowel
/ɑ/	*hot*, *rock*, *Boston*	Low-back, tense, and unrounded vowel
/aɪ/	*light*, *five*, *eye*	Diphthong (low-back to mid-/high-front)
/aʊ/	*now*, *out*, *brown*	Diphthong (low/low-mid back to mid-back/high-mid-back)
/eɪ/	*say*, *eight*, *bait*	Diphthong (mid-front to high-mid front)
/oʊ/	*go*, *home*, *boat*	Diphthong (mid-back to high-mid-back)
/ɔɪ/	*boy*, *join*, *coy*	Diphthong (low-mid-back/mid-back to mid-to-high-front position)

SCREENING THE CLIENT'S HEARING

When conducting a thorough diagnostic evaluation, a hearing screening test should be included. Pure tone air conduction testing, administered in a quiet room with a portable audiometer, is typical. Test procedures may vary depending on state licensing standards. Guidelines for hearing screening procedures for the SLP are based on recommendations from government agencies, the American Academy of Audiology, and the American Speech-Language-Hearing Association (ASHA).

When to Refer

This overview describes a hearing screening for a cooperative client using pure tones, a portable audiometer, and earphones. The SLP should refer the client to a certified audiologist in cases of:

- Newborn screening/testing
- Very young children (birth to 3 years) and/or difficult testing with children requiring sound-field (not earphones) testing or play audiometry
- A client of any age with a known hearing loss or a history of ear disorders (e.g., frequent ear infections)
- Failure of the hearing screening (see below)

Patient Performance

Prior to placement of the earphones, the SLP explains the test procedure and how the client should respond. The client is asked to respond when the tone is (faintly) heard. Typical responses include (1) raise a finger or hand, (2) say yes or nod, or (3) press a button.

What to Test

A hearing screening determines whether or not the client hears various tones (frequencies) in each ear (left and right ears assessed separately) at predetermined intensity levels (dB HL). The frequencies and intensity levels to assess may vary depending on the age of the client, the test environment, and other work-setting and/or state guidelines. In general, the following screening guidelines should be considered:

- Screen clients age 3 (chronologically and developmentally) and older.
- For ages 3 to 40 or 50 years, test frequencies 500 (optional), 1,000, 2,000, and 4,000 Hz at 20 dB HL.
- For adults 50 and older, test frequencies 1,000, 2,000, and 4,000 Hz at 25 dB HL.

Note: Tympanometry (middle ear) testing is within the scope of practice for SLPs. When tympanometry is included, the selection of test frequencies may be adjusted.

What Constitutes Failure

Screenings are either pass or fail. The client fails the hearing screening when he or she does not hear even one test frequency in one or both ears. The client should be referred to an audiologist for an audiological evaluation.

HEARING-RELATED QUESTIONS TO ASK THE PARENT OF A CLIENT

During the case history interview for a child being evaluated for a possible speech-language disorder, the clinician should ask the parent or guardian the following questions about the child's hearing ability:

1. Have you been concerned about your child's hearing?
2. Does your child currently have an ear infection? How frequently does your child have an ear infection?
3. Is there a history of hearing loss in tour family? Describe.
4. When your child is sleeping in a quiet room, does a loud noise cause him or her to awaken?
5. Does your child turn his or her head directly toward a loud sound?
6. Does your child respond to his or her name being spoken and turn to look at the speaker?
7. Is your child beginning to repeat some of the sounds that you make?
8. Did your child receive a newborn hearing screening? Is so, what were the results?
9. Has your child suffered from any of the following: head injury, mumps, meningitis, encephalitis, cerebral palsy, or birth defects?
10. Was your child in an intensive care nursery after birth?
11. Were there issues at birth (Apgar scores of 0 to 4 at 1 minute or 0 to 6 at 5 minutes)?
12. What medications does your child take? What medications has your child taken? (Check for ototoxicity.)

AUDITORY PROCESSING DISORDER CONSIDERATIONS

An auditory processing disorder (APD), previously known as a central auditory processing disorder (CAPD), remains a controversial, if not missed, diagnosis. Often there is no hearing acuity problem, or there is only a mild deficit, in children with APD. Rather than hearing, the issue in APD is more listening, or "what is done" with the incoming auditory signal; hence, the emphasis is on processing. The disorder is difficult to define and there is no consensus on whether its basis is auditory-phonological or cognitive-linguistic. It is accepted that a poor auditory signal at the peripheral level (ear) can result in poor representation in the central auditory nervous system (brain). In this manner, the child with repeated otitis media (middle ear infections) often has difficulties in processing auditory stimuli, particularly if the speech-language is presented rapidly and/or with competing background noise (or other degraded conditions). The child with APD has trouble listening and learning in the classroom. Academic failure is one of the reasons a child is brought by the parent for an evaluation. It is clear that a modality-general approach to assessment (more than just auditory) is needed with this population of children. However, findings often mimic other conditions and may make a differential diagnosis difficult. Some symptoms of APD may be similar to those of other language-based issues, learning disabilities, attention deficit disorder (ADD), attention deficit hyperactivity disorder (ADHD), Asperger syndrome and other spectrum disorders, dyslexia, and specific language impairments. Even when APD is diagnosed, some school districts do not consider it a qualifying diagnosis for services; thus, school-age children may be treated under other diagnoses, such as a receptive language disorder. Common symptoms of APD may include the following (the first two are considered core APD features):

- Increased difficulty listening in a noisy background
- Difficulty processing speech-language that is temporally altered (e.g., fast)
- Intermittent inability to process verbal information
- Difficulty following complex verbal instructions
- Increased difficulty with verbal skills–based curricula (e.g., reading, learning second language, math), and other so-called left hemisphere functions

APD is difficult to detect and relies on subjective symptoms (like those listed above), which are usually noticed by teachers, parents, and others. Such concerns lead to a specialized evaluation. A team approach to diagnosis and intervention is important. Typically, the child suspected of having an APD is evaluated by a neurologist. Children with APD often have no evidence of neurological disease, however, and so the diagnosis is made on the basis of performance on behavioral tests that tap the child's ability to interpret sounds and verbal information. To date, there is no consensus on testing for APD, although common themes of evaluation exist among audiologists and speech-language pathologists, and perhaps school psychologists.

A hearing assessment, not just a screening, is needed. An audiologist should also perform specialized central auditory nervous system testing, such as temporal processing, speech comprehension in noise, dichotic listening, and ability to comprehend degraded speech (speech that is filtered to reduce high frequencies or that is rapid in speed).

The SLP's role in assessing APD includes administering a thorough language test. Supplementary testing that we like to use includes the follwing:

- *Test of Auditory Processing Skills* (TAP-3) (Gardner, 2005)
- *Revised Token Test* (McNeil & Prescott, 1978)
- Selected oral language subtests from the *Woodcock-Johnson IV* (Schrank, McGrew, Mather, & Woodcock, 2014)

READING PASSAGES USEFUL IN ASSESSING SPEECH AND LANGUAGE

Reading passages have long been used in the various assessments of speech, language, voice, and fluency. The following passages are considered standard in clinical practice, and some are appropriate for different grade-level reading abilities:

- The Rainbow
- The Zoo
- My Grandfather
- The Caterpillar
- The Night Sky

These passages are provided next.

THE RAINBOW PASSAGE *(Reading Level: Adult) The Rainbow passage is attributed to Grant Fairbanks (1960) and is in the public domain. The Rainbow passage, particularly its popular first paragraph, is said to contain all English sounds in proportion to usage in the* *language; however, the representativeness of phonetic frequency has been challenged (Zurinskas, 2009). The Rainbow has become one of the most widely used reading passages, not only in the field of communication disorders but also among other healthcare professionals and educators. SLPs find the 100-word passage (including title) useful for quick calculations of percentage errors. Percentage of disfluent words is an example. For use in assessing resonance, note that the passage contains 11.5% nasal consonants.*

The Rainbow

When the sunlight strikes raindrops in the air, they act like a prism and form a rainbow. A rainbow is the division of white light into many beautiful colors. These take the shape of a large, round arch, with its path high above and its two ends apparently beyond the horizon. There is, according to legend, a boiling pot of gold at one end. People look but no one ever finds it. When a man looks for something beyond his reach, his friends say he is looking for the pot of gold at the end of the rainbow.

Source: FAIRBANKS, GRANT, VOICE ARTICULATION DRILLBOOK, 1st Ed., c1960. Reprinted and Electronically reproduced by permission of Pearson Education, Inc., Upper Saddle River, New Jersey.

THE ZOO PASSAGE *(Reading Level: Child, Grade Not Specified) Since its introduction, the Zoo passage (Fletcher, 1978) has been a popular reading sample in the assessment of resonance. It provides a 71-word sample of speech that is devoid of any normally nasal consonants. This facilitates perceptual listening for hypernasality on vowels (not influenced by nasal consonants). Also, the passage is used in instrumental analysis of the voice with the KayPENTAX Nasometer (www.kaypentax.com).*

Zoo

Look at this book with us. It's a story about a zoo. That is where bears go. Today it's very cold out of doors, but we see a cloud overhead that's a pretty white fluffy shape. We hear that straw covers the floor of cages to keep the chill away; yet a deer walks through the trees with her head high. They feed seeds to birds so they're able to fly.

Source: FLETCHER, SAM, DIAGNOSING SPEECH DISORDERS FROM CLEFT PALATE, c1978. Reprinted under Fair Use.

MY GRANDFATHER PASSAGE *(Reading Level: Adult or Child, Grade 5) Often falsely attributed to another, Van Riper (1963) created the now-standard reading passage of My Grandfather for his early books on speech correction. Content of the passage recently has been linked to the author's love of Sherlock Holmes novels (Reilly & Fisher, 2012). Over the years this passage has become popular for speech assessments in stuttering, aphasia, reading disorders, and motor speech disorders (the later bolstered by its use at the Mayo Clinic). According to Reilly and Fisher (2012), the passage contains a diverse sample of English speech sounds "in isolation and in improbable clusters (e.g., frock, zest)" that present the reader with articulatory, semantic, and syntactic demands likely to challenge the patient and unmask problems. Attributes of the passage, according to Patel et al. (2013), include 133 words, 177 syllables, a 1.33 word:syllable ratio, 15.9 mean length of utterance, and a fifth-grade reading level.*

My Grandfather

You wish to know all about my grandfather. Well, he is nearly 93 years old, yet he still thinks as swiftly as ever. He dresses himself in an ancient, black frock coat, usually minus several buttons.

A long, flowing beard clings to his chin, giving those who observe him a pronounced feeling of the utmost respect. When he speaks his voice is just a bit cracked and quivers a trifle. Twice each day he plays skillfully and with zest upon a small organ.

Except in the winter when the snow or ice prevents, he slowly takes a short walk in the open air each day. We have often urged him to walk more and smoke less but he always answers, "Banana oil!" Grandfather likes to be modern in his language.

Source: VAN RIPER, SPEECH CORRECTION: PRINCIPLES & METHODS, 4th Ed., c1963. Reprinted and Electronically reproduced by permission of Pearson Education, Inc., Upper Saddle River, New Jersey.

THE CATERPILLAR PASSAGE (*Reading Level: Child, Grade 5*) *A novel reading passage was developed for the assessment and differentiation of motor speech disorders by Patel et al. (2013). The Caterpillar purports to distinguish between and among speech errors typical of dysarthria versus apraxia of speech. This is based on the passage's complexity, words of increasing length, word repetitions, prosody fluctuations, and the like. The authors state that the 197-word passage contains 261 syllables, a 1.33 word:syllable ratio, 13.4 mean length of utterance, and a fifth-grade reading level.*

The Caterpillar

Do you like amusement parks? Well, I sure do. To amuse myself, I went twice last spring. My most MEMORABLE moment was riding on the Caterpillar, which is a gigantic rollercoaster high above the ground. When I saw how high the Caterpillar rose into the bright blue sky I knew it was for me. After waiting in line for thirty minutes, I made it to the front where the man measured my height to see if I was tall enough. I gave the man my coins, asked for change, and jumped on the cart. Tick, tick, tick, the Caterpillar climbed slowly up the tracks. It went SO high I could see the parking lot. Boy was I SCARED! I thought to myself, "There's no turning back now." People were so scared they screamed as we swiftly zoomed fast, fast, and faster along the tracks. As quickly as it started, the Caterpillar came to a stop. Unfortunately, it was time to pack the car and drive home. That night I dreamt of the wild ride on the Caterpillar. Taking a trip to the amusement park and riding on the Caterpillar was my MOST memorable moment ever!

Source: Republished with permission of American Speech-Language-Hearing Association, from "The caterpillar": A novel reading passage for assessment of motor speech disorders, R. Patel et al., American Journal of Speech-Language pathology, 22(1), 1–9, 2013; permission conveyed through Copyright Clearance Center, Inc.

THE NIGHT SKY PASSAGE (*Reading Level: Grade 2*) *This expository reading passage is part of a reading skill inventory, level 2. It consists of 125 words, with an assortment of nasal and nonnasal sounds.*

The Night Sky

Look up at the sky at night. If it is a clear night, you will see stars. How many stars are there? No one knows for sure. But there is one star that you know by name. You can see it in the daytime. It is our sun. The sun is a star. All stars are suns. Our sun is so close that we cannot see other stars in the day. We only see the other suns at night.

Stars are made up of very hot gas, and they seem to twinkle because of the air moving across them. Even though we can't always see them, they are always in the sky, even in the daytime.

Source: COOTER, ROBERT B.; FLYNT, E. SUTTON; COOTER, KATHLEEN SPENCER, THE FLYNT/COOTER COMPREHENSIVE READING INVENTORY-2: ASSESSMENT OF K–12 READING SKILLS IN ENGLISH & SPANISH, 2nd Ed., c2014. Reprinted and Electronically reproduced by permission of Pearson Education, Inc., Upper Saddle River, New Jersey.

Appendix C

Early Child Language Assessment Interview Protocol

GENERAL INFORMATION
Pertinent History

- Referral source:
- Parent's statement of the problem:
- History of prior assessments:
- History of prior treatments:
- Parental treatment attempts:
- Daycare/preschool status:
- Number and relationships of people living at home:

BIOLOGICAL PREREQUISITES FOR COMMUNICATION DEVELOPMENT
Birth and General Health

- Pregnancy:
- Birth:
- History of childhood illnesses:
- Present state of child's health:

Auditory Status

- History of frequent colds:
- History of earaches and ear infections:
- Parent's estimation of hearing acuity:

Neurological Status

- Concussions/unconsciousness:
- Seizures:
- Has the child been seen by a neurologist? For what condition?
- Does the child evidence any motor difficulties?

GENERAL DEVELOPMENT

- Concern about self-help skills?
- Concern about fine and gross motor development?
- Concern about social development?
- Concern about communication development?

SOCIAL PREREQUISITES FOR COMMUNICATION DEVELOPMENT

- Approximate time spent in social interaction on typical day:
- Who are the persons the child frequently interacts with?
- What are the activities associated with social interactions?
- Does the child exhibit any antisocial or socially inappropriate behaviors (avoiding interactions, consistent playing alone)?
- Does the child exhibit any self-stimulating behaviors (e.g., rocking, flapping arms, etc.)?
- Does the child maintain eye contact?
- Does the child regulate an adult's behavior nonverbally through gestures or physical manipulation?
- Does the child use objects or repeat actions to get an adult's attention?
- Does the child vocalize during his or her social interactions?
- Does the child joint-reference with the caretaker?
- Describe the child's typical day in detail:

COGNITIVE PREREQUISITES TO COMMUNICATION DEVELOPMENT

Does the child exhibit play routines and behavior that would indicate the following attainments (specify example activity):

- Object permanence:
- Means–end:
- Immediate imitation:
- Functional use of objects:
- Deferred imitation:
- Symbolic play with own body:
- Symbolic play with objects:
- Symbolic play with surrogate objects:
- Distal pointing:
- Combining more than one object at a time in play:
- What are the child's most frequent play activities?

COMMUNICATION DEVELOPMENT

- Does the child exhibit phonetically consistent forms?
- Parent estimation of the number of single words used expressively:
- Parent estimation of mean length of utterance (MLU):
- Reports of presyntactic devices?
- Parent's report of semantic relation types:
- Parent's estimate of language comprehension:
- Parent estimate of child's intelligibility:

Appendix D

Coding Sheet for Early Multiword Analysis

Child   *Post–Stage I*

Utterance	Semantic Relation	Function	Initiation	Element
"Pushing car"	Action + object	Regulate action	Child initiated	*-ing*
"Push it"	Action + object	Regulate action	Child initiated	
"Car going"	Instrument + action	Label/ comment	Child initiated	*-ing*
"More car"	Recurrence + X	Regulate action	Child initiated	
"Car all gone?"	X + disappearance	Questioning	Child initiated	
"Juice up there"	Entity + locative	Elicited imitation	Adult initiated	
"Gimme juice"	Action + object	Regulating action	Child initiated	
"That truck"	Nomination + X	Answering	Adult initiated	
"Ball"	Personal/social	Label/ comment	Child initiated	
"Me ball"	Possessor + possession	Protest	Child initiated	
"No"	Personal/social	Protest	Child initiated	
"Mommy throw"	Agent + action	Regulating action	Child initiated	
"Throw it"	Action + object	Regulating action	Child initiated	
"Go there"	Action + locative	Answering	Adult initiated	
"Horsie"	General nominal	Answering	Adult initiated	
"Big horsie"	Attribute + entity	Spontaneous imitation	Child initiated	

434

Child   *Post–Stage I*

Utterance	Semantic Relation	Function	Initiation	Element
"Me riding"	Agent + action	Label/ comment	Child initiated	*-ing*
"More ride"	Recurrence + X	Questioning	Child initiated	
"Please"	Personal/social	Regulating action	Child initiated	
"Put on table"	Action + locative	Regulating action	Child initiated	*on*

Appendix E

Summary Sheet for Early Multiword Analysis

Child: _____ Age: _____ Birth Date: _____ Sample Date: _____

Context of sample (include people and objects present):

Length of sample in time:

Activities performed during sample:

Mean length of utterance (column 1 of coding sheet):

Total number of child utterances (column 1 of coding sheet):

Longest utterance in morphemes (column 1 of coding sheet):

Number of single-word responses (column 1 of coding sheet):

Semantic relations evident in sample (column 2 of coding sheet):

Functions evident in sample (column 3 of coding sheet):

Percentages of child- and adult-initiated utterances (column 4 of coding sheet):

Post–stage I elements noted (column 5 of coding sheet):

Semantic relations missing from sample:

Functions missing from sample:

Appendix F

Data Consolidation in Limited Language Evaluations

IDENTIFYING INFORMATION

Name: Address:
Telephone: Parents:
Date of Evaluation: Date of Birth: Age:

DATA OBTAINED IN EVALUATION

Case history

Reports from professionals

Hearing screening
Oral peripheral

Behavioral observation of caretaker—
  Child interaction

Behavioral observation of clinician—
  Child interaction

Parental checklist (lexicon)

Adaptive behavior scale

General developmental battery

Spontaneous communication sample

Nonstandardized tasks

Cognitive scale

Comprehension test

Language battery

Other

ANALYSES PERFORMED ON DATA

Mean length of utterance (MLU)

Distributional analysis

Early multiword analysis (semantic
  relations/functions)

Communicative gesture analysis
  Cognitive analysis of play

Vocalization analysis
  Phonetic inventory

Phonological analysis

Caretaker–child interaction analysis

Scoring of standardized measurements

Analysis of social behavior (e.g.,
  turntaking, joint referencing)

Scoring of nonstandardized procedures

Other

AREAS OF STRENGTH (+) AND CONCERN (−)

Biological
Hearing _____
Neurological _____
Medical _____
Anatomical _____

Adaptive Behavior
Self-help _____
Gross motor _____
Fine motor _____
Social _____

Early Multiword Combinations
Variety _____
Productivity _____
MLU _____

Cognitive
Play level _____
SM substage _____
Symbolic play _____

Communicative Intent
Imperatives
Declaratives
Level _____
Rate _____

Phonology
Phonetic inventory _____
Processes _____

Social
Reciprocity _____
Play partner _____

Single Words
Number _____
Variety _____
Functions _____

Caretaker Strategies
Joint referencing _____
Model _____

RECOMMENDATIONS

Referrals:
Further testing by SLP:
Prognosis:
Treatment directions:

References

Aase, D., Hovre, C., Krause, K., Schelfhout, S., Smith, J., & Carpenter, L. (2000). *Contextual test of articulation* [Measurement instrument]. Eau Claire, WI: Thinking Publications.

Accardo, P. J., & Capute, A. J. (2005). *The Capute scales: Cognitive adaptive test and clinical linguistic & auditory milestone scale* [Measurement instrument]. Baltimore, MD: Brookes.

Adamovich, B., & Henderson, J. (1992). *Scales of cognition ability for traumatic brain injury* [Measurement instrument]. Chicago, IL: Riverside.

Adams, M. (1977). A clinical strategy for differentiating the normally nonfluent child and the incipient stutterer. *Journal of Fluency Disorders, 2,*141–148.

Adler, S. (1990). Multicultural clients: Implications for the SLP. *Language, Speech, and Hearing Services in Schools, 21,* 135–139.

Adler, S. (1991). Assessment of language proficiency of limited English proficient speakers: Implications for the speech-language specialist. *Language, Speech, and Hearing Services in Schools, 22*(2), 12–18.

ADVANCE. (2010). Landmark study suggests verbal apraxia symptoms are part of larger syndrome. *ADVANCE for Speech-Language Pathologists & Audiologists, 20*(1), 20.

Allen, D., Bliss, L., & Timmons, J. (1981). Language evaluation: Science or art? *Journal of Speech and Hearing Disorders, 46,* 66–68.

Als, H., Lester, B., Tronick, E., & Brazelton, T. (1982). Toward a research instrument for the assessment of preterm infants' behavior (APIB)." In H. Fitzgeralt, B. Lester, & M. Yogman (Eds.), *Theory and research in behavioral pediatrics* (Vol. 1, pp. 35–63). New York, NY: Plenum Press.

Ambrose, N., & Yairi, E. (1994). The development of awareness of stuttering in preschool children. *Journal of Fluency Disorders, 19,* 229–245.

Ambrose, N., & Yairi, E. (1999). Normative disfluency data for early childhood stuttering. *Journal of Speech, Language, and Hearing Research, 42,* 895–909.

American Speech-Language-Hearing Association. (2004a). *ASHA Supplement No. 222, 7,* 73–87.

American Speech-Language-Hearing Association. (2004b). Preferred practice patterns for the profession of speech-language pathology. Retrieved from http://www.asha.org/members/

American Speech-Language-Hearing Association. (2005). Evidence-based practice in communication disorders [Position statement]. Retrieved from http://www.asha.org/members/deskref-journals/deskref/default

American Speech-Language-Hearing Association. (2007). Childhood apraxia of speech: Ad hoc committee on apraxia of speech in children. Retrieved from http://www.asha.org/docs/html/TR2007-00278.html

American Speech-Language-Hearing Association. (2014). Phonemic inventories across languages. Retrieved from http://www.asha.org/Practice-Portal/Templates/

Amir, O., & Ezrati-Vinacour, R. (2002). Stuttering in a volatile society—Israel. *Newsletter for the ASHA Special Interest Division 14: Perspectives on Communication Disorders and Sciences in Culturally and Linguistically Diverse Populations, 8*(2), 13–14.

Ammer, J. J., & Bangs, T. (2000). *Birth to three assessment and intervention system* (2nd ed.) [Measurement instrument]. Austin, TX: Pro Ed.

Ammons, R., & Johnson, W. (1944). Studies in the psychology of stuttering: XVIII. The construction and application of a test of attitude toward stuttering. *Journal of Speech Disorders, 9,* 39–49.

Anastasi, A. (1976). *Psychological testing.* New York, NY: Macmillan.

Anastasi, A. (1997). *Psychological testing* (7th ed.). Upper Saddle River, NJ: Prentice Hall.

Andersson, L. (2005). Determining the adequacy of tests of children's language. *Communication Disorders Quarterly, 26*(4), 207–225.

Andrews, G., & Cutler, J. (1974). Stuttering therapy: The relationship between changes in symptom level and attitudes. *Journal of Speech and Hearing Disorders, 39,* 312–319.

Antonios, N., Carnaby-Mann, G., Crary, M., Miller, L., Hubbard, H., Hood, K., . . . Silliman, S. (2010). Analysis of a physician tool for evaluating dysphagia on an inpatient stroke unit: The Modified Mann Assessment of Swallowing Ability. *Journal of Stroke and Cerebrovascular Diseases, 19*(1), 49–57.

Apel, K. (1999). An introduction to assessment and intervention with older students with language-learning impairments: Bridges from research to clinical practice. *Language, Speech, and Hearing Services in Schools, 30,* 228–230.

Applebee, A. (1978). *The child's concept of a story: Ages 2 to 17.* Chicago, IL: University of Chicago Press.

Aram, D., & Nation, J. (1980). Preschool language disorders and subsequent language and academic difficulties. *Journal of Communication Disorders, 13,* 159–170.

Arndt, J., & Healey, E. C. (2001). Concomitant disorders in school-age children who stutter. *Language, Speech, and Hearing Services in Schools, 32,* 68–78.

Arvedson, J. C. (1993). Oral-motor and feeding assessment. In J. C. Arvedson & L. Brodsky (Eds.), *Pediatric swallowing and feeding: Assessment and Management.* San Diego, CA: Singular Publishing.

Arvedson, J. C., & Brodsky, L. (2002). *Pediatric swallowing and feeding: Assessment and management.* San Diego, CA: Thomson Delmar.

Atkins, C., & Cartwright, L. (1982). An investigation of the effectiveness of three language elicitation procedures on Head Start children. *Language, Speech, and Hearing Services in Schools, 13,* 33–36.

Avery-Smith, W., Rosen, A. B., & Dellarosa, D. (1997). *Dysphagia Evaluation Protocol* [Measurement instrument]. Boston, MA: Pearson.

Aviv, J. E., Kim, T., Sacco, R., Kaplan, S., Goodhart, K., Diamond, B., Close, L. G. (1998). FEESST: A new bedside endoscopic test of the motor and sensory component of swallowing. *Annals of Otology, Rhinology, and Laryngology, 107*(5), 378–387.

Awan, S. N. (2000). *The voice diagnostic protocol: A practical guide to the diagnosis of voice disorders.* Austin, TX: Pro-Ed.

Awan, S., & Roy, N. (2009). Outcome measures in voice disorders: Application of an acoustic index of dysphonia severity. *Journal of Speech, Language, and Hearing Research, 52,* 482–499.

Bailey, D., & Simeonsson, R. (1988). *Family assessment in early intervention.* Columbus, OH: Merrill.

Bain, B., & Olswang, L. (1995). Examining readiness for learning two word utterances by children with specific expressive language impairment: Dynamic assessment validation. *American Journal of Speech-Language Pathology, 4,* 81–91.

Baines, K. A., Heeringa, H. M., & Martin, A. (1999). *Assessment of language-related functional activities* [Measurement instrument]. Austin, TX: Pro-Ed.

Bakker, K., & Myers, F. L. (2011). *Cluttering severity instrument* [Measurement instrument]. Retrieved from http://associations.missouristate.edu/ica/Resources/Resources%20and%20Links%20pages/CSI%20software%20ALL/CSI_Software.htm

Balason, D., & Dollaghan, C. (2002). Grammatical morpheme production in 4-year-old children. *Journal of Speech, Language, and Hearing Research, 45,* 961–969.

Ball, M., & Gibbon, F. (2012). *Handbook of vowels and vowel disorders.* Oxford, UK: Taylor & Francis.

Baltaxe, C., & Simmons, J. (1975). Language in childhood psychosis: A review. *Journal of Speech and Hearing Disorders, 40,* 439–458.

Bankson, N., & Bernthal, J. (1990). *Bankson-Bernthal test of phonology* [Measurement instrument]. Austin, TX: Pro-Ed.

Barlow, J. (2002). Recent advances in phonological theory and treatment: Part II. *Language, Speech, and Hearing Services in Schools, 33,* 4–8.

Barnes, E., Roberts, J., Long, S., Martin, G., Berni, M., Mandulak, K., & Sideris, J. (2009). Phonological accuracy and intelligibility in connected speech of boys with fragile X syndrome or Down syndrome. *Journal of Speech, Language, and Hearing Research, 52,* 1048–1061.

Barrie-Blackley, S., Musselwhite, C., & Rogister, S. (1978). *Clinical oral language sampling.* Danville, IL: Interstate.

Bartko, J. (1976). On various intraclass correlation reliability coefficients. *Psychological Bulletin, 83*(5), 762–765.

Bashir, A., Kuban, K., Kleinman, S., & Scavuzzo, A. (1983). Issues in language disorders: Considerations of cause, maintenance and change. In J. Miller, D. Yoder, & R. Shiefelbusch (Eds.), *ASHA Report No. 12.* Rockville, MD: American Speech-Hearing-Language Association.

Bates, E. (1976). *Language in context.* New York, NY: Academic Press.

Bates, E. (1979). *The emergence of symbols: Cognition and communication in infancy.* New York, NY: Academic Press.

Bates, E., Benigni, L., Bretherton, I., Camaioni, L., & Volterra, V. (1979). *The emergence of symbols: Cognition and communication in infancy.* New York, NY: Academic Press.

Bates, E., Bretherton, I., & Snyder, L. (1988). *From first words to grammar.* Cambridge, MA: Cambridge University Press.

Battle, J. (1992). *Culture-free self-esteem inventories* (2nd ed.) [Measurement instrument]. Austin, TX: Pro-Ed.

Battle, D. E. (2012). *Communication disorders in multicultural and international populations* (4th ed.). Maryland Heights, MO: Mosby.

Bauman-Waengler, J. (2012). *Articulation and phonological impairments: A clinical focus* (4th ed.). Boston, MA: Pearson.

Baumgartner J., & Duffy J. (1997). Psychogenic stuttering in adults with and without neurologic disease. *Journal of Medical Speech-Language Pathology, 5*(2), 75–95.

Bayles, K. A., & Tomoeda, C. K. (1993). *Arizona battery for communication disorders of dementia* [Measurement instrument]. Austin, TX: Pro-Ed.

Bayles, K. A., & Tomoeda, C. K. (1994). *The functional linguistic communication inventory* [Measurement instrument]. Tucson, AZ: Canyonlands Publishing.

Bayles, K. A., & Tomoeda, C. K. (2007). *Communication disorders of dementia.* San Diego, CA: Plural.

Bayley, N. (2006). *Bayley scales of infant and toddler development* (3rd ed.) [Measurement instrument]. San Antonio, TX: Harcourt Assessment.

Beard, R. (1969). *An outline of Piaget's developmental psychology for students and teachers.* New York, NY: Basic Books.

Bedrosian, J. (1985). An approach to developing conversational competence. In D. Ripich & F. Spinelli (Eds.), *School discourse problems.* San Diego, CA: College-Hill Press.

Beitchman, J. H., Wilson, B., Brownlie, E. B., Walters, H., & Lancee, W. (1996). Long-term consistency in speech/language profiles: I. Developmental and academic outcomes. *Journal of the American Academy of Child and Adolescent Psychiatry, 35*(6), 804–814.

Beitchman, J. H., Wilson, B., Brownlie, E. B., Walters, H., Inglis, A., & Lancee, W. (1996). Long-term consistency in speech/language profiles: II. Behavioral, emotional, and social outcomes. *Journal of the American Academy of Child & Adolescent Psychiatry, 35*(6), 815–825.

Belafsky, P. C., Mouadeb, D. A., Rees, C. J., Pryor, J. C., Postma, G. N., Allen, J., & Leonard, R. J. (2008). Validity and reliability of the Eating Assessment Tool (EAT-10). *Annals of Otology, Rhinology, and Laryngology, 117*(12), 919–924.

Benedict, H. (1975). Early lexical development: Comprehension and production. *Journal of Child Language, 6,* 183–200.

Benton, A. L., Hamsher, K., & Sivan, A. (1994). *Multilingual aphasia examination* [Measurement instrument]. Lutz, FL: Psychological Assessment Resources.

Berkowitz, S. (2013). *Cleft lip and palate: Diagnosis and management* (3rd ed.). New York, NY: Springer.

Bernhardt, B., & Holdgrafer, G. (2001). Beyond the basics II: Supplemental sampling for in-depth phonological analysis. *Language, Speech, and Hearing Services in Schools, 32,* 28–37.

Bernthal, J., Bankson, N., & Flipsen, P. (2013). *Articulation and phonological disorders* (7th ed.). Boston, MA: Pearson.

Beukelman, D., & Mirenda, P. (1992). *Augmentative and alternative communication.* Baltimore, MD: Paul H. Brookes.

Beukelman, D., & Mirenda, P. (2013). *Augmentative and alternative communication: Supporting children and adults with complex communication needs* (4th ed.). Baltimore, MD: Paul H. Brookes.

Biddle, A., Watson, L., Hooper, C., Lohr, K. N., & Sutton, S. F. (2002). Criteria for determining disability in speech-language disorders. *AHRQ Publication No. 02-E010.* Rockville, MD: Agency for Healthcare Research and Quality.

Bird, E. K., Cleave, P., Trudeau, N., Thordardottir, E., Sutton, A., & Thorpe, A. (2005). The language abilities of bilingual children with Down syndrome. *American Journal of Speech-Language Pathology, 14,* 187–199.

Bird, J., Bishop, D., & Freeman, N. (1995). Phonological awareness and literacy development in children with expressive phonological impairments. *Journal of Speech and Hearing Research, 38,* 446–462.

Bishop, D. V. M. (2006). *Children's communication checklist* (2nd ed.) [Measurement instrument]. San Antonio, TX: Pearson.

Blagden, C., & McConnell, N. (1983). *Interpersonal language skills assessment* [Measurement instrument]. Moline, IL: Linguisystems.

Blake, M. L. (2011). Cognitive-communicative deficits associated with right hemisphere brain damage. In M. Kimbarow (Ed.), *Cognitive communication disorders* (pp. 119–168). San Diego, CA: Plural.

Blakeley, R.W. (2000). *Screening test for developmental apraxia of speech* (2nd ed.) [Measurement instrument]. Austin, TX: Pro-Ed.

Blakely, R. W. (2001). Treatment of developmental apraxia of speech. In W. H. Perkins (Ed.), *Dysarthria and apraxia: Current therapy of communication disorders.* New York, NY: Thieme-Stratton.

Blodgett, E., & Cooper, E. (1987). *Analysis of the language of learning: The practical test of metalinguistics.* Moline, IL: Linguisystems.

Blood, G., Blood, I., Kreiger, J., & O'Connor, S. (2009). Double jeopardy for children who stutter: Race and coexisting disorders. *Communication Disorders Quarterly, 30*(3), 131–141.

Blood, G., & Conture, E. (1998). Outcomes measurement issues in fluency disorders. In C. Frattali (Ed.), *Measuring outcomes in speech-language pathology.* New York, NY: Thieme.

Bloodstein, O., & Ratner, N. (2008). *A handbook on stuttering* (6th ed.). Clifton Park, NY: Delmar.

Bloom, C., & Cooperman, D. K. (1999). *Synergistic stuttering therapy: A holistic approach.* Boston, MA: Butterworth Heinemann.

Bloom, L. (1970). *Language development: Form and function in emerging grammars.* Cambridge, MA: MIT Press.

Bloom, L. (1973). *One word at a time: The use of single word utterances before syntax.* The Hague: Mouton.

Bloom, L., & Lahey, M. (1978). *Language development and language disorders.* New York, NY: Wiley.

Bloom, L., Lightbrown, P., & Hood, L. (1975). Structure and variation in child vanguage. *Monographs of the Society for Research in Child Development, 40,* 1–41.

Blosser, J. (2011). *School programs in speech-language pathology organization and service delivery* (5th ed.). San Diego, CA: Plural.

Blosser, J. L., & Neidecker, E. A. (2010). *School programs in speech-language pathology: Organization and service delivery* (5th ed.). Boston, MA: Plural.

Boehm, A. E. (2000). *Boehm test of basic concepts* (3rd ed.) [Measurement instrument]. San Antonio, TX: Pearson.

Bondy, A., & Frost, L. (1998). The Picture Exchange Communication System. *Seminars in Speech and Language, 19,* 373–389.

Boone, D. (1993). *Boone voice program for children* (2nd ed.) [Measurement instrument]. Austin, TX: Pro-Ed.

Boone, D. (2000). *Boone voice program for adults* (3rd ed.) [Measurement instrument] Austin, TX: Pro-Ed.

Boone, D., McFarlane, S. C., Von Berg, S., & Zraich, R. (2014). *The voice and voice therapy* (8th ed.). Boston, MA: Allyn & Bacon.

Bopp, K., Brown, K., & Mirenda, P. (2004). Speech-language pathologists' roles in the delivery of positive behavior support for individuals with developmental disabilities. *American Journal of Speech-Language Pathology, 13,* 5–19.

Bopp, K., Mirenda, P., & Zumbo, B. (2009). Behavior predictors of language development over 2 years in children with autism spectrum disorders. *Journal of Speech, Language, and Hearing Research, 52,* 1106–1120.

Bornbaum, C., Day, A., & Doyle, P. (2014). Examining the construct validity of the V-RQOL in speakers who use alaryngeal voice. *American Journal of Speech-Language Pathology, 23,* 196–202.

Bornstein, M., Tal, J., & Tamis-Lemonda, C. (1991). Parenting in cross-cultural perspective: The United States, France and Japan. In M. Bornstein (Ed.), *Cultural approaches to parenting.* Hillsdale, NJ: Lawrence Erlbaum Associates.

Bornstein, M., Tamis-Lemonda, C., Pecheux, M., & Rahn, C. (1991). Mother and infant activity and interaction in France and the United States: A comparative study. *International Journal of Behavioral Development, 14,* 21–43.

Borsel, J. A., Maes, E., & Foulon, S. (2001). Stuttering and bilingualism: A review. *Journal of Fluency Disorders, 26,* 179–205.

Borson, S., Scanlan, J. M., Chen, P., & Ganguli, M. (2003). The Mini-Cog as a screen for dementia: Validity in a population-based sample. *Journal of the American Geriatrics Society, 51*(10), 141–145.

Boscolo-Rizzo, P., Maronato, F., Marchiori. C., Gava, A., & Mosto, M. C. (2008). Long-term quality of life after total laryngectomy and postoperative radiotherapy versus concurrent chemoradiotherapy for laryngeal preservation. *Laryngoscope, 118,* 300–306.

Boseley, M., Cunningham, M., Volk, M., & Hartnick, C. (2006). Validity of the Pediatric Voice-Related Quality-of-Life Survey. *Archives of Otolaryngology, Head and Neck Surgery, 132*(7), 717–720.

Boseley, M. E., & Hartnick, C. J. (2004). Assessing the outcome of surgery to correct velopharyngeal insufficiency with pediatric outcomes surgery. *International Journal of Pediatric Otorhinolaryngology, 68*(11), 1429–1433.

Bosone, Z. (1999). Tracheoesophageal speech: Treatment considerations before and after surgery. In S. Salmon (Ed.), *Alaryngeal speech rehabilitation* (2nd ed., pp. 105–150). Austin, TX: Pro-Ed.

Bothe, A. K. (2004). *Evidence-based treatment of stuttering.* Mahwah, NJ: Erlbaum.

Bothe, A. K., Davidow, J. H., Bramlett, R. E., & Ingham, R. J. (2006). Stuttering treatment research 1970–2005: I. Systematic review incorporating trial quality assessment of behavioral, cognitive, and related approaches. *American Journal of Speech-Language Pathology, 15*(4), 321–341.

Boudreau, D. (2005). Use of a parent questionnaire in emergent and early literacy assessment of preschool children. *Language, Speech, and Hearing Services in Schools, 36,* 33–47.

Boudreau, D., & Hedberg, N. (1999). A comparison of early literacy skills in children with specific language impairment and their typically developing peers. *American Journal of Speech-Language Pathology, 8,* 249–260.

Bowerman, M. (1973). Structural relationships in children's utterances: Syntactic or semantic? In T. Moore (Ed.), *Cognitive development and the acquisition of language* (pp. 197–213). New York, NY: Academic Press.

Bowers, L., Barrett, M., Huisingh, R., Orman, J., & LoGiudice, C. (2007). *Test of problem solving-2 adolescent* [Measurement instrument]. East Moline, IL: LinguiSystems.

Bowers, L., & Huisingh, R. (2010). *LinguiSystems articulation test* [Measurement instrument]. East Moline, IL: LinguiSystems.

Bowers, L., Huisingh, R., & LoGiudice, C. (2005). *Test of problem solving-3 elementary* [Measurement instrument]. East Moline, IL: LinguiSystems.

Bowers, L., Huisingh, R., & LoGiudice, C. (2008). *Social language development test elementary* [Measurement instrument]. East Moline, IL: LinguiSystems.

Bowers, L., Huisingh, R., & LoGiudice, C. (2010). *Social language developmental test adolescent* [Measurement instrument]. East Moline, IL: LinguiSystems.

Bowers, L., Huisingh, R., LoGiudice, C., & Orman, J. (2002). *Test of semantic skills—Primary* [Measurement instrument]. East Moline, IL: LinguiSystems.

Brackenbury, T., & Pye, C. (2005). Semantic deficits in children with language impairments: Issues for clinical assessment. *Language, Speech, and Hearing Services in Schools, 36,* 5–16.

Brady, N., Marquis, J., Fleming, K., & McLean, L. (2004). Prelinguistic predictors of language growth in children with developmental disabilities. *Journal of Speech, Language, and Hearing Research, 47,* 663–677.

Brady, W. A., & Hall, D. E. (1976). The prevalence of stuttering among school-age children. *Language, Speech, and Hearing Services in Schools, 7*(2), 75–81.

Braine, M. (1963). The ontogeny of English phrase structure: The first phrase. *Language, 39,* 1–14.

Braine, M. (1976). Children's first word combinations. *Monographs of the Society for Research in Child Development, 41,* 1–104.

Bransford, J., & Nitsch, K. (1978). Coming to understand things we could not previously understand. In J. Kavanagh & W. Strange (Eds.), *Speech and language in the laboratory, school and clinic* (pp. 267–307). Cambridge, MA: MIT Press.

Brazelton, T. B., & Nugent, J. K. (2011). *Neonatal behavior assessment scale* (5th ed.). London, England: Mac Keith Press.

Brice, A.E. (2002). *The Hispanic child.* Boston, MA: Allyn & Bacon.

Bricker, D. (2002). *Assessment, evaluation, and programming system for infants and children* (2nd ed.) [Measurement instrument]. Baltimore, MD: Brookes.

Brinton, B., & Fujiki, M. (1984). Development of topic manipulation skills in discourse. *Journal of Speech and Hearing Research, 27,* 350–358.

Brinton, B., & Fujiki, M. (1989). *Conversational management with language-impaired children.* Rockville, MD: Aspen.

Bronfenbrenner, U. (1979). *The ecology of human development.* Cambridge, MA: Harvard University Press.

Brook, I. (2013). *The laryngectomee guide.* Washington, DC: MedStar Health.

Brown, L., Sherbenou, R., & Johnson, S. (2010). *Test of nonverbal intelligence* (4th ed.) [Measurement instrument]. Austin, TX: Pro-Ed.

Brown, R. (1973). *A first language: The early stages.* Cambridge, MA: Harvard University Press.

Brown, R., & Fraser, C. (1963). The acquisition of syntax. In C. Cofer & B. Musgrave (Eds.), *Verbal behavior and learning: Problems and processes* (pp. 158–209). New York, NY: McGraw-Hill.

Brownell, R. (2010). *Expressive one-word picture vocabulary test-4* [Measurement instrument]. Novato, CA: Academic Therapy Publications.

Brownell, R. (2010). *Receptive one-word picture vocabulary test* (4th ed.) [Measurement instrument]. Novato, CA: Academic Therapy Publications.

Bruner, J. (1981). The social context of language acquisition. *Language & Communication, 1*(2),155–178.

Brunson, K., & Haynes, W. (1991). Profiling teacher/child classroom communication: Reliability of an alternating time sampling procedure. *Child Language Teaching and Therapy, 7*(2), 192–212.

Brutten, E., & Dunham, S. (1989). The Communication Attitude Test: A normative study of grade school children. *Journal of Fluency Disorders, 14,* 371–377.

Brutten, E., & Shoemaker, D. (1974). *Southern Illinois behavior checklist* [Measurement instrument]. Carbondale, IL: Southern Illinois University.

Brutten, G., & Vanrychkeghem, M. (2003). *Behavior Assessment Battery: A multi-dimensional and evidence-based approach to diagnostic and therapeutic decision making for children who stutter.* Destelbergen, Belgium: Stichting Integratie Gehandicapten & Acco Publishers.

Bryan, K. L. (1995). *The right-hemisphere language battery* (2nd ed.) [Measurement instrument]. London, England: Whurr.

Bryant, B. R., Wiederholt, J. L., & Bryant, D. P. (2004). *Gray diagnostic reading tests* (2nd ed.) [Measurement instrument]. Austin, TX: Pro-Ed.

Bunting, G. (2004). Voice following laryngeal cancer surgery: troubleshooting common problems after tracheoesophageal voice restoration. *Otolaryngologic Clinics of North America, 37*(3), 597–612.

Burke, B. L., Arkowitz, H., & Menchola, M. (2003). The efficacy of motivational interviewing: A meta-analysis of controlled clinical trials. *Journal of Consulting and Clinical Psychology, 71*(5), 843–861.

Burns, M. (1997). *Burns brief inventory of communication and cognition* [Measurement instrument]. Boston, MA: Pearson.

Burrus, A. E., & Willis. L.B. (2013). *Professional communication in speech-language pathology: How to write, talk, and act like a clinician.* San Diego, CA: Plural.

Butt, P., & Bucks, R. (2004). *Butt non-verbal reasoning test* [Measurement instrument]. London, UK: Speechmaker.

Bzoch, K. (2004). *Communicative disorders related to cleft lip and palate* (5th ed.). Austin, TX: Pro-Ed.

Bzoch, K. R., League, R., & Brown, V. L. (2003). *Receptive-expressive emergent language test* (3rd ed.) [Measurement instrument]. Austin, TX: Pro-Ed.

Bzoch, K. R., League, R., & Brown, V. L. (2003). *Receptive-Expressive Emergent Language Test: Examiner's manual.* Austin, TX: Pro-Ed.

Cabell, S., Justice, L., Zucker, T., & Kilday, C. (2009). Validity of teacher report for assessing the emergent literacy skills of at-risk preschoolers. *Language, Speech, and Hearing Services in Schools, 40,* 161–173.

Calandrella, A., & Wilcox, M. (2000). Predicting language outcomes for young prelinguistic children with developmental delay. *Journal of Speech, Language, and Hearing Research, 43,* 1061–1071.

Canning, B., & Rose, M. (1974). Clinical measurements of the speed of tongue and lip movements in British children with normal speech. *British Journal of Disorders of Communication, 9,* 45–50.

Capone, N., & McGregor, K. (2004). Gesture development: A review for clinical and research practices. *Journal of Speech, Language, and Hearing Research, 47,* 173–186.

Carding, P., & Horsley, I. A. (1992). An evaluation study of voice therapy in non-organic dysphonia. *International Journal of Language and Communication Disorders, 27*(2), 137–158.

Carew, L., Dacakis, G., & Oates, J. (2007). The effectiveness of oral resonance therapy on the perception of femininity of voice in male-to-female transsexuals. *Journal of Voice, 21*(5), 591–603.

Carl, L., & Johnson, P. (2006). *Drugs and dysphagia: How medicines can affect eating and swallowing.* Austin, TX: Pro-Ed.

Carlson, S. M., Mandell, D. J., & Williams, L. (2004). Executive function and theory of mind: Stability and prediction from ages 2 to 3. *Developmental Psychology, 40*(6), 1105–1122.

Carnaby, G. D., & Crary, M. (2014). Development and validation of a cancer-specific swallowing assessment tool: MASA-C. *Support Care Cancer, 22*(3), 595–602.

Carpenter, M. (1999). Treatment decisions in alaryngeal speech. In S. Salmon (Ed.), *Alaryngeal speech rehabilitation* (2nd ed., pp. 55–77). Austin, TX: Pro-Ed.

Carpenter, R. L. (1987). Play scale. In L. Olswang, C. Stoel-Gammon, T. Coggins, & R. Carpenter (Eds.), *Assessing prelinguistic and early behaviors in developmentally young children* (pp. 44–77). Seattle, WA: University of Washington Press.

Carrow-Woolfolk, E. (1998). *Test for auditory comprehension of language* (3rd ed.) [Measurement instrument]. Austin, TX: Pro-Ed.

Carrow-Woolfolk, E. (1999). *Comprehensive assessment of spoken language* [Measurement instrument]. Torrance, CA: Western Psychological Services.

Carrow-Woolfolk, E. (2011). *Oral and written language scales* (2nd ed.) [Measurement instrument]. Torrance, CA: Western Psychological Services.

Carrow-Woolfolk, E., & Lynch, J. I. (1982). *An integrative approach to language disorders in children.* New York, NY: Grune & Stratton.

Casby, M. W. (2003). Developmental assessment of play: A model for early intervention. *Communication Disorders Quarterly, 24*(4), 175–183.

Casby, M. W. (2011). An examination of the relationship of sample size and mean length of utterance for children with developmental language impairment. *Child Language Teaching & Therapy, 27*(3), 286–293.

Case-Smith, J. (1988). An efficacy study of occupational therapy with high-risk neonates. *The American Journal of Occupational Therapy, 42,* 499–506.

Catts, H. (1993). The relationship between speech-language impairments and reading disabilities. *Journal of Speech and Hearing Research, 36,* 948–958.

Catts, H. (1997). The early identification of language-based reading disabilities. *Language, Speech, and Hearing Services in Schools, 28,* 86–89.

Catts, H., Fey, M., Zhang, X., & Tomblin, J. B. (2001). Estimating the risk of future reading difficulties in kindergarten children: A research based model and its clinical implications. *Language, Speech, and Hearing Services in Schools, 32,* 38–50.

Catts, H. W., Fey, M. E., Tomblin, J. B., & Zhang, X. (2002). A longitudinal investigation of reading outcomes in children with language impairments. *Journal of Speech, Language, and Hearing Research, 45*(6), 1142–1157.

Cazden, C. (1970). The neglected situation of child language research and education. In F. Williams (Ed.), *Language and Poverty: Perspectives on a Theme* (pp. 81–101). Chicago, IL: Rand-McNally.

Chabon, S., Udolf, L., & Egolf, D. (1982). The temporal reliability of Brown's mean length of utterance measure with post stage V children. *Journal of Speech and Hearing Research, 25,* 124–128.

Chafe, W. (1970). *Meaning and the structure of language.* Chicago, IL: University of Chicago Press.

Channell, R. (2003). Automated developmental sentence scoring using computerized profiling software. *American Journal of Speech-Language Pathology, 12*, 369–375.

Chapey, R. (2014). Cognitive stimulation: Stimulation of recognition/comprehension, memory, and convergent, divergent and evaluative thinking. In R. Chapey (Ed.), *Language intervention strategies in aphasia and related neurogenic communication disorders* (5th ed., pp. 469–506). Baltime, MD: Lippincott Williams & Wilkins.

Chapman, R. (1978). Comprehension strategies in children. In J. Kavanagh & W. Strange (Eds.), *Speech and language in the laboratory, school and clinic* (pp. 308–327). Cambridge, MA: MIT Press.

Chapman, R. (1981). Exploring children's communicative intents. In J. Miller (Ed.), *Assessing language production in children: Experimental procedures* (pp. 11–136). Baltimore: University Park Press.

Chen, A., Frankowski, F., Bishop-Leone, J., Herbert, T., Leyk, S., Lewis, J., & Goepfert, H. (2001). The development and validation of a dysphagia-specific quality-of-life questionnaire for patients with head and neck cancer. *Archives of Otolaryngology–Head and Neck Surgery, 127*(7), 870–876.

Cheng, L., (1989). Service delivery to Asian/Pacific LEP children: A cross-cultural framework. *Topics in Language Disorders, 9*, 1–14.

Cherney, L. R., Pannelli, J. J., & Cantiere, C. A. (1994). Clinical evaluation of dysphagia in adults. In L. R. Cherney (Ed.), *Clinical management of dysphagia in adults and children* (2nd ed., pp. 49–69). Gaithersburg, MD: Aspen Publishers.

Chiat, S., & Roy, P. (2007). The Preschool Repetition Test: An evaluation of performance in typically developing and clinically referred children. *Journal of Speech, Language, and Hearing Research, 50*, 429–443.

Chomsky, N., & Halle, M. (1968). *The sound pattern of English.* New York, NY: Harper & Row.

Clark, D. (1989). Neonates and infants at risk for hearing and speech-language disorders. *Topics in Language Disorders, 10*(1), 1–12.

Clune, C., Paolella, J., & Foley, J. (1979). Free play behavior of atypical children: An approach to assessment. *Journal of Autism and Developmental Disorders, 9*, 61–72.

Coggins, T., & Carpenter, R. (1978). Categories for coding prespeech intentional communication. Unpublished manuscript, University of Washington, Seattle.

Cohen, S., Jacobson, B., Garrett, C. G., Noordzij, J. P., Stewart, M., Attia, A., . . . Cleveland, T. (2007,). Creation and validation of the Singing Voice Handicap Index. *Annals of Otology, Rhinology & Laryngology, 116*(6), 402–406.

Cole, E., & St. Clair-Stokes, J. (1984). Caregiver-child interactive behavior: A videotape analysis procedure. *Volta Review, 86*, 200–217.

Common Core State Standards Initiative. (2010a). *Common Core State Standards for English Language Arts and Literacy in History/Social Studies, Science, and Technical Subjects.* Retrieved from http://www.corestandards.org

Common Core State Standards Initiative. (2010b). *Common Core State Standards for Mathematics.* Retrieved from http://www.corestandards.org

Conti-Ramsden, G., & Durkin, K. (2008). Language and independence in adolescents with and without a history of specific language impairment (SLI). *Journal of Speech, Language, and Hearing Research, 51*, 70–83.

Conti-Ramsden, G., Mok, P. L., Pickles, A., & Durkin, K. (2013). Adolescents with a history of specific language impairment (SLI): Strengths and difficulties in social, emotional and behavioral functioning. *Research in Developmental Disabilities, 34*(11), 4161–4169.

Conture, E. (2001). *Stuttering: Its nature, diagnosis and treatment.* Boston, MA: Allyn & Bacon.

Conture, E., & Curlee, R. (2008). *Stuttering and related disorders of fluency* (3rd ed.). New York, NY: Thieme.

Cooper, E. B. (1973). The development of a stuttering chronicity prediction checklist: A preliminary report. *Journal of Speech and Hearing Disorders, 38*(2), 215–223.

Cooper, E. B., & Cooper, C. S. (2003). *Personalized fluency control therapy* (3rd ed.). Austin, TX: Pro-Ed.

Cooper, E. B., & Cooper, C. (2004). *Personalized fluency control therapy for children* [Measurement instrument]. Austin, TX: Pro-Ed.

Cooter, R., Flynt, E. S., & Cooter, K. (2014). *The Flynt-Cooter comprehensive reading inventory–2: Assessment of K–12 reading skills in English & Spanish* [Measurement instrument]. Boston, MA: Pearson.

Coplan, J. (1993). *Early language milestone scale* (2nd ed.). Austin, TX: Pro-Ed.

Cordier, R., Munro, N., Wilkes-Gillan, S., Speyer, R., & Pearce, W. M. (2014). Reliability and validity of the Pragmatics Observational Measure (POM): A new observational measure of pragmatic language for children. *Research in Developmental Disabilities, 35*(7), 1588–1598.

Cosby, M., & Ruder, K. (1983). Symbolic play and early language development in normal and mentally retarded children. *Journal of Speech and Hearing Research, 25*, 404–411.

Courtney, B., & Flier, L. (2009). RN dysphagia screening, a stepwise approach. *Journal of Neuroscience Nursing, 41*(1), 28–38.

Craig, H., & Evans, J. (1993). Pragmatics and SLI: Within-group variations in discourse behaviors. *Journal of Speech and Hearing Research, 36*, 777–789.

Crais, E. (1995). Expanding the repertoire of tools and techniques for assessing the communication skills of infants and toddlers. *American Journal of Speech-Language Pathology, 4*, 47–59.

Crais, E., Douglas, D., & Campbell, C. (2004). The intersection of the development of gestures and intentionality. *Journal of Speech, Language, and Hearing Research, 47*, 678–694.

Crais, E., & Roberts, J. (1991). Decision making in assessment and early intervention planning. *Language, Speech, and Hearing Services in Schools, 22*, 19–30.

Crais, E., Watson, L., & Baranek, G. (2009). Use of gesture development in profiling children's prelinguistic communication skills. *American Journal of Speech-Language Pathology, 18*, 95–108.

Crary, M., Haak, N. J., & Malinsky, A. (1989). Preliminary psychometric evaluation of an acute aphasia screening protocol. *Aphasiology, 3*, 611–618.

Crary, M., Mann, G., & Groher, M. (2005). Initial psychometric assessment of a functional oral intake scale for dysphagic stroke patients. *Archives of Physical Medicine and Rehabilitation, 86*, 1516.

Crary, M. A. (1988). A multifaced perspective on developmental apraxia of speech. Speech & Hearing Association of Alabama Conference. Presentation conducted from Orange Beach, AL.

Crystal, D., Fletcher, P., & Garman, M. (1976). *The grammatical analysis of language disability: A procedure for assessment and remediation.* London, England: Edward Arnold.

Cunningham, R., Farrow, V., Davies, C., & Lincoln, N. (1995). Reliability of the Assessment of Communicative Effectiveness in Severe Aphasia. *European Journal of Disorders of Communication, 30*, 1–16.

Curcio, F. (1978). Sensorimotor functioning and communication in mute autistic children. *Journal of Autism and Childhood Schizophrenia, 8*, 281–292.

Dabul, B. (2000). *Apraxia battery for adults* [Measurement instrument]. Austin, TX: Pro-Ed.

Dale, P. (1980). Is early pragmatic development measureable? *Journal of Child Language, 7*, 1–12.

Dale, P. S. (1991). The validity of a parent report measure of vocabulary and syntax at 24 months. *Journal of Speech, Language, and Hearing Research, 34*(3), 565–571.

Daly, D. (1996). *The source for stuttering and cluttering.* East Moline, IL: LinguiSystems, Inc.

Daly, D. A. (2006). *Predictive cluttering inventory* [Measurement instrument]. Ann Arbor, MI: Author.

Damico, J. (1985). Clinical discourse analysis: A functional approach to language assessment. In C. S. Simon (Ed.), *Communication Skills and Classroom Success: Assessment of language-learning disabled students* (pp. 165–204). San Diego: College-Hill press.

Damico, J., & Oller, J. (1980). Pragmatic versus morphological/syntactic criteria for language referrals. *Language, Speech, and Hearing Services in Schools, 11,* 85–94.

Damico, J. S., Oller, J. W., & Tetnowski, J. (1999). An investigation of the inter-observer reliability of a direct observational language assessment tool. *Advances in Speech Language Pathology, 1,* 77–94.

Dawson, J., Stout, C., & Eyer, J. (2005). *Structured photographic expressive language test-3* [Measurement instrument]. DeKalb, IL: Janelle.

Dawson, J., & Tattersall, P. (2001). *Structured photographic articulation test II featuring Dudsberry* [Measurement instrument]. DeKalb, IL: Janelle.

Deal, J. L. (1982). Sudden onset of stuttering: A case report. *Journal of Speech and Hearing Disorders, 47,* 301–304.

Deary, I. J., Wilson, J. A., Carding, P. N., & Mackenzie, L. (2003). VoiSS—A patient-derived voice system scale. *Journal of Psychosomatic Research, 54*(5), 483–489.

Delis, D., Kaplan, E., & Kramer, J. (2001). *Delis-Kaplan executive function system* [Measurement instrument]. Boston, MA: PsychCorp.

De Nil, L. F., Jokel, R., & Rochon, E. (2007). Stuttering associated with acquired neurological disorders: Review, assessment and intervention. In E. G. Conture & R. F. Curlee (Eds.), *Stuttering and related disorders of fluency* (3rd ed., pp. 326–343). New York, NY: Thieme.

Depippo, K., Holas, M., & Reding, M. (1992). Validation of the 3-oz water swallowing test for aspiration following stroke. *Archives of Neurology, 49,* 1259–1261.

Dodd, B., Hua, Z., Crosbie, S., Holm, A., & Ozanne, A. (2006). *Diagnostic evaluation of articulation and phonology* [Measurement instrument]). Boston, MA: Pearson.

Doesborgh, S. J., van de Sandt-Koenderman, W. M., Dippel, D. W., van Harskamp, F., Koudstaal, P. J., & Visch-Brink, E. G. (2003). Linguistic deficits in the acute phase of stroke. *Journal of Neurology, 250,* 977–982.

Donaldson, M. (1978). *Children's minds.* London, England: Fontana.

Dore, J. (1975). Holophrases, speech acts and language universals. *Journal of Child Language, 2,* 21–40.

Dore, J., et al. (1976). Transitional phenomena in early language acquisition. *Journal of Child Language, 3,* 13–28.

Drummond, S. S. (1993). *Dysarthria examination battery* [Measurement instrument]. San Antonio, TX: Communication Skill Builders.

Duchan, J., & Weitzner-Lin, B. (1987). Nurturant-naturalistic intervention for language impaired children: Implications for planning lessons and tracking progress. *Journal of the American Speech and Hearing Association, 29*(7), 45–49.

Duffy, J. R. (2013). *Motor speech disorders: Substrates, differential diagnosis, and management* (3rd ed.). St. Louis, MO: Elsevier Mosby.

Duffy, M. C., Proctor, A., & Yairi, E. (2004). Prevalence of voice disorders in African American and European American preschoolers. *Journal of Voice, 18*(3), 348–353.

Dunn, L. M., & Dunn, D. M. (2007). *Peabody picture vocabulary Test* (4th ed.) [Measurement instrument]. San Antonio,TX: Pearson.

Dunst, C. (1980). *A clinical and educational manual for use with the Uzigiris and Hunt Scales of Infant Psychological Development.* Baltimore, MD: University Park Press.

Durkin, K., & Conti-Ramsden, G. (2007). Language, social behavior, and the quality of friendships in adolescents with and without a history of specific language impairment. *Child Development, 78*(5), 1441–1457.

Dwivedi, R. C., St. Rose, S., Chisholm, E. J., Georgalas, C., Bisase, B., Amen, F., . . . Kazi, R. (2012). Evaluation of swallowing by Sydney Swallowing Questionnaire (SSQ) in oral and oropharyngeal cancer patients treated with primary surgery. *Dysphagia, 27*(4), 491–497.

Dworkin, J. P., & Culatta, R. A. (1996). *Dworkin-Culatta oral mechanism examination and treatment system* [Measurement instrument]. Nicholasville, KY: Edgewood Press.

Dworkin, J., Marurick, M., & Krouse, J. (2004). Velopharyngeal dysfunction: Speech characteristics, variable etiologies, evaluation techniques, and differential treatments. *Language, Speech, and Hearing Services in Schools, 35*(4), 333–352.

Dwyer, C., Robb, M., & O'Beirne, G. (2009). The influence of speaking rate on nasality in the speech of hearing-impaired individuals. *Journal of Speech, Language, and Hearing Research, 56,* 1321–1333.

Dykes, R. L. (1995). Prevalence of stuttering among African-American school-age children in the South: A survey of speech-language pathologists' caseloads. Unpublished doctoral dissertation, Auburn University, AL.

Dyson, A. (1988). Phonetic inventories of 2- and 3-year-old children. *Journal of Speech and Hearing Disorders, 53*(1), 89–93.

Eadie, T. L., Day, A. M., Sawin, D. E., Lamvik, K., & Doyle, P. C. (2013). Auditory-perceptual speech outcomes and quality of life after total laryngectomy. *Otolaryngology–Head & Neck Surgery, 148*(1), 82–88. doi:10.1177/0194599812461755

Earnest, M. (2001). *Preschool motor speech evaluation and intervention* [Measurement instrument]. Austin, TX: Pro-Ed.

Edmonds, P., & Haynes, W. (1988). Topic manipulation and conversational participation as a function of familiarity in school-age language-impaired and normal language peers. *Journal of Communication Disorders, 21,* 209–228.

Edmonston, N., & Thane, N. (1992). Children's use of comprehension strategies in response to relational words: Implications for assessment. *American Journal of Speech-Language Pathology, 1,* 30–35.

Edwards, M. (1992). In support of phonological processes. *Language, Speech, and Hearing Services in Schools, 23,* 233–240.

Edwards, S., Letts, C., & Sinka, I. (2011). *The new Reynell Developmental Language Scales* (4th ed.) [Measurement instrument]. London, UK: GL Assessment.

Egan, G. (2014). *The skilled helper: A problem-management and opportunity-development approach to helping.* Belmont, CA: Brooks/Cole Cengage Learning.

Ehlers, P., & Cirrin, F. (1983). Topic relevancy abilities of language-impaired children. Paper presented at the annual convention of the American Speech-Language-Hearing Association, Cincinnati, OH.

Ehren, B. (1993). Eligibility, evaluation and the realities of role definition in the schools. *American Journal of Speech Language Pathology, 2*(1), 20–23.

Ehren, B. J., Blosser, J., Roth, F. P., Paul, D. R., & Nelson, N. W. (2012). Core commitment. *The ASHA Leader, 17*(4), 10–13.

Ehren, B. J., Montgomery, J., Rudebusch, J., Whitmire, K. (2007). *Responsiveness to intervention: New roles for speech-language pathologists.* Retrieved from http://www.asha.org/slp/schools/prof-consult/NewRolesSLP.htm

Eickhoff, J., Betz, S. K., & Ristow, J. (2010). Clinical procedures used by speech-language pathologists to diagnose SLI. Poster session presented at the Symposium on Research in Child Language Disorders, Madison, WI.

Eisenberg, S. (2005). When conversation is not enough: Assessing infinitival complements through elicitation. *American Journal of Speech-Language Pathology, 14,* 92–106.

Eisenberg, S., Fersko, T., & Lundgren, C. (2001). The use of MLU for identifying language impairment in preschool children: A review. *American Journal of Speech-Language Pathology, 10,* 323–342.

Eisenberg, S., Ukrainetz, T., Hsu, J., Kaderavek, J., Justice, L., & Gillam, R. (2008). Noun phrase elaboration in children's spoken stories. *Language, Speech, and Hearing Services in Schools, 39*, 145–157.

Elmiyeh, B., Dwivedi, R, Jallali, N., Chisholm, E., Kari, R., Clarke, P., & Rhys-Evans, P. (2010). Surgical voice restoration after total laryngectomy: An overview. *Indian Journal of Cancer, 47*(3), 239–247. doi:10.4103/0019-509X.64707

Emerick, L. (1984). *Speaking for ourselves: Self-portraits of the speech or hearing handicapped,* Danville, IL: Interstate.

Enderby, P., & Palmer, R. (2008). The standardized assessment of dysarthria is possible. In W. R. Berry (Ed.), *Clinical Dysarthria* (pp. 86–101). Austin, TX: Pro-Ed.

Enderby, P., Wood, V., & Wade, D., (2006). *Frenchay aphasia screening test* (2nd ed.) [Measurement instrument]. Hoboken, NJ: Wiley.

Engler, L., Hannah, E., & Longhurst, T. (1973). Linguistic analysis of speech samples: A practical guide for clinicians. *Journal of Speech and Hearing Disorders, 38*, 192–204.

Epstein, R., Hiran, S. P., Stygall, J., & Newman, S. P. (2009). How do individuals cope with voice disorders? Introducing voice disability coping questionnaire. *Journal of Voice, 23*(2), 209–217.

Ettema, S. L., Kuehn, D. P., Perlman, A. L., & Alperin, N. (2002). Magnetic resonance imaging of the levator veli palatini muscle during speech. *The Cleft Palate-Craniofacial Journal, 39*, 130–144.

Evard, B., & Sabers, D. (1979). Speech and language testing with distinct ethnic-racial groups: A survey for improving test validity. *Journal of Speech and Hearing Disorders, 44*, 271–281.

Ezrati-Vinacou, R., & Levin, I. (2004). The relationship between anxiety and stuttering: A multidimensional approach. *Journal of Fluency Disorders, 29*(2), 135–148.

Fagan, J., & Isaacs, S. (2002). Tracheoesophageal speech in a developing world community. *Archives of Otolaryngology—Head and Neck Surgery, 128*, 50–53.

Fagundes, D., Haynes, W., Haak, N., & Moran, M. (1998). Task variability effects on the language test performance of southern lower socioeconomic class African-American and Caucasian five-year-olds. *Language, Speech, and Hearing Services in Schools, 29*, 148–157.

Fairbanks, G. (1960). *Voice and articulation drillbook* (2nd ed.). New York, NY: Harper & Row.

Featherstone, H. (1980). *A difference in the family: Life with a disabled child.* New York, NY: Basic Books.

Felsenfeld, S., Broen, P., & McGue, M. (1994). A 28-year follow-up of adults with a history of moderate phonological disorder: Educational and occupational results. *Journal of Speech and Hearing Research, 37*, 1341–1353.

Fenson, L., Marchman, V., Thal, D., Dale, P., Reznick, J., & Bates, E. (2006). *MacArthur-Bates communicative development inventories.* Baltimore, MD: Paul H. Brookes.

Fenson, L., Marchman, V. A., Thal, D. J., Dale, P., Reznick, S., & Bates, E. (2007). *MacArthur-Bates communicative development inventories* (2nd ed.) [Measurement instrument]. Baltimore, MD: Brookes.

Fey, M. (1986). *Language intervention with young children.* San Diego, CA: College-Hill.

Fey, M., & Leonard, L. (1983). Pragmatic skills of children with specific language impairment. In T. Gallagher & C. Prutting (Eds.), *Pragmatic Assessment and Intervention Issues in Language* (pp. 65–82). San Diego, CA:College-Hill.

Fillmore, C. (1968). The case for case. In E. Bach & R. Harms (Eds.), *Universals in linguistic theory* (pp. 1–87). New York, NY: Holt, Rinehart, and Winston.

Finan, D. S. (2010). Get hip to the data acquisition scene: Principles of digital signal recording. *Sig 5 Perspectives on Speech Science and Orofacial Disorders, 20*, 6–13.

Finkelstein, Y., Wexler, D. B., Nachmani, A., & Ophir, D. (2002). Endoscopic partial adenoidectomy for children with submucous cleft. *The Cleft Palate-Craniofacial Journal, 39*, 479–486.

Fisher, H., & Logemann, J. (1971). *The Fisher-Logemann test of articulation competence* [Measurement instrument]. Boston, MA: Houghton-Mifflin.

Flamand-Roze, C., Falissard, B., Roze, E., Maintigneux, L., Beziz, J., Chacon, A., . . . Denier, C. (2011). Validation of a new language screening for patients with acute stroke: The Language Screening Test. *Stroke, 42*, 1224–1229.

Fleming, V. (2014). Early detection of cognitive-linguistic changes associated with mild cognitive impairment. *Communicative Disorders Quarterly, 35*(3), 146–157.

Fletcher, S. (1972). Time-by-count measurement of diadochokinetic syllable rate. *Journal of Speech and Hearing Research, 15*, 763–770.

Fletcher, S. (1978). *Diagnosing speech disorders from cleft palate.* New York, NY: Grune & Stratton.

Flipsen, P., Hammer, J., & Yost, K. (2005). Measuring severity of involvement in speech delay: Segmental and whole-word measures. *American Journal of Speech-Language Pathology, 14*, 298–312.

Fluharty, N. (2000). *Fluharty preschool speech and language screening test* (2nd ed.) [Measurement instrument]. Austin, TX: Pro-Ed.

Fogel, A., Toda, S., & Kawai, M. (1988). Mother-infant face-to-face interaction in Japan and the United States: A laboratory comparison using 3-month-old infants. *Developmental Psychology, 24*, 398–406.

Folger, J., & Chapman, R. (1978). A pragmatic analysis of spontaneous imitations. *Journal of Child Language, 5*, 25–38.

Folstein, M. F., & Folstein, S. E. (2009). Mini-Mental State: A practical method for grading the cognitive state of patients for the clinician. *Journal of Psychiatric Research, 12*, 189–198.

Folstein, M. F., & Folstein, S. E. (2010). *Mini–Mental State Examination* (2nd ed.). [Measurement instrument]. Lutz, FL: PAR.

Foster, W., & Miller, M. (2007). Development of the literacy achievement gap: A longitudinal study of kindergarten through third grade. *Language, Speech, and Hearing Services in Schools, 38*, 173–181.

Fox, D., & Johns, D. (1970). Predicting velopharyngeal closure with a modified tongue-anchor technique. *Journal of Speech and Hearing Disorders, 35*, 248–251.

Frankenburg, W., & Drumwright, A. (1973). *Denver articulation screening exam* [Measurement instrument]. Denver, CO: Denver Developmental Materials.

Frattali, C., Thompson, C. K., Holland, A., Wohl, C. B., & Ferketig, M. M. (1997). *ASHA functional assessment of communication skills for adults* [Measurement instrument]. Rockville, MD: American Speech-Language-Hearing Association.

Freed, D. B. (2012). *Motor speech disorders: Diagnosis and treatment* (2nd ed.). San Diego, CA: Singular.

Fuchs, D., Fuchs, L., Dailey, A., & Power, M. (1985). The effect of examiner's personal familiarity and professional expertise on handicapped children's test performance. *Journal of Educational Research, 78*, 3–14.

Fudala, J. (2000). *Arizona articulation proficiency scale* (3rd revision) [Measurement instrument]. Torrance, CA: Western Psychological Services.

Fudala, J., & Reynolds, W. (1993). *Arizona articulation proficiency scale* (2nd ed.) [Measurement instrument]. Los Angeles, CA: Western Psychological Services.

Fujiki, M., Brinton, B., & Todd, C. (1996). Social skills of children with specific language impairment. *Language, Speech, and Hearing Services in Schools, 27*, 195–202.

Fujiki, M., et al. (2001). Social behaviors of children with language impairment on the playground: A pilot study. *Language, Speech, and Hearing Services in Schools, 32*, 101–113.

Furey, J., & Watkins, R. (2002). Accuracy of online language sampling: A focus on verbs. *American Journal of Speech-Language Pathology, 11,* 434–439.

Gallagher, L. (2010). The impact of prescribed medication on swallowing: An overview. *SIG 13 Perspectives on Swallowing and Swallowing Disorders, 19,* 98–102.

Gallagher, T. (1983). Preassessment: A procedure for accomodating language use variability. In T. Gallagher & C. Prutting (Eds.), *Pragmatic assessment and intervention issues in language* (pp. 1–28). San Diego, CA: College-Hill.

Gardner, M. (2005). *Test of auditory processing skills* (3rd ed.) [Measurement instrument]. Novato, CA: Academic Therapy.

Garrett, K., & Lasker, J. (2007). *Multimodal communication screening test for persons with aphasia* [Measurement instrument]. Academic Communication Associates: Oceanside, CA. Retrieved in multiple parts from http://aac.unl.edu/screen/screen.html; http://aac.unl.edu/screen/pictures.pdf; http://aac.unl.edu/screen/score.pdf

Garrett, K., & Moran, M. (1992). A comparison of phonological severity measures. *Language, Speech, and Hearing Services in Schools, 23,* 48–51.

Garvey, C. (1977a). The contingent query: A dependent act in conversation. In M. Lewis & L. Rosenblum (Eds.), *Interaction, conversation, and the development of language* (Vol. 5, pp. 63–93). New York, NY: Wiley.

Garvey, C. (1977b). Play with language and speech. In S. Ervin-Tripp & C. Mitchell-Kernan (Eds.), *Child discourse* (pp. 22–47). New York, NY: Academic Press.

Gazella, J., & Stockman, I. (2003). Children's story retelling under different modality and task conditions: Implications for standardizing language sampling procedures. *American Journal of Speech-Language Pathology, 12,* 61–72.

Gelfer, M., & Pazera, J. (2006). Maximum duration of sustained /s/ and /z/ and the s/z ratio with controlled intensity. *Journal of Voice, 20*(3), 369–379.

German, D. J. (1990). *The test of adolescent and adult word-finding* [Measurement instrument]. Austin, TX: Pro-Ed.

Ghirardi, A. C., Ferreira, L. P., Giannini, S. P., & Latorre, M. (2013). Screening Index for Voice Disorders (SIVD): Development and validation. *Journal of Voice, 27*(2), 195–200.

Gibbon, F. E., & Crampin, L. (2002). Labial-lingual double articulations in speakers with cleft palate. *The Cleft Palate-Craniofacial Journal, 39,* 40–49.

Gierut, J. (2007). Phonological complexity and language learnability. *American Journal of Speech-Language Pathology, 16,* 6–17.

Gierut, J., Elbert, M., & Dinnsen, D. (1987). A functional analysis of phonological knowledge and generalization learning in misarticulating children. *Journal of Speech and Hearing Research, 30*(4), 462–479.

Gilbertson, M., & Bramlett, R. (1998). Phonological awareness screening to identify at-risk readers: Implications for practitioners. *Language, Speech, and Hearing Services in Schools, 29,* 109–116.

Gillam, R., & Pearson, N. (2004). *Test of narrative language* [Measurement instrument]. Austin, TX: Pro-Ed.

Gillam, R. B., Logan, K. J., & Pearson, N. A. (2009). *Test of childhood stuttering* [Measurement instrument]. Austin, TX: Pro-Ed.

Gillam, S., Fargo, J., & Robertson, K. (2009). Comprehension of expository text: Insights gained from think-aloud data. *American Journal of Speech-Language Pathology, 18,* 82–94.

Gilliam, J. A., & Miller, L. (2006). *Pragmatic language skills inventory* [Measurement instrument]. Austin, TX: Pro-Ed.

Ginsburg, H., & Opper, S. (1969). *Piaget's theory of intellectual development: An introduction.* Englewood Cliffs, NJ: Prentice-Hall.

Glascoe, F. P. (2006). *Parents' evaluation of developmental status* [Measurement instrument]. Nashville, TN: Ellsworth & Vandermeer.

Glaspey, A., & Stoel-Gammon, C. (2005). Dynamic assessment in phonological disorders. *Topics in Language Disorders, 25,* 220–230.

Glennen, S. (2007). Predicting language outcomes for internationally adopted children. *Journal of Speech, Language, and Hearing Research, 50,* 529–548.

Gliklich, R. E., Glovsky, R. M., & Montgomary, W. W. (1999). Validation of a voice outcome survey for unilateral vocal cord paralysis. *Otolaryngology-Head & Neck Surgery, 120*(2), 153–158.

Glover, M. E., Preminger, J. L., & Sanford, A. R. (1995). *Early learning accomplishment profile for developmentally young children: Birth to 36 months* [Measurement instrument]. Lewisville, NC: Kaplan Press.

Goh, S., & O'Kearney, R. (2012). Emotional and behavioural outcomes later in childhood and adolescence for children with specific language impairment: Meta-analyses of controlled prospective studies. *Journal of Child Psychology and Psychiatry, 54*(5), 516–524.

Goldfarb, R., & Serpanos, C. (2013). *Professional writing in speech-language pathology and audiology* (2nd ed.). San Diego, CA: Plural.

Golding-Kushner, K. J., Argamaso, R. V., Cotton, R. T., Grames, L. M., Henningsson, G., Jones, D. L., . . . Marsh, J. L. (1990). Standardization for the reporting of nasopharyngoscopy and multiview videofluoroscopy: A report from an international working group. *Cleft Palate Journal, 27*(4), 337–348.

Goldman, R., & Fristoe, M. (2000). *Goldman-Fristoe test of articulation* (2nd ed.) [Measurement instrument]. Boston, MA: Pearson.

Goldstein, B. (2000). *Cultural and linguistic diversity resource guide for speech-language pathologists.* San Diego, CA: Singular Publishing Group, Inc.

Goldstein, B., & Iglesias, A. (2006). *Contextual probes of articulation competence–Spanish* [Measurement instrument]. Greenville, SC: Super Duper.

Goodglass, H., Gleason, J. B., Bernholtz, N. D., & Hyde, M. R. (1972). Some linguistic structures in the speech of a Broca's aphasic. *Cortex, 8,* 191–212.

Goodglass, H., Kaplan, E., & Barresi, N. (2000). *Boston Diagnostic Examination of Aphasia and Related Disorders* (3rd ed.). Austin, TX: Pro-Ed.

Gordon, P., & Luper, H. (1992). The early identification of beginning stuttering, I: protocols. *American Journal of Speech-Language Pathology, 1,* 43–53.

Gordon-Brannan, M., & Hodson, B. (2000). Intelligibility/severity measurements of prekindergarten children's speech. *American Journal of Speech-Language Pathology, 9,* 141–150.

Gowie, C., & Powers, J. (1979). Relations among cognitive, semantic and syntactic variables in children's comprehension of the minimal distance principle: A two-year developmental study. *Journal of Psycholinguistic Research, 8,* 29–41.

Graham, S., & Harris, K. (1999). Assessment and intervention in overcoming writing difficulties: An illustration from the self-regulated strategy development model. *Language, Speech, and Hearing Services in Schools, 30,* 255–264.

Greenslade, K., Plante, E., & Vance, R. (2009). The diagnostic accuracy and construct validity of the Structured Photographic Expressive Language Test–Preschool, second edition. *Language, Speech, and Hearing Services in Schools, 40,* 150–160.

Grice, H. (1975). Logic and conversation. In P. Cole & J. Morgan (Eds.), *Studies in syntax, semantics and speech acts* (Vol. 3, pp. 41–58). New York, NY: Academic Press.

Groher, M., & Crary, M. (2010). *Dysphagia clinical management in adults and children.* Maryland Heights, MO: Mosby Elsevier.

Grunwell, P. (1988). *Clinical phonology.* Baltimore, MD: Williams & Wilkins.

Guitar, B. (2006). *Stuttering: An integrated approach to its nature and treatment* (3rd ed.). Baltimore, MD: Lippincott/Williams & Wilkins.

Guitar, B. (2013). *Stuttering: An integrated approach to its nature and treatment* (4th ed.). Baltimore, MD: Lippincott, Williams & Wilkins.

Guitar, B., & Grims, S. (1977, November). Developing a scale to assess communication attitudes in children who stutter. Paper presented at the Annual Meeting of the American Speech Language and Hearing Association, Atlanta, GA.

Gummersall, D., & Strong, C. (1999). Assessment of complex sentence production in a narrative context. *Language, Speech, and Hearing Services in Schools, 30,* 152–164.

Gutierrez-Clellen, V., & Pena, E. (2001). Dynamic assessment of diverse children: A tutorial. *Language, Speech, and Hearing Services in Schools, 32,* 212–224.

Gutierrez-Clellen, V. F., & Quinn, R. (1993). Assessing narratives of children from diverse cultural/linguistic groups. *Language, Speech, and Hearing Services in Schools, 24*(1), 2–9.

Hall, K. M. (1992). Overview of functional assessment scales in brain injury rehabilitation. *NeuroRehabilitation, 2,* 98–113.

Hall, N. (2004). Lexical development and retrieval in treating children who stutter. *Language, Speech, and Hearing Services in Schools, 35,* 57–69.

Hall, P., & Tomblin, J. (1978). A follow-up study of children with articulation and language disorders. *Journal of Speech and Hearing Disorders, 43,* 227–241.

Hall, P. K., Hardy, J. C., & LaVelle, W. E. (1990). A child with signs of developmental apraxia of speech with whom a palatal lift prosthesis was used to manage palatal dysfunction. *Journal of Speech and Hearing Disorders, 55,* 454–460.

Halliday, M. (1975). *Learning how to mean: Explorations in the development of language.* New York, NY: Elsevier.

Halliday, M., & Hasan, R. (1976). *Cohesion in English.* London, England: Longman.

Halper, A. S., Cherney, L. R., & Burns, M. S. (2010). *Rehabilitation Institute of Chicago clinical management of right hemisphere dysfunction* (3rd ed.). Chicago, IL: Rehabilitation Institute of Chicago.

Hammill, D. D., Brown, V. L., Larsen, S. C., & Wiederholt, J. L. (1994). *Test of adolescent and adult language* (3rd ed.) [Measurement instrument]. Austin, TX: Pro-Ed.

Hammill, D. D., & Larsen, S. C. (2009). *Test of written language* (4th ed.) [Measurement instrument]. Austin, TX: Pro-Ed.

Hammill, D. D., & Newcomer, P. L. (2008). *Test of language development—Intermediate* (4th ed.) [Measurement instrument]. Austin, Tx: Pro Ed.

Hanna, E., Sherman, A., Cash, D., Adams, F., Vural, E., Fan, C. Y., & Suen, J. (2004). Quality of life for patients following total laryngectomy vs. chemoradiation for laryngeal preservation. *Archives of Otolaryngology—Head & Neck Surgery, 130*(7), 875–879.

Hardin-Jones, M., Chapman, K., & Scherer, N. (2006, June 13). Early intervention in children with cleft palate. *The ASHA Leader, 11,* 8–9, 32.

Hardy, E. (1995). *Bedside evaluation of dysphagia* [Measurement instrument]. Austin, TX: Pro-Ed.

Harrison, L., & McLeod, S. (2010). Risk and protective factors associated with speech and language impairment in a nationally representative sample of 4- to 5-year-old children. *Journal of Speech, Language, and Hearing Research, 53,* 508–529.

Harrison, P. L., Kaufman, A. S., Kaufman, N. L., Bruininks, R., Rynders, J., Ilmer, S., . . . Cicchetti, D. (1990). *Early screening profile* [Measurement instrument]. San Antonio, TX: Pearson.

Harrison, P. L., & Oakland, T. (2003). *Manual for the Adaptive Behavior Assessment System.* San Antonio, TX: Harcourt Assessment.

Hartnick, C. J., Volk, M., & Cunningham, M. (2003). Establishing normal voice-related quality of life scores with the pediatric population. *Archives of Otolaryngology, Head and Neck Surgery, 29*(10), 1090–1093.

Haskill, A., & Tyler, A. (2007). A comparison of linguistic profiles in subgroups of children with specific language impairment. *American Journal of Speech-Language Pathology, 16,* 209–221.

Hay, I., Oates, J., Giannini, A., Berkowiz, R., & Rotenberg, B. (2009). Pain perception of children undergoing nasendoscopy for investigation of voice and resonance disorders. *Journal of Voice, 23*(3), 380–388.

Hayden, D., & Square, P. (1999). *Verbal motor production assessment for children* [Measurement instrument]. Boston, MA: Pearson.

Haynes, W., Haynes, M., & Jackson, J. (1982). The effects of phonetic context and linguistic complexity on /s/ misarticulation in children. *Journal of Communication Disorders, 15,* 287–297.

Haynes, W., & McCallion, M. (1981). Language comprehension testing: The influence of cognitive tempo and three modes of test administration. *Language, Speech, and Hearing Services in Schools, 12,* 74–81.

Haynes, W., Moran, M., & Pindzola, R. (2012). *Communication disorders in educational and medical settings: An introduction for speech-language pathologists, teachers, and allied health professionals.* Boston, MA: Jones & Bartlett Learning.

Haynes, W., & Oratio, A. (1978). A study of clients' perceptions of therapeutic effectiveness. *Journal of Speech and Hearing Disorders, 43*(1), 21–33.

Haynes, W., Purcell, E., & Haynes, M. (1979). A pragmatic aspect of language sampling. *Language, Speech, and Hearing Services in Schools, 10,* 104–110.

Heath, S. (1983). *Ways with words.* Cambridge, UK: Cambridge University Press.

Heath, S. (1989). The learner as a cultural member. In M. Rice & R. Schiefelbusch (Eds.), *The teachability of language* (pp. 333–350). Baltimore, MD: Brookes.

Hebbeler, K., & Rooney, R. (2009). Accountability for services for young children with disabilities and the assessment of meaningful outcomes: The role of the speech-language pathologist. *Language, Speech, and Hearing Services in Schools, 40,* 446–456.

Hegde, M. (1987). *Clinical research in communication disorders.* Boston, MA: Little, Brown.

Heilmann, J., Miller, J., & Nockerts, A. (2010). Using language sample databases. *Language, Speech, and Hearing Services in Schools, 41,* 84–95.

Heilmann, J., Miller, J., Nockerts, A., & Dunaway, C. (2010). Properties of the narrative scoring scheme using narrative retells in young school-age children. *American Journal of Speech-Language Pathology, 19,* 154–166.

Heilmann, J., Nockerts, A., & Miller, J. F. (2010). Language sampling: Does the length of the transcript matter? *Language, Speech, and Hearing Services in Schools, 41,* 393–404.

Heilmann, J., Weismer, S., Evans, J., & Hollar, C. (2005). Utility of the MacArthur-Bates Communicative Development Inventory in identifying language abilities of late-talking and typically developing toddlers. *American Journal of Speech-Language Pathology, 14,* 40–51.

Helm-Estabrooks, N. (1992). *Aphasia diagnostic profiles* [Measurement instrument]. Austin, TX: Pro-Ede.

Helm-Estabrooks, N. (1999). Stuttering associated with acquired neurological disorders. *Stuttering and Related Disorders of Fluency, 2,* 255–268.

Helm-Estabrooks, N. (2001). *Cognitive linguistic quick test* [Measurement instrument]. Boston, MA: Pearson.

Helm-Estabrooks, N., Albert, M., & Nicholas, M. (2014). *Manual of aphasia and aphasia therapy* (3rd ed.). Austin, TX: Pro-Ed.

Helm-Estabrooks, N., & Hotz, G. (1991). *Brief test of head injury* [Measurement instrument]. Austin, TX: Pro-Ed.

Helm-Estabrooks, N., Ramsberger, G., Morgan, A. R., & Nicholas, M. (1989). *Boston assessment of severe aphasia* [Measurement instrument]. Austin, TX: Pro-Ed.

Henley, J., & Souliere, C. (2009). Tracheoesophageal speech failure in the laryngectomee: The role of constrictor myotomy. *The Laryngoscope, 96*(9), 1016–1020.

Henry, L. A., Messer, D. J., & Nash, G. (2012). Executive functioning in children with specific language impairment. *Journal of Child Psychology and Psychiatry, 53*(1), 37–45.

Hester, E. (1996). Narratives of young African American children. In A. Kamhi, K. Pollock, & J. Harris (Eds.), *Communication development and disorders in African American children* (pp. 227–245). Baltimore, MD: Brookes.

Hickley, J., & Nash (2007). Cognitive assessment and aphasia severity. *Brain and Language, 103*, 195–196.

Hickman, L. (1997). *The apraxia profile* [Measurement instrument]. Boston, MA: Pearson.

Hilari, K., Byng, S., Lamping, D., & Smith, S. (2003). Stroke and Aphasia Quality of Life Scale–39 (SAQOL–39): Evaluation of acceptability, reliability, and validity. *Stroke, 34*, 1944–1950.

Hirano, M. (1981). *Clinical examination of voice*. Vienna, Austria: Springer-Verlag.

Hixon, T. J., & Hoit, J. D. (1998). Physical examination of the diaphragm by the speech-language pathologist. *American Journal of Speech-Language Pathology, 7*, 37–45.

Hixon, T. J., & Hoit, J. D. (1999). Physical examination of the abdominal wall by the speech-language pathologist. *American Journal of Speech-Language Pathology, 8*, 335–345.

Hodson, B. (2003). *Hodson computerized analysis of phonological patterns* [Measurement instrument]. Wichita, KS: PhonoComp Software.

Hodson, B. (2004). *Hodson assessment of phonological patterns* (3rd ed.) [Measurement Instrument]. Austin, TX: Pro-Ed.

Hodson, B., & Paden, E. (1991). *Targeting intelligible speech: A phonological approach to remediation* (2nd ed.). Austin, TX: Pro-Ed.

Hoffman, H. T., Porter, K., Karnell, L. H., Cooper, J. S., Weber, R. S., Langer, C. J., . . . Robinson, R. A. (2006). Laryngeal cancer in the United States: Changes in demographics, patterns of care, and survival. *The Laryngoscope, 116*(9 Pt. 2 Suppl. 111), 1–13.

Hogikyan, N. D., & Sethurama, G. (1999). Validation of an instrument to measure voice-related quality of life (V-RQOL). *Journal of Voice, 13*, 557–569.

Holland, A. (1975). Language therapy for children: Some thoughts on context and content. *Journal of Speech and Hearing Disorders, 40*, 514–523.

Holland, A., Frattali, C., & Fromm, D. (1999). *Communication activities of daily living* (2nd ed.). Austin, TX: Pro-Ed.

Holland, A., & Thompson, C. (1998). Outcomes measures in aphasia. In C. Frattali (Ed.), *Measuring outcomes in speech-language pathology* (pp. 245–266). New York, NY: Thieme.

Howard, S., & Lohmander, A. (2011). *Cleft palate speech assessment and intervention*. New York, NY: John Wiley & Sons.

Howe, C. (1976). The meanings of two-word utterances in the speech of young children. *Journal of Child Language, 3*, 29–47.

Hresko, W. P., Reid, D. K., & Hammill, D. D. (1999). *Test of early language development* (3rd ed.) [Measurement instrument]. Austin, TX: Pro Ed.

Huang, R., Hopkins, J., & Nippold, M. (1997). Satisfaction with standardized language testing: A survey of speech-language pathologists. *Language, Speech, and Hearing Services in Schools, 28*, 12–23.

Hubbell, R. (1981). *Children's language disorders: An integrated approach*. Englewood Cliffs, NJ: Prentice Hall.

Hubbell, R. (1988). *A handbook of English grammar and language sampling*. Englewood Cliffs, NJ: Prentice Hall.

Huer, M. B., & Miller, L. (2011). *Test of early communication and emerging language* [Measurement instrument]. Austin, TX: Pro-Ed.

Hughes, C. (2002). Executive functions and development: Emerging themes. *Infant and Child Development, 11*(2), 201–209.

Hughes, D., Fey, M., & Long, S. (1992). Developmental sentence scoring: Still useful after all these years. *Topics in Language Disorders, 12*, 1–12.

Humes, K., Jones, N. A., & Ramirez, R. R. (2011). *Overview of race and Hispanic origin, 2010*. Washington, DC: US Department of Commerce, Economics and Statistics Administration, US Census Bureau.

Hutchinson, T. (1996). What to look for in the technical manual: Twenty questions for users. *Language, Speech, and Hearing Services in Schools, 27*, 109–121.

Hux, K., Morris-Friehe, M., & Sanger, D. (1993). Language sampling practices: A survey of nine states. *Language, Speech, and Hearing Services in Schools, 24*, 84–91.

Ingham, R. (2005). Clinicians deserve better: Observations on a clinical forum titled "What child language research may contribute to the understanding and treatment of stuttering (2004)." *Language, Speech, and Hearing Services in Schools, 36*(2), 152–155.

Ingram, D. (1976). *Phonological disability in children*. New York, NY: Elsiever.

Ingram, D. (1981). *Procedures for the phonological analysis of children's language*. Baltimore, MD: University Park Press.

Ingram, D., & Ingram, K. (2001). A whole word approach to phonological analysis and intervention. *Language, Speech, and Hearing Services in Schools, 32*, 271–283.

Ireton, H. (1990). *Child development review parent questionnaire* [Measurement instrument]. Minneapolis, MN: Behavior Science Systems.

Isshiki, N., Yanigahara, N., & Morimoto, H. (1966). Approach to the objective diagnosis of hoarseness. *Folia Phoniatrica, 18*, 393–400.

Ivanova, M., & Hallowell, B. (2013). A tutorial on aphasia test development in any language: Key substantive and psychometric considerations. *Aphasiology, 27*(8), 891–920.

Iverson, J. M., & Thal, D. J. (1998). Communicative transitions: There's more to the hand than meets the eye. In A. M. Wetherby, S. F. Warren, & J. Reichle (Eds.), *Transitions in prelinguistic communication: Preintentional to intentional and presymbolic to symbolic* (pp. 59–86). Baltimore, MD: Paul H. Brookes.

Jackson, S., Pretti-Frontczak, K., Harjusola-Webb, S., Grisham-Brown, J., & Romani, J. (2009). Response to intervention: Implications for early childhood professionals. *Language, Speech, and Hearing Services in Schools, 40*, 424–434.

Jacobson, B., Johnson, A., Grywalski, C., Silbergleit, A., Jacobson, B., & Benninger, S. (1997). The Voice Handicap Index (VHI): Development and validation. *American Journal of Speech-Language Pathology, 6*(3), 66–70.

Jelm, J. M. (1990). *Oral-motor feeding rating scale* [Measurement instrument]. Boston, MA: Pearson.

Jelm, J. M. (2001). *Verbal dyspraxia profile* [Measurement instrument]. DeKalb, IL: Janelle.

John, A., Sell, D., Sweeney, T., Harding-Bell, A., & Williams, A. (2006). The cleft audit protocol for speech–augmented: A validated and reliable measure for auditing cleft speech. *Cleft Palate–Cranifacial Journal, 43*(3), 272–288.

Johns, V., & Haynes, W. (2002). Dynamic assessment and predicting children's benefit from narrative training. Paper presented at the convention of the American Speech-Language-Hearing Association, Atlanta, GA.

Johnson, J. (1982) Narratives: A new look at communication problems in older language-disordered children. *Language, Speech, and Hearing Services in Schools, 13*, 144–155.

Johnson, C. (1995). Expanding norms for narration. *Language, Speech, and Hearing Services in Schools, 26*, 326–341.

Johnson, C., Beitchman, J., & Brownlie, E. (2010). Twenty-year follow-up of children with and without speech-language impairments: Family, educational, occupational, and quality of life outcomes. *American Journal of Speech-Language Pathology, 19*, 51–65.

Johnson, C., Weston, A., & Bain, B. (2004). An objective and time-efficient method for determining severity of childhood speech delay. *American Journal of Speech-Language Pathology, 13*, 55–65.

Johnson-Martin, N. M., Attermeier, S. M., & Hacker, B. J. (2004). *The Carolina curriculum for infants and toddlers with special needs* (3rd ed.) [Measurement instrument]. Baltimore, MD: Brookes.

Johnston, J. (1982). Narrative: A new look at communication problems in older language-disordered children. *Language, Speech, and Hearing Services in Schools, 13,* 144–155.

Johnston, J. (2001). An alternate MLU calculation: Magnitude and variability of effects. *Journal of Speech, Language, and Hearing Research, 44,* 156–164.

Johnston, J. (2006) *Thinking about child language: Research to practice.* Eau Claire, WI: Thinking Publications.

Johnston, J., Miller, J., Curtiss, S., & Tallal, P. (1993). Conversations with children who are language impaired: Asking questions. *Journal of Speech and Hearing Research, 36,* 973–978.

Jokel, R., De Nil, L., & Sharpe, K. (2007). Speech disfluencies in adults with neurogenic stuttering associated with stroke and traumatic brain injury. *Journal of Medical Speech-Language Pathology, 15*(3), 243–261.

Justice, L. (2006). Evidence-based practice response to intervention and the prevention of reading difficulties. *Language, Speech, and Hearing Services in Schools, 37,* 284–297.

Justice, L. (2010). *Communication sciences and disorders: A contemporary perspective* (2nd ed). Boston, MA: Pearson.

Justice, L., Bowles, R., Kaderavek, J., Ukrainetz, T., Eisenberg, S., & Gillam, R. (2006). The index of narrative microstructure: A clinical tool for analyzing school-age children's narrative performances. *American Journal of Speech-Language Pathology, 15,* 177–191.

Justice, L., & Ezell, H. (2004). Print referencing: An emergent literacy enhancement strategy and its clinical applications. *Language, Speech, and Hearing Services in Schools, 35,* 185–193.

Justice, L., Invernizzi, M., & Meier, J. (2002). Designing and implementing an early literacy screening protocol: Suggestions for the speech-language pathologist. *Language, Speech, and Hearing Services in Schools, 33,* 84–101.

Justice, L., & Kaderavek, J. (2004). Embedded-explicit emergent literacy intervention I: Background and description of approach. *Language, Speech, and Hearing Services in Schools, 35,* 201–211.

Kaderavek, J., & Justice, L. (2004). Embedded-explicit emergent literacy intervention II: Goal selection and implementation in the early childhood classroom. *Language, Speech, and Hearing Services in Schools, 35,* 212–228.

Kaderavek, J., & Sulzby, E. (1998). Parent–child joint book reading: An observational protocol for young children. *American Journal of Speech-Language Pathology, 7,* 33–47.

Kaderavek, J., & Sulzby, E. (2000). Narrative production by children with and without specific language impairment: Oral narratives and emergent readings. *Journal of Speech, Language, and Hearing Research, 43,* 38–49.

Kadushin, A. (1972). The social work interview. New York, NY: Columbia University Press.

Kahn, J. (1984). Cognitive training and initial use of referential speech. *Topics in Language Disorders, 5,* 14–18.

Kahn, L., & James, S. (1980). A method for assessing the use of grammatical structures in language-disordered children. *Language, Speech, and Hearing Services in Schools, 11,* 188–197.

Kahn, L., & Lewis, N. (2002). *Kahn-Lewis phonological analysis-2* [Measurement instrument]. Boston, MA: Pearson.

Kamhi, A., & Johnston, J. (1982). Towards an understanding of retarded children's linguistic deficiencies. *Journal of Speech and Hearing Research, 25,* 435–445.

Kamhi, A., Pollock, K., & Harris, J. (1996). *Communication development and disorders in African-American children.* Baltimore, MD: Paul H. Brookes.

Kander, M., & Satterfield, L. (2014). Changes ahead for speech generating device reimbursement. *The ASHA Leader, 19*(5), 25–27.

Kaplan, N., & Dreyer, D. (1974). The effect of self-awareness training on student speech pathologist–client relationships. *Journal of Communication Disorders, 7,* 329–342.

Kaplan, E., Goodglass, H., & Weintraub, S. (2001). *Boston naming test* (2nd ed.) [Measurement instrument]. Philadelphia, PA: Lippencott Williams & Wilkins.

Kaplan, N., & Dreyer, D. (1974). The effect of self-awareness training on student speech pathologist–client relationships. *Journal of Communication Disorders, 7,* 329–342.

Karnell, M., Melton, S., Childes, J., Coleman, T., Dailey, S., & Hoffman, H. (2007). Reliability of clinician-based (GRBAS and CAPE-V) and patient-based (V-RQOL and IPVI) documentation of voice disorders. *Journal of Voice, 21*(5), 576–590.

Katz, R. C. (2001). Computer applications in aphasia treatment. In R. Chapey (Ed.), *Language intervention strategies in aphasia and related neurogenic communication disorders* (4th ed., pp. 718–741). Philadelphia, PA: Lippincott Williams & Wilkins.

Kaufman, N. (1995). *Kaufman speech praxis test for children* [Measurement instrument]. Austin, TX: Pro-Ed.

Kay, J., Lesser, R., & Coltheart, M. (1997). *Psycholinguistic assessments of language processing in aphasia* [Measurement instrument]. Hove, UK: Psychology Press.

Kayser, H. (1995). *Bilingual speech and language pathology: An Hispanic focus.* San Diego, CA: Singular.

Kazi, R., De Cordova, J., Kanagalingam, J., Venkitaraman, R., Nutting, C. M., Clarke, P., . . . Harrington, K. J. (2007). Quality of Life following total laryngectomy: Assessment using the UW-QOL Scale. *Journal for Oto-Rhino-Laryngology, Head and Neck Surgery, 69*(2), 100–106.

Keenan, E., & Schieffelin, B. (1976). Topic as a discourse notion: A study of topic in the conversations of children and adults. In C. Li (Ed.), *Subject and Topic* (pp. 335–384). New York, NY: Academic Press.

Keenan, J., & Brassell, E. (1975). *Aphasia language performance scales* [Measurement instrument]. Murfreesboro, TN: Pinnacle Press.

Kempster, G., Gerratt, B., Verdolini-Abbott, K., Barkmeier-Kraemer, J., & Hillman, R. (2009). Consensus auditory-perceptual evaluation of voice: Development of a standardized clinical protocol. *American Journal of Speech-Language Pathology, 18,* 124–132.

Kenny, D., Koheil, R., Greenberg, J., Reid, D., Milner, M., Roman, R., & Judd, P. (1989). Development of a multidisciplinary feeding profile for children who are dependent feeders. *Dysphagia, 4,* 16–28.

Kent, L., & Chabon, S. (1980). Problem-oriented records in a university speech and hearing clinic. *Journal of the American Speech and Hearing Association, 22,* 151–158.

Kent, R., Miolo, G., & Bloedel, S. (1994). The intelligibility of children's speech: A review of evaluation procedures. *American Journal of Speech-Language Pathology, 3,* 81–95.

Kertesz, A. (2006). *Western aphasia battery* (Revised edition) [Measurement instrument]. Boston, MA: Pearson.

Khan, L., & Lewis, N. (2002). *Khan-Lewis phonological analysis* (2nd ed.) [Measurement instrument]. Boston, MA: Pearson.

Kimbarow, M. (2011). *Cognitive communication disorders.* San Diego, CA: Plural.

King, R., Jones, C., & Lasky, E. (1982). In retrospect: A fifteen-year follow-up report of speech-language disorders in children. *Language, Speech, and Hearing Services in Schools, 13,* 24–32.

Kirk, S., & Kirk, W. (1971). *Psycholinguisic learning disabilities.* Urbana, IL: University of Illinois Press.

Kirkwood, T. (2000). *Time of our lives: The science of human aging.* Oxford, England: Oxford University Press.

Klassen, A. F., Tsangaris, E., Forrest, C. R., Wong, K. W., Pusic, A. L., Cano, S. L., . . . Goodacre, T. (2012). Quality of life of children treated for cleft lip and/or palate: A systematic review. *Journal of Plastic, Reconstructive & Aesthetic Surgery, 65*(5), 547–557.

Klecan-Aker, J., & Hedrick, D. (1985). A study of the syntactic language skills of normal school-age children. *Language, Speech, and Hearing Services in Schools, 16,* 187–198.

Klee, T., Pearce, K., & Carson, D. (2000). Improving the positive predictive value of screening for developmental language disorder. *Journal of Speech, Language and Hearing Research, 43,* 821–833.

Kleiman, L. (2003). *Functional communication profile* (Revised edition) [Measurement instrument]. East Moline, IL: LinguiSystems.

Klein, H., & Liu-Shea, M. (2009). Between word simplification patterns in the continuous speech of children with speech sound disorders. *Language, Speech, and Hearing Services in Schools, 40,* 17–30.

Klein, M., & Briggs, M. (1987). Facilitating mother–infant communicative interactions in mothers of high-risk infants. *Journal of Childhood Communication Disorders, 10*(2), 95–106.

Klinger, L., & Dawson, G. (1992). Facilitating early social and communicative development in children with autism. In S. Warren & J. Reichle (Eds.), *Causes and Effects in Communication and Language Intervention* (pp. 157–186). Baltimore, MD: Brookes.

Kramer, P. (1977). Young children's free responses to anomalous commands. *Journal of Experimental Child Psychology, 24,* 219–234.

Kratcoski, A. (1998). Guidelines for using portfolios in assessment and evaluation. *Language, Speech, and Hearing Services in Schools, 29,* 3–10.

Kuhl, P. (2004). Early language acquisition: Cracking the speech code. *Nature, 5,* 831–843.

Kummer, A. (2005). Ankyloglossia: To clip or not to clip: That's the question. *The ASHA Leader, 10*(17), 6–7, 30.

Kummer, A. (2013a). *Cleft palate and craniofacial anomalies: Effects on speech and resonance* (3rd ed.). Clifton Park, NJ: Delmar.

Kummer, A. (2013b). School matters: Options for affordable, low-tech intervention with resonance disorders. *The ASHA Leader, 18*(4), 28–29.

Kummer, A., & Lee, L. (1996). Evaluation and treatment of resonance disorders. *Language, Speech, and Hearing Services in Schools, 27,* 271–281.

Kwan, K. L. K., Gong, Y., & Maestas, M. (2010). Language, translation, and validity in the adaptation of psychological tests for multicultural counseling. In J. G. Ponterotto, J. M. Casas, L. A. Suzuki, & C. M. Alexander (Eds.), *Handbook of Multicultural Counseling* (2nd ed. pp. 397–412). Los Angeles, CA: Sage Publications.

Kwiatkowski, J., & Shriberg, L. (1992). Intelligibility assessment in developmental phonological disorders: Accuracy of caregiver gloss. *Journal of Speech and Hearing Research, 35,* 1095–1104.

LaBorgne, W. (2011). *Rating laryngeal videostroboscopy and acoustic recordings: Normal and pathologic samples.* San Diego, CA: Plural.

Lahey, M. (1988). *Language disorders and language development.* New York, NY: Macmillan.

Lahey, M., & Edwards, J. (1995). Specific language impairment: Preliminary investigation of factors associated with family history and with patterns of language performance. *Journal of Speech and Hearing Research, 38,* 643–657.

Lambert, N., Nihira, K, & Leland, H. (1993). *Adaptive behavior scale–school* (2nd ed.) [Measurement instrument]. Austin, TX: Pro-Ed.

Lanyon, R. I. (1967). The measurement of stuttering severity. *Journal of Speech, Language, and Hearing Research, 10*(4), 836–843.

LaParo, K., Justice, L., Skibbe, L., & Pianta, R. (2004). Relations among maternal, child and demographic factors and the persistence of preschool language impairment. *American Journal of Speech-Language Pathology, 13,* 291–303.

LaPointe, L., & Eisenson, J. (2008). *Examining for aphasia: Assessment of aphasia and related impairments* (4th ed.). Austin, TX: Pro-Ed.

LaPointe, L., & Horner, J. (1998). *Reading comprehension battery for aphasia-2* [Measurement instrument]. Austin, TX: Pro-Ed.

Larsen, S. C., Hammill, D., & Moats, L. (2013). *Test of written spelling* (5th ed.) [Measurement instrument]. Austin, TX: Pro-Ed.

Larson, V., & McKinley, N. (1995). *Language disorders in older students: Preadolescents and adolescents.* Eau Claire, WI: Thinking Publications.

Lau, C., & Kesnierczyk, I. (2001). Quantitative evaluation of infant's nonnutritive and nutritive sucking. *Dysphagia, 16,* 58–67.

Lauder, E. (1978). *Self-help for the laryngectomee.* San Antonio, TX: Lauder Enterprises.

Lawrence, C. (1992). Assessing the use of age-equivalent scores in clinical management. *Language, Speech, and Hearing Services in Schools, 23,* 6–8.

Least-Heat-Moon, W. (1982). *Blue highways: A journey into America.* Boston, MA: Atlantic—Little, Brown.

Leavitt, R. R. (1974). *The Puerto Ricans: Cultural change and language deviance.* Tucson, AZ: University of Arizona Press.

LeBorgne, W. (2011). *Rating laryngeal videostroboscopy and acoustic recordings: Normal and pathologic samples.* San Diego, CA: Plural.

Lee, L. (1966). Developmental sentence types: A method for comparing normal and deviant syntactic development. *Journal of Speech and Hearing Disorders, 31,* 311–330.

Lee, L. (1974). *Developmental sentence analysis.* Evanston, IL: Northwestern University Press.

Lee, L., Koenigsknecht, R., & Mulhern, S. (1975). *Interactive language development teaching.* Evanston, IL: Northwestern University Press.

Lee, L., Stemple, J., Glaze, L., & Kelchner, L. (2004). Quick screen of voice and supplemental documents for identifying pediatric voice disorders. *Language, Speech, and Hearing Services in Schools, 35,* 308–319.

Lefton-Greif, M. A. (1994). Diagnosis and management of pediatric feeding and swallowing disorders: Role of the speech-language pathologist. In D. N. Tuchman & R. S. Walter (Eds.), *Disorders of feeding and swallowing in infants and children: Pathophysiology, diagnosis, and treatment* (pp. 97–113). San Diego, CA: Singular.

Leonard, L. (1975). On differentiating syntactic and semantic features in emerging grammars: Evidence from empty form usage. *Journal of Psycholinguistic Research, 4,* 357–364.

Leonard, L. (1976). *Meaning in child language: Issues in the study of early semantic development.* New York, NY: Grune and Stratton.

Leonard, L. (2009). Is expressive language disorder an accurate diagnostic category? *American Journal of Speech-Language Pathology, 18,* 115–123.

Leonard, L., Prutting, C., Perozzi, C., &d Berkley, R. (1978). Nonstandardized approaches to the assessment of language behaviors. *Journal of the American Speech and Hearing Association,* May, 371–379.

Leonard, L., Steckol, K., & Panther, K. (1983). Returning meaning to semantic relations: Some clinical applications. *Journal of Speech and Hearing Disorders, 48,* 25–35.

Leonard, L., Weismer, S., Miller, C., Francis, D., Tomblin, J., & Kail, R. (2007). Speed of processing, working memory and language impairment in children. *Journal of Speech, Language, and Hearing Research, 50,* 408–428.

Levin, H. S., O'Donnell, V. M., & Grossman, R. G. (1979). The Galveston Orientation and Amnesia Test: A practical scale to assess cognition after head injury. *Journal of Nervous System and Mental Disorders, 167,* 675–684.

Lewis, J. (1999). Tracheoesophageal communication: Beyond traditional speech treatment. In S. Salmon (Ed.), *Alaryngeal Speech Rehabilitation* (2nd ed., pp. 193–224). Austin, TX: Pro-Ed.

Lewis, B., & Freebairn, L. (1992). Residual effects of preschool phonology disorders in grade school, adolescence and adulthood. *Journal of Speech and Hearing Research, 35,* 819–831.

Lewis, B., Freebairn, L., Hansen, A., Miscimarra, L., Iyengar, S., & Taylor, H. (2007). Speech and language skills of parents of children with speech sound disorders. *American Journal of Speech-Language Pathology, 16*, 108–118.

Lewis, V., & Boucher, J. (1998). *Test of pretend play* [Measurement instrument]. London, UK: Psychological Corporation.

Lidz, C. (1991). *A practitioner's guide to dynamic assessment.* New York, NY: Guilford Press.

Lifter, K., Edwards, G., Avery, D., Anderson, S., & Sulzer-Azaroff, B. (1988). Developmental assessment of children's play: Implications for intervention. Paper presented at the convention of the American Speech-Language-Hearing Association, Boston, MA.

Liles, B. (1985). Cohesion in the narratives of normal and language-disordered children. *Journal of Speech and Hearing Research, 28*, 123–133.

Liles, B. (1993). Narrative discourse in children with language disorders and children with normal language: A critical review of the literature. *Journal of Speech and Hearing Research, 36*, 868–882.

Linder, T. W. (2008). *Transdisciplinary play-based assessment and intervention* (Revised edition) [Measurement instrument]. Baltimore, MD: Brookes.

Lindsay, G., & Dockrell, J. (2013). *The relationship between speech, language and communication needs (SLCN) and behavioral, emotional and social difficulties (BESD).* Department for Education, London:*DFE-RR247-BCRP6*.

Loban, W. (1976). *Language development: Kindergarten through grade twelve.* Research Report No. 18. Urbana, IL: National Councils of Teachers of English.

Logemann, J. A., Veis, S., & Colangelo, L. (1999). A screening procedure for oropharyngeal dysphagia. *Dysphagia, 14*, 44–51.

Lohmander, A., Willadsen, E., Persson, C., Henningsson, G., Bowden, W., & Hutters, B. (2009). Methodology for speech assessment in the Scandcleft project—an international randomized clinical trial on palatal surgery: Experience from a pilot study. *Cleft Palate–Craniofacial Journal, 46*(4), 347–362.

Lomas, J., Pickard, L., Bester, S., Elbard, H., Finlayson, A., & Zoghaib, C. (1989). The Communicative Effectiveness Index: Development and psychometric evaluation of a functional communication measure for adult aphasia. *Journal of Speech and Hearing Disorders, 54*, 113–124.

Lombardino, L. J., Lieberman, R. J., & Brown, J. C. (2005). *Assessment of literacy and language* [Measurement instrument]. San Antonio, TX: Pearson.

Long, S., & Channell, R. (2001). Accuracy of four language analysis procedures performed automatically. *American Journal of Speech-Language Pathology, 10*, 180–188.

Long, S., Fey, M., & Channell, R. (2002). *Computerized profiling*, Version 9.4.1. Retrieved from http://www.computerizedprofiling.org

Longhurst, T., & File, J. (1977). A comparison of developmental sentence scores for Head Start children in four conditions. *Language, Speech, and Hearing Services in Schools, 8*, 54–64.

Longhurst, T., & Grubb, S. (1974). A comparison of language samples collected in four situations. *Language, Speech, and Hearing Services in Schools, 5*, 71–78.

Longhurst, T., & Schrandt, T. (1973). Linguistic analysis of children's speech: A comparison of four procedures. *Journal of Speech and Hearing Disorders, 38*, 240–249.

Lord, C., Rutter, M., DiLavore, P. C., Risi, S., Gotham, K., & Bishop S. (2012). *Autism diagnostic observation schedule* (2nd ed.). Torrance, CA: Western Psychological Services.

Love, R. J. (2000). *Childhood motor speech disability* (2nd ed.). Needham Heights, MA: Allyn & Bacon.

Lowe, M., & Costello, A. (1988). *Symbolic play test* (2nd ed.) [Measurement instrument]. Windsor, England: Nfer-Nelson.

Lucas, E. (1980). *Semantic and pragmatic language disorders.* Rockville, MD: Aspen.

Ludlow, C. (1983). Identification and assessment of aphasic patients for language intervention. In J. Miller, D. Yoder, & R. Schiefelbusch (Eds.), *Contemporary issues in language intervention.* Rockville, MD: American Speech-Language-Hearing Association.

Lukens, C. T., & Linscheid, T. R. (2008). Development and validation of an instrument to assess mealtime behavior problems in children with autism. *Journal of Autism and Developmental Disorders, 38*, 342–352.

Lum, J. A., Conti-Ramsden, G., Page, D., & Ullman, M. T. (2012). Working declarative and procedural memory in specific language impairment. *Cortex, 48*(9), 1138–1154.

Lund, N., & Duchan, J. (1988). *Assessing children's language in naturalistic contexts* (2nd ed.). Englewood Cliffs, NJ: Prentice Hall.

Lund, N., & Duchan, J. (1993). *Assessing children's language in naturalistic contexts* (3rd ed.). Englewood Cliffs, NJ: Prentice Hall.

Luterman, D. (1979). *Counseling parents of hearing-impaired children.* Boston, MA: Little, Brown.

Lutz, K. C., & Mallard, A. R. (1986). Disfluencies and rate of speech in young adult nonstutterers. *Journal of Fluency Disorders, 11*, 307–316.

Luyster, R., Qiu, S., Lopez, K., & Lord, C. (2007). Predicting outcomes of children referred for autism using the MacArthur-Bates Communicative Development Inventory. *Journal of Speech, Language, and Hearing Research, 50*, 667–681.

Lynch, E. (1998). Developing cross-cultural competence. In E. Lynch & M. Hanson (Eds.), *Developing cross-cultural competence* (2nd ed., pp. 47–90). Baltimore, MD: Brookes.

Ma, E., & Yiu, E. (2001). Voice activity and participation profile: Assessing the impact of voice disorders on daily activities. *Journal of Speech, Language, and Hearing Research, 44*(3), 511–524.

MacDonald, J., & Carroll, J. (1992). A social partnership model for assessing early communication development: An intervention model for preconversational children. *Language, Speech, and Hearing Services in Schools, 23*, 113–124.

MacDonald, S. (2005). *Functional assessment of verbal reasoning and executive strategies* [Measurement instrument]. Ontario, Canada: CCD.

Mahr, G., & Leith, W. (1992). Psychogenic stuttering of adult onset. *Journal of Speech and Hearing Research, 35*, 283–286.

Mann, G. (2002). *Mann assessment of swallowing ability* [Measurement instrument]. Clifton Park, NJ: Delmar Cengage Learning.

Manning, W. (2010). *Clinical decision making in fluency disorders.* Clifton Park, NY: Delmar.

Manning, W. H. (1994). The SEA-Scale: Self-efficacy scaling for adolescents who stutter. In *Presentation to the Annual meeting of the American Speech-Language-Hearing Association*, New Orleans, LA.

Manning, W. H. (2009). *Clinical decision making in fluency disorders.* New York, NY: Cengage Learning.

Mansson, H. (2000). Childhood stuttering: Incidence and development. *Journal of Fluency Disorders, 25*, 47–57.

Marks, I. M. (1987). *Fears, phobias and rituals.* New York, NY: Oxford University Press.

Martin, N., & Brownell, R. (2005). *Test of auditory processing skills-3* [Measurement instrument]. Novato, CA: Academic Therapy.

Martin, N., & Brownell, R. (2010). *Receptive one-word picture vocabulary test* (4th ed.) (ROWPVT-4). Novato, CA: ATP Assessments.

Martin, S., & Lockhart, M. (2005). *Voice impact profile* [Measurement instrument]. London, England: Speechmark.

Martino, R., Pron, G., & Diamant, N. (2000). Screening for oropharyngeal dysphagia in stroke: Insufficient evidence for guidelines. *Dysphagia, 15*, 19–30.

Martino, R., Silver, F., Teasell, R., Bayley, M., Nicholson, G., Streiner, D. L., & Diamant, N. E. (2009). The Toronto Bedside Swallowing Screening Test (TOR-BSST): Development and validation of a dysphagia screening tool for patients with stroke. *Stroke, 40*(2), 555–561.

Massey, R., & Jedlicka, D. (2002). The Massey bedside swallowing screen. *Journal of Neuroscience Nursing, 34*(5), 252–257.

Masterson, J. J., & Apel, K. (2000). Spelling assessment: Charting a path to optimal intervention. *Topics in Language Disorders, 20*(5), 50–65.

Masterson, J. J., & Apel, K. (2010). The spelling sensitivity score: Noting developmental changes in spelling knowledge. *Assessment for Effective Intervention, 36*(1), 35–45.

Masterson, J. J., Apel, K., & Wasowicz, J. (2006). *Spelling performance evaluation for language and literacy* (2nd ed.) [Measurement instrument]. Evanston, IL: Learning by Design.

Masterson, J., & Bernhardt, B. (2001). *Computerized articulation and phonology evaluation system* (Version 1.0.1) [Measurement instrument]. San Antonio, TX: Psychological Corporation.

Masterson, J., Bernhardt, B., & Hofheinz, M. (2005). A comparison of single words and conversational speech in phonological evaluation. *American Journal of Speech-Language Pathology, 14*, 229–241.

Masterson, J., & Crede, L. (1999). Learning to spell: Implications for assessment and intervention. *Language, Speech, and Hearing Services in Schools, 30*, 243–254.

Mattes, L. (1994). *Spanish articulation measures* (Revised edition) [Measurement instrument]. Oceanside, CA: Academic Communication Associates.

Mattes, L. J., & Santiago, G. (1985). *Bilingual language proficiency questionnaire* [Measurement instrument]. Oceanside, CA: Academic Communication Associates.

Mattis, S. (2001). *Dementia rating scale-2* [Measurement instrument]. Lutz, FL: Psychological Assessment Resources.

Maxwell, S., & Wallach, G. (1984). The language-learning disabilities connection: Symptoms of early language disability change over time. In G. Wallach & K. Butler (Eds.), *Language Learning Disabilities in School-Age Children* (pp. 15–34). Baltimore, MD: Williams and Wilkins.

McCabe, A., Bliss, L., Barra, G., & Bennett, M. (2008). Comparison of personal versus fictional narratives of children with language impairment. *American Journal of Speech-Language Pathology, 17*, 194–206.

McCathren, R., Warren, S., & Yoder, P. (1996). Prelinguistic predictors of later language development. In K. Cole, P. Dale, & D. Thal (Eds.), *Assessment of communication and language* (pp. 57–75). Baltimore, MD: Brookes.

McCauley, R. (1996). Familiar strangers: Criterion referenced measures in communication disorders. *Language, Speech, and Hearing Services in Schools, 27*, 122–131.

McCauley, R., & Strand, E. (2008). A review of standardized tests of nonverbal oral and speech motor performance in children. *American Journal of Speech-Language Pathology, 17*, 81–91.

McCauley, R., Strand, E., Lof, G., & Schooling, T. (2009). Evidence-based systematic review: Effects of nonspeech oral motor exercises on speech. *American Journal of Speech-Language Pathology, 18*, 343–360.

McCauley, R., & Swisher, L. (1984a). Psychometric review of language and articulation tests for preschool children. *Journal of Speech and Hearing Disorders, 49*, 34–42.

McCauley, R., & Swisher, L. (1984b). Use and misuse of norm-referenced tests in clinical assessment: A hypothetical case. *Journal of Speech and Hearing Disorders, 49*, 338–348.

McCollum, J., & Stayton, V. (1985). Social interaction assessment/intervention. *Journal of the Division for Early Childhood, 9*, 125–135.

McCullough, G. H., Wertz, R. T., Rosenbek, R. C., & Dinneen, C. (1999). Clinicians' preferences and practices in conducting clinical/bedside and videofluoroscopic swallowing examinations in an adult, neurogenic population. *American Journal of Speech Language Pathology, 8*, 149–163.

McCune, L. (1995). A normative study of representational play at the transition to language. *Developmental Psychology, 31*, 198–206.

McCurtin, A., & Murray, G. (2000). *The manual of AAC assessment*. Chesterfield, UK: Winslow.

McEachern, D., & Haynes, W. (2004). Gesture-speech combinations as a transition to multiword utterances. *American Journal of Speech-Language Pathology, 13*, 227–236.

McFadden, T. (1996). Creating language impairments in typically achieving children: The pitfalls of "normal" normative sampling. *Language, Speech, and Hearing Services in Schools, 27*, 3–9.

McFadin, S. (2006). *Auditory discrimination and lip reading skills inventory* [Measurement instrument]. Greenville, SC: Super Duper.

McGhee, R. L., Ehrler, D. J., & DiSimoni, F. (2007). *Token test for children* (2nd ed.). [Measurement instrument]. Austin, TX: Pro-Ed.

McGinty, A., & Justice, L. (2009). Predictors of print knowledge in children with specific language impairment: Experimental and developmental factors. *Journal of Speech, Language, and Hearing Research, 52*, 81–97.

McGowan, R., McGowan R., Denny, M., & Nittrouer, S. (2014). A longitudinal study of very young children's vowel production. *Journal of Speech, Language, and Hearing Research, 57*(1), 1–15.

McHorney, C. A., Bricker, D. E., Robbins, J., Kramer, A. E., Rosenbek, J. C., & Chignell, K. A. (2000). The SWAL-QOL outcomes tool for oropharyngeal dysphagia in adults: II item reduction and preliminary scaling. *Dysphagia, 15*, 122–133.

McLean, J. E., McLean, L. K., Brady, N. C., & Etter, R. (1991). Communication profiles of two types of gesture using nonverbal persons with severe to profound mental retardation. *Journal of Speech, Language, and Hearing Research, 34*(2), 294–308.

McLean, J., & Snyder-Mclean, L. (1978). *A transactional approach to early language training*. Columbus, OH: Merrill.

McLeod, S., Harrison, L., & McCormack, J. (2012). The intelligibility in context scale: Validity and reliability of a subjective rating measure. *Journal of Speech, Language, and Hearing Research, 55*(2), 648–656.

McLeod, S., Van Doorn, J., & Reed, V. (2001). Normal acquisition of consonant clusters. *American Journal of Speech-Language Pathology, 10*, 99–110.

McNeil, M., & Prescott, T. (1978). *Revised token test* [Measurement instrument]. Austin, TX: Pro-Ed.

McNeil, M. R., Robin, D. A., & Schmidt, R. A. (2008). Apraxia of speech: Definition, differentiation, and treatment. In M. R. McNeil (Ed.), *Clinical management of sensorimotor speech disorders* (2nd ed.). New York, NY: Thieme.

McNeill, D. (1970). *The acquisition of language: The study of developmental psycholinguistics*. New York, NY: Harper & Row.

Meisels, S. J., Dombro, A. L., Marsden, D. B., Weston, D. R., & Jewkes, A. M. (2003). *Ounce scale* [Measurement instrument]. New York, NY: Pearson Early Learning.

Merrell, A., & Plante, E. (1997). Norm referenced test interpretation in the diagnostic process. *Language, Speech, and Hearing Services in Schools, 28*, 50–58.

Merritt, D., & Liles, B. (1989). Narrative analysis: Clinical applications of story generation and story retelling. *Journal of Speech and Hearing Disorders, 54*, 438–447.

Messick, S. (1975). The standard problem: Meaning and values in measurement and evaluation. *American Psychologist, 30*, 955–966.

Messick, S. (1980). Test validity and the ethics of assessment. *American Psychologist, 35*, 1012–1027.

Messner, A. H., & Lalakea, M. L. (2002). The effect of ankyloglossia on speech in children. *Otolaryngology, Head and Neck Surgery, 127*, 539–545.

Miles, S., Chapman, R., & Sindberg, H. (2006). Sampling context affects MLU in the language of adolescents with Down syndrome. *Journal of Speech, Language, and Hearing Research, 49*, 325–337.

Millen, K., & Prutting, C. (1979). Consistencies across three language comprehension tests for specific grammatical features. *Language, Speech, and Hearing Services in Schools, 10*, 162–170.

Miller, J. (1981). *Assessing language production in children: Experimental procedures.* Baltimore, MD: University Park Press.

Miller, J., & Chapman, R. (1981). The relation between age and mean length of utterance in morphemes. *Journal of Speech and Hearing Research, 24,* 154–161.

Miller, J., & Chapman, R. (2008). *Systematic analysis of language transcripts* (Version 8—computer software). Madison, WI: University of Wisconsin–Madison, Waisman Center, Language Analysis Laboratory.

Miller, J., & Paul, R. (1995). *The clinical assessment of language comprehension.* Baltimore, MD: Brookes.

Miller, L., Gillam, R., & Pena, E. (2001). *Dynamic assessment and intervention: Improving children's narrative abilities.* Austin, TX: Pro-Ed.

Miller, W. R., & Rollnick, S. (1991). *Motivational interviewing: Preparing people for change.* New York, NY: Guilford Press.

Miller, W. R., & Rollnick, S. (2002). *Motivational interviewing: Preparing people for change* (2nd ed.). New York, NY: Guilford Press.

Mimura, M., Kato, M., Sano, Y., Kojima, T., Naesar, M., & Kashima, H. (1998). Prospective and retrospective studies of recovery in aphasia: Changes in cerebral blood flow and language function. *Brain, 121,* 2083–2094.

Miyake, A., Friedman, N. P., Emerson, M. J., Witzki, A. H., & Howeter, A. (2000). The unity and diversity of executive functions and their contributions to complex "frontal lobe" tasks: A latent variable analysis. *Cognitive Psychology, 41,* 49–100.

Montes, J., & Erickson, J. G. (1990). Bilingual stuttering: Exploring a diagnostic dilemma. *Ethnotes, 1,* 14–15.

Montgomery, J., & Evans, J. (2009). Complex sentence comprehension and working memory in children with specific language impairment. *Journal of Speech, Language, and Hearing Research, 52,* 269–288.

Montgomery, J., Magimairaj, B., & Finney, M. (2010). Working memory and specific language impairment: An update on the relation and perspectives on assessment and treatment. *American Journal of Speech-Language Pathology, 19,* 78–94.

Montgomery, J. K. (2008). *Montgomery assessment of vocabulary acquisition* [Measurement instrument]. Greenville, SC: Super Duper.

Morehead, D., & Morehead, A. (1974). From signal to sign. In *Language perspectives—Acquisition, retardation and intervention* Baltimore, MD: University Park Press.

Morgan, D. L., & Guilford, A. M. (1984). *Adolescent language screening test* [Measurement instrument]. Austin, TX: Pro-Ed.

Morris, N., & Crump, W. (1982). Syntactic and vocabulary development in the written language of learning disabled and non-disabled students at four age levels. *Learning Disability Quarterly, 5,* 163–172.

Morris, S. (2009). Test-retest reliability of independent measures of phonology in the assessment of toddlers' speech. *Language, Speech, and Hearing Services in Schools, 40,* 46–52.

Morris, S. (2010). Clinical application of the mean babbling level and syllable structure level. *Language, Speech, and Hearing Services in Schools, 41,* 223–230.

Morris, S., & Klein, M. D. (2000). *Pre-feeding skills* (2nd ed.). Austin, TX: Pro-Ed.

Morrison, M. (1998). *Let evening come: Reflections on aging.* New York, NY: Random House.

Mulac, A., Prutting, C., & Tomlinson, C. (1978). Testing for a specific syntactic structure. *Journal of Communication Disorders, 11,* 335–347.

Mullen, E. M. (1995). *Mullen scales of early learning* (AGS edition) [Measurement instrument]. San Antonio, TX: Pearson.

Muma, J. (1973a). Language assessment: The co-occurring and restricted structure procedure. *Acta Symbolica, 4,* 12–29.

Muma, J. (1973b). Language assessment: Some underlying assumptions. *Journal of the American Speech and Hearing Association, 15,* 331–338.

Muma, J. (1975). The communication game: Dump and play. *Journal of Speech and Hearing Disorders, 40,* 296–309.

Muma, J. (1978). *Language handbook: Concepts, assessment, intervention.* Englewood Cliffs, NJ: Prentice Hall.

Muma, J. (1981). *Language primer.* Lubbock, TX: Natural Child Publisher.

Muma, J. (1983). Speech language pathology: Emerging clinical expertise in language. In T. Gallagher & C. Prutting (Eds.), *Pragmatic assessment and intervention issues in language* (pp. 195–214). San Diego, CA: College-Hill Press.

Muma, J. (1984). Semel and Wiig's CELF: Construct validity? *Journal of Speech and Hearing Disorders, 49,* 101–104.

Muma, J. (1985). "No news is bad news": A response to McCauley and Swisher. *Journal of Speech and Hearing Disorders, 50,* 290–293.

Muma, J. (1998). *Effective speech-language pathology: A cognitive socialization approach.* Mahwah, NJ: Erlbaum.

Muma, J. (2002). Construct validity: The essence of language assessment. Unpublished manuscript.

Muma, J., Lubinski, R., & Pierce, S. (1982). A new era in language assessment: Data or evidence? In N. Lass (Ed.), *Speech and language* (Vol. 7, pp. 135–138). New York, NY: Academic Press.

Mundy, P., Hogan, A., & Doehring, P. (1996). *A preliminary manual for the abridged Early Social-Communication Scales.* Coral Gables, FL: University of Miami.

Munoz-Sandoval, A., Cummins, J., Alvarado, C. G., & Ruef, M. L. (2005). *Bilingual verbal ability tests–normative update* [Measurement instrument]. Rolling Meadows, IL: Riverside.

Murray, D., Ruble, L., Willis, H., & Molloy, C. (2009). Parent and teacher report of social skills in children with autism spectrum disorders. *Language, Speech, and Hearing Services in Schools, 40,* 109–115.

Musselwhite, C., & Barrie-Blackley, S. (1980). Three variations of the imperative format of language sample elicitation. *Language, Speech, and Hearing Services in Schools, 11,* 56–67.

Myers, F. (1996). Cluttering a matter of perspective. *Journal of Fluency Disorders, 21,* 175–186.

Myers, F., & St. Louis, K. (1996). *Cluttering: A clinical perspective.* San Diego, CA: Singular.

Myers, P. S. (2008). Communication disorders associated with right hemisphere damage. In R. Chapey (Ed.), *Language intervention strategies in aphasia and related neurogenic communication disorders* (5th ed.). Philadelphia, PA: Lippincott Williams and Wilkins.

Nagy, A., Steele, C., & Pelletier, C. (2014). Barium versus nonbarium stimuli: Differences in taste intensity, chemesthesis, and swallowing behavior in healthy adult women. *Journal of Speech, Language, and Hearing Research, 57,* 758–767.

Nakase-Thompson, R., Manning, E., Sherer, M., Yablon, S. A., Gontkovsky, S. L., & Vickery, C. (2005). Brief assessment of severe language impairments: Initial validation of the Mississippi Aphasia Screening Test. *Brain Injury, 19,* 685–691.

Nasreddine, Z. (2003). *Montreal cognitive assessment* [Measurement instrument]. Montreal, Quebec Canada: McGill University and Sherbrooke University.

National Association of State Directors of Special Education. (2005). Retrieved from http://www.nasdse.org

National Center for Learning Disabilities (n.d.). *IDEA parent guide.* Retrieved from http://www.ncld.org/parents-child-disabilities/idea-guide

Nelson, K. (1973). Structure and strategy in learning to talk. *Monographs of the Society for Research in Child Development, 38,* 11–56.

Nelson, K. (1974). Concept, word and sentence: Interrelations in acquisition and development. *Psychological Review, 81,* 267–285.

Nelson, N. (2010). *Language and literacy disorders: Infancy through adolescence.* Boston, MA: Allyn & Bacon.

Newborg, J. (2004). *Battelle developmental inventory* (2nd ed.) [Measurement instrument]. Rolling Meadows, IL: Riverside.

Newcomer, P., & Barenbaum, E. (2003). *Test of phonological awareness skill* [Measurement instrument]. Austin, TX: Pro-Ed.

Newcomer, P. L., & Hammill, D. D. (2008). *Test of language development–Primary* (4th ed.) [Measurement instrument]. Austin, TX: Pro Ed.

Newhoff, M., & Leonard, L. (1983). Diagnosis of developmental language disorders. In I. Meitus & B. Weinberg (Eds.), *Diagnosis in speech-language pathology* (pp. 140–162). Baltimore, MD: University Park Press.

Newman, R., & McGregor, K. (2006). Teachers and laypersons discern quality differences between narratives produced by children with or without SLI. *Journal of Speech, Language, and Hearing Research, 49,* 1022–1036.

Nicholas, J., & Geers, A. (2008). Expected test scores for preschoolers with a cochlear implant who use spoken language. *American Journal of Speech-Language Pathology, 17,* 121–138.

Nippold, M. (1993). Developmental markers in adolescent language: Syntax, semantics and pragmatics. *Language, Speech, and Hearing Services in Schools, 24,* 21–28.

Nippold, M. (2007). *Later language development: School-age children, adolescents, and young adults* (3rd ed.). Austin, TX: Pro-Ed.

Nippold, M. (2009). School-age children talk about chess: Does knowledge drive syntactic complexity? *Journal of Speech, Language, and Hearing Research, 52,* 856–871.

Nippold, M. (2014). *Language sampling with adolescents: Implications for intervention* (2nd ed.). San Diego, CA: Plural Press.

Nippold, M., Mansfield, T., Billow, J., & Tomblin, J. (2008). Expository discourse in adolescents with language impairments: Examining syntactic development. *American Journal of Speech-Language Pathology, 17,* 356–366.

Nippold, M., Mansfield, T., Billow, J., & Tomblin, J. (2009). Syntactic development in adolescents with a history of language impairments: A follow-up investigation. *American Journal of Speech-Language Pathology, 18,* 241–251.

Nippold, M., Schwarz, I., & Undlin, R. (1992). Use and understanding of adverbial conjuncts: A developmental study of adolescents and young adults. *Journal of Speech and Hearing Research, 35,* 108–118.

Norcross, J. C. (Ed.). (2011). *Psychotherapy relationships that work: Evidence-based responsiveness.* New York, NY: Oxford University Press.

Norcross, J. C., & Wampold, B. E. (2011). Evidence-based therapy relationships: Research conclusions and clinical practices. *Pshychotherapy, 48*(1), 98–102.

Norris, J. (1995). Expanding language norms for school-age children and adolescents: Is it pragmatic? *Language, Speech, and Hearing Services in Schools, 26,* 342–352.

Nuffield Speech and Hearing Center. (2004). *Nuffield Center Dyspraxia Programme* (3rd ed.) [Measurement instrument]. Eton, UK: The Miracle Factory.

Nyqvist, K. H., Rubertsson, C., Ewald, U., & Sjödén, P. O. (1996). Development of the Preterm Infant Breastfeeding Behavior Scale (PIBBS): A study of nurse-mother agreement. *Journal of Human Lactation, 12*(3), 207–219.

Oetting, J., Cleveland, L., & Cope, R. (2008). Empirically derived combinations of tools and clinical cutoffs: An illustrative case with a sample of culturally/linguistically diverse children. *Language, Speech, and Hearing Services in Schools, 39,* 44–53.

Olswang, L., Rodriguez, B., & Timler, G. (1998). Recommending intervention for toddlers with specific language learning difficulties: We may not have all the answers, but we know a lot. *American Journal of Speech-Language Pathology, 7,* 23–32.

Olswang, L., Stoel-Gammon, C., Coggins, T., & Carpenter, R. (1987). *Assessing prelinguistic and early linguistic behaviors in developmentally young children.* Seattle, WA: University of Washington Press.

Omark, A. (1981). *Communication assessment of the bilingual, bicultural child: Issues and guidelines.* Baltimore, MD: Pro-Ed.

Omori, K. (2011). Diagnosis of voice disorders. *Japanese Medical Association Journal, 54*(4), 248–253.

O'Neill, D. (2007). The Language Use Inventory for Young Children: A parent-report measure of pragmatic language development for 18–47-month-old children. *Journal of Speech, Language, and Hearing Research, 50,* 214–228.

Onslow, M. (1996). *Behavioral management of stuttering.* San Diego, CA: Singular.

Opitz, V. (1982). Pragmatic analysis of the communicative behavior of an autistic child. *Journal of Speech and Hearing Disorders, 47,* 99–108.

Ornstein, A., & Manning, W. H. (1985). Self-efficacy scaling by adult stutterers. *Journal of Communication Disorders, 18,* 313–320.

Overby, M., Trainin, G., Smith, A. B., Bernthal, J., & Nelson, R. (2012). Preliterate speech sound production skill and literacy outcomes: A study using the Templin Archive. *Language, Speech, and Hearing Services in Schools, 43,* 97–115.

Owens, R. (2004). *Language disorders: A functional approach to assessment and intervention* (4th ed.). Boston, MA: Allyn & Bacon.

Owens, R. (2012). *Language development: An introduction* (8th ed.). Needham Heights, MA: Allyn & Bacon.

Owens, R. (2014). *Language disorders: A functional approach to assessment and intervention* (6th ed.). Needham Heights, MA: Allen & Bacon.

Palisano, R., Rosenbaum, P. L., Walter, S., Russell, D., Woods, E., & Galuppi, B. (1997). Development and reliability of a system to classify gross motor function in children with cerebral palsy. *Developmental Medicine and Child Neurology, 39,* 214–223.

Palmer, M. M., Crawley, K., & Blanco, I. (1993). Neonatal Oral-Motor Assessment Scale: A reliability study. *Journal of Perinatology, 13,* 28–35.

Pannbacker, M., Middleton, G., Vekovius, G., & Sanders, K. (2001). *Report writing for speech-language pathologists and audiologists.* Austin, TX: Pro-Ed.

Paradis, M. (2011). Principles underlying the Bilingual Aphasia Test (BAT) and its uses. *Clinical Linguistics & Phonetics, 25*(6–7), 427–443.

Patel, R., Connaghan, K., Franco, D., Edsall, E., Forgit, D., Olsen, L., . . . Russel, S. (2013). "The Caterpillar": A novel reading passage for assessment of motor speech disorders. *American Journal of Speech-Language Pathology, 22*(1), 1–9.

Paul, R. (2001). *Language disorders from infancy through Adolescence: Assessment and Intervention.* St. Louis, MO: Mosby.

Paul, R. (2007). *Language disorders from infancy through adolescence: Assessment and intervention* (3rd ed). St. Louis, MO: Mosby.

Paul, R. (2012). *Language disorders from infancy through adolescence: Assessment and intervention* (4th ed.). St. Louis, MO: Mosby.

Paul, R., & Alforde, S. (1993). Grammatical morpheme acquisition in 4-year-olds with normal, impaired and late developing language. *Journal of Speech and Hearing Research, 36,* 1271–1275.

Paul, R., & Jennings, P. (1992). Phonological behavior in toddlers with slow expressive language development. *Journal of Speech and Hearing Research, 35,* 99–107.

Pena, E. (1996). Dynamic assessment: The model and its language applications. In P. Cole, P. Dale, & D. Thal (Eds.), *Assessment of communication and language* (pp. 281–307). Baltimore, MD: Brookes.

Pena, E., Gillam, R., Malek, M., Ruiz-Felter, R., Resendiz, M., Fiestas, C., & Sabel, T. (2006). Dynamic assessment of school-age children's narrative ability: An experimental investigation of classification accuracy. *Journal of Speech, Language, and Hearing Research, 49,* 1037–1057.

Pena, E., Quinn, R., & Iglesias, A. (1992). The application of dynamic assessment to language assessment: A non-biased procedure. *Journal of Special Education, 26,* 269–280.

Pennington, B. F., & Bishop, D. V. (2009). Relations among speech, language, and reading disorders. *Annual Review of Psychology, 60,* 283–306.

Pendergast, K., Dickey, S., Selmar, J., & Soder, A. (1997). *Photo-articulation test* (3rd ed.) [Measurement instrument]. Austin, TX: Pro-Ed.

Perlin, W. S., & Boner, M. M. (1994). Clinical assessment of feeding and swallowing in infants and children. In L. R. Cherney (Ed.), *Clinical management of dysphagia in adults and children.* Gaithersburg, MD: Aspen.

Perry, L. (2001). Screening swallowing function of patients with acute stroke part I: Identification, implementation and initial evaluation of a screening tool for use by nurses. *Journal of Clinical Nursing, 10,* 463–473.

Petersen, R., Smith, G., Waring, S., Ivnik, R., Tangalos, E., & Kokmen, E. (1999). Mild cognitive impairment: Clinical characterization and outcome. *Archives of Neurology, 56*(3), 303–308.

Peterson, C., & McCabe, A. (1983). *Developmental psycholinguistics: Three ways of looking at a child's narrative.* New York, NY: Plenum Press.

Peterson, R. L., Pennington, B. F., Shriberg, L. D., & Boada R. (2009). What influences literacy outcome in children with speech sound disorder? *Journal of Speech, Language, and Hearing Research, 52,* 1175–1188.

Peterson-Falzone, S. (1982). Resonance disorders in structural defects. In N. Lass, L. McReynolds, J. Northern, & D. Yoder (Eds.), *Speech, language and hearing, Vol. 2: Pathologies of speech and language.* Philadelphia, PA: W. B. Saunders.

Phelps-Terasaki, D., & Phelps-Gunn, T. (2007). *Test of pragmatic language* (2nd ed.) [Measurement instrument]. Austin, TX: Pro-Ed.

Piaget, J. (1952). *The origins of intelligence in children.* New York, NY: International Universities Press.

Pigott, T., Barry, J., Hughes, B., Eastin, D., Titus, P., Stensel, H., . . . Porter, B. (1985). *Speech-Ease screening inventory (K–1)* [Measurement instrument]. Danville, IL: Interstate Printers.

Pimental, P. A., & Knight, J. (2004). *Mini inventory of right brain injury* (2nd ed.) [Measurement instrument]. Austin, TX: Pro-Ed.

Pindzola, R. H. (1987). *A voice assessment protocol for children and adults* [Measurement instrument]. Austin, TX: Pro-Ed.

Pindzola, R. H. (1988). *Stuttering intervention program: Age 3 to grade 3.* Austin, TX: Pro-Ed.

Pindzola, R. H., Jenkins, M., & Lokken, K. (1989). Speaking rates of young children. *Language, Speech, and Hearing Services in Schools, 20,* 133–138.

Pindzola, R. H., & White, D. (1986). A protocol for differentiating the incipient stutterer. *Language, Speech, and Hearing Services in Schools, 17,* 2–15.

Plante, E., & Vance, R. (1994). Selection of preschool language tests: A data-based approach. *Language, Speech, and Hearing Services in Schools, 25,* 15–24.

Plante, E., & Vance, R. (1995). Diagnostic accuracy of two tests of preschool language. *American Journal of Speech-Language Pathology, 4,* 70–76.

Plexico, L. W., Sandage, M. J., & Faver, K. Y. (2011). Assessment of phonation threshold pressure: A critical review and clinical implications. *American Journal of Speech-Language Pathology, 20,* 348–366.

Poburka, P. (1999). A new stroboscopy rating form. *Journal on Voice, 13*(3), 403–413.

Polmanteer, K., & Turbiville, V. (2000). Family-responsive individualized family service plans for speech-language pathologists. *Language, Speech, and Hearing Services in Schools, 31,* 4–14.

Popham, J. (1981). *Modern educational measurement.* Englewood Cliffs, NJ: Prentice Hall.

Porch, B. (1981). *Porch index of communicative ability* (Revised edition) [Measurement instrument]. Albuquerque, NM: PICA Programs.

Porch, B. (2001). *Porch index of communicative ability: Revised.* Austin, TX: Pro-Ed.

Powell, L., & Courtice, K. (1983). *Alzheimer's disease.* Reading, MA: Addison-Wesley.

Powell, T. (1995). A clinical screening procedure for assessing consonant cluster production. *American Journal of Speech Language Pathology, 4,* 59–65.

Prathanee, B. (1998). Oral diadochokinetic rate in adults. *Journal of the Medical Association of Thailand, 81*(10), 784–788.

Prathanee, B. (2010). Cleft palate-speech evaluation. In M. Blouin & J. Stone (Eds.), *International Encyclopedia of Rehabilitation.* Retrieved from http://cirrie.buffalo.edu/encyclopedia/en/article/261/

Prathanee, B., Thanaviratananich, S., Pongjunyakul, A., & Rengpatanakij, K. (2003). Nasalance scores for speech in normal Thai children. *Scandinavian Journal of Plastic and Reconstructive Surgery and Hand Surgery, 37*(6), 351–355.

Prather, E., Hedrick, D., & Kern, C. (1975). Articulation development in children aged 2 to 4 years. *Journal of Speech and Hearing Disorders, 40,* 179–191.

Prather, E. M., Van Audsal Breecher, S., Stafford, M. L., & Wallace, E. M. (1980). *Screening test of adolescent language* (Revised edition) [Measurement instrument]. Torrance, CA: Western Psychological Services.

Prelock, P., Beatson, J., Bitner, B., Broder, C., & Ducker, A. (2003). Interdisciplinary assessment of young children with autism spectrum disorder. *Language, Speech, and Hearing Services in Schools, 34,* 194–202.

Preston, J., & Edwards, M. (2010). Phonological awareness and types of sound errors in preschoolers with speech sound disorders. *Journal of Speech, Language, and Hearing Research, 53,* 44–60.

Price, L., Hendricks, S., & Cook, C. (2010). Incorporating computer-aided language sample analysis into clinical practice. *Language, Speech, and Hearing Services in Schools, 41,* 206–222.

Prins, D., & Ingham, R. J. (2009). Evidence-based treatment and stuttering—historical perspective. *Journal of Speech, Language, and Hearing Research, 52*(1), 254–263.

Prizant, B., & Wetherby, A. (1988). Providing services to children with autism (ages 0 to 2 years) and their families. *Topics in Language Disorders, 9*(1), 1–23.

Proctor, A. (1989). Stages of normal noncry vocal development in infancy: A protocol for assessment. *Topics in Language Disorders, 10,* 26–42.

Proctor, A., Duffy, M. C., Patterson, A., & Yairi, E. (2001). Stuttering in African American and European American preschoolers. *ASHA Leader, 6*(15), 141.

Provence, S., Erikson, J., Vater, S., & Palmeri, S. (1995). *Infant-toddler developmental assessment* [Measurement instrument]. Rolling Meadows, IL: Riverside.

Prutting, C. A., & Kirchner, D. M. (1987). A clinical appraisal of the pragmatic aspects of language. *Journal of Speech and Hearing Disorders, 52,* 105–119.

Puntil-Sheltman, J. (2002). Medically fragile patients. *The ASHA Leader, 18,* 14–15.

Puranik, C., Lombardino, L., & Altmann, L. (2008). Assessing the microstructure of written language using a retelling paradigm. *American Journal of Speech-Language Pathology, 17,* 107–120.

Purdy, M. (2011). Executive function: Theory, assessment, and treatment. In M. Kimbarow (Ed.), *Cognitive communication disorders* (pp. 77–118). San Diego, CA: Plural.

Rabidoux, P., & Macdonald, J. (2000). An interactive taxonomy of mothers and children during storybook interactions. *American Journal of Speech-Language Pathology, 9,* 331–344.

Rafaat, S., Rvachew, S., & Russell, R. (1995). Reliability of clinician judgments of severity of phonological impairment. *American Journal of Speech Language Pathology, 4,* 39–46.

Ramsay, M., Martel, C., Porporino, M., & Zygmuntowicz, C. (2011). The Montreal Children's Hospital Feeding Scale: A brief bilingual screening tool for identifying feeding problems. *Paediatrics & Child Health, 16*, 142–151.

Raposo-do-Amaral, C. E., Kuczynski, E., & Alonso, N. (2011). Quality of life among children with cleft lip and palate: A critical review of measurement instruments. *Revista Brasileira de Cirurgia Plastica, 26*(4). Retrieved from http://www.scielo.br/scielo.php?pid=S1983-51752011000400017&script=sci_arttext&tlnp

Ratner, N. R. (2004). Caregiver–child interactions and their impact on children's fluency implications for treatment. *Language, Speech, and Hearing Services in Schools, 35*, 46–56.

Ray, B., & Baker, B. (2002). *Hypernasality modification program: A systematic approach*. Austin, TX: Pro-Ed.

Realica, R. M., Smith, M. K., Glover, A. L., & Yu, J. C. (2000). A simplified pneumotachometer for the quantitative assessment of velopharyngeal incompetence. *Annals of Plastic Surgery, 44*(2), 163–166.

Reardon, N. A., & Yaruss, J. S. (2004). *The source for stuttering: Ages 7–18*. East Moline, IL: LinguiSystems.

Rees, N., & Shulman, M. (1978). I don't understand what you mean by comprehension. *Journal of Speech and Hearing Disorders, 43*, 208–219.

Reid, D. K., Hresko, W. P., & Hammill, D. D. (2001). *Test of early reading ability* (3rd ed.) [Measurement instrument]. Austin, TX: Pro-Ed.

Reilly, J., & Fisher, J. L. (2012). Sherlock Holmes and the strange case of the missing attribution: A historical note on "The Grandfather Passage." *Journal of Speech, Language, and Hearing Research 55*(1), 84–88.

Reisberg, B., Ferris, S. H., & Crook, T. (1982). Signs, symptoms, and course of age-associated cognitive decline. In S. Corkin, K. L. Davis, J. H. Growdon, E. Usdin, & R. L. Wurtman (Eds.), *Aging, Vol. 19, Alzheimer's Disease: A Report of Progress*. New York, NY: Raven Press.

Reitan, R. M., & Wolfson, D. (1985). *The Halstead-Reitan Neuropsychological Test Battery: Theory and clinical interpretation*. Tucson, AZ: Neuropsychology Press.

Reitzes, P. (2014). The powered-up parent. *The ASHA Leader, 19*(7), 50–56.

Relic, A., Mazemja, P., Arens, C., Koller, M., & Ganz, H. (2001). Investigating quality of life and coping resources after laryngectomy. *European Archives of Oto-Rhino-Laryngology, 258*(10), 514–517.

Remacle, A., Morsomme, D., & Finck, C. (2014). Comparison of vocal loading parameters in kindergarten and elementary school teachers. *Journal of Speech, Language, and Hearing Research, 57*, 406–415.

Remine, M. D., Care, E., & Brown, P. M. (2008). Language ability and verbal and nonverbal executive functioning in deaf students communicating in spoken English. *Journal of Deaf Studies and Deaf Education, 13*(4), 531–545.

Rescorla, L. (1989). The Language Development Survey: A screening tool for delayed language in toddlers. *Journal of Speech and Hearing Disorders, 54*, 587–599.

Rescorla, L. (2002). Language and reading outcomes to age 9 in late talking toddlers. *Journal of Speech, Language, and Hearing Research, 45*, 360–371.

Rescorla, L. (2009). Age 17 language and reading outcomes in late-talking toddlers: Support for a dimensional perspective on language delay. *Journal of Speech, Language, and Hearing Ressearch, 52*, 16–30.

Rescorla, L., & Alley, A. (2001). Validation of the Language Development Survey (LDS): A parent report tool for identifying language delay in toddlers. *Journal of Speech, Language, and Hearing Research, 44*, 434–445.

Rescorla, L., Alley, A., & Christine, J. (2001). Word frequencies in toddlers' lexicons. *Journal of Speech, Language, and Hearing Research, 44*, 598–609.

Rescorla, L., & Goossens, M. (1992). Symbolic play development in toddlers with expressive specific language impairment (SLI-E). *Journal of Speech and Hearing Research, 35*, 1290–1302.

Rescorla, L., Ratner, N., Jusczyk, P., & Jusczyk, A. (2005). Concurrent validity of the Language Development Survey: Associations with the MacArthur-Bates Communicative Development Inventories—Words and Sentences. *American Journal of Speech-Language Pathology, 14*, 156–163.

Rescorla, L., Ross, G., & McClure, S. (2007). Language delay and behavioral/emotional problems in toddlers: Findings from two developmental clinics. *Journal of Speech, Language, and Hearing Research, 50*, 1063–1078.

Retherford, K. (2000). *Guide to analysis of language transcripts*. Eau Claire, WI: Thinking Publications.

Rey, G., Sivan, A., & Benton, A. (1994). *Multilingual aphasia examination–Spanish* [Measurement instrument]. Lutz, FL: Psychological Assessment Resources.

Reynolds, C., & Horton, A. (2007). *Test of verbal comprehension and fluency* [Measurement instrument]. Austin, TX: Pro-Ed.

Rhyner, P., Kelly, D., Brantley, A., & Krueger, D. (1999). Screening low-income African American children using the BLT-2S and the SPELT-P. *American Journal of Speech-Language Pathology, 8*, 44–52.

Riccio, C., Imhoff, B., Hasbrouck, J., & Davis, G. N. (2004). *Test of phonological awareness in Spanish* [Measurement instrument]. Austin, TX: Pro-Ed.

Rice, M., Sell, M., & Hadley, P. (1990). The Social Interactive Coding System (SICS): An on-line, clinically relevant descriptive tool. *Language, Speech, and Hearing Services in Schools, 21*, 2–14.

Rice, M., Smolik, F., Perpich, D., Thompson, T., Rytting, N., & Blossom, M. (2010). Mean length of utterance levels in 6-month intervals for children 3 to 9 years with and without language impairments. *Journal of Speech, Language, and Hearing Research, 53*, 333–349.

Richard, G. J., & Hanner, M. A. (2005). *Language processing test 3: Elementary* [Measurement instrument]. East Moline, IL: LinguiSystems.

Richardson, W. S., Wilson, M. C., & Guyatt, G. (2002). The process of diagnosis. Users' guides to the medical literature: *A manual for evidence-based clinical practice* (2nd ed.). New York, NY: McGraw-Hill. Retrieved from http://medicine.ucsf.edu/education/resed/articles/jama6_the_process.pdf

Riley, G. D. (1981). *Stuttering prediction instrument for young children* [Measurement instrument]. Austin, TX: Pro-Ed.

Riley, G. D. (2009). *Stuttering severity instrument* (4th ed.) [Measurement instrument]. Austin, TX: Pro-Ed.

Roberts, J., Martin, G., Moskowitz, L., Harris, A., Foreman, J., & Nelson, L. (2007). Discourse skills of boys with fragile X syndrome in comparison to boys with Down syndrome. *Journal of Speech, Language, and Hearing Research, 50*, 475–492.

Robertson, C (2007). *The phonological awareness Test II* [Measurement instrument]. East Moline, IL: LinguiSystems.

Robinson, T. L. (2012). Cultural diversity and fluency disorders. In K. Faulk & J. Gower (Eds.), *Communication disorders in multicultural populations* (pp. 164–173). St. Louis, MO: Elsevier Mosby.

Roebers, C. M., & Schneider, W. (2005). Individual differences in young children's suggestibility: Relations to event memory, language abilities, working memory, and executive functioning. *Cognitive Development, 20*(3), 427–447.

Rogers, B., Arvedson, J., Buck, G., Smart, P., & Msall, M. (1994). Characteristics of dysphagia in children with cerebral palsy. *Dysphagia, 9*, 69–73.

Rogers, S. (1977). Characteristics of the cognitive development of profoundly retarded children. *Child Development, 48*, 837–843.

Rogers, S., El-Sheikha, J., & Lowe, D. (2009). The development of a Patients Concerns Inventory (PCI) to help reveal patients concerns in the head and neck clinic. *Oral Ontology, 45*(7), 555–561.

Roseberry-McKibbin, C. (1994). *Bilingual classroom communication profile* [Measurement instrument]. Oceanside, CA: Academic Communication Associates.

Rosen, C., Lee, A., Osborne, J., Zullo, T., & Murry, T. (2004). Development and validation of the Voice Handicap Index-10. *The Laryngoscope, 114*(9), 1549–1556.

Rosenbek, J., LaPointe, L., & Wertz, T. (1989). *Aphasia: A clinical approach.* Boston, MA: College-Hill.

Rosenbek, J., Robbins, J., Roecker, E., Coyle, M., & Wood, J. (1996). A penetration-aspiration scale. *Dysphagia, 11*(2), 93–98.

Ross-Swain, D., & Fogle, P. (2011). *Ross information processing assessment–Geriatric* (2nd ed.) [Measurement instrument]. Austin, TX: Pro-Ed.

Ross-Swain, D., & Kipping, P. (2003). *Swallowing ability and function evaluation* [Measurement instrument]. Austin, TX: Pro-Ed.

Rossetti, L. M. (2006). *Rossetti infant-toddler language scale* [Measurement instrument]. East Moline, IL: LinguiSystems.

Roth, F. P., & Worthington, C. K. (2005). *Treatment resource manual for speech-language pathology.* Clifton Park, NY: Delmar.

Rubak, S., Sandbaek, A., Lauritzen, T., & Christensen, B. (2005). Motivational interviewing: A systematic review and meta-analysis. *British Journal of General Practice, 55,* 305–312.

Rubin, J., Sataloff, R. T., & Korovin, G. (2006). *Diagnosis and treatment of voice disorders* (3rd ed.). San Diego, CA: Plural.

Rutter, M. (1978). Diagnosis and definition of childhood autism. *Journal of Autism and Childhood Schizophrenia, 8,* 139–169.

Rvachew, S., & Bernhardt, B. (2010). Clinical implications of dynamic systems theory for phonological development. *American Journal of Speech-Language Pathology, 19,* 34–50.

Rvachew, S., Chiang, P., & Evans, N. (2007). Characteristics of speech errors produced by children with and without delayed phonological awareness skills. *Language, Speech, and Hearing Services in Schools, 38,* 60–71.

Ryan, B. (1974). *Programmed therapy for stuttering in children and adults.* Springfield, IL: Charles C. Thomas.

Sabers, D. (1996). By their tests we will know them. *Language, Speech, and Hearing Services in Schools, 27,* 102–121.

Sachs, J., & Devin, J. (1976). Young children's use of age appropriate speech styles in social interaction and role playing. *Journal of Child Language, 3,* 81–98.

Sackett, D., Straus, S., Richardson, W., Rosenberg, W., & Haynes, R. (2000). *Evidence-based medicine: How to practice and teach EBM* (2nd ed.). Edinburgh, UK: Churchill Livingstone.

Salmon, S. J. (1999). *Alaryngeal speech rehabilitation* (2nd ed.). Austin, TX: Pro-Ed.

Salter, K., Jutai, J., Foley, N., Hellings, C., & Teasell, R. (2006). Identification of aphasia post stroke: A review of screening assessment tools. *Brain Injury, 20*(6), 559–568.

Salvia, J., & Ysseldyke, J. (1981). *Assessment in special and remedial education.* Boston, MA: Houghton-Mifflin.

Salvia, J., & Ysseldyke, J. (2004). *Assessment: In special and inclusive education* (9th ed.). Boston, MA: Houghton Mifflin.

Salvia, J., Ysseldyke, J., & Bolt, S. (2010). *Assessment: In special and inclusive education* (11th ed.). Stamford, CT: Cengage Learning.

Sapienza, C., & Ruddy, B. H. (2013). *Voice disorders* (2nd ed.). San Diego, CA: Plural.

Saville-Troike, M. (1986). Anthropological considerations in the study of communication. In O. Taylor (Ed.), *Nature of Communication Disorders in Culturally Diverse Populations* (pp. 47–72). San Diego, CA: College Hill Press.

Schensul, S. L., Schensul, J. J., & LeCompte, M. D. (2013). *Initiating ethnographic research: A mixed methods approach* (Vol. 2). Lanham, MD: Rowman & Littlefield.

Schieffelin, B. (1985). The acquisition of Kaluli. In D. Slobin (Ed.), *The Cross-Linguistic Study of Language Acquisition* (Vol. 1., pp. 525–593). Hillsdale, NJ: Lawrence Erlbaum Associates.

Schindler, J. S., & Kelly, J. H. (2002). Swallowing disorders in the elderly. *The Laryngoscope, 112,* 589–602.

Schlesinger, I. (1974). Relational concepts underlying language. In R. Schiefelbusch & L. Lloyd (Eds.), *Language perspectives—Acquisition, retardation and intervention* (pp. 129–151). Baltimore, MD: University Park Press.

Schlosser, R., & Wendt, O. (2008). Effects of augmentative and alternative communication intervention on speech production in children with autism: A systematic review. *American Journal of Speech-Language Pathology, 17,* 212–230.

Schrank, F., McGrew, K., Mather, N., & Woodcock, R. (2014). *Woodcock-Johnson IV* [Measurement instrument]. Rolling Meadows, IL: Houghton Mifflin Harcourt-Riverside.

Schuele, C., & Boudreau, D. (2008). Phonological awareness intervention: Beyond the basics. *Language, Speech, and Hearing Services in Schools, 39,* 3–20.

Schuell, H. (1973). *The Minnesota test for differential diagnosis of aphasia* [Measurement instrument]. Minneapolis, MN: University of Minnesota Press.

Sclan, S., & Reisberg, B. (1992). Functional assessment staging (FAST) in Alzheimer's disease: Reliability, validity, and ordinality. *International Psychogeriatrics, 4*(3), 55–69.

Scott, C. (1988). Spoken and written syntax. In M. Nippold (Ed.), *Later Language Development: Ages Nine through Nineteen* (pp. 45–95). Austin, TX: Pro-Ed.

Scott, C., & Stokes, S. (1995). Measures of syntax in school-age children and adolescents. *Language, Speech, and Hearing Services in Schools, 26,* 309–319.

Scott, K., Roberts, J., & Krakow, R. (2008). Oral and written language development of children adopted from China. *American Journal of Speech-Language Pathology, 17,* 150–160.

Seaver, E. J., Dalston, R. M., Leeper, H. A., & Adams, L. E. (1991). A study of nasometric values for normal nasal resonance. *Journal of Speech & Hearing Research, 34*(4), 715–721.

Secord, W., & Shine. R. (1997). *Secord contextual articulation test* [Measurement instrument]. Greenville, SC: Super Duper.

Seiverling, L., Hendy, H. M., & Williams, K. (2011). The Screening Tool of Feeding Problems Applied to Children (STEP-CHILD): Psychometric characteristics and association with child and parent variables. *Research in Developmental Disabilities, 32,* 1122–1129. doi: 10.1016/j.ridd.2011.01.012

Semel, E, Wiig, E. H., & Secord, W. A. (2013). *Clinical evaluation of language fundamentals* (5th ed.) [Measurement instrument]. San Antonio, TX: Harcourt Assessment.

Seymour, H. (1992). The invisible children: A reply to Lahey's perspective. *Journal of Speech and Hearing Research, 15,* 640–641.

Seymour, H., Roeper, T., DeVilliers, J., & DeVilliers, P. (2005). Treating child language disorders: Lessons from African-American English. Paper presented at the convention of the American Speech-Language-Hearing Association, Atlanta, GA.

Shadden, B. B., & Toner, M.A. (2011). Counseling and clinical interactions with older clients and caregivers. In *Aging and Communication: For Clinicians by Clinicians* (2nd ed., pp. 299–320). Austin, TX: Pro-Ed.

Shapiro, D. A. (2011). *Stuttering intervention: A collaborative journey to fluency freedom* (2nd ed.). Austin, TX: Pro-Ed.

Sharf, D. (1972). Some relationships between measures of early language development. *Journal of Speech and Hearing Disorders, 37,* 64–74.

Sheehy, G. (1996). *New passages: Mapping your life across time.* New York, NY: Random House.

Shine, R. (1980). Direct management of the beginning stutterer. *Seminars in Speech, Language and Hearing, 1*(4), 339–350.

Shine, R. (1988). *Systematic fluency training for young children* (3rd ed.) [Measurement instrument]. Austin, TX: Pro-Ed.

Shine, R. E. (1988). *Systematic fluency training for children.* Austin, TX: Pro-Ed.

Shipley, K. G. (1990). *Systematic assessment of voice* [Measurement instrument]. Oceanside, CA: Academic Communication Associates.

Shipley, K. G., & McAfee, J. G. (2009). *Assessment in speech-language pathology: A resource manual.* Clifton Park, NY: Delmar Cengage Learning.

Shorr, D. (1983). Grammatical comprehension assessment: The picture avoidance strategy. *Journal of Speech and Hearing Disorders, 48,* 89–92.

Shriberg, L. (1993). Four new speech and prosody voice measures for genetics research and other studies in developmental phonological disorders. *Journal of Speech and Hearing Research, 36,* 105–140.

Shriberg, L., & Kwiatkowski, J. (1980). *Natural process analysis.* New York, NY: John Wiley.

Shriberg, L., & Kwiatkowski, J. (1982a). Phonological disorders, I: A diagnostic classification system. *Journal of Speech and Hearing Disorders, 47,* 226–241.

Shriberg, L., & Kwiatkowski, J. (1982b). Phonological disorders, III: A procedure for assessing severity of involvement. *Journal of Speech and Hearing Disorders, 47,* 256–270.

Shriberg, L., & Kwiatkowski, J. (1994). Developmental phonological disorders, I: A clinical profile. *Journal of Speech and Hearing Research, 37*(5), 1100–1126.

Shriberg, L., Lohmeier, H., Campbell, T., Dollaghan, C., Green, J., & Moore, C. (2009). A nonword repetition task for speakers with misarticulations: The syllable repetition task (SRT). *Journal of Speech, Language, and Hearing Research, 52,* 1189–1212.

Shulman, B. (1986). *Test of pragmatic skills* (Revised ed.). Tucson, AZ: Communication Skill Builders.

Siegel, G. (1975). The use of language tests. *Language, Speech, and Hearing Services in Schools, 6,* 211–217.

Silverman, F. (1984). *Speech language pathology and audiology.* Columbus, OH: Merrill.

Silverman, F. (1995). *Communication for the speechless.* Needham Heights, MA: Allyn & Bacon.

Silverman, S., & Ratner, N. B. (2002). Measuring lexical diversity in children who stutter: Application of *VOCD. Journal of Fluency Disorders, 27,* 289–304.

Simms-Hill, S., & Haynes, W. (1992). Language performance in low-achieving elementary school students. *Language, Speech, and Hearing Services in Schools, 23,* 169–175.

Simon, C. (1987). Out of the broom closet and into the classroom: The emerging SLP. *Journal of Childhood Communication Disorders, 11,* 41–66.

Simon, C. (1989). *Classroom communication screening procedure for early adolescents (CCSPEA).* Tempe, AZ: Communi-Cog Publications.

Simon, C. (1994). *Evaluating communicative competence* [Measurement instrument]. Tempe, AZ: Communi-Cog.

Singer, M., & Blom, E. (1980). An endoscopic technique for restoration of voice after laryngectomy. Presentation at the Annual American Laryngologic Association Conference, Palm Beach, FL.

Singleton, N., & Shulman, B. (2014). *Language development: Foundations, processes, and clinical applications.* Boston, MA: Jones & Bartlett.

Siric, L., Sos, D., Rosso, M., & Stevanovic, S. (2012). Objective assessment of tracheoesophageal and esophageal speech using acoustic analysis of voice. *Colegium Antropologicum, 36*(2), 111–114.

Skahan, S., Watson, M., & Lof, G. (2007). Speech-language pathologists' assessment practices for children with suspected speech sound disorders: Results of a national survey. *American Journal of Speech-Language Pathology, 16,* 246–259.

Skarakis-Doyle, E., Campbell, W., & Dempsey, L. (2009). Identification of children with language impairment: Investigating the classification accuracy of the MacArthur-Bates Communicative Development Inventories, Level III. *American Journal of Speech-Language Pathology, 18,* 277–288.

Skarakis-Doyle, E., & Dempsey, L. (2008). The detection and monitoring of comprehension errors by preschool children with and without language impairment. *Journal of Speech, Language, and Hearing Research, 51,* 1227–1243.

Skarakis-Doyle, E., Dempsey, L., & Lee, C. (2008). Identifying language comprehension impairment in preschool children. *Language, Speech, and Hearing Services in Schools, 39,* 54–65.

Skibbe, L. E., Moody, A. J., Justice, L. M., & McGinty, A. S. (2010). Socio-emotional climate of storybook reading interactions for mothers and preschoolers with language impairment. *Reading and Writing, 23*(1), 53–71.

Sklar, M. (1983). *Sklar aphasia scale* [Measurement instrument]. Los Angeles, CA: Western Psychological Services.

Smith, V., Mirenda, P., & Zaidman-Zait, A. (2007). Predictors of expressive vocabulary growth in children with autism. *Journal of Speech, Language, and Hearing Research, 50,* 149–160.

Snow, C. (1977). The development of conversation between mothers and babies. *Journal of Child Language, 4,* 1–22.

Snyder, L. (1978). Communicative and cognitive disabilities in the sensorimotor period. *Merrill Palmer Quarterly, 24,* 161–180.

Snyder, L. (1981). Assessing communicative abilities in the sensorimotor period: Content and context. *Topics in Language Disorders, 1,* 31–46.

Sonies, B. C., Weiffenbach, J., Atkinson, J. C., Brahim, J., Macynski, A., & Fox, P. C. (1987). Clinical examination of motor and sensory functions of the adult oral cavity. *Dysphagia, 1,* 4.

Sparks, S. (1989). Assessment and intervention with at-risk infants and toddlers: Guidelines for the speech-language pathologist. *Topics in Language Disorders, 10*(1), 43–56.

Sparrow, S. S., Cicchetti, D. V., & Balla, D. A. (2005). *Vineland adaptive behavior scales* (2nd ed.) [Measurement instrument]. Livonia, MN: Pearson Assessments.

Sparrow, S., Cicchetti, D., & Balla, D. (2005). *Vineland-II: Vineland adaptive behavior scales: Survey forms manual.* Minneapolis, MN: NCS Pearson.

Spaulding, T., Plante, E., & Farinella, K. (2006). Eligibility criteria for language impairment: Is the low end of normal always appropriate? *Language, Speech, and Hearing Services in Schools, 37,* 61–72.

Spaulding, T. J. (2010). Investigating mechanisms of suppression in preschool children with specific language impairment. *Journal of Speech, Language, and Hearing Research, 53*(3), 725–738.

Speyer, R., Bogaardt, H., Passos, V. L., Boodenburg, N., Zumach, A., Heijnen, M., . . . Brunings, J. (2010). Maximum phonation time: Variability and reliability. *Journal of Voice, 24*(3), 281–284.

Spies, R. (2010). Buros Mental Measurements Yearbook. In I. B. Weiner & W. E. Craighead (Eds.), *The Corsini Encyclopedia of Psychology* (pp. 945–946). Hoboken, NJ : John Wiley & Sons.

Spradley, J. P. (1979). *The ethnographic interview.* New York, NY: Holt, Rinehart & Winston.

Square, P., & Weidner, W. E. (1981). Differential diagnosis of developmental apraxia. Speech and Hearing Association Conference, Birmingham, AL.

Squires, J., & Bricker, D. (2009). *Ages and stages questionaire: A parent-completed child monitoring system* (3rd ed.) [Measurement instrument]. Baltimore, MD: Brookes.

St. Clair, M. C., Pickles, A., Durkin, K., & Conti-Ramsden, G. (2011). A longitudinal study of behavioral, emotional and social difficulties in individuals with a history of specific lan-guage impairment (SLI). *Journal of Communication Disorders, 44*(2), 186–199.

St. Louis, K., & Ruscello, D. (2000). *The oral speech mechanism examination* (3rd ed.) [Measurement instrument]. Austin, TX: Pro-Ed.

Staab, C. (1983). Language functions elicited by meaningful activities: A new dimension in language programs. *Language, Speech, and Hearing Services in Schools, 14,* 164–170.

Stark, R., Bernstein, L., & Demorest, M. (1993). Vocal communication in the first 18 months of life. *Journal of Speech and Hearing Research, 36,* 548–558.

Starkweather, C. W., Gottwald, S. R., & Halfond, M. M. (1990). *Stuttering prevention: A clinical method.* Englewood Cliffs, NJ: Prentice Hall.

State University of New York at Buffalo. (1993a). *Guide for the uniform data set for medical rehabilitation (Adult FIM), version 4.0.* Buffalo, NY: Author.

State University of New York at Buffalo. (1993b). *Guide for the Functional Independence Measure for Children (WeeFIM) of the uniform data system for medical rehabilitation, version 4.0–Community/Outpatient.* Buffalo, NY: Author.

Steckol, K., & Leonard, L. (1981). Sensorimotor development and the use of prelinguistic performatives. *Journal of Speech and Hearing Research, 24,* 262–268.

Stein-Rubin, C., & Fabus, R. (2012). *A guide to clinical assessment and professional report writing in speech-language pathology.* Clifton Park, NY: Delmar Cengage Learning.

Stemple, J. C., Roy, N., & Klaben, B. (2010). *Clinical voice pathology: Theory and management* (5th ed.). San Diego, CA: Plural.

Stevens, N., & Isles, D. (2001). *Phonological screening assessment* [Measurement instrument]. London, UK: Speechmark.

Stiegler, L. (2007). Discovering communicative competencies in a non-speaking child with autism. *Language, Speech, and Hearing Services in Schools, 38,* 400–413.

Stocker, B., & Goldfarb, R. (1995). *Stocker probe for fluency and language* (3rd ed.) [Measurement instrument] Norcross, GA: The Speech Bin.

Stockman, I. (2010). A review of developmental and applied language research on African American children: From a deficit to difference perspective on dialect differences. *Language, Speech, and Hearing Services in Schools, 41,* 23–38.

Stoel-Gammon, C. (1987). Phonological skills in 2-year-olds. *Language, Speech, and Hearing Services in Schools, 18,* 323–329.

Stoel-Gammon, C. (1996). Phonological assessment using a hierarchial framework. In K. Cole, P. Dale, & D. Thal (Eds.), *Assessment of communication and language* (Vol. 6). Baltimore, MD: Paul H. Brookes.

Stoel-Gammon, C., & Dunn, C. (1985). *Normal and disordered phonology in children.* Baltimore, MD: University Park Press.

Stokes, S., & Klee, T. (2009). The diagnostic accuracy of a new test of early nonword repetition for differentiating late talking and typically developing children. *Journal of Speech, Language, and Hearing Research, 52,* 872–882.

Stover, S., & Haynes, W. (1989). Topic manipulation and cohesive adequacy in conversations of normal adults between the ages of 30 and 90. *Clinical Linguistics and Phonetics, 3,* 137–149.

Strand, E., McCauley, R., Weigand, S., Stoeckel, R., & Baas, B. (2013). A motor speech assessment for children with severe speech disorders: Reliability and validity evidence. *Journal of Speech and Hearing Research, 56*(2), 505–520.

Strandberg, T., & Griffith, J. (1969). A study of the effects of training in visual literacy on verbal language behavior. *Journal of Communication Disorders, 2,* 252–263.

Strominger, A., & Bashie, A. (1977). A nine-year follow-up of language delayed children. Paper presented at the convention of the American Speech-Language-Hearing Association, Chicago, IL.

Strong, C. J. (1998). *The Strong narrative assessment procedure* [Measurement instrument]. Eau Claire, WI: Thinking.

Sturner, R., Heller, J., Funk, S., & Layton, T. (1993). The Fluharty preschool speech and language screening test: A population-based validation study using sample-independent decision rules. *Journal of Speech and Hearing Research, 36,* 738–745.

Sturner, R., Layton, T., Evans A., Heller J., Funck S., & Machton, M. (1994). Preschool speech and language screening: A review of currently available tests. *American Journal of Speech-Language Pathology, 35,* 25–36.

Swain, D. R., & Long, N. (2004). *Auditory processing abilities test* [Measurement instrument]. Novato, CA: Academic Therapy.

Swanson, L. A., Fey, M. E., Mills, C. E., & Hood, L. S. (2005). Use of narrative-based language intervention with children who have specific language impairment. *American Journal of Speech-Language Pathology, 14,* 131–141.

Swigert, N. (1998). *The source for pediatric dysphagia* (2nd ed.). East Moline, IL: LinguiSystems.

Swigert, N. (2006). Clinical documentation, coding, and billing. *Seminars in Speech and Language, 27*(2), 101–118.

Swigert, N. (2007). *The source for dysphagia* (3rd ed.). East Moline, IL: LinguiSystems.

Syder, D., Body, E., Parker, M., & Boddy, M. (1993). *Sheffield screening test for acquired language disorders* [Measurement instrument]. Windsor, England: NFER-Nelson.

Tade, W. J., & Slosson, S. W. (1986). *Slosson articulation, language test with phonology* [Measurement instrument]. East Aurora, NY: Slosson Educational.

Tager-Flusberg, H., Rogers, S., Cooper, J., Landa, R., Lord, C., Paul, R., Rice, M., Stoel-Gammon, C., Wetherby, A., & Yoder, P. (2009). Defining spoken language benchmarks and selecting measures of expressive language development for young children with autism spectrum disorders. *Journal of Speech, Language, and Hearing Research, 52,* 643–652.

Tanner, D. (1994). *Pragmatic stuttering intervention for children* (2nd ed.) [Measurement instrument]. Oceanside, CA: Academic Communication Associates.

Tanner, D., & Culbertson, W. (1999). *Quick assessment for apraxia of speech* [Measurement instrument]. Oceanside, CA: Academic Communication Associates.

Tanner, D., (1990). *Assessment of stuttering behaviors* [Measurement instrument]. Oceanside, CA: Academic Communication Associates.

Tanner, D. (2001). The brave new world of the cyber speech and hearing clinic. *The ASHA Leader, 6,* 6–7.

Tanner, D., Belliveau, W., & Siebert, G. (1995). *Pragmatic stuttering intervention for adolescents and adults* [Measurement instrument]. Oceanside, CA: Academic Communication Associates.

Tanner, D., & Culbertson, W. (1999). *Quick assessment for aphasia* [Measurement instrument]. Oceanside, CA: Academic Communication Associates.

Tanner, D., & Culbertson, W. (1999). *Quick assessment for dysarthria* [Measurement instrument]. Oceanside, CA: Academic Communication Associates.

Taylor, O., & Payne, K. (1983). Culturally valid testing: A proactive approach. *Topics in Language Disorders, 3,* 8–20.

Taylor, O., & Payne, K. (1994). Culturally valid testing: A proactive approach. In K. Butler (Ed.), *Cross-cultural perspectives in language assessment and intervention.* Gaithersburg, MD: Aspen Publications.

Teoh, A. P., & Chin, S. B. (2009). Transcribing the speech of children with cochlear implants: Clinical application of narrow phonetic transcriptions. *American Journal of Speech-Language Pathology, 18,* 388–401.

Terkel, S. (1980). *American dreams: Lost and found.* New York, NY: Pantheon.

Terkel, S. (1986). *Hard times: An oral history of the Great Depression.* New York, NY: Random House.

Terkel, S. (1993). *Race: How Blacks and Whites think and feel about the American obsession.* New York, NY: Anchor Press.

Terkel, S. (2001). *Will the circle be unbroken? Reflections on death, rebirth and hunger for a faith.* New York, NY: New Press.

Thal, D., DesJardin, J., & Eisenberg, L. (2007). Validity of the MacArthur-Bates Communicative Development Inventories for measuring language abilities in children with cochlear implants. *American Journal of Speech-Language Pathology, 16,* 54–64.

Thal, D., O'Hanlon, L., Clemmons, M., & Franklin, L. (1999). Validity of a parent report measure of vocabulary and syntax for preschool children with language impairment. *Journal of Speech, Language, & Hearing Disorders, 42,* 482–496.

Thal, D., & Tobias, S. (1992). Communicative gestures in children with delayed onset of oral expressive vocabulary. *Journal of Speech and Hearing Research, 35,* 1281–1289.

Thommessen, B., Thoressen, G. E., Bautz-Holter, E., & Laake, K. (1999). Screening by nurses for aphasia in stroke—the Ullevaal Aphasia Screening (UAS) test. *Disability and Rehabilitation, 21,* 110–115.

Thompkins, C., & Lehman, M. (1998). Outcomes measurement in cognitive communication disorders: Right hemisphere brain damage. In C. Frattali (Ed.), *Measuring outcomes in speech-language pathology* (pp. 281–292). New York, NY: Thieme.

Thompkins, C. A. (1995). *Right hemisphere communication disorders: Theory and management.* San Diego, CA: Singular.

Thoyre, S., Pados, B., Park, J., Estrem, H., Hodges, E., McComish, C., . . . Murdoch, K. (2014). Development and content validation of the Pediatric Easting Assessment Tool (Pedi-EAT). *American Journal of Speech-Language Pathology, 23,* 46–59.

Tian, W., Yin, H., Redett, R. Shi, B., Shi, J., Zhang, R., & Zheng, Q. (2010). Magnetic resonance imaging assessment of velopharyngeal mechanism at rest and during speech in children. *Journal of Speech Language Hearing Research, 53,* 1595–1615.

Tieu, D. D., Gerber, M. E., Miczuk, H. A., Parikh, S. R., Perkins, J. A., Yoon, P. J., & Sie, K. C. (2012). Generation of consensus in the application of a rating scale to nasendoscopic assessment of velopharyngeal function. *Archives of Otolaryngology–Head and Neck Surgery, 38*(10), 923–928.

Tomik, B., & Guiloff, R. J. (2010). Dysarthria in amyotrophic lateral sclerosis: A review. *Amyotrophic Lateral Sclerosis, 11,* 4–15.

Toner, M. A., Shadden, B., & Gluth, M. (2011). *Aging and communication* (2nd ed.). Austin, TX: Pro-Ed.

Torgensen, J., & Bryant, B. (2004). *Test of phonological awareness PLUS* (2nd ed.) [Measurement instrument]. Austin, TX: Pro-Ed.

Tough, J. (1977). *The development of meaning.* New York, NY: Halsted Press.

Trapl, M., Enderle, P., Nowotny, M., Teuschl, Y., Matz, K., Dachenhausen, A., & Brainin, M. (2007). Dysphagia bedside screening for acute-stroke patients: The Gugging Swallowing Screen. *Stroke, 38*(11), 2948–2952.

Trost-Cardamone, J. E., & Bernthal, J. E. (1993). Articulation assessment procedures and treatment decisions. In K. T. Moller & C. D. Starr (Eds.), *Cleft palate: Interdisciplinary issues and treatments.* Austin, TX: Pro-Ed.

Tyack, D., & Gottsleben, R. (1974). *Language sampling, analysis and training: A Handbook for teachers and clinicians.* Palo Alto, CA: Consulting Psychologists Press.

Ukrainetz, T. (2006). The Implications of RTI and EBP for SLPs: Commentary on L. M. Justice. *Language, Speech, and Hearing Services in Schools, 37,* 298–303.

Ukrainetz, T., & Gillam, R. (2009). The expressive elaboration of imaginative narratives by children with specific language impairment. *Journal of Speech, Language, and Hearing Research, 52,* 883–898.

Uzigiris, I., & Hunt, J. (1975). *Assessment in infancy.* Urbana, IL: University of Illinois Press.

Van Borsel, J., Maes, L., & Foulon, S. (2001). Stuttering and bilingualism: A review. *Journal of Fluency Disorders, 26,* 179–205.

Van Borsel, J. V. (1997). Neurogenic stuttering: A review. *Journal of Clinical Speech and Language Studies, 7,* 16–33.

Van Gilder, J., & Street-Tobin, S. (2011). Supervision: Assessing diagnostic report writing. *SIG 11 Perspectives on Administration and Supervision, 21,* 103–111.

Van Lierde, K. M., Muyts, F. L., Bonte, K., & Van Cauwenberge, P. (2007). The Nasality Severity Index: An objective measure of hyponasality based on a multiparameter approach, a pilot study. *Folio Phoniatrica et Logopaedica, 59*(1), 31–38.

Van Riper, C. (1963). *Speech correction: Principles and methods* (4th ed.). Englewood Cliffs, NJ: Prentice-Hall.

Van Riper, C., & Emerick, L. (1984). *Speech correction: An introduction to speech pathology and audiology.* Englewood Cliffs, NJ: Prentice Hall.

Vanryckeghem, M., & Brutten, G. J. (2007). *KiddyCat: Communication attitude test for preschool and kindergarten children who stutter* [Measurement instrument]. San Diego, CA: Plural.

Vanryckeghem, M., Hylebos, C., Brutten, G., & Peleman, M. (2001). The relationship between communication attitude and emotion of children who stutter. *Journal of Fluency Disorders, 26,* 1–15.

Vaughn-Cook, F. (1986). The challenge of assessing the language of nonmainstream speakers. In O. Taylor (Ed.), *Treatment of Communication Disorders in Culturally and Linguistically Diverse Populations* (pp. 23–48). San Diego, CA: College Hill Press.

Velleman, S., & Vihman, M. (2002). Whole-word phonology & templates: Trap, bootstrap, or some of each? *Language, Speech, and Hearing Services in Schools, 33,* 9–23.

Vitali, G. (1986). *Test of oral structures and functions* [Measurement instrument]. East Aura, NY: Slosson.

Vogel, A., Ibrahim, H., Reilly, S., & Kilpatrick, N. (2009). A comparative study of two acoustic measures of hypernasality. *Journal of Speech, Language, and Hearing Research, 52,* 1640–1651.

Vygotsky, L. (1978). *Mind in society: The development of higher psychological processes.* Cambridge, MA: Harvard University Press.

Wade, K., & Haynes, W. (1989). Dynamic assessment of spontaneous language and cue responses in adult-directed and child-directed play: A statistical and descriptive analysis. *Child Language Teaching and Therapy, 5,* 157–173.

Wagner, R., Togersen, J., & Rashotte, C. (1999). *Comprehensive test of phonological Processing* [Measurement instrument]. Austin, TX: Pro-Ed.

Wall, L., Ward, E., Cartmill, B., & Hill, A. (2013). Physiological changes to the swallowing mechanism following (chemo)radiotherapy for head and neck cancer: A systematic review. *Dysphagia, 28,* 481–493.

Wallace, G., & Hammill, D. D. (2013). *Comprehensive receptive and expressive vocabulary test* (3rd ed.) [Measurement instrument]. Austin, TX: Pro-Ed.

Wallach, G., & Miller, L. (1988). *Language intervention and academic success.* Boston, MA: College-Hill Press.

Ward, D., & Scott, S. K. (2011). *Cluttering: Research, intervention and education.* East Sussex, UK: Psychology Press.

Ward, E., Crombie, J., Trickey, M., Hill, A., Theodoros, D., & Russell, T. (2009). Assessment of communication and swallowing post-laryngectomy: A telerehabilitation trial. *Journal of Telemedicine and Telecare, 15,* 232–237.

Ward, S., & Birkett, D. (1994). *Ward infant language screening test, assessment, acceleration, and remediation* [Measurement instrument]. Manchester: Manchester Health Care Trust.

Watson, B. U., & Thompson, R. W. (1983). Parent's perception of diagnostic reports and conferences. *Language, Speech, and Hearing Services in Schools, 14,* 114–120.

Watson, J. B. (1988). A comparison of stutterers' and nonstutterers' affective, cognitive, and behavioral self-reports. *Journal of Speech and Hearing Research, 31*(3), 377–385.

References   **461**

Watson-Gegeo, K., & Gegeo, D. (1986). Calling out and repeating routines in Kwara'ae children's language socialization. In B. Schieffelin & E. Ochs (Eds.), *Language and Socialization Across Cultures* (pp. 17–50). Cambridge, UK: Cambridge University Press.

Weismer, S., Branch, J., & Miller, J. (1994). A prospective longitudinal study of language development in late talkers. *Journal of Speech and Hearing Research, 37,* 852–867.

Weiss, A. (2004). Why we should consider pragmatics when planning treatment for children who stutter. *Language, Speech, and Hearing Services in Schools, 35,* 34–45.

Weiss, A., Leonard, L., Rowan, L., & Chapman, K. (1983). Linguistic and nonlinguistic features of style in normal and language-impaired children. *Journal of Speech, and Hearing Disorders, 48,* 154–163.

Weisz, J., & Zigler, E. (1979). Cognitive development in retarded and nonretarded persons: Piagetian tests of the similar sequence hypothesis. *Psychological Bulletin, 86,* 831–851.

Wepman, J. M., MacGhan, J. A., Rickard, J. C., & Shelton, N. W. (1953). The objective measurement of progressive esophageal speech development. *Journal of Speech & Hearing Disorders, 18,* 247–251.

Wertz, R. T., LaPointe, L. L., & Rosenbek, J. C. (1984). *Apraxia of speech in adults: The disorder and its management.* New York, NY: Grune & Stratton.

West, J., Sands, E., & Ross-Swain, D. (1998). *Bedside evaluation screening test* (2nd ed.) [Measurement instrument]. Austin, TX: Pro-Ed.

Westby, C. (1980). Assessment of cognitive and language abilities through play. *Language, Speech, and Hearing Services in Schools, 11,* 154–168.

Weston, A., & Shriberg, L. (1992). Contextual and linguistic correlates of intelligibility in children with developmental phonological disorders. *Journal of Speech and Hearing Research, 35,* 1316–1332.

Wetherby, A., Cain, D., Yonclas, D., & Walker, V. (1988). Analysis of intentional communication of normal children from the prelinguistic to the multiword stage. *Journal of Speech and Hearing Research, 31,* 240–252.

Wetherby, A., & Prizant, B. (1992). Profiling young children's communicative competence. In S. Warren & J. Reichle (Eds.), *Causes and effects in communication and language intervention* (pp. 217–251). Baltimore, MD: Brookes.

Wetherby, A., & Prizant, B. (1998). *Communication and symbolic behavior scales—Developmental profile* [Measurement instrument]. Chicago, IL: Applied Symbolix.

Wetherby, A., & Prizant, B. (2002a). *Communication and symbolic behavior scales.* Baltimore, MD: Brookes.

Wetherby, A., & Prizant B. (2002b). *Infant-toddler checklist* [Measurement instrument]. Baltimore, MD: Brookes.

Wetherby, A., & Prutting, C. (1984). Profiles of communicative and cognitive-social abilities in autistic children. *Journal of Speech and Hearing Research, 27,* 364–377.

Wetherby, A., & Rodriguez, G. (1992). Measurement of communicative intentions in normally developing children during structured and unstructured contexts. *Journal of Speech and Hearing Research, 35,* 130–138.

Wetherby, A., Yonclas, D., & Bryan, A. (1989). Communicative profiles of preschool children with handicaps: Implications for early intervention. *Journal of Speech and Hearing Disorders, 54,* 148–158.

Whitehill, T. L. (2002). Assessing intelligibility in speakers with cleft palate: A critical review of the literature. *The Cleft Palate-Craniofacial Journal, 39,* 50–62.

Whurr, R. (1999). *Children's acquired aphasia screening test* [Measurement instrument]. London, England: Whurr.

Whurr, R. (2011). *Aphasia screening test* (3rd ed.) [Measurement instrument]. London, England: Speechmark.

Wiederholt, J. L., & Blalock, G. (2000). *Gray silent teading tests* [Measurement instrument]. Austin, TX: Pro-Ed.

Weiderholt, J. L., & Bryant, B. R. (2012). *Gray oral reading tests* (5th ed.) [Measurement instrument]. Austin, TX: Pro-Ed.

Wiig, E. (2004). *Wiig assessment of basic concepts* [Measurement instrument]. Greenville, SC: Super Duper.

Wiig, E., & Secord, W. (2006). *Emerging literacy and language assessment* [Measurement instrument]. Greenville, SC: Super Duper.

Wiig, E., & Secord, W. (2011). *HearBuilder phonological awareness test* [Measurement instrument]. Greenville, SC: Super Duper.

Wiig, E. H., & Secord, W. (1989). *Test of language competence* (Expanded edition) [Measurement instrument]. San Antonio, TX: Pearson.

Wiig, E. H., & Secord, W. (1992). *Test of word knowledge* [Measurement instrument]. San Antonio, TX: Pearson.

Wiig, E. H., Semel E., & Secord, W.A. (2013). *Clinical evaluation of language fundamentals screening test* (5th ed.) [Measurement instrument]. Bloomington, MN: Pearson.

Wilcox, M. (1984). Developmental language disorders: Preschoolers. In A. Holland (Ed.), *Language disorders in children: Recent advances* (pp. 101–128. San Diego, CA: College-Hill.

Williams, D. E., Darley, F. L., & Spriestersbach, D. C. (1978). *Diagnostic methods in speech pathology* (2nd ed.). New York, NY: Harper & Row.

Williams, K. (2007). *Expressive vocabulary test* (2nd ed.) [Measurement instrument]. Boston, MA: Pearson.

Wilson, B. A., Alderman, N., Burgess, P. W., Emslie, H., & Evans, J. J. (1996). *Behavioural assessment of the dysexecutive syndrome* [Measurement instrument]. St. Edmunds, UK: Thomas Valley Test Company.

Wilson, D. K. (1987). *Voice problems in children* (3rd ed.). Baltimore, MD: Williams & Wilkins.

Wilson, K., Blackmon, R., Hall, R., & Elcholtz, G. (1991). Methods of language assessment: A survey of California public school clinicians. *Language, Speech, and Hearing Services in Schools, 22,* 236–241.

Wise, J., Sevcik, R., Morris, R., Lovett, M., & Wolf, M. (2007). The relationship among receptive and expressive vocabulary, listening comprehension, pre-reading skills, word identification skills and reading comprehension by children with reading disabilities. *Journal of Speech, Language, and Hearing Research, 50,* 1093–1109.

Wolf, M., & Denckla, M. B. (2005). *Rapid automatized naming and rapid alternating stimulus tests* [Measurement instrument]. Norcross, GA: The Speech Bin.

Wolfus, B., Moscovitch, M., & Kinsbourne, M. (1980). Subgroups of developmental language impairment. *Brain and Language, 10,* 152–171.

Woodcock, R. W. (2011). *Woodcock reading mastery tests* (3rd ed.) [Measurement instrument]. San Antonio, TX: Pearson.

Woods, J., & Wetherby, A. (2003). Early identification of and intervention for infants and toddlers who are at risk for autism spectrum disorder. *Language, Speech, and Hearing Services in Schools, 34,* 180–193.

Woolf, G. (1967). The assessment of stuttering as struggle, avoidance and expectancy. *British Journal of Disorders of Communication, 2,* 158–171.

World Health Organization. (2002). Toward a common language for functioning, disability and health (ICF). Retrieved from http:www3 .who.int/icf/

World Health Organization. (2002). *The world health report: 2002: Reducing the risks, promoting healthy life.* New York, NY: Author.

Wright, L., & Ayre, A. (2000). *Wright and Ayre stuttering self-rating profile* [Measurement instrument]. Bichester, UK: Speechmark.

Wuyts, F. L., DeBodt, M. S., Molenberghs, G., Remacle, M., Heylen, L., Millet, B., . . . Van de Heyning, P. H. (2000). The Dysphonia Severity Index: An objective measure of vocal quality based on a multiparameter approach. *Journal of Speech, Language, and Hearing Research, 43*(3), 796–809.

Wyatt, T. (1998). Assessment issues with multicultural populations. In D. E. Battle (Ed.), *Communication disorders in multicultural populations* (2nd ed., pp. 379–425). Boston, MA: Butterworth-Heinemann.

Wyatt, T. A. (2002). Assessing the communicative abilities of clients from diverse cultural and language backgrounds. In D. E. Battle (Ed.), *Communication disorders in multicultural populations* (3rd ed., pp. 415–459). Boston, MA: Butterworth-Heinemann.

Yairi, E. (1997). Home environments of stuttering children. In R. Curlee & G. Siegel (Eds.), *Nature and treatment of stuttering*. Needham Heights, MA: Allyn & Bacon.

Yairi, E., & Ambrose, N. (1992). Onset of stuttering in preschool children: Selected factors. *Journal of Speech and Hearing Research, 35*(4), 782–788.

Yairi, E., & Ambrose, N. G. (2005). *Early childhood stuttering for clinicians by clinicians*. Austin, TX: Pro-Ed.

Yairi, E., Ambrose, N., & Niermann, R. (1993). The early months of stuttering: A developmental study. *Journal of Speech and Hearing Research, 36*, 521–528.

Yairi, E., Ambrose, N., Paden, E., & Throneburg, R. (1996). Predictive factors of persistence and recovery: Pathways of childhood stuttering. *Journal of Communication Disorders, 29*, 51–77.

Yairi, E., & Lewis, B. (1984). Disfluencies at the onset of stuttering. *Journal of Speech and Hearing Research, 27*, 155–159.

Yairi, E., & Seery, C. (2011). *Stuttering foundations and clinical approaches*. Boston, MA: Pearson.

Yairi, E. H., & Seery, C. H. (2014). *Stuttering: Foundations and clinical applications* (2nd ed.). San Antonio, TX: Pearson.

Yaruss, J. S. (1999). Current status of academic and clinical education in fluency disorders at ASHA-accredited training programs. *Journal of Fluency Disorders, 24*, 169–184.

Yaruss, J. S. (2000). Converting between word and syllable counts in children's conversational speech samples. *Journal of Fluency Disorders, 25*, 305–316.

Yaruss, J. S., & Logan, K. J. (2002). Evaluating rate, accuracy, and fluency of young children's diadochokinetic productions: A preliminary investigation. *Journal of Fluency Disorders, 27*, 65–86.

Yaruss, J. S., & Quesal, R. W. (2002). Academic and clinical education in fluency disorders: An update. *Journal of Fluency Disorders, 27*, 43–63.

Yaruss, J. S., Quesal, R. W., & Coleman, C. (2010). *Overall assessment of the speaker's experience of stuttering* [Measurement instrument]. San Antonio, TX: Pearson.

Yaruss, J. S., Quesal, R. W., & Coleman, C. (2010). *Overall assessment of the speaker's experience of stuttering*. Boston, MA: Pearson.

Yavas, M., & Goldstein, B. (1998). Phonological assessment and treatment of bilingual speakers. *American Journal of Speech-Language Pathology, 7*(2), 49–60.

Yiu, E. M. (2002). Impact and prevention of voice problems in the teaching profession: Embracing the consumer's view. *Journal of Voice, 16*, 215–228.

Yoder, P., Warren, S., & McCathren, R. (1998). Determining spoken language prognosis in children with developmental disabilities. *American Journal of Speech-Language Pathology, 7*, 77–87.

Yont, K., Hewitt, L., & Miccio, A. (2000). A coding system for describing conversational breakdowns in preschool children. *American Journal of Speech-Language Pathology, 9*, 300–309.

Yorkston, K., Beukelman, D., Stand, E., & Hakel, E. (2010). *Management of motor speech disorders in children and adults*. Austin, TX: Pro-Ed.

Yorkston, K., Beukelman, D., & Traynor, C. (1984). *Assessment of intelligibility of dysarthric speech* [Measurement instrument]. Austin, TX: Pro-Ed.

Yorkston, K., Spencer, K. A., & Duffy, J. R. (2003). Behavioral management of respiratory/phonatory dysfunction from dysarthria: A systematic review of the evidence. *Journal of Medical Speech-Language Pathology, 11*(2), xiii–xxxviii.

Yoss, K., & Darley, F. L. (1974). Developmental apraxia of speech in children with defective articulation. *Journal of Speech and Hearing Research, 17*, 399–416.

Young, A. R., Beitchman, J. H., Johnson, C., Douglas, L., Atkinson, L., Escobar, M., & Wilson, B. (2002). Young adult academic outcomes in a longitudinal sample of early identified language impaired and control children. *Journal of Child Psychology and Psychiatry, 43*(5), 635–645.

Zimmerman, I., Steiner, V., & Pond, R. (2011). *Preschool language scale* (5th ed.) [Measurement instrument]. San Antonio, TX: Psychological Corporation.

Zur, K., Cotton, S., Kelchnor, L., Baker, S., Weinrich, B., & Lee, L. (2007). Pediatric Voice Handicap Index (pVHI): A new tool for evaluating pediatric dysphonia. *International Journal of Pediatric Otorhinolaryngology, 71*(1), 77–82.

Zurinskas, T. (2009, November 2). Is the Rainbow Passage representative of phoneme frequencies? Message posted to https:groups.yahoo.com/neo/groups/truespel/conversations/topics/547

Zuur, J., Muller, S., de Jongh van Zandwijk, N., & Hilger, F. (2006). The physiological rationale of heat and moisture exchangers in post-laryngectomy pulmonary rehabilitation: A review. *European Archives of Oto-Rhino-Laryngology, 263*(1), 1–8. doi: 10.1007/soo405-005-0969-3

Index

MCI (mild cognitive impairment), aphasia versus, 267–268
McKinley, N., 183
McLean, J., 98, 109, 122
McLean, J. E., 107
McLean, L., 94
McLean, L. K., 107
McLeod, S., 188, 288
McNeil, M., 261, 264, 268, 429
McNeil, M. R., 279, 283
McNeill, D., 121
MCST-A (Multimodal Communication Screening Test for Persons with Aphasia), 259
MDADI (M.D. Anderson Dysphagia Inventory), 304, 310
Mean Babbling Level (MBL), 198–199
Mean flow rate (MFR), 338, 339–340
Mean length of response (MLR), 124–125
Mean length of utterance (MLU), 124–126, 152, 153, 154
Measurement
   dynamic assessment, 9–1
   evidence-based practice, 4–7
   functional, importance of, 11–14
   importance in current trends, 4–11
   response to intervention, 7–9
Medicaid, 415
Medical settings, reports, 394–395, 410–411
Medicare Part B, 416
Medications affecting swallowing, 303
Meier, J., 181
Meisels, S. J., 115
Memory, issues in language disorders, 176–178
Menchola, M., 51
Merrell, A., 77
Merritt, D., 169
Messer, D. J., 178
Messick, S., 58, 59
Messner, A. H., 420
MET (xaximum exhalation time), 338, 339
Metalinguistic skills, 180
Metcalf, K., 195
Meyers, F. L., 225
MFP (Multidisciplinary Feeding Profile), 314, 315
MFR (mean flow rate), 338, 339–340
Miccio, A., 175
Microstructure, 172
Middleton, G., 394
Mild cognitive impairment (MCI), aphasia versus, 267–268
Miles, S., 172
Millen, K., 90, 108, 158
Miller, C., 177
Miller, J., 118, 120, 123, 124, 125, 126, 151, 152, 156, 157, 159, 160, 161, 162, 165, 166
Miller, L., 10, 117, 147, 170, 179
Miller, M., 179
Miller, W. R., 51
Mills, C., 172
Mimura, M., 254
Mini Inventory of Right Brain Injury (MIRBI-2), 265
Mini-Cog, 264
Mini-Mental State Examination (MMSE-2), 264
Mini-tour questions, 50
Minnesota Test for Differential Diagnosis of Aphasia (MTDDA), 260
Miolo, G., 216
MIRBI-2 (Mini Inventory of Right Brain Injury), 265
Mirenda, P., 94, 99, 131, 132, 295
Misarticulations
   classification of, 186–187
   factors affecting, 192–193
Mississippi Aphasia Screening Test, 259
Mixed dysarthria, 291
Mixed vocal resonance, 349
Miyake, A., 178
MLR (mean length of response), 124–125
MLU (mean length of utterance), 124–126, 152, 153, 154
MMSE-2 (Mini-Mental State Examination), 264
Moats, L., 181
MoCA (Monterey Cognitive Assessment), 264

Modal level of play, 105–106
Modified barium swallow (MBS), 307–308, 315
Modified Erickson Scale of Communication Attitudes (S-24), 236
Mok, P. L., 141, 201
Molloy, C., 99
Monterey Cognitive Assessment (MoCA), 264
Montes, J., 249
Montgomery, J., 8, 177, 177
Montgomery, J. K., 146
Montgomery, W. W., 328, 329
Montgomery Assessment of Vocabulary Acquisition (MAVA), 146
Montreal Children's Hospital Feeding Scale, 314, 315
Moody, A. J., 98
Moran, M., 216
Moran, M., 79, 101
Morehead, A., 102
Morehead, D., 102
Morgan, D. L., 142, 145
Morimoto, H., 337
Morphemes, in utterance analysis, 127
Morphology, language disorder symptoms and, 139
Morris, N., 155
Morris, R., 179
Morris, S., 198, 208, 314
Morris-Friehe, M., 138
Morrison, M., 27
Morsome, D., 319
Moscovitch, M., 88
Moskowitz, L., 175
MOST (Marshalla Oral Sensorimotor Test), 288
Motivational interviewing, 51
Motor assessment, 287
Motor speech assessment, 287
Motor speech disorders
   adult dysarthrias, 288–293
   aphasia versus, 263
   apraxia of speech, 278–288. See also Apraxia of speech (AOS)
   augmentative and alternative communication needs, assessing, 295–296
   cerebral palsy and dysarthria in children, 293–294
Motor Speech Evaluation, 282–283
Motor Speech Evaluation template (ASHA), 280, 291, 422
MPT (maximum phonation time), 338, 339, 390
MTDDA (Minnesota Test for Differential Diagnosis of Aphasia), 260
Mulac, A., 150
Mulhern, S., 161
Mullen, E. M., 115
Mullen Scales of Early Learning: AGS Edition, 115
Muller, S., 389
Multicultural considerations/issues
   assessment, 132–133
   bias, standardized testing, 79–80
   cancer prevalence, SEER study, 372
   client interview, 37, 38–39
   dialectical variation, 191
   fluency disorders, 248–250
   language disorders, 121
   language sampling, 153
   literacy evaluation, 179
   nonverbal communication, 42
   population demographics, 78–82
   testing considerations, 78–82
Multidisciplinary Feeding Profile (MFP), 314, 315
Multilingual Aphasia Examination (MAE-3), 260
Multilingual Aphasia Examination, Spanish (MAE-S), 260
Multimodal Communication Screening Test for Persons with Aphasia(MCST-A), 259
Multi-Speech, 333
Multiword communicators, 85–87
   Coding Sheet for Early Multiword Analysis, 434–435
   Summary Sheet for Early Multiword Analysis, 436
Muma, J., 56, 58, 59, 76, 78, 83, 90, 123, 126, 154, 160, 162, 166

Mundy, P., 107
Munoz-Sandoval, A., 260
Munro, N., 167
Murray, D., 99
Murray, G., 295
Murry, T., 328
Musselwhite, C., 150, 152
Muyts, F. L., 363, 364
My Grandfather passage, 292, 430–431
Myers, F., 224
Myers, P. S., 264

Nachmani, A., 354
Nagy, A., 307
Nakase-Thompson, R., 259
Narrative Assessment Profile, 172
Narrative development, Applebee's stages of, 171
Narrative production, assessment of, 168–174
Narrative Scoring Scheme (NSS), 172, 173–174
Nasal emission, 348, 355–356
Nasal resonance, assessment, 360
Nasal rustle, 348
Nasal snort, 355
Nasality Severity Index (NSI), 364–365
NASDSE (National Association of State Directors of Special Education), 7
Nash, G., 178, 264
Nasometer, 363, 430
Nasometry, 363–364
Nasopharyngoscopy, 365
Nasreddine, Z., 264
Nation, J., 139, 178
National Association of State Directors of Special Education (NASDSE), 7
National Cancer Institute, 371, 372
National Center for Learning Disabilities, 412
National Outcomes Measurement System (NOMS), 12, 13, 411, 417
National Stuttering Association, 232
Natural Process Analysis, 198, 204
NCLB (No Child Left Behind), 8
NDP3 (Nuffield Center Dyspraxia Programme, Third Edition), 288
Nelson, K., 86, 102, 118, 119
Nelson, L., 175
Nelson, N., 17, 50, 52, 87, 91, 130, 144, 182
Nelson, N. W., 143
Neonatal Behavioral Assessment Scale, Fourth Edition, 128
Neonatal Oral-Motor Assessment Scale (NOMAS), 314, 315
Nestlé Nutrition Institute, 304
Neurogenic stuttering, 223–224
Neurolinguistic analysis, 262
Neurologic Speech and Language Examination, 281, 291
Neuropsychological analysis, 262
"New test" syndrome, 21
Newborg, J., 112
Newcomer, P., 211
Newcomer, P. L., 148
Newhoff, M., 87
Newman, R., 170
Newman, S. P., 329
Nicholas, J., 119
Nicholas, M., 252
Niermann, R., 226
Night Sky passage, 431
Nihira, K., 101
Nippold, M., 56, 151, 153, 155
Nitsch, K., 156
Nittrouer, S., 188
No Child Left Behind (NCLB), 8
Nockerts, A., 154, 165, 172
Noise
   artificial larynx speech, 381–382
   esophageal speech, 384
NOMAS (Bottle-Breast Feeding: Neonatal Oral Motor Assessment Scale), 314
NOMAS (Neonatal Oral-Motor Assessment Scale), 314, 315